10.17.18

62059

Gift

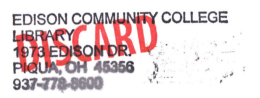

Clinical Chemistry
A Laboratory Perspective

Clinical Chemistry
A Laboratory Perspective

Wendy Arneson, MS, MT(ASCP)
Biodetection Lab Manager
Emergency Medicine Section, Biodetection
  Laboratory
University of Oklahoma – Tulsa
Tulsa, Oklahoma

Jean Brickell, EdD, MT(ASCP)
Associate Professor
Department of Clinical Laboratory Sciences
University of Texas Medical Branch
Galveston, Texas

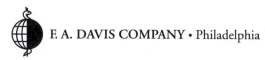
F. A. DAVIS COMPANY • Philadelphia

F. A. Davis Company
1915 Arch Street
Philadelphia, PA 19103
www.fadavis.com

Copyright © 2007 by F. A. Davis Company

Printed in the United States of America

Last digit indicates print number: 10 9 8 7 6 5 4 3 2 1

Acquisitions Editor: Christa A. Fratantoro
Manager of Content Development: Deborah J. Thorp
Developmental Editor: Molly Connors
Art and Design Manager: Carolyn O'Brien

As new scientific information becomes available through basic and clinical research, recommended treatments and drug therapies undergo changes. The author(s) and publisher have done everything possible to make this book accurate, up to date, and in accord with accepted standards at the time of publication. The author(s), editors, and publisher are not responsible for errors or omissions or for consequences from application of the book, and make no warranty, expressed or implied, in regard to the contents of the book. Any practice described in this book should be applied by the reader in accordance with professional standards of care used in regard to the unique circumstances that may apply in each situation. The reader is advised always to check product information (package inserts) for changes and new information regarding dose and contraindications before administering any drug. Caution is especially urged when using new or infrequently ordered drugs.

Library of Congress Cataloging-in-Publication Data

Clinical chemistry : a laboratory perspective / [edited by] Wendy Arneson, Jean Brickell.
   p. ; cm.
  Includes bibliographical references and index.
  ISBN-13: 978-0-8036-1498-7
  ISBN-10: 0-8036-1498-5
  1. Clinical chemistry—Laboratory manuals.   I. Arneson, Wendy.   II. Brickell, Jean.
  [DNLM: 1. Clinical Chemistry Tests.   QY 90 C6413 2007]
  RB40.C5693 2007
  616.07′56—dc22   2006039688

Dedication

I would like to thank the many people who have contributed to my knowledge of clinical laboratory science and dedicate this book to my mentors: Mary Haven, Dr. Denise Kolbet, Phyllis Muellenberg, Dr. Thomas Williams and Ruth Sibilia. I would also like to thank my family for their patience and devotion.
W.A.

I dedicate my efforts in this text to Reed Foster for his shining example of perseverance in the face of significant obstacles and to Ruth McArthur in appreciation of her years of service for our profession.
J.B.

Preface

Years ago, when one of the authors fearfully asked her phlebotomy instructor if she could just review the text one more time before she performed her first phlebotomy, the instructor replied, "There is nothing like experience." In a modification of that motto, the theme of this book is that the way to learn clinical chemistry is to explore real-life scenarios of everyday practice in clinical chemistry.

While teaching in a variety of programs over the past 20 years, we have seen a trend for clinical chemistry textbooks to move away from clinical laboratory applications and procedures and toward increased emphasis on physiology, biochemistry, and pathology. The case studies provided in these textbooks are presented from the perspective of the first provider, such as the physician, in the style and language that might be taught to medical students and residents while on grand rounds. Although these case studies present an abundance of laboratory data, the goal is making a diagnosis based on clinical signs and symptoms (which are not gathered by the laboratorian) and the laboratory results. This emphasis creates the expectation for the clinical laboratory science (CLS) student that the role and purpose of the clinical laboratory scientist is predominantly diagnosis.

Although today's textbooks have moved away from the perspective of the clinical chemist, they remain written in the style familiar to the language of the "baby boomer" faculty who are currently teaching. The majority of the student body are "generation Y" or "millennium generation" learners. Educational researchers report that these learners prefer to be presented with a problem first, see the value or relevance in the situation, and then focus on the knowledge needed to solve the problem through application and critical thinking skills.

Given the language and organization of most clinical chemistry textbooks, we have noticed a trend in CLS students to resist using them for more than a brief overview of reading assignments, They often do not recognize their value during the clinical experience and sometimes return them to the bookstore long before graduation. In other words, there seems to be great resistance for students to use and keep the clinical chemistry textbook.

In response to the needs of the current generation of learners, this textbook has a different look than most other clinical chemistry textbooks. Following the introduction of general topics, the remaining topics and chapters are organized as applications of laboratory tests for management of diseases or conditions. We purposely organized the course information around Case Scenarios from the perspective of the laboratorian. Each chapter has key words highlighted and defined where first used to facilitate reading and understanding. Sidebars provide additional pertinent information to the accompanying text and include The Team Approach, Common Sense Check, and Clinical Correlation. Test Methodologies, with a focus on principle, sources of interferences, preanalytical aspects, specimen characteristics, and reference ranges, are provided in each chapter so that learners can relate this methodology to automated systems of analyses. Frequent cross references to other chapters are provided when background or more detailed information on a similar topic is needed. Finally, many illustrations and tables are provided to further illuminate the concepts presented in the text.

Wendy Arneson and Jean Brickell

Acknowledgments

We would like to acknowledge Diana Mass for her contributions to certification, licensure, and the scope of practice of clinical laboratory scientists. Marian Cavagnaro contributed to our understanding of body fluid collection, processing, and role in clinical chemistry testing. We would like to thank Meg Crellin for her extensive contribution to quality assessment, quality control, and statistical analysis. Vicki Freeman supported us throughout the preparation of this textbook with her expertise, her encouragement, and her time. We also wish to thank Josh Schuetz for his expertise and contribution to respiratory function testing. We would like to acknowledge Linda Gorman's sense of humor as exhibited in her chapter describing cardiovascular disorders. That sense of humor is, ultimately, the basis of a sense of relevance. We would like to thank Maria G. Boosalis, a Registered Dietitian, for her willingness to "cross the hall" and collaborate with clinical laboratory scientists. Camellia St. John and Michelle Kanuth contributed to multiple myeloma and breast cancer tumor markers and we would like to acknowledge their contributions. We would like to acknowledge Karen Chandler for her contribution to basic information in endocrinology and adrenal cortical function testing. We would like to thank Dean Arneson for his knowledge and expertise in therapeutic drug monitoring.

Reviewers

Bernadette Bekken, BS, MT(ASCP)BB, CLS(NCA)
Program Director
Clinical Laboratory Science
Augusta Medical Center
Fisherville, Virginia

Patricia Russo Castro, MS, MT(ASCP)BB
Program Director and Professor
Health Sciences
Community College of Southern Nevada
Las Vegas, Nevada

Russell Cheadle, MLT, CLT
Program Director and Associate Professor
Medical Laboratory Technology
University of Rio Grande
Rio Grande, Ohio

Judith E. Colver, MMS, PA-C
Associate Chair and Physician Assistant
Physician Assistant Studies
University of Texas Health Science Center
San Antonio, Texas

Muneeza Esani, MHA, MT(ASCP)
Assistant Professor
Medical Laboratory Sciences
University of Texas Southwestern Medical Center
Dallas, Texas

Glenn Flodstrom, MS, MT(ASCP)
Assistant Professor
Medical Laboratory
Northern Virginia Community College
Springfield, Virginia

Kevin F. Foley, PhD, MT
Assistant Professor
Medical Laboratory and Radiation Sciences
The University of Vermont
Burlington, Vermont

Vicki S. Freeman, PhD
Chair and Professor
Clinical Laboratory Sciences
University of Texas Medical Branch
Galveston, Texas

Margaret J. Hall, PhD
Professor
Medical Technology
University of Southern Mississippi
Hattiesburg, Mississippi

Audrey E. Hentzen, PhD, MT(ASCP)
Instructor
Phlebotomy Department
Casper College
Casper, Wyoming

Susan A. K. Higgins, MS, MT(ASCP)SC
Clinical Assistant Professor
Allied Health
Indiana University Northwest
Gary, Indiana

Stephen M. Johnson, MS, MT(ASCP)
Program Director
Medical Technology
St. Vincent Health Center
Erie, Pennsylvania

Pam Kieffer, BS, MS, CLS(NCA)
Program Director
Clinical Laboratory Sciences
Rapid City Regional Hospital
Rapid City, South Dakota

Martin H. Kroll, MD
Director
Pathology and Laboratory Medicine
North Texas VA Medical Center
Dallas, Texas

Marguerite E. Neita, PhD, MT(ASCP)
Chair and Program Director
Clinical Laboratory Sciences
Howard University
Washington, DC

Jennifer D. Perry, BS, MS, MT(ASCP)
Assistant Professor
Clinical Laboratory Sciences
Marshall University
Huntington, West Virginia

Valerie Polansky, MEd, MT(ASCP)
Program Director
Medical Laboratory Technology
St. Petersburg College
St. Petersburg, Florida

Joan Radtke, MS, MT(ASCP)SC, CLS(NCA)
Assistant Professor
Clinical Laboratory Sciences
Rush Presbyterian–St. Luke's
Chicago, Illinois

Jan C. Rogers, MS, MT(ASCP)
Associate Professor
Biology
Morrisville State College
Morrisville, New York

Lauren I. Strader, MEd, MT(ASCP)
MLT Program Director
Allied Health Department Chair
North Georgia Technical College
Clarkesville, Georgia

Contributors

Dean L. Arneson, Pharm D, PhD
Associate Dean
College of Pharmacy
University of Oklahoma
Tulsa, Oklahoma

Maria G. Boosalis, PhD, MPH, RD, LD
Associate Professor
Clinical Laboratory Sciences
University of Kentucky
Lexington, Kentucky

Marian Cavagnaro, MS, MT(ASCP)DLM
Laboratory Director
Memorial Hospital West
Pembroke Pines, Florida

Karen Chandler, MS, MT(ASCP), CLS(NCA)
Assistant Dean
College of Health Sciences and Human Services
University of Texas Pan American
Edinburg, Texas

Margaret Crellin, BS, MT(ASCP)
Medical Technologist Master
Chandler Medical Center
University of Kentucky
Lexington, Kentucky

Vicki Freeman, PhD, MT(ASCP)SC, CLS(NCA)
Department Chair
Clinical Laboratory Sciences
University of Texas Medical Branch
Galveston, Texas

Linda S. Gorman, PhD, MT(ASCP)
Director of Graduate Studies
Clinical Laboratory Science
University of Kentucky
Lexington, Kentucky

Michelle Kanuth, PhD, MT(ASCP)SBB
Associate Professor
Clinical Laboratory Sciences
University of Texas Medical Branch
Galveston, Texas

Diana Mass, MA, MT(ASCP)
Program Director and Clinical Professor
Clinical Laboratory Science
Arizona State University
Tempe, Arizona

Joshua R. Schuetz, RRT, MEd, RCP
Assistant Clinical Professor and Director of Clinical
Education in Respiratory Care
University of Texas Medical Branch
Galveston, Texas

Camellia St. John, MEd, MT(ASCP)SDB
Associate Professor
Clinical Laboratory Sciences
University of Texas Medical Branch
Galveston, Texas

Contents

Case Scenario Contents

Clinical chemistry is a science, a service, and an industry.

Overview of Clinical Chemistry

Jean Brickell, Wendy Arneson, and Diana Mass

Clinical chemistry is a science, a service, and an industry. As a science, clinical chemistry links the knowledge of general chemistry, organic chemistry, and biochemistry with an understanding of human physiology. As a service, the clinical chemistry laboratory produces objective evidence from which medical decisions may be made. As an industry, clinical laboratories are businesses, which operate under the regulations and practices that guide commerce in the United States.

This textbook introduces the student of clinical chemistry to the organization of the discipline of clinical chemistry and presents the elements of clinical chemistry as they will be practiced. Each chapter presents laboratory situations that are pertinent to the role of the clinical laboratory in assessment of health and disease. By working through the scenarios as they are presented, the student will gain knowledge about the correlation of the assessment of human physiology and disease with the measurement of biochemical markers. Each scenario allows the student to examine the laboratory assessment process, including the impact of preanalytical factors, such as specimen collection and handling; the effects of variation on the analytical procedure; and the importance of postanalytical factors, such as communication of results. There is a focus on the analysis phase in each chapter, including test methodologies for many of the common clinical chemistry analytes. The procedures emphasize the chemical reaction and detection, sources of reaction interference, the types of specimens used, calculations as they pertain to determining reportable results, and reference ranges to compare patient results with those expected in healthy populations. The student will explore the role of the laboratory professional in providing the laboratory results that aid in diagnosis and monitoring of clinical disorders. The side boxes in each chapter provide common sense tips, definitions of terms, brief descriptions of pathophysiology, and clinical correlations as well as reminders of the team approach in health care. Text boxes within the chapter outline methodology for laboratory assessment of physiological function.

OBJECTIVES

Upon completion of this chapter, the student will have the ability to

- Describe the regulatory guidelines that define the practice of clinical chemistry in the United States.
- Discuss measures for ensuring competency of clinical laboratory professionals.
- Describe specific biochemical markers of disease, including carbohydrates, lipids, proteins, and hormones.
- Associate biochemical markers of disease with the organ or tissue location of the disease.

Clinical Chemistry Is a Service and an Industry

CASE SCENARIO 1-1

The New Class

The instructor addressed a clinical chemistry class of future clinical laboratory scientists.

REGULATORY GUIDELINES

outcome - consequence, conclusion, or result

Clinical chemistry laboratories are judged upon **outcome** measures. The most obvious outcome of laboratory testing is the laboratory test report. Information that is provided to physicians on this report must be accurate, timely, and relevant. As a third-party payer of health-care dollars, the U.S. government requires assurance of quality for laboratory outcome. The **Clinical Laboratory Improvement Amendments (CLIA) of 1988** outline the minimum requirements by which a clinical laboratory may operate in order to receive government funds, such as Medicaid and Medicare dollars.

CLIA '88 defines clinically laboratories broadly. A clinical laboratory is defined as any facility that performs laboratory testing on specimens derived from humans for the purpose of providing information for the diagnosis, prevention, or treatment of disease, or impairment of or assessment of health. Sites such as hospitals, clinics, physician's offices, nursing homes, and dialysis centers in which laboratory testing is performed are brought under the **regulatory** guidelines of CLIA as clinical laboratories. Two levels of regulation, **waived** and **nonwaived**, are defined by the complexity of the tests that are performed in the laboratory. Additionally, laboratories in which the health-care provider examines specimens directly via microscopy are considered as a separate category, the provider-performed microscopy laboratory. Waived tests are simple laboratory examinations and procedures that are cleared by the U.S. Food and Drug Administration (FDA) for home use. They employ methodologies that are sufficiently simple and accurate as to render the likelihood of erroneous results negligible or pose no reasonable risk of harm to the patient if the test is performed incorrectly.[1] Examples of waived tests are the *Streptococcus* antigen test and the fecal occult blood test. Nonwaived tests are moderately and highly complex tests as defined by the requirements for operator skill, reagent preparation, and automation and the difficulty of interpretation of results.

The more complicated the test, the more stringent the requirements. Laboratories that perform nonwaived testing are regulated under guidelines that cover quality standards for **proficiency testing** (PT), patient test management, quality control, personnel qualifications, and quality assurance. The regulatory process is outcome oriented, with PT as the principle outcome measure. PT consists of five challenges three times a year for each test that the laboratory offers. Several organizations have obtained **deemed status** from the federal government in order to offer approved PT programs. Although there are specific sanctions for failing PT challenges, the intent of regulation is educational, rather than **punitive**. Improvement of laboratory medicine is the goal.

Additionally, laboratories may be inspected for quality. The laboratory may be inspected by the state regulatory agency or by an agency that has been granted deemed status to perform inspections. Daily quality control and documentation of quality assessment are key areas for inspection. CLIA '88 provides guidelines for both daily quality control and systemic quality assurance of the testing process from ordering the test to reporting the test. Data indicate that CLIA '88 has helped to improve the quality of testing in the United States. A review of PT data shows that the failure rate has decreased.[2] The educational value of PT in laboratories has been the most effective force for change.

Clinical Laboratory Improvement Amendments of 1988 (CLIA) - quality standards for all clinical laboratories to ensure the accuracy, reliability, and timeliness of patient test results regardless of where the test was performed; the Centers for Medicare and Medicaid Services regulates all laboratory testing (except research) performed on humans in the United States

regulatory - relating to rules or directives

waived - tests that are very simple or pose no reasonable risk of harm to the patient if the test is performed incorrectly

nonwaived - complex tests that require skill to perform and interpret and are therefore regulated

proficiency testing - a method of monitoring accurate outcome; in which test samples from an external source are analyzed and results compared to those of reference laboratories and scored for accuracy

deemed status - permission given to an external second party to act as the agent of the first party

punitive - relating to punishment

Case Scenario 1-1 The New Class

The New Class Discusses Safety Issues

The clinical laboratory science instructor asked if anyone had questions about safety concerns for working in the medical laboratory. James had some concerns about working with blood and reagents such as acids since he had heard about laboratory workers getting injured or sick.

Safety Regulations

In the clinical chemistry laboratory, local, state, and federal regulations, including the Occupational Safety and Health Act (OSHA), provide guidelines for safe operation of testing processes. Regulations include guidelines for operating safety equipment and identifying, handling, and storing chemical hazards. Table 1–1 outlines the types of safety equipment that may be necessary to operate a clinical chemistry laboratory safely. Table 1–2 outlines proper identification of chemicals within the laboratory through the use of **material safety data sheet** (MSDS) sys-

material safety data sheet - documents produced by the manufacturer of the chemical to provide safety information

TABLE 1-1
Safety Equipment

Equipment	Description	Use
PERSONAL PROTECTIVE EQUIPMENT		
Glasses or goggles	Unbreakable eye shields that surround the eye area	Protects exposed skin and clothes that may be worn outside the laboratory
Work shields	Spatter protection for exposed skin	
Gloves	Latex or vinyl cover for hands	
Coat or apron	Cover for clothes that will be worn outside the laboratory	
FUME HOOD	Ventilation system that operates at 100–120 ft/min at the sash; system must be monitored regularly	Reduces the risk of inhaling caustic chemicals; respirators with HEPA filters may be used when fume hoods are not available
STORAGE UNITS		
Explosion-proof refrigerators	Refrigerators that can contain the force of a chemical explosion	Reduce the risk of unwanted chemical reactions; reduce the danger of injury from chemical reactions
Compressed gas storage	Reinforcement straps or chains for storing compressed gas containers vertically	
Storage cabinets	Separate cabinets for storing: Flammable solids Organic acids Oxidizers Water-reactive substances	
FIRE EXTINGUISHERS		
Class A	Pressurized water	Wood, paper, cloth fires
Class B	Carbon dioxide	Flammable liquid, paint, oil fires
Class C	Dry chemical	Electrical fires
Class ABC	Dry chemical	All fires
SAFETY SHOWER	Drench-type safety shower	Remove chemical spills from clothing, skin, or eyes
EYEWASHES	Fountain that can be used to drench the eye with water	
SPILL KITS	Commercial kits that may be used to collect spills of specific substances such as acids or mercury	Restrict the spill to a localized area; collect the spill in a safe container for disposal

TABLE 1-2

Material Safety Data Sheet (MSDS) Information

Identification of chemical	Reactivity data
Hazardous ingredients	Spill, leak, and disposal procedures
Physical data	Personal protection information
Fire and explosion data	Special precautions and comments
Health hazard information	

tems. Clinical chemistry laboratory personnel must adhere to the general **blood-borne pathogens** safety protection procedures that are in place throughout the clinical laboratory.[3] The laboratory must have a safety manual in which work practices, procedures, and policies for providing a safe environment are listed. At minimum, the manual should include the following items:

1. Basic rules and procedures
2. Chemical procurement, distribution, and storage
3. Environmental monitoring
4. Housekeeping, maintenance, and inspections
5. Health hazards and medical treatment options
6. Personal protective apparel and equipment
7. Records, including MSDSs
8. Requirements for signs and labels
9. Procedures and documentation for spills and accidents
10. Requirements for training
11. Waste disposal

All chemical substances in the laboratory should be labeled. The safety diamond is one method for labeling chemicals. The diamond pictured in Figure 1–1 indicates the severity of hazard by increased number (0 = no danger, 4 = most severe

blood-borne - carried or transmitted by blood

pathogens - causative agents of disease

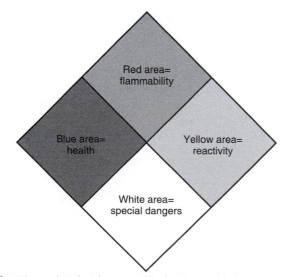

Figure 1–1. Safety Diamond. Colored areas within the diamond indicate types of danger: red area (top) = flammability, blue area (left) = health; yellow area (right) = reactivity; and white area (bottom) = special dangers.

danger). Colored areas within the diamond indicate types of danger: red area = flammability, blue area = health; yellow = reactivity; and white = special dangers. The Safety Diamond is used in conjunction with the MSDS for each chemical. Each chemical in the laboratory must have an MSDS on file. The MSDS must be available in an area that would be accessible if a spill or accident occurred in the laboratory.

Only small amounts of chemicals that will be used within a short amount of time should be stored in the clinical chemistry laboratory. The best safety procedures in the laboratory are attention to the job, good housekeeping procedures, and common sense.

> **THE TEAM APPROACH**
> Laboratory safety regulations are in place to protect those who work in the laboratory as well as those who come to the laboratory for specimen collection, laboratory results, or inspections or for other reasons. A team approach involving many different personnel of the health-care facility is needed to develop, implement, and maintain safety practices.

Case Scenario 1-1 The New Class

Final Comments on Safety Policies and Procedures

James had some concerns about working with blood and reagents such as acids since he had heard about laboratory workers getting injured or sick. The students learned that the laboratory is required to have and use procedures that list the safety hazards encountered with each procedure. In addition, general safety policies are provided, and taught to all laboratory workers, concerning the proper handling and disposal of needles, blood and body fluids, contaminated supplies and equipment, and other aspects of biohazard, chemical, fire, and electrical safety. James and his fellow students were assured that these procedures would be taught in the student laboratory as well as the clinical laboratory. Also, MSDS information would be available for all chemicals encountered in the laboratory that would provide specific policies for handling, disposal, and treating accidental exposure. Thus, safe practices would be taught and implemented to limit hazardous conditions in the laboratory. ●

CASE SCENARIO 1-2

The New Class Discusses the Scope of Practice

After the instructor introduced the role of the clinical laboratory as a business subject to federal, state, and local regulations, she asked the students if there were any questions about what clinical laboratory scientists do in the laboratory. Suzanne asked this question: "Will I be making a diagnosis?" John asked if they will take an examination for **licensure** after graduation.

> **licensure -** the process by which an agency of a state government grants permission to persons meeting predetermined qualifications to engage in a given occupation and/or to use a particular title; individuals who are not licensed cannot practice in that state

LICENSURE AND REGISTRY

Clinical laboratory sciences is a complex field that includes clinical chemistry as one discipline within laboratory practice. This challenging field is constantly changing as it responds to new technologies as well as to economic and societal pressure. Thus, the roles of clinical laboratory scientists develop and expand on a continuous basis. In 1981, the American Society for Medical Technology (now the American Society for Clinical Laboratory Science [ASCLS]) published its Scope of Practice, which describes in general terms services provided by clinical laboratory scientists (Table 1–3).[4] In basic terms, the clinical laboratory science profession

TABLE 1-3

Scope of Practice: General Services Provided by Clinical Laboratory Scientists

Clinical laboratory personnel, as members of the health-care team, are responsible for

1. Assuring reliable test results that contribute to the prevention, diagnosis, prognosis, and treatment of physiological and pathological conditions. This assurance requires
   A. Producing accurate test results.
   B. Correlating and interpreting test data.
   C. Assessing and improving existing laboratory test methods.
   D. Designing, evaluating, and implementing new methods.
2. Designing and implementing cost-effective administrative procedures for laboratories, including their services and personnel.
3. Designing, implementing, and evaluating processes for education and continued education of laboratory personnel.
4. Developing and monitoring a quality assurance system to include
   A. Quality control of services.
   B. Competence assurance of personnel.
5. Promoting an awareness and understanding of the services they render to the consumer, the public, and other health-care professionals.

provides information based on the analytical tests performed on body substances to detect evidence of or to prevent disease or impairment, and to promote and monitor good health.

Although clinical laboratory scientists do not directly make a diagnosis on a patient, the clinical laboratory scientist can confer and consult with the clinician. Based on patient history and symptoms, the proper tests to order and the interpretation of the test results are essential diagnostic activities in the proper utilization of laboratory services. These activities are responsibilities as described in the preanalytical and postanalytical processes of the total testing process as defined by CLIA '88. Therefore, it is important that students learn the diagnostic process in order to assume this type of role, which will improve patient safety outcomes—a quality indicator.

Another method of regulating quality in the health-care industry is through occupational licensure laws. Unfortunately, the clinical laboratory industry is not uniform in this regard. Fewer than 15 states have any type of personnel licensure for individuals who work in the clinical laboratory. Instead, most laboratory personnel are certified. Standards established by the profession specify what individuals must meet to be licensed or certified. In states without licensure, the employer can employ noncertified individuals, thus hiring individuals who do not meet the profession's established personnel standards. While licensure is mandated by state law, **certification** is voluntary. An individual does not need a certificate to practice. Thus, in terms of upholding quality, licensure is the preferred gatekeeper to prevent incompetent people from practicing.

Both licensure and certification require predetermined qualifications that include the completion of a professional academic program and passing an examination. While some states have individual examinations, other states accept a national certification examination as equivalent.

Other related concepts for standards of laboratory practice by laboratory personnel include **registration** and **credentialing**. *Registration* is the process by which qualified individuals are listed on an official roster maintained by a governmental or

certification - the process by which a nongovernmental agency or association grants recognition to an individual who has met certain predetermined qualifications specified by that agency or association

registration - the process by which qualified individuals are listed on an official roster maintained by a governmental or nongovernmental agency

credentialing - the processes involved in identifying those institutions and individuals meeting acceptable standards in areas of accreditation, certification, or licensure

nongovernmental agency. *Credentialing* is a collective term that refers to the processes involved in identifying those institutions and individuals meeting acceptable standards in areas of **accreditation**, certification, or licensure. *Accreditation* is the process by which an agency or an organization evaluates and recognizes a program of study or an institution as meeting certain predetermined qualifications or standards. Accreditation applies only to institutions and programs. Clinical laboratories are accredited by different standards and agencies than educational programs. Educational programs for clinical laboratory sciences have their own accrediting agency, the National Accrediting Agency for Clinical Laboratory Sciences.[5]

As mentioned before, the clinical laboratory science field is constantly changing, and personnel must maintain their competence. One way to maintain quality personnel is to encourage the learning process through continuing education. Today, various continuing education requirements must be met to maintain licensure or certification.

accreditation - the process by which an agency or an organization evaluates and recognizes a program of study or an institution as meeting certain predetermined qualifications or standards; applies only to institutions and programs

---

Case Scenario 1-2 The New Class Discusses the Scope of Practice

Scope of Practice: Additional Questions

The instructor asked the clinical laboratory science students for further questions about what clinical laboratory scientists do in the laboratory. Suzanne had asked this question: "Will I be making a diagnosis?" It was discussed that clinical laboratory scientists do not directly diagnose a patient; however, the clinical laboratory scientist confers and consults with the clinician. The physician or other clinical staff member determines patient history and symptoms and orders tests. However, laboratory personnel can be helpful in their decisions as to the proper utilization of laboratory services. Federal regulations laid out by CLIA '88 include the laboratory in these responsibilities.

John had asked if they would take an examination for licensure after graduation. It was discussed that few states currently require licensure for laboratory personnel, including clinical laboratory scientists. Requirements for licensure in these states typically involve completion of a professional program and passing a standardized examination. Certification is a voluntary process in which individuals choose to have their academic credentials reviewed and often sit for a standardized examination in order to meet the profession's established personnel standards. All graduating students are encouraged to take a certification examination, even if they reside in a state that does not require licensure, in order to indicate they meet professional personnel standards and to be more competitive in the job market. ●

Clinical Chemistry Is a Science

THE BIOCHEMISTRY OF DISEASE

The clinical chemistry laboratory measures change in biochemical compounds as an indicator of health status or disease processes. Because the biochemical changes of compounds are not uniform in tissue and organs in response to disease, the measurement of selected **biochemical markers** can be used to monitor diseases processes as they occur in specific living cell systems. For instance, an increase in the concentration of urea nitrogen in the blood may indicate kidney failure and increased concentration of blood cholesterol may indicate increased risk of cardiac disorders.

The clinical chemistry laboratory provides accurate, precise measurements of selected biochemical markers, accompanied by reference, or comparison, ranges of the concentration of these biochemical markers in healthy individuals.

Biochemical marker analysis is one factor in the assessment of the patient. Physicians also gather history and symptoms of the complaint; examination findings, such as blood pressure; and testing by other health-care team members in ancillary fields, such as radiology and respiratory therapy. The physician uses all data to assess the patient and implement a plan for treatment.

Four categories of organic biochemical markers are used for assessment and diagnosis of disease: carbohydrates, lipids, proteins, and nucleic acids and the derivatives of these markers. The assessment of inorganic chemicals, such as ions, minerals, and dissolved gases, provide a measure of **homeostasis** in the body. In addition to the measurement of these **endogenous** substances, the clinical chemistry laboratory provides measurement of chemicals that are **exogenous** to the body—both beneficial chemicals, such as therapeutic drugs, and harmful substances, such as poisons.

biochemical marker - any biochemical compound, such as an antigen, antibody, abnormal enzyme, or hormone, that is sufficiently altered in a disease to serve as an aid in diagnosing or in predicting susceptibility to the disease

homeostasis - the state of dynamic equilibrium of the internal environment of the body that is maintained by processes of feedback and regulation in response to external or internal changes

endogenous - originating inside the body

exogenous - originating outside an organ or part of the body

Carbohydrates

Carbohydrates are chemical substances that contain only carbon, hydrogen, and oxygen. Often carbohydrate molecules consist of one H_2O molecule per carbon, hence the nomenclature "carbohydrate," or hydrate of carbon. The simplest carbohydrates are monosaccharides, which usually contain 3 to 6 carbons. Monosaccharides are the units that make up more complex carbohydrates. Glucose, fructose, ribose, and galactose are common monosaccharides of living organisms.

Monosaccharides bind together covalently through glycosidic linkages to form disaccharides (two sugars) and polysaccharides (large polymers of monosaccharides). Lactose, maltose, and sucrose are common disaccharides of living cells. Starch, cellulose, and glycogen are common polysaccharides of living cells. Plants store glucose as starch and cellulose. Animals store glucose as long, branching polymers called *glycogen*. Structures for the carbohydrate molecules are reviewed in Figure 1–2.

Carbohydrates are excellent sources of immediate energy and resources of energy storage in polysaccharide form. Carbohydrates that are conjugated to proteins or lipids—glycoproteins or glycolipids, respectively—make up a diverse group of structural components of cells and organs. The roles of conjugated carbohydrates include antigen markers, nerve sheathing, and lubricants.

Several chemical properties of carbohydrates are important to the clinical chemist in the identification and measurement of carbohydrates in body fluids. Carbohydrates that have an active ketone or aldehyde functional group can act as reducing substances. This property is used in many methods in the determination of glucose, fructose, maltose, galactose, and lactose. Some carbohydrates are nonreducing substances. The ketone or aldehyde groups of these carbohydrates have been used to form the glycosidic bond. Sucrose is an example of these carbohydrates.

The digestion of dietary polysaccharides starts in the mouth with the catalysis of glycosidic bonds of the carbohydrate polymers by amylase. The disaccharides that are produced by this reaction are further digested in the duodenum. Disaccharides are split into monosaccharides by disaccharide enzymes (such as lactase) that are located on the microvilli of the intestine. These monosaccharides are then actively absorbed into the lymph and bloodstream and travel to tissue cells.

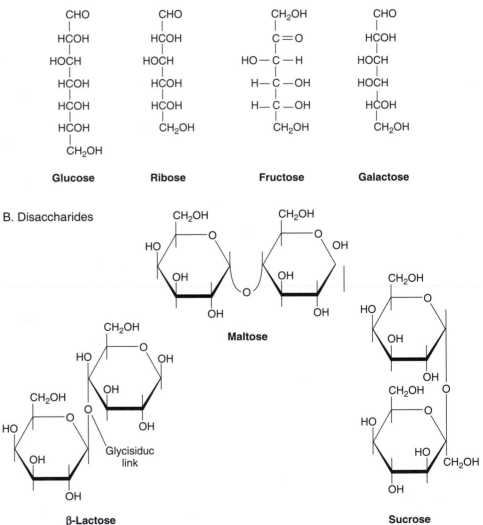

Figure 1–2. Carbohydrate structures.

C.Polysaccharides

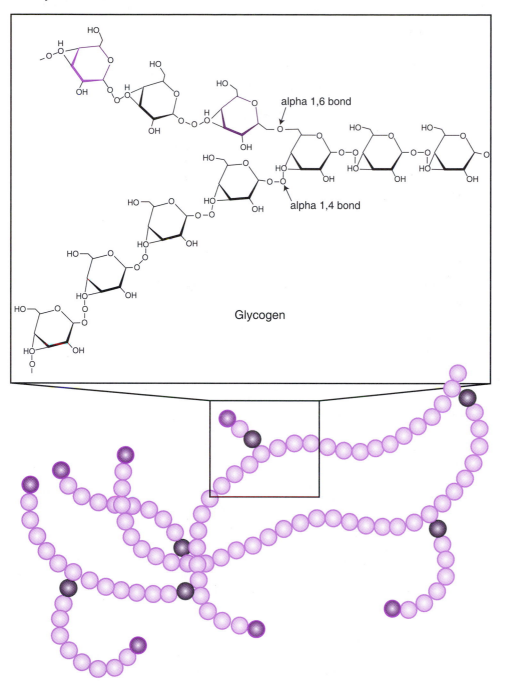

alpha 1,6 bond

alpha 1,4 bond

Glycogen

Figure 1–2. *(continued)*

C.Polysaccharides

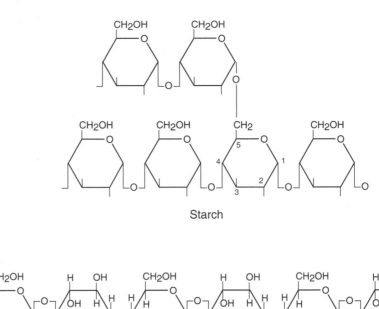

Starch

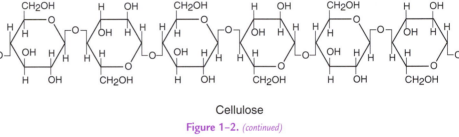

Cellulose

Figure 1–2. *(continued)*

Prokaryotic and eukaryotic living cells use diverse metabolic processes for breaking down carbohydrates and building molecules from carbohydrates. The pathways of carbohydrate metabolism are shown diagrammatically in Figure 1–3. Almost all living cells have the necessary enzymes to oxidize glucose through glycolysis, or the Embden-Meyerhof metabolic pathway. The 6-carbon monosaccharide glucose undergoes **catabolism** to two 3-carbon molecules of pyruvate. As glucose is oxidized, coenzymes are reduced and adenosine triphosphate (ATP) is produced. ATP stores energy within its high-energy phosphate bonds. Many catabolic reactions produce energy that is transferred to the bonds of ATP for storage and for use in the energy-consuming reactions of anabolic metabolism.

Pyruvate that is produced through glycolysis may be consumed through anaerobic fermentation or may undergo further **oxidation** through the tricarboxylic, or Krebs, cycle. Pyruvate is converted to acetylcoenzyme A, which condenses with intermediates of the cycle. Products of the cycle include CO_2, which represents the complete oxidation of glucose, reduced coenzymes, and a small amount of ATP. Not all cells produce the specific enzymes that are needed for each metabolic process. Diverse bacteria ferment sugars to alcohol, mixed acids, and other products. Other cells, including some animal cells, oxidize glucose completely to CO_2. Some living organisms also have the components that are necessary to oxidize the reduced coenzymes and couple the release of energy from these reactions to phosphorylation of adenosine diphosphate in the production of ATP. Production of ATP through this process is called *oxidative phosphorylation*. Some cells transfer

catabolism - the destructive phase of metabolism

oxidation - combining with oxygen; increasing the positive valence of a molecule by loss of electrons

Carbohydrate Metabolism

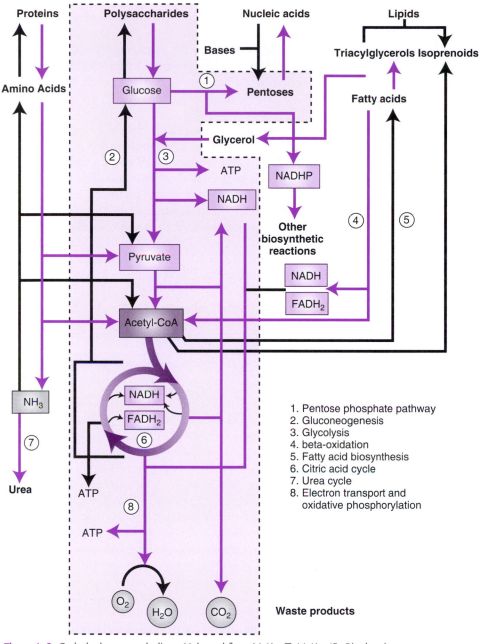

Figure 1–3. Carbohydrate metabolism. (Adapted from McKee T, McKee JR: Biochemistry: The Molecular Basis of Life, ed 3. New York: McGraw-Hill, 2003.)

energy to O_2 in the last step of the reaction, so the process is termed *aerobic respiration*. Other cells transfer energy to molecules other than O_2 in the last step of the reaction; these processes are termed *anaerobic respiration*.

Carbohydrate metabolism includes several other processes. Glucose may be converted to ribose via the pentose phosphate, or hexose monophosphate, pathway.

The pentose phosphate pathway does not produce energy in the form of ATP; however, its products are useful in biosynthetic reactions. Ribose is a component of nucleic acid productions, and NADPH (reduced nicotinamide adenine dinucleotide phosphate), another product of the pathway, is a source of reducing power for biosynthetic processes.

The polysaccharide glycogen is produced in the glycogenesis pathway. Glucose is converted to glycogen for storage of glucose units. Liver and muscle are the major tissues involved in carbohydrate storage. When glucose is needed by the body, glycogen is cleaved to its glucose subunits by the breakdown of glycogen, or *glycogenolysis.*

Some cells, such as liver hepatocytes, produce the necessary enzymes to convert pyruvate to glucose. This process is an example of **anabolism** and is termed *gluconeogenesis,* the birth of new glucose. Carbohydrates may also be formed from the other noncarbohydrate sources, such as fatty acids or amino acids.

Carbohydrate metabolism is regulated by substrate availability, enzyme modification, and hormone control. Two pancreatic hormones, insulin and glucagon, provide regulation for carbohydrate metabolism. The actions of these hormones oppose each other. Insulin is normally released when glucose levels are high and not released when glucose levels are decreased. Insulin is the only hormone that decreases glucose concentration levels in the blood and is referred to as a hypoglycemic agent.

Insulin decreases glucose blood concentration by

- increasing glycogenesis
- increasing glycolysis
- increasing the entry of glucose into muscle and adipose cells via nonspecific receptors
- inhibiting glycogenolysis

Glucagon is released in times of stress and in fasting states. Glucagon increases glucose concentration in the blood and is referred to as a hyperglycemic agent. It increases glucose levels by

- increasing glycogenolysis in liver
- increasing gluconeogenesis

Two hormones that are produced by the adrenal gland also affect carbohydrate metabolism. Epinephrine release is stimulated by physical or emotional stress (the "fight or flight" response). Epinephrine increases blood glucose concentration by

- inhibiting insulin secretion
- increasing glycogenolysis

Cortisol, another adrenal hormone, also increases plasma glucose levels by

- increasing gluconeogenesis
- increasing intestinal absorption of glucose
- increasing glucose entry into the cell

The thyroid hormone thyroxine increases plasma glucose levels by

- increasing glycogenolysis
- increasing gluconeogenesis
- increasing intestinal absorption of glucose

anabolism - the constructive phase of metabolism

Carbohydrates as Biochemical Markers of Disease

The most common carbohydrate disorder in humans is diabetes mellitus. This disease is caused by an inability to produce or to respond to the hormone insulin. Laboratory tests of body fluids of individuals with this disease show increased concentrations of glucose. The laboratory tests for ketones, acids, and glycosylated proteins provide measures of disease severity.

Lipids

Lipids are, by definition, organic compounds that are poorly soluble in solutions such as water and soluble in organic solutions such as ether. As a group of molecules that is defined functionally by solubility, lipids consist of diverse chemical structures. Chemically, lipids are either compounds that yield fatty acids when hydrolyzed or complex alcohols that can combine with fatty acids to form **esters**. Only a limited number of lipids are clinically important. This group includes fatty acids, triacylglycerols (or triglycerides), cholesterol, and phospholipids. The structures for some lipids molecules are reviewed in Figure 1–4.

ester - compound formed by combination of an organic acid and an alcohol with elimination of water

The various types of lipids differ in their chemical and physical properties and in their physiological roles. Some lipids are structural and functional elements of cell membranes. Other lipids serve as precursors for other essential compounds or act as a sources or storage of energy. Lipids are important insulators against heat loss and organ damage and allows for nerve conduction in the central nervous system. When conjugated with proteins, lipids compounds are called *lipoproteins*, the transport form of lipids in aqueous substances such as blood. Apolipoproteins are the protein moieties associated with plasma lipoproteins.

Lipids are classified as *simple lipids*, esters of the fatty acids with various alcohols; *conjugated lipids*, esters of the fatty acids containing groups in addition to an alcohol and fatty acid; and *derived lipids*, substances derived from the above groups by hydrolysis.

Simple lipids are the esters of the fatty acids with various alcohols. For example, triacylglycerols or triglycerides are the esters of the fatty acids with glycerol. The **acyl moiety** of triacylglycerols may be saturated (i.e., they contain no double bonds) or unsaturated (i.e., they contain one or more double bonds). Such chemical structure will influence physical properties such as melting point. Simple lipids may be hydrolyzed by strong alkalis or acids or by enzymes known as lipases to liberate free fatty acids and glycerol. Most triacylglycerol molecules are stored in adipose tissue and degraded by **lipolysis** only when needed.

acyl - the radical derived from an organic acid when the hydroxyl group is removed

moiety - a portion of something that has been divided

lipolysis - the catabolic degradation of triacylglycerol

Phospholipids are conjugated lipids that contain phosphoric acid and nitrogen. The primary importance of phospholipids is their role in the structure of the cell membrane. Lecithin, cephalin, and sphingomyelin are all examples of phospholipids. Glycolipids are conjugated lipids that contain a carbohydrate and nitrogen, but do not contain phosphoric acid. Cerebrosides, sphingolipids, and sphingosine are examples of glycolipids. Of the sphingolipids, sphingomyelin is of primary importance in the structure of cell membranes and the central nervous system.

Lipoproteins are lipid-protein complexes that contain varying amounts and types of lipids, proteins, and phosphates. Chylomicrons are the major carrier of exogenous triacylglycerols. Other lipoproteins include very low-density lipoprotein (VLDL), low-density lipoprotein (LDL), intermediate-density lipoprotein (IDL), and high-density lipoprotein (HDL).

Lipid Structures

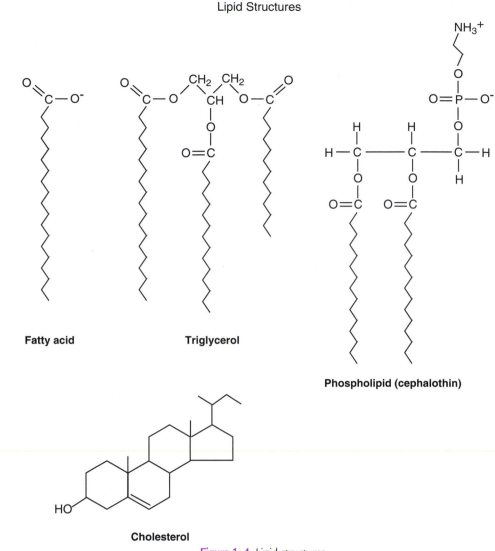

Figure 1–4. Lipid structures.

Derived lipids are substances that are derived from simple or conjugated lipids by hydrolysis. Fatty acids, straight-chain carboxylic acids, are examples of derived lipids. Fatty acids are a source of energy when the energy from carbohydrate metabolism is unavailable. Fatty acids are also the precursors of prostaglandins, a group of molecules that function in many regulatory events in human metabolism.

Fatty acids contain highly reduced hydrocarbons that may be oxidized to produce reduced coenzymes in a process called *beta-oxidation*. Just as the reduced coenzymes of glycolysis and the Krebs cycle may be coupled to the production of ATP through oxidative phosphorylation, the reduced coenzymes that are produced through beta-oxidation may be used to produce ATP. In some disorders, large quantities of fatty acids are oxidized for energy. Intermediate molecules of the degradation process accumulate as the ketone bodies acetoacetate, hydroxybutyrate, and acetone. The production of ketone bodies from the breakdown of lipids is characteristic of severe consequences of diabetes mellitus, in which glucose cannot be utilized for energy and abnormally high concentrations of lipids are degraded. Fatty acids are stored as triacylglycerols, as acyl residues attached to a glycerol molecule through three ester bonds.

Sterols are alcohol derivatives of lipids. The primary sterol derivative, cholesterol, is used to produce bile acids, steroid hormones, and vitamins, such as vitamin D. Cholesterol also modulates cell membrane fluidity. Cholesterol is a ringed structure that can be produced endogenously in the liver or may enter the body through diet.

Lipid Metabolism

Humans are able to produce some lipids endogenously and receive some lipids through the diet. Most dietary lipids are digested in the intestine. Bile salts emulsify or break up the large dietary triacylglycerol molecules into very small particles that can be acted upon by digestive enzymes. Pancreatic and intestinal enzymes digest cholesterol and the emulsified triglycerides so that they can enter the intestinal mucosal cell as small aggregates called *micelles*. Once in the mucosal cell of the intestine, a reassembly process regenerates the triacylglycerol and cholesterol molecules and releases these molecules into circulation in two forms: chylomicrons and free fatty acids that are bound to albumin. Chylomicrons are transported to all tissues in the body, heavily laden with triacylglycerols that are rapidly taken up by cells of adipose tissue.

In tissues cells other than liver cells, chylomicrons are hydrolyzed by an enzyme yielding a remnant particle that is relatively poor in triacylglycerol and rich in cholesterol. In the liver, chylomicron remnants are degraded to VLDL. VLDL is released into bloodstream, where it transfers some of its lipid content to tissue cells, resulting in an IDL particle. IDL is recognized by the liver and degraded to LDL.

LDL is recognized by receptors on the membranes of hepatocytes and peripheral tissue cells. The cholesterol-rich LDL is engulfed by cells (including smooth muscle cells), leading to deposits of cholesterol in the cytoplasm of tissue cells. Smooth muscle accumulation of LDL cholesterol results in atherosclerotic plaques in arterial walls.

HDL is produced in both the liver and intestinal wall (and peripheral circulation). This lipoprotein serves to transport cholesterol away from tissues and thus provides some protection against coronary artery disease.

In the cell, lipids may be oxidized for energy or used as precursors for lipid derivatives or structural properties of cells. Lipid metabolism is also carefully regulated through regulation of the enzymes that catalyze its metabolic reactions and through hormonal control. Lipid metabolism, including fatty acid metabolism, is reviewed in Figure 1–5.

Lipids as Biochemical Markers of Disease

Clinical chemistry laboratories offer many tests for lipid disorders. One of the most common tests is the lipid profile. This panel of tests includes measures of triacylglycerol and cholesterol in the form of lipoprotein-cholesterol molecules, low-density lipoprotein cholesterol (LDL-C) and high-density lipoprotein cholesterol (HDL-C). The results of testing for these lipids provide measures of risk for coronary artery disease.

Although the concentration of cholesterol in blood is dependent on many factors such as genetics, age, sex, diet, and physical activity, total cholesterol measurement is used clinically to monitor disease. In addition to its role as a risk factor for

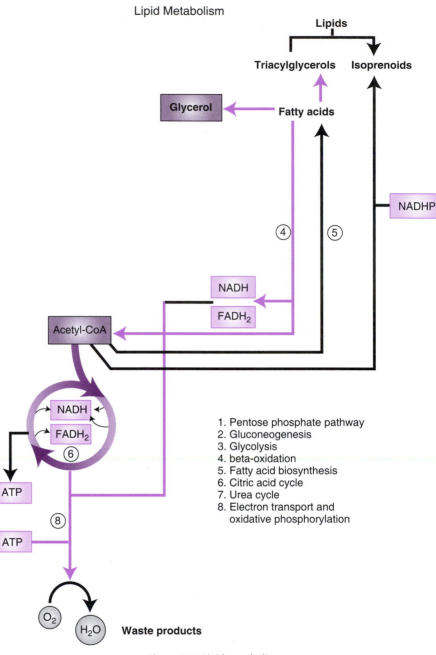

Figure 1–5. Lipid metabolism.

The lipid panel includes measures of triacylglycerol and cholesterol in the form of lipoprotein-cholesterol molecules, low-density lipoprotein cholesterol (LDL-C), and high-density lipoprotein cholesterol (HDL-C). The results of testing for these lipids provide measures of risk for coronary artery disease.

coronary artery disease, increased cholesterol concentration may be the result of hypothyroidism, liver disease, renal disease, or diabetes. Decreased cholesterol concentration may be the result of hyperthyroidism, digestive malabsorption, or impaired liver function. Factors that increase HDL-C include increased estrogen in women, increased exercise, and the effects of certain blood pressure medicines. Factors that decrease HDL-C include increased progesterone, obesity, smoking, and diabetes. Increased triacylglycerol may be the result of pancreatitis, diabetes mellitus, acute alcohol consumption, or certain liver diseases. In addition, triacylglycerol may be increased artifactually in nonfasting blood samples.

Proteins and Amino Acids

The human body requires 20 amino acids as the building blocks of proteins. Humans make some of these amino acids but must gain the rest, as **essential nutrients**, through the diet. Plants and bacteria produce the essential amino acids and many others.

The production of proteins from amino acid building blocks is directed by a template that is produced by the **DNA** of the cell. Therefore, the amino acid sequence of protein is a reflection of the genetic information of the cell. Most enzymes are proteins that are able to catalyze reactions. Through regulation of reactions via enzymes, the genetic information directs the diverse metabolic reactions of the cell. In addition to their function as an energy source and in catalysis, amino acids and proteins are used as transport molecules, structural components of cells and tissues, hormones, clotting agents, and immune agents.

Proteins and amino acids have unique structures (Fig. 1–6) and participate in characteristic chemical reactions. Proteins are polymers consisting of amino acid units. Amino acid units within the protein are joined by peptide bonds. Each amino acid unit contains a unique R group. The amino acid unit on the carboxyl end of the protein contains a free carboxyl group that does not participate in peptide bond formation. The amino acid unit on the amino end of the protein contains a free amino group that does not participate in peptide bond formation.

The carboxyl end may become charged when a hydrogen ion is lost. The amino end may become charged when a hydrogen ion is gained. The peptide bond consists of the covalent linkage of an amino group from one amino acid and a carboxyl group of another amino acid. Proteins are *ampholytes;* that is, in aqueous solutions they may have positive and negative charges on the same molecule. This property

essential nutrients - molecules that are required for metabolism but cannot be produced endogenously; required in the diet

DNA - deoxyribonucleic acid; in the eukaryote and some prokaryotes, the chemical that transmits inherited characteristics of an organism to its progeny

Amino Acid and Protein Structure

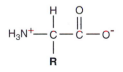

Amino acid

(**R** = unique portion of molecule for each amino acis)

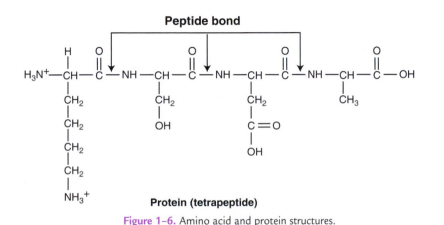

Protein (tetrapeptide)

Figure 1–6. Amino acid and protein structures.

of proteins is used to separate protein molecules during electrophoresis. The *pH* (hydrogen ion concentration) of the solution determines the net charge of the molecule. At different pH environments, hydrogen ions will be gained or lost from the carboxyl and amino ends and from functional groups of R residues of the amino acids. Since proteins are composed of different amino acids, different proteins will gain or lose hydrogen ions at different pH environments.

Each peptide has a pH at which the net loss and gain of hydrogen ions is equal. This pH is called the *pI*, or isoelectric point, and is unique for each protein. The pI is unique for each protein because each protein has a unique chemical makeup and structure.

In addition to the properties of proteins as ampholytes, proteins also have other representative structural properties. Fibrous proteins usually function as structural components of the body, such as fibrinogen and collagen. Most plasma proteins and enzymes are globular proteins. Fibrous proteins are insoluble. The structure of fibrous proteins imbues strength to tissue through its linear configuration. Globular proteins play many roles in the body. Globular proteins contain intricate folding sequences. Subgroups within globular proteins interact through noncovalent bonding. Noncovalent interaction is an important character of enzyme proteins.

Proteins may be characterized by the sequence of the amino acids that compose them, the chemical interaction of the components of the protein strand, the regular pattern of folding within the strand, and, finally, the interaction of several protein strands that make up the functional protein. *Primary structure* refers to the sequence of amino acid units that make up the protein strand. The amino acid sequence is coded from DNA information of the cell in which the protein was created. *Secondary structure* refers to the folds of the protein strand. Sections of the protein strand may be folded into regular structures, such as alpha helixes and beta pleats. *Tertiary structure* refers to folds of sections of the protein. Hydrogen bonds, disulfide bridges, and hydrophobic interactions between functional groups of the protein strand may stabilize tertiary structure. *Quaternary structure* refers to the association of two or more peptide strands to form one functioning protein.

Several protein fractions may be found in normal serum:

Prealbumin, also called *transthyretin*, is a transport protein. Prealbumin is important in the transport of the thyroid hormones thyroxine and triiodothyronine. Prealbumin concentration is used as a measurement of nutritional status.

Albumin has an important role in maintaining colloidal oncotic pressure and preventing edema. Since water moves freely through cell membranes and into the intravascular space by osmosis, the high concentration of proteins in intravascular fluid allows movement of water into vessels, and normal blood pressure and cardiac output allow circulation to evenly distribute the fluids. If the concentration of albumin is significantly decreased, fluids accumulate in interstitial spaces and cause edema. Normal protein concentration in blood vessels allows fluid to flow freely from intracellular to interstitial to intravascular spaces. Albumin also serves as a transport molecule for various substances.

Alpha$_1$ antitrypsin is a serine proteinase inhibitor that inhibits elastase. Elastase breaks down elastin in such tissues as the tracheobroncial tree. Alpha$_1$ antitrypsin is an acute-phase protein.

Alpha$_1$ acid glycoprotein is a conjugated protein that consists of 45% carbohydrate. Alpha$_1$ acid glycoprotein inactivates lipophilic hormones. It is an acute-phase protein.

Alpha₁ fetoprotein is a conjugated protein that consists of 4% carbohydrate. Alpha₁ fetoprotein is the predominant plasma protein of the fetus. It is a fetal albumin analog.

Haptoglobin is a glycoprotein that consists of four protein chains. Haptoglobin transports free hemoglobin through the blood to the liver for degradation. Haptoglobin is an acute-phase protein.

Alpha₂ macroglobulin is a proteinase inhibitor and acute-phase reactant.

Ceruloplasmin is a copper-containing alpha₂ globulin. Ceruloplasmin is involved in **reduction** and oxidation reactions in cellular metabolism. Ceruloplasmin is an acute-phase protein and transports copper.

Transferrin is a transport protein for iron.

C4 is a complement protein that plays roles in the antibody-antigen response and in the destruction of bacteria and viruses. C4 is an acute-phase protein.

C3 is a complement protein that plays roles in the antibody-antigen response and in the destruction of bacteria and viruses. C3 is an acute-phase protein.

Beta₂ microglobulin is the light chain of the human leukocyte antigen (HLA) molecule.

Beta lipoprotein is a conjugated protein that transports lipids, primarily cholesterol.

Gamma globulin proteins contain two light and two heavy chains. Variations of amino acid sequences on the heavy chains distinguish the immunoglobulin (Ig) classes. IgG is produced in response to specific infections to destroy toxins and foreign invaders of the body. IgA is the secretory immunoglobulin protecting the mucosal surfaces. IgM is the first antibody produced in response to an infection.

C-reactive protein is an acute-phase protein; that is, it appears in the blood following infection or tissue damage.

Amino acids can be *deaminated* to organic intermediates of carbohydrate and lipid metabolism and used as energy. The amino group that results from deamination may be used to produce other amino acids in a reaction called *transamination.* Free amino groups may be converted to ammonia molecules, a toxic compound. Mammals convert ammonia to urea in the liver and excrete the urea via the kidney.

Total Serum/Plasma Proteins and Plasma Albumin as Biochemical Markers of Disease

Plasma proteins have functions in many organ and tissue systems. They are carrier molecules, receptor chemicals, immune response agents, and enzymes or catalytic proteins. Total plasma protein is a measure of nutrition, the status of many organs and tissues that are involved in protein metabolism, and the process of breakdown and excretion of protein metabolites. The measurement of plasma protein fractions provides more specific evidence for diagnosis and assessment of disorders. Because of its importance in maintaining osmotic pressure, the measure of albumin concentration is a reflection of this pressure. As a transport protein, the measurement of albumin monitors the ability of the body to transport such diverse substances as bilirubin, fatty acids, and calcium through the blood. Measurement of the transport proteins of a specific substance provides information about the metabolism of that substance. For example, the measurement of transferrin is helps the physician understand the metabolic processes involving iron.

Most amino acids are broken down in the liver and then excreted through the kidney. Therefore, blood and urine tests that measure the concentration of these

reduction - losing oxygen; increasing the negative valence of a molecule by gain of electrons

metabolites monitor both liver and urine function. The urea nitrogen test is an indicator of renal disorders and may be used to determine the source of the disorder: prerenal, renal or postrenal. Other breakdown products, such as ammonia, are measured as toxic compounds of metabolism.

Enzymes

An enzyme is a protein catalyst that accelerates the speed of a chemical reaction by binding specifically to a substrate, forming a complex. This complex lowers the activation energy in the reaction without the enzyme becoming consumed or without changing the equilibrium of the reaction.

Enzyme analysis is used to aid in diagnosis and treatment of disease. In particular, enzymes synthesized intracellularly carry out their functions within cells, and are released into body fluids when those cells become diseased. Thus, an increase in enzyme activity when compared to the reference range can indicate pathological changes in certain cells and tissues. Enzyme activity levels in body fluids can reflect leakage from cells due to cellular injury, or changes in enzyme production rate, or actual enzyme induction due to metabolic or genetic states or proliferation of neoplasms. In the latter case, increased enzyme activity can be used as a tumor marker.

One aspect of enzyme activity that must be considered when it is used to indicate tissue pathology is the relative time frame in which the enzyme activity appears and then remains in circulation in relationship with the disorder. For example, some enzymes found in plasma due to tissue necrosis or inflammation rise at such a slow rate that they are not useful for early detection or treatment of the disease. Other enzymes rapidly decline in circulation because of inactivation or metabolism. The clinical utility of enzyme activity in relationship to specific tissue pathology and clinical signs is enhanced when the enzyme activity quickly rises following the onset of the disorder and remains elevated for an adequate time frame, particularly when other clinical signs and symptoms are not sufficient to provide a diagnosis.

Enzymes as Biochemical Markers of Disease

Damage to tissue can release different types of enzymes based on their location. For example, mild inflammation of the liver reversibly increases the permeability of the cell membrane and releases cytoplasmic enzymes such as lactate dehydrogenase (LD), alkaline phosphatase (ALP), and aspartate transaminase (AST), while necrosis will release mitochondrial sources of alanine transaminase (ALT) as well as AST. Distribution of these enzymes within specific types of hepatic tissues varies. ALP and gamma-glutamyltransferase (GGT) are more concentrated in the biliary tree or **canalicular** tissues, while AST, ALT, and LD are found in **parenchymal** hepatic cells. Multiple forms of enzymes (isoenzymes) exist and are distributed in several different tissue types. For example, ALP is found in **hepatobiliary** tissues and also found in all cytoplasmic membranes of all cells of the body, especially in **osteoblasts** of the bone, intestinal mucosa, placenta, and renal tubules.

Classes of Enzymes

There are six classes of enzymes, describing the type of reaction involved: oxidoreductases, transferases, hydrolases, lyases, ligases, and isomerases. Enzyme nomenclature has evolved into a standardized system to include a systematic name with numerical designation for each enzyme as well as a trivial or practical name.

canalicular - within canals or small ducts

parenchymal - part of the main structure of the organ

hepatobiliary - relating to bile ducts and ducts within the liver

osteoblasts - young active cells of the bone

The following descriptions are relevant to enzyme analysis:

Enzyme: a protein catalyst that accelerates the speed of a chemical reaction by complexing specifically to a substrate, forming a complex that lowers the activation energy in the reaction without becoming consumed or without changing the equilibrium of the reaction.

Activity: rate of product produced or substrate consumed per unit of time; dependent on enzyme activity, substrate, activator, and coenzyme concentrations; temperature; pH; and other reaction conditions.

Substrate: precursor to a product that combines with an enzyme at a unique attachment site and becomes transformed to affect the reaction rate of product formation. Concentration of substrate plays a significant role in enzyme activity for formation of product.

International unit (U) of activity: quantity of enzyme able to convert one micromole (1 μmol) of substrate per minute to product; often expressed as units per liter (U/L) or microunits per liter (mU/L). The formula for determining U/L is

$$\Delta A/min \times ([1/micromolar\ absorptivity\ of\ product] \times total$$
$$volume\ [mL])/volume\ of\ sample\ (mL) = \mu mol/min/L\ or\ U/L$$

Activator: substance, such as a metal, that promotes formation of enzyme-substrate complex and may affect enzyme activity for the formation of product.

Coenzyme: complex molecule, such as dinucleotide (involved in electron transfer), that acts along with the substrate to aid in formation of product in a primary reaction or as the actual substrate in a secondary reaction.

Michaelis constant: K_m, the equilibrium coefficient that is one-half maximum velocity ($^1/_2\ V_{max}$).

Inhibitors: different types of interferences with the function of an enzyme that may be reversible or irreversible and lower the reaction rate of product formation.

Competitive inhibitors: compete with the substrate for the active site of the enzyme and prevent formation of product, but have a higher K_m than the preferred substrate and can be overcome by addition of more substrate.

Noncompetitive inhibitors: bind on a different active site of the enzyme than the substrate and so cannot be overcome by addition of more substrate, but prevent formation of product despite the enzyme-substrate complex.

Uncompetitive inhibitors: bind to the enzyme-substrate complex and prevent the formation of product. This type of inhibition is also reversible.

Aspects of enzyme kinetics (where S = substrate, E = enzyme, and P = product):

$$S \rightarrow P\ requires\ more\ energy$$
$$S + E \rightarrow SE \rightarrow P + E\ requires\ less\ energy$$

First-Order and Zero-Order Enzyme Kinetics

First-order kinetics is described in the following manner: as substrate concentration increases, the rate of product formation increases hyperbolically as it combines with available enzyme and, thus, rate of product formation depends on both substrate and enzyme concentration. Zero-order kinetics is described as enzyme activity at maximum velocity (V_{max}) due to excess substrate concentration. Increasing

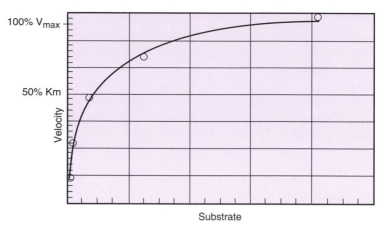

Figure 1–7. Michaelis-Menton curve: substrate concentration versus rate of product formation.

substrate concentration will not increase the velocity of product formation in this circumstance. For analysis of enzyme levels and determining activity of enzymes in serum or other body fluids, maintaining the conditions with substrate concentration in excess is necessary.

As substrate concentration increases for a particular enzyme, the rate of product formation increases hyperbolically and up to V_{max}. The equilibrium coefficient that represents the likelihood of a particular enzyme-substrate complex to dissociate and form product is the Michaelis constant, K_m. This is unique for a particular enzyme-substrate complex and is determined as $^{1}/_{2} V_{max}$ of the Michaelis-Menton curve. Figure 1–7 depicts this relationship. K_m can be useful to determine the preferred substrate for a particular enzyme since it is lowest for the preferred substrate. It is also useful when characterizing the type of enzyme inhibition that may be present in a system. Lineweaver and Burk created a linear transformation of this kinetic conversion of substrate to product that helps to identify the effect of inhibition more easily. Figure 1–8 shows the Lineweaver-Burk relationship of substrate concentration to velocity.

When substrate is in excess and pH, temperature, and activator concentrations are held at optimum conditions, the velocity of the enzyme catalysis of substrate to product is dependent only on enzyme activity. Temperature has a major effect on the outcome of enzyme kinetic analyses. Increasing the temperature of the reaction conditions will increase movement of the enzyme and substrate molecules, allowing for the rate of product formation to increase. For example, increasing the temperature by 10°C will double the reaction rate. Thus, reference ranges for enzymes

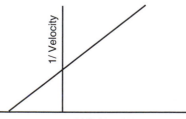

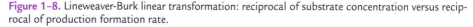

Figure 1–8. Lineweaver-Burk linear transformation: reciprocal of substrate concentration versus reciprocal of production formation rate.

need to be based on the temperature at which the analysis occurs and often are set for 37°C.

Integration of Metabolism

All metabolic processes in the body are interconnected (Fig. 1–9). Carbohydrate molecules can be used to produce proteins; the carbon skeleton of amino acids can be converted to certain carbohydrates. Lipid structures such as glycerol may be

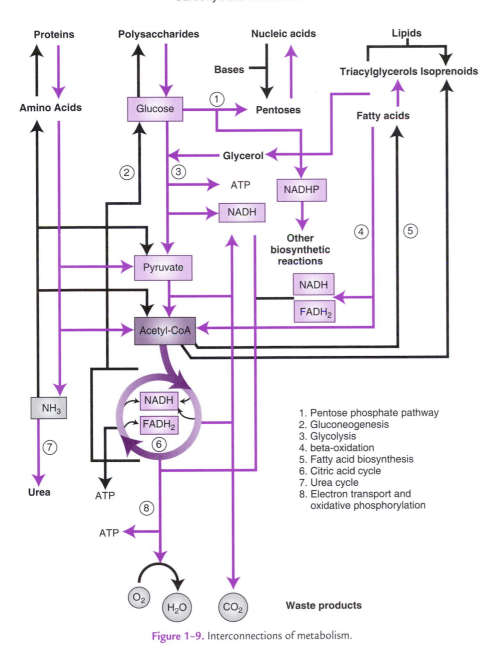

Figure 1–9. Interconnections of metabolism.

used as intermediate molecules for gluconeogenesis. Enzymes catalyze the metabolic reactions of carbohydrate, lipid, and protein biochemical markers. The impact of the interconnection on disease is that a disorder that originates in one biochemical marker category, such as carbohydrates, will eventually impact on the metabolism of other categories of biochemical markers.

Clinical chemistry laboratory scientists use their knowledge of biochemistry as the basis for understanding clinical disorders that involve metabolic processes. Laboratory assessment is designed to detect concentration changes of enzymes, proteins, lipids, carbohydrates, and their derivatives from the "normal" concentration range of a healthy population (reference range). Laboratory assessment may also include measurement of change in concentration of markers that may be altered in disease, such as electrolytes and vitamins.

The correlation of change in selected biochemical markers and the assessment of disease are based on research studies of healthy and diseased individuals over time. The more commonly known research studies that are used to support correlation of biochemical marker concentrations to disease processes include the Diabetes Research Group study and the Framingham cardiac risk study. The Diabetes Research Group studies include examination of the effects of diabetes mellitus on the concentration of blood glucose and glycolated hemoglobin. The results of the studies are published in *Diabetes Care* and are used by scientists and clinicians to determine threshold concentration values for diagnosis of diabetes and assessment of the risk for severe consequences of the disease.[7]

The Framingham study measured selected biochemical markers in the blood of hundreds of individuals over time. The study showed that those individuals who had increased blood lipids were at greater risk for cardiac disorders than those individuals with lower concentrations of blood lipids over time.[8–10]

Genetic Metabolism

Metabolism of the cell is ultimately directed by the genetic components, DNA and **RNA**, of the cell. DNA is composed of antiparallel polymers of nucleotide units. The nucleotides of each polymer strand are bound together covalently by phosphodiester bonds, while the two polymer strands are held together by hydrogen bonds. This loose attraction of hydrogen bonding allows separation and **replication** of the strands by enzymes to occur more easily than would be possible if the bonds were covalent.

DNA may also be transcribed to another form of nucleic acid, RNA, for transport of the genetic message to cell cytoplasm. Through the **transcription** of intermediate messages of RNA, the nucleic acids of the nucleus are synthesized into proteins by **translation**. Ribosomal RNA directs the production of cell proteins in the **endoplasmic reticulum**.

Proteins, the products of this process, are further modified by the cells to form essential elements of the cell. Some proteins, the enzymes, form the catalysts of metabolic reactions. These enzymes regulate metabolism of the cell, the tissue, and the organism. The **genome** of the cells directs the production of the **proteome** of the cell and organism.

Genetic Markers as Biochemical Markers of Disease

Molecular diagnostics laboratories perform testing to detect nucleic acids that code for specific proteins, or specific sequences of proteins, that are associated with diseases such as malignancies. The major testing done by these laboratories involves

RNA - ribonucleic acid; serves as a messenger of inherited nucleic acid from the nucleus template and translates that message into protein; in some prokaryotes, it is the chemical that serves as the inherited message

replication - duplication of DNA

transcription - synthesis of RNA from a DNA template

translation - synthesis of protein

endoplasmic reticulum - cell organelle that serves as a compartment for numerous chemical reactions

genome - the complete set of genetic information produced by the cell

proteome - the complete set of proteins produced by the cell

polymerase chain reaction (PCR), reverse transcriptase–PCR (RT-PCR), and fluorescent in-situ hybridization (FISH). FISH methodology is discussed in this textbook as it relates to tumor marker measurement.

As a reflection of the fundamental character of the cell, analysis of the proteome of the cell may provide information about pathological processes of the organism. Growing interest in an examination of the post-translation modification of the proteome as it is related to disease and health is contributing to the implementation of methods in **proteomics** in the clinical laboratory. The future of the clinical chemistry laboratory may lie in the science of proteomics.

> ■■ **CLINICAL CORRELATION**
> ■■
> Molecular diagnostics laboratories perform testing to detect nucleic acids that code for specific proteins, or specific sequences of proteins, that are associated with diseases such as malignances.

proteomics - analysis of the proteome

Case Scenario 1-2 The New Class Discusses the Scope of Practice

Scope of Practice: Final Comments

The instructor continues, "The clinical laboratory uses analysis of biochemicals to provide evidence of function or dysfunction of body systems. Use your knowledge of anatomy and physiology to offer specific laboratory test results for directed diagnosis and treatment."

THE CLINICAL CHEMISTRY LABORATORY AND ORGAN SYSTEMS

Cardiovascular Circulatory System

The heart is enclosed in a two-layered sac, or pericardium. The inner layer surrounds the heart; the outer layer holds a serous fluid that helps reduce friction as the heart beats. The heart is composed of the epicardium, an outer fibrous layer; the myocardium, a layer of muscle; and an inner epithelium, or endocardium. The four chambers of the heart contract rhythmically to pump blood to cells of the body. The chambers on the right, the right atrium and ventricle, pump blood to the lungs and the chambers on the left, the left atrium and ventricle, pump blood to other body cells. Deoxygenated blood enters the right atrium and is pumped to the lungs by the right ventricle. Blood is oxygenated in the lungs and returns to the left atrium and leaves the heart to be pumped to tissue cells by the left ventricle. A pair of coronary arteries supplies oxygenated blood to the heart muscles. Heart muscle damage and chest pain are caused by decreased blood flow through these arteries. Two pair of large and small veins carry deoxygenated blood away from the muscles of the body and into the venous circulation. Figure 1–10 depicts the heart, arteries, and veins.

Arteries conduct blood away from the heart under high pressure. The arteries are thicker than veins and may be aided by smooth muscle. Veins return blood back to the heart under lower pressure. Veins are more elastic than arteries and are aided less by muscle action. At certain points of the venous system, valves within the endothelium prevent backward flow of blood. Capillaries are thin endothelial tubes that allow exchange of nutrients and gases to and from tissue cells by diffusion. The veins in the crook of the arm (formed when the elbow is slightly bent) are commonly used to obtain blood samples for testing in the clinical laboratory. Figure 1–11 depicts the location of the systemic veins and the vena cava.

Within the blood, specific cells perform many functions. Red blood cells contain hemoglobin, an iron-containing protein that transports oxygen and carbon dioxide to body cells. As blood passes through the lungs, oxygen molecules attach to the hemoglobin. As the blood passes through the body's tissue, the hemoglobin

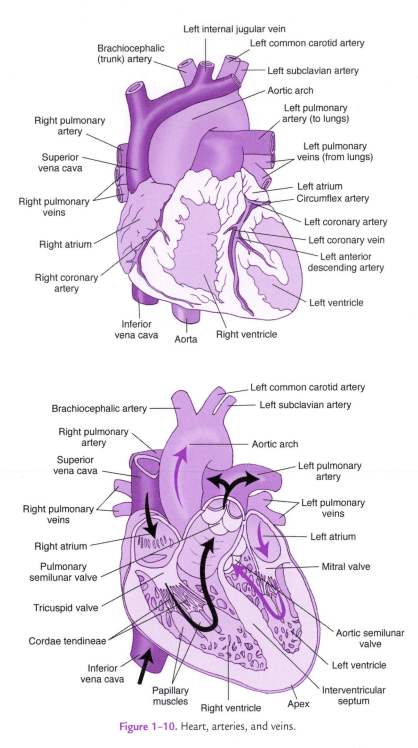

Figure 1–10. Heart, arteries, and veins.

releases the oxygen to the cells. Hemoglobin molecules then bond with carbon dioxide, a waste product of metabolism, and transport it back to the lungs.

The laboratory provides information about the function of the heart muscle, the condition of the arteries and veins that transport blood, and the ability of hemoglobin to transport gases. The clinical chemistry laboratory offers analysis of

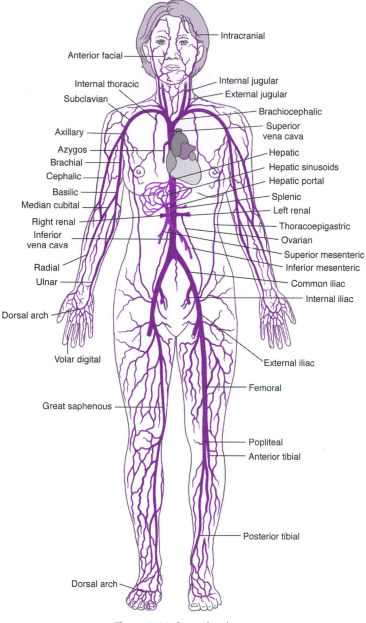

Figure 1-11. Systemic veins.

biochemicals for the assessment of acute myocardial infarction, congestive heart failure and coronary artery disease. The laboratory offers measurement of lipids as predictive factors for the development of heart disease. Measurement of arterial blood gases helps assess the acid-base and oxygenation status of the patient.

Respiratory Tract

The function of the respiratory tract is to transfer gases from the environment to tissue cells and from tissues cells to the environment. The respiratory system also

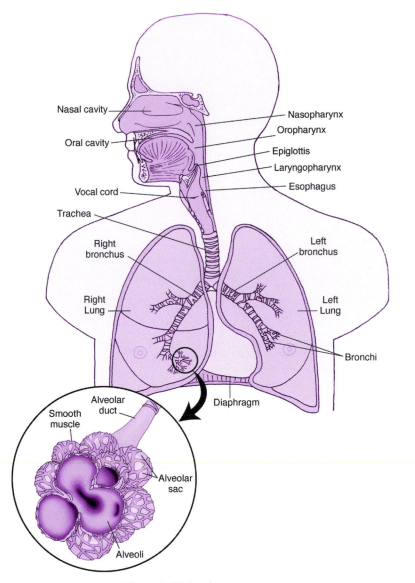

Figure 1–12. Respiratory tract.

helps maintain the acid-base balance in the body. The respiratory tract includes the air passages of the nasal cavity, trachea, bronchi, bronchioles, alveolar ducts, and air sacs or alveoli. (The singular forms of bronchi and alveoli are *bronchus* and *alveolus*.) Oxygen from the environment travels through the bronchioles to alveolar ducts and into the alveoli, where it is absorbed into blood, while carbon dioxide is released from blood to the environment along the reverse route. Figure 1–12 depicts the respiratory system.

Measurement of arterial blood gases helps assess the function of the respiratory system, as well as the circulatory system. Blood oxygenation and pH are dependent upon the uptake of oxygen by hemoglobin and removal of carbon dioxide from red blood cells. The assessment of diseases such as chronic obstructive pulmonary disease is dependent upon the measurement of partial pressures of oxygen and carbon dioxide in arterial blood to monitor the function of the lungs.

Liver

The two lobes of the liver contain lobules that are highly vascularized by the portal blood system. Blood filters into the **sinusoids** of the lobules and into hepatocytes. Here nutrients are metabolized. The gallbladder stores the bile that is produced by the liver and delivers it into the small intestine via the common bile duct. Bile is composed of water, salts, pigments, and fatty acids that have been processed by the liver. Bile emulsifies fats into small particles to make them more digestible by intestinal enzymes.

The liver regulates most chemical levels in the blood and excretes bile, which remove waste products from the body. The many function of the liver include

- production of bile, which helps remove waste (especially fat-soluble waste) through the digestive tract
- production of plasma proteins
- production of endogenous cholesterol
- production and storage of glycogen for storage glucose units
- breakdown of amino acids and conversion of the toxic breakdown product, ammonia, to urea
- conjugation of bilirubin
- biotransformation of **xenobiotics**, including drugs

sinusoid - a large, permeable capillary

xenobiotic - a biochemical that is not produced in the body

These substances serve as biochemical markers of liver disease. The laboratory provides measurement of the waste products of degradation of proteins, such as ammonia and urea, and the waste product of the degradation of heme (bilirubin) to assess liver function. The clinical chemistry laboratory offers a plethora of tests that provide information about specific diseases of the liver. Measurement of the concentration of the enzyme alanine transaminase (ALT) provides information about hepatitis. Measurement of the enzyme alkaline phosphatase (ALP) provides information about biliary tract disorders. Analysis of the concentrations of proteins that are made in the liver provides information about the ability of the liver to perform this function.

Renal System

The urinary-renal system (Fig. 1–13) includes the kidneys, ureters, urinary bladder, and urethra. The kidneys filter blood in a process that maintains acid-base balance, preserves water volume, and conserves the concentration of chemicals in blood. Through a **filtration** and **resorption** system, ions and metabolic chemicals are kept in narrow concentrations in the blood, with the renal system at times excreting a chemical or conserving the chemical as needed to maintain balance.

The functional unit of the kidney, the nephron, filters chemicals from the blood through the glomerulus and resorbs some chemicals back into the blood through the nephron tubule in a highly regulated process that establishes the homeostasis of the blood.

The kidneys filter blood plasma and excrete waste, including urea, creatinine, uric acid, metabolites of drugs, and other foreign substances. They are also the site of reabsorption of some of these same substances, nutrients, and electrolytes. The kidneys regulate blood pH by conserving or excreting ions such as ammonia and carbonate. They are the site for the maintenance of blood pressure by regulating blood and urine water content.

filtration - the process of removing particles from a solution by passing the solution through a membrane or other barrier

resorption - to soak up or take in again

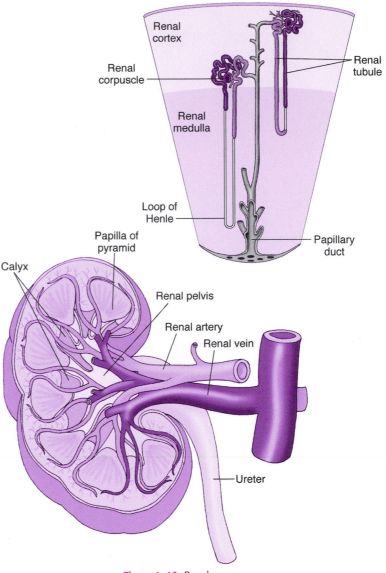

Figure 1–13. Renal system.

The clinical chemistry laboratory offers many tests for different biochemical markers of renal function, including electrolytes, minerals, and protein metabolic waste products. These biochemical markers are measured in serum, urine, and other body fluids.

Digestive System

The digestive system is a tube that runs through the body, starting with the oral cavity and continuing to the anal canal. The liver and pancreas have ducts that empty into the digestive system. The function of the digestive system is to break down and prepare nutrients for absorption into the blood for transport to tissue cells. Food is pulverized in the oral cavity; the salivary glands secrete amylase into the pulverized food, beginning the chemical breakdown of the carbohydrates.

In the stomach, food is broken down mechanically and enzymatically. Protein is digested by the enzyme pepsin, which is secreted into the stomach by **chief cells**. Hydrochloric acid that is secreted by **parietal cells** further breaks down nutrients. The stomach also secretes intrinsic factor that acts in the small intestine to influence the absorption of vitamin B$_{12}$. Most digestion of nutrients occurs in the small intestine. Secretions from the pancreas and liver, via the gallbladder, digest carbohydrates, lipids, and proteins into their constituent units. The pancreas secretes the enzymes lipase and amylase into the small intestine to degrade triacylglycerol and polysaccharides, respectively, into units that can pass through enterocyes of the small intestine. These nutrients cross the mucosa of the small intestine into blood. In the large intestine, only water, minerals, and some vitamins are absorbed. Nutrient-laden blood is transported by the hepatic portal circulatory system to the liver, where nutrients are altered and metabolized to be sent out to the body as nutrient components are needed. Figure 1–14 depicts the organs of the digestive system.

chief cells - secretory cells that line the gastric glands and secrete pepsin or its precursor, pepsinogen

parietal cells - cells of the stomach that secrete hydrochloric acid and intrinsic factor

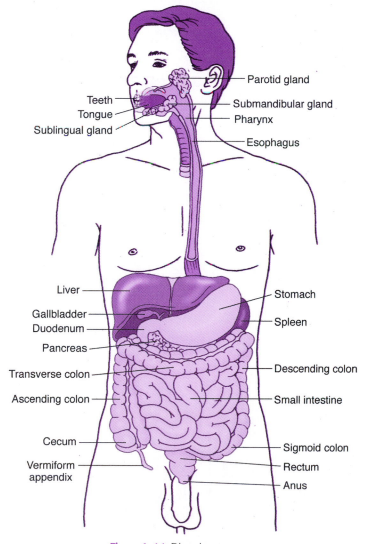

Teeth
Tongue
Sublingual gland

Parotid gland
Submandibular gland
Pharynx
Esophagus

Liver
Gallbladder
Duodenum
Pancreas
Transverse colon
Ascending colon
Cecum
Vermiform appendix

Stomach
Spleen
Descending colon
Small intestine
Sigmoid colon
Rectum
Anus

Figure 1–14. Digestive system.

The clinical chemistry laboratory provides information about nutritional status, intestinal absorption, and function of the pancreas and other organs of the digestive tract. The concentration of proteins of varying **half-life** helps establish the length of time of nutritional deficiency. Analysis of gastric fluid assesses the ability of the stomach to secrete acid. Measurement of serum concentrations of lipase and amylase monitors the exocrine function of the pancreas.

half-life - one-half of the time between synthesis and degradation of a compound

Endocrine System

The endocrine glands consist of secretory cells that are supported by connective tissue. The endocrine glands do not contain hormone-secreting ducts; rather, they secrete hormones directly into the blood, where the hormones are taken to tissue cells that are receptive to their effects. The glands of the pituitary, thyroid, parathyroid, adrenals, pancreas, ovaries, and testes all have endocrine function. In addition, the kidney, gastrointestinal tract, and placenta produce chemicals that have hormone function. Figure 1–15 depicts the glands of the endocrine system.

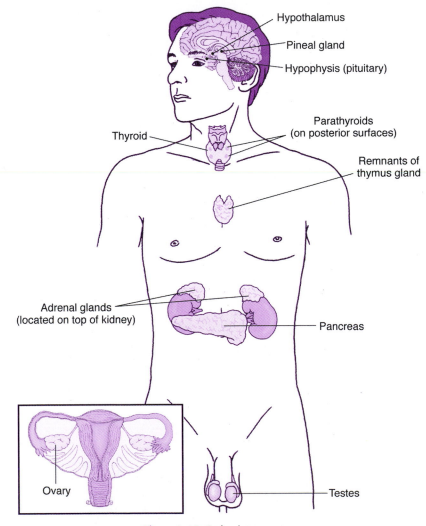

Hypothalamus

Pineal gland

Hypophysis (pituitary)

Parathyroids
(on posterior surfaces)

Thyroid

Remnants of
thymus gland

Adrenal glands
(located on top of kidney)

Pancreas

Ovary

Testes

Figure 1–15. Endocrine system.

Hormones differ in chemical structure. An endocrine hormone is a chemical substance that is produced by an endocrine gland that has a regulatory effect on the cells of tissue other than the tissue in which it is synthesized. Growth hormone, antidiuretic hormone, and adrenocorticotropic hormone (corticotropin) are all examples of hormones that are peptides in chemical structure. Cortisol, testosterone, and estrogen are examples of steroid hormones. The chemical structure of the hormone directs the method by which it is transported in blood, its action on its target cell, and the length of its life.

The clinical laboratory measures the concentrations of some hormones. For the assessment of other hormones that vary in concentration over a 24-hour period or are too labile to measure with accuracy, the laboratory scientist establishes hormonal function by measuring the concentration of the metabolites of hormone degradation or the process that the hormone regulates. Clear understanding of specimen collection and handling is essential for offering useful laboratory tests results of hormonal function.

Bone

Bone is living tissue that uses oxygen and gives off waste products in metabolism. Bone requires a blood supply and a source of nutrients to grow and develop. The functions of bone include protection of soft tissue and support for mechanical activity. Bones protect the nervous system, the respiratory system, and the heart. Within the red marrow of bones, **hematopoiesis**, the formation of blood cells, occurs. Figure 1–16 depicts a long bone and the location of marrow in the medullary (inner central) cavity.

hematopoiesis - the production and development of blood cells

Bones are dependent upon a source of calcium and phosphorus, which make up the intercellular matrix of bone structure. Calcium and phosphorus are continually stored in bone and resorbed into blood as nutrients are available.

The clinical chemistry laboratory offers the health-care provider several measures for the assessment of bone. Serum calcium and phosphate concentrations provide a measure of the resorption of these chemicals from bone. The measurement of parathyroid hormone assesses hormone regulation of bone development. Analysis of vitamin D concentration provides a measure of the ability of the body to absorb dietary calcium through the small intestine.

Central Nervous System

The central nervous system consists of the brain, spinal cord, and neuron processes. The central nervous system is surrounded by membranes of the meninges. The outer covering is a thick membrane consisting mostly of collagen. The ventricles or chambers produce the cerebrospinal fluid, which circulates to the **subarachnoid space** where it cushions and feeds the brain. This clear fluid, with a volume of approximately 100 ml, exchanges chemicals with blood to feed the cells of the nervous system and carry away waste products. Figure 1–17 illustrates the region in which cerebrospinal fluid is produced and circulates.

subarachnoid space - space between the membranes of the covering of the central nervous system that contains the cerebrospinal fluid

The brain directs most metabolic processes in the body. Brain cells are not energy producers, but have a constant need for energy. Under normal conditions, the brain uses glucose as its sole source of energy. When glucose levels are low, the brain can use some ketones as energy sources.

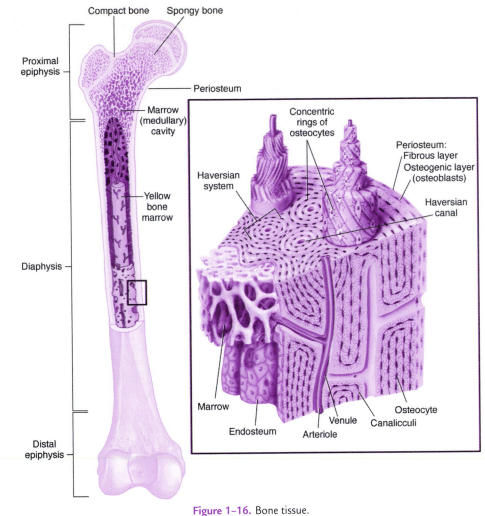

Figure 1–16. Bone tissue.

Chemical analysis of cerebrospinal fluid provides information about trauma, infection, and demyelinating diseases. Most commonly, glucose and total protein are measured in spinal fluid. However, laboratory tests for lactate, immunoglobulin proteins, and other biochemicals are available.

SUMMARY

The clinical chemistry laboratory operates under the guidelines of local, state, and federal regulations. Laboratory personnel may hold a license and/or certification that defines their level of practice based on state or professional standards. The chemical analytes that are chosen for measurement in the clinical laboratory are substances that have been shown by research to exhibit an association with a particular disease or risk for disease. Clinical chemistry tests are carefully chosen to provide diagnostic, prognostic, and therapeutic information upon which medical decisions can be made. Laboratory personnel must have an understanding of both

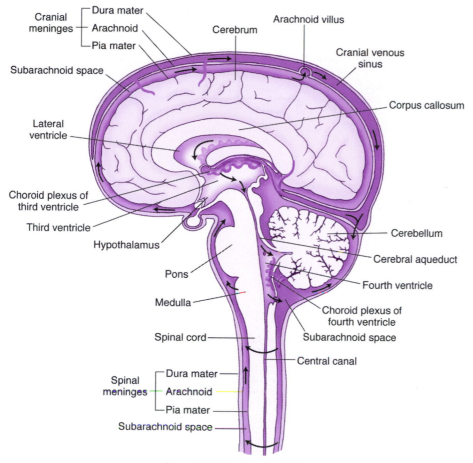

Figure 1–17. Cerebrospinal fluid.

the biochemistry and the anatomy of disease to provide sensitive and specific information for medical decision-making.

EXERCISES

As you consider the scenarios presented in this chapter, answer the following questions:

1. List the regulations that guide the practice of clinical chemistry laboratory testing.
2. What is the purpose of federal regulation of clinical laboratory testing?
3. What measures are used for ensuring competency of a clinical laboratory professional?
4. List and describe five examples of safety equipment that will be found in the clinical chemistry laboratory.
5. What information may be found in an MSDS?
6. What information is provided by a Safety Diamond?

7. How are the following used as biochemical markers of disease?
Carbohydrates
Lipids
Total serum/plasma proteins and plasma albumin
Enzymes
Genetic markers

8. Describe the functions of the following:
Cardiovascular system
Respiratory system
Liver
Renal system
Digestive system
Endocrine system
Bone
Central nervous system

References

1. CLIA program; categorization of tests and personnel modifications—HCFA. Final rule with comment period. *Fed Regist* 1995; 60(78):20035–20051.
2. Ehrmeyer SS, Laessig RH: Has compliance with CLIA requirements really improved quality in US clinical laboratories? *Clin Chim Acta* 2004; 346:37–43.
3. Occupational exposure to hazardous chemicals in laboratories: 1910. *http:// www.osha. gov/pls/oshaweb/owastand.display_standard_group?p_toc_level=1&p_part_number=1910*
4. Fiorella BJ, Maturen A: Statements of competence for practitioners in the clinical laboratory sciences. *Am J Med Technol* 1981; 47:647–652.
5. Spence HA, Bering NM: Credentialing in the clinical laboratory sciences. *Am J Med Technol* 1978; 44(5):393–397.
6. Venes D (ed): *Tabor's Cyclopedic Medical Dictionary*, ed 19. Philadelphia: FA Davis. 2001.
7. The Diabetes Control and Complications Trial Research Group: The effect of intensive treatment of diabetes on the development and progression of long-term complications in insulin-dependent diabetes mellitus. *N Engl J Med* 1993; 329:977–986.
8. Kannel WB, Castelli WP, Gordon T: Cholesterol in the prediction of atherosclerotic disease: New perspectives based on the Framingham study. *Ann Intern Med* 1979; 90:85–91.
9. Kannel WB, Gordon T: Physiological and medical concomitants of obesity: The Framingham Study. In Bray GA (ed): *Obesity in America*. Bethesda, MD: Public Health Service, 1979, pp 125–163.
10. Kannel WB, et al: An investigation of coronary heart disease in families: The Framingham Offspring Study. *Am J Epidemiol* 1979; 110:281–290.

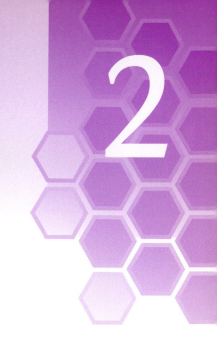

The goal of laboratory analysis is to provide the reliable laboratory data to the health-care provider in order to assist in clinical decision-making.

Quality Assessment

Margaret Crellin, Marian Cavagnaro, and Wendy Arneson

The assurance of high-quality laboratory results relies on a commitment to all aspects of the testing system, including attention to preanalytical, analytical, and postanalytical factors. Preanalytical factors are those factors that affect the laboratory results due to handling of the specimen sample prior to analysis. Postanalytical factors include timely and accurate laboratory result reporting and other aspects that occur after the analysis phase. The analytical phase includes verification of instrument linearity, **precision**, **accuracy**, and overall reliability through the use of standard materials, **quality control (QC) samples**, procedures, and QC rules. Management of high-quality laboratory testing systems must include the use of QC procedures, which measure the validity of the analysis and also consider all aspects of the process of laboratory testing prior to and after analysis. This atten-

precision - how closely measured results compare with each other

accuracy - how closely a measured value agrees with a true or expected value

quality control sample - sample with a matrix similar to patient specimens with known concentration

tion to the total quality of the system is referred to as total quality management (TQM), continuous quality improvement (CQI), or other similar phrases. This chapter will discuss QC in the context of quality assessment (QA). *Quality assessment* is the term recognized by federal laboratory standards; this concept was formerly referred to as *quality assurance*. The side boxes in this chapter provide common sense tips, definitions of terms, brief descriptions of pathophysiology, and clinical correlations as well as reminders of the team approach in health care. Text boxes within the chapter outline methodology for laboratory assessment of method reliability.

OBJECTIVES

Upon completion of this chapter, the student will have the ability to

- Define the following: precision, accuracy, linearity, mean, preanalytical errors, standard deviation, quality control sample, QC, QA, and postanalytical errors.
- Calculate mean, standard deviation, and coefficient of variation.
- Discuss the acceptance or rejection of an analysis based on QC rules, including modified Westgard QC rules.
- Describe the typical specimen collection, transport, and storage requirements for routine clinical chemistry testing to include glucose, electrolytes, and enzymes.
- List two common preanalytical variations and describe their effect on the results of clinical chemistry testing.

QUALITY ASSESSMENT VERSUS QUALITY CONTROL

Quality assessment (QA) is a complete system of creating and following procedures and policies to aim for providing the most reliable patient laboratory results and to minimize errors in the preanalytical, analytical, and postanalytical phases. QA also includes analyzing known samples called quality control (QC) samples along with unknown (patient) samples to test for analytical problems. When QC samples do not produce accurate and precise results, it can be assumed that any patient results obtained at the same time are also erroneous. Following a set of guidelines for acceptance or rejection of patient results based on the QC results helps to assure reliability of the analysis. Specific rules for assuring quality regarding the patient specimen through collection, analysis, and reporting are also important aspects of QA. Thus, preanalytical, analytical, and postanalytical variables need to be considered and minimized in order to have valid test results. *Quality assessment* is the term recognized by federal laboratory standards from the Clinical Laboratory Improvement Amendment of 1988 (CLIA '88) Final Rule.

Until recently the abbreviation QA was used to represent quality assurance, which implied assuring quality but may not have placed emphasis on assessing and managing laboratory results. In the most recent interpretation of the CLIA '88 Final Rule, it was recommended that the term *quality assessment* be adopted since it places the focus on assessment of testing performance through all phases. The new interpretation of CLIA '88 rules also places an emphasis on establishing and following written polices and procedures, taking corrective action, and making changes in policies and procedures to prevent problems from reoccurring. Assessment actually leads to assuring quality when actions taken to correct problems become permanent changes in policies, procedures, and behaviors. Similar terms that have been used in the past to represent quality assessment include *total quality management* (TQM) and *continuous quality improvement* (CQI). These terms may also be more descriptive than the term *quality assurance* since they relate to assessing practices and applying management skills to aim for improvement in quality of laboratory work.

Many of the practices for assessing quality of laboratory results have been adopted from principles used in business and manufacturing. Thus, QC, TQM, and QCI may be familiar to you as a consumer. Another recent laboratory management procedure that has been borrowed and adapted from business is the Six Sigma process. The Six Sigma process is client oriented and uses facts and data to help make decisions about improving service. In the case of the laboratory, the patient, physician, other laboratory professionals, and other members of the health-care team are all considered clients depending on the situation. The main focus of Six Sigma is to help reduce turnaround time and provide better service with a focus on the patient to create a more satisfied health-care team through these processes.[1] It is another TQM program that includes cost and waste reduction along with other aspects of QA. Aspects of Six Sigma include defining client needs and values with a focus on quality, cost, process, people, and accountability.[2]

Overview of Preanalytical Variables

Preanalytical refers to everything creating an impact on the patient specimen before it is tested for the analyte. Many things can go wrong with the specimen while it is collected from the patient and sent to the laboratory for testing. If the patient and the specimen aren't correctly identified, and the specimen isn't collected or handled properly, the specimen won't be worthy of testing. Suitable transport conditions such as in ice water or with protection from light may be necessary in order to preserve certain analytes in the specimen prior to testing. Other aspects of the preanalytical phase include training of personnel for proper collecting and handling of samples, including adherence to specific steps and maintaining turnaround time involving sample receiving and accessioning. Use of well-written procedures and policies can help to minimize preanalytical errors.[3] Specific information about avoiding preanalytical errors while collecting, transporting, and processing blood and other body fluid specimens will be discussed later in this chapter.

Overview of Analytical Variables

Chemical analysis involves many steps and components. These include specimen measurement, sample pretreatment, reagent volume measuring, sample and reagent mixing, incubation, reaction timing, reaction analysis, calculations, and result reporting. Accuracy and reproducibility of the analysis involves following precise steps within a procedure, maintaining the function of an instrument, and testing known or QC samples along with unknown samples. QC practices include the use of QC samples, which are analyzed in conjunction with patient samples and following specific rules for acceptance and rejection of analytical runs. Using analytical methods with a high degree of accuracy and precision as well as maintaining optimal operational conditions of instruments also help to minimize analytical errors. The use of QC samples, following a program of error detection, statistical calculation, error correction, and method evaluation, will be discussed in more detail later in this chapter.

Overview of Postanalytical Variables

Postanalytical variables are those that affect the patient results in the reporting stage. These include reporting the patient results in a timely manner and in an accepted format that can be understood and correctly interpreted by health-care providers. Maintaining and monitoring records of patient results also sustains QA practices. Postanalytical factors, including setting up and using reference ranges, medical decision limits, and critical values, will be discussed in the latter portion of this chapter.

PREANALYTICAL ERRORS AND SPECIMEN PROBLEMS

Some specimen variations can be controlled through proper patient identification, collection, and handling and strict rejection policies. Light, heat, evaporation, and exposure to the atmosphere will change many substances in routine clinical chemistry testing. Examples include the photodegradation of bilirubin by light exposure and the heat lability of enzymes. Exposure of plasma samples to high temperatures can significantly lower potassium concentrations.[4]

hemolysis - rupture of erythrocyte cell membranes causing release of intracellular contents

The laboratory or health-care team can be trained to avoid misidentification, **hemolysis**, atmospheric exposure to light and heat, and evaporation of blood specimens. Accurate patient identification, specimen identification, and sample aliquot identification are necessary from the time of collection until testing is completed and the result is reported. If there is any question as to the integrity or identification of the sample, the laboratory should reject the sample and request that it be recollected. Supervision of policy adherence and periodic training may be necessary in order to implement and maintain laboratory specimen QA.

Specimen collection and handling procedures must be explained to all parties involved in the processing of specimens. It has become increasingly common for nursing personnel, physician assistants, and health-care professionals other than laboratory personnel to collect blood samples. Although laboratory personnel may not be directly involved in the collection of specimens, they are responsible for minimizing preanalytical errors based on acceptance or rejection of the received specimens. Laboratory personnel are also responsible for training other personnel involved in specimen collection and transport and for communicating effectively in order to maintain optimal quality of specimens for laboratory testing. Since preanalytical errors seem to make up the majority of most laboratory test problems, proper training is an important area to address.[5]

Some preanalytical problems may or may not be controlled directly by laboratory personnel, but information about such problems should be made available to health-care providers. These problems include patient-related factors such as ambulation, lying down or standing prior to collection, and biological differences, such as time of day, age, gender, and intake of certain foods or herb supplements. Ambulation prior to specimen collection can impact upon total proteins, lipids, and other protein-bound substances. Levels of cortisol and many other hormones vary throughout the day, so collection needs to be timed according to physician orders so as to provide the most accurate information. Intake of food greatly impacts on glucose, triglycerides, certain hormones, and electrolytes, so length of fasting prior to specimen collection is a preanalytical factor that is commonly addressed prior to specimen collection and testing.[6] Intake of certain foods or herbs may impact on therapeutic drug testing or other laboratory results but often is not within the control of laboratory personnel prior to specimen collection.[7] The age of the patient may be an important variable for the test result. For example, bilirubin and alkaline phosphatase values are different in pediatric patients than in adult populations, so coordinated reference intervals are needed. This variation is addressed through the use of age-appropriate reference ranges, but the information on patient age is often obtained at specimen collection, in the preanalytical phase.

Blood Specimens

The body fluid most commonly analyzed in the clinical laboratory is blood. Whole blood can be allowed to clot in a clean plastic collection tube and then be centrifuged and the serum removed for testing in clinical chemistry. Conversely, clotting can be prevented by allowing the whole blood to mix with an anticoagulant such as lithium heparin so that it can be measured as whole blood or centrifuged to obtain the plasma for analysis. Other types of testing performed in the clinical laboratory, such as the complete blood count, require anticoagulated, well-mixed whole blood.

Serum specimens obtained from venous circulation are most commonly used in clinical chemistry. Therefore, proper collection technique is needed in order to obtain an acceptable specimen, which minimizes preanalytical errors. Standards of practice in blood collection are found in other resources as those published by the Clinical Laboratory Standards Institute (CLSI; formerly the National Committee for Clinical Laboratory Standards [NCCLS]). A **tourniquet** typically is used in order to cause short-term venous occlusion, allowing **palpation** of the veins in the **antecubital fossa** prior to venipuncture. If the tourniquet is maintained longer than 1 minute, a relative **hemoconcentration** occurs due to fluid changes. Low molecular weight compounds such as potassium leave the capillaries and pool in the interstitial fluid region during hemoconcentration, while proteins tend to be increased in the remaining plasma. Clenching of the fist prior to venipuncture is a common technique. However, the technique should be avoided prior to collection of specimens for clinical laboratory analysis due to the changes that can be initiated. Fist clenching tends to increase lactate, phosphate, and potassium as well as lower pH. Secondarily, ionized calcium increases due to the transient lactic acidosis.[6]

tourniquet - band used on arm to cause the veins to distend

palpation - simple technique in which a physician presses lightly on the surface of the body to feel the organs or tissues underneath

antecubital fossa - area in the crook of the arm

hemoconcentration - relative increase in the number of red blood cells resulting from a decrease in the volume of plasma

CASE SCENARIO 2-1

Hemolysis: Why Is the Potassium Level So High Today?

A physician called the laboratory to inquiry about a specimen collected from his patient. The plasma potassium concentration had been reported as 5.9 mmol/L. This value was abnormally high when compared to the reference range (3.5 to 4.5 mmol/L) for potassium. The physician was concerned that hemolysis had falsely elevated the potassium result. The technologist checked the sample and assured the physician that there were no visible signs of hemolysis.

Hemolysis

Hemolysis is generally a preanalytical problem that can be avoided. It is graded based on visible presence of hemoglobin, when greater than 20 mg/dL, and it is often graded as mild, moderate, or gross hemolysis.[6] Gross hemolysis will often impact on almost every test method due to release of intracellular constituents into the serum and colorimetric interference due to pigments.

Grossly hemolyzed specimens should always be rejected. Lysis of blood cells makes a serious impact on many chemistry tests. For intracellular chemicals such as potassium, phosphates, lactate dehydrogenase (LD), and aspartate transaminase (AST), hemolysis will directly increase serum levels. For other analytes such as creatinine kinase, glucose, and bilirubin, hemolysis will cause chemical interference, which may increase or decrease the results. Mild to moderate hemolysis may necessitate specimen rejection or at least a qualification statement for particular test results that are positively or negatively impacted. Older whole blood or clotted blood samples will become hemolyzed within 24 hours of the collection time, especially at 24°C and warmer temperatures.[6]

Hemolysis can be caused by a variety of conditions during the collection and processing steps. Difficulty with **phlebotomy** procedures can cause hemolysis. Examples include poor placement of the needle into the vein, pulling back the plunger on a syringe too quickly, and allowing air leakage due to a poorly fitted needle. Poor specimens are likely to be obtained and should be discarded when the blood container is only partially filled or fills slowly. Problems during specimen processing can also lead to hemolyzed samples. For example, wringing out a blood clot prior to or after centrifugation or rough handling during transport are common causes of hemolysis.[6] Using a small-bore needle when compared to the size of the evacuated tube or forcing blood through a stopper into the evacuated tube is likely to cause hemolysis as well.

Sample **indices** are measured by some automated chemistry analyzers and can be used to estimate the amount of free hemoglobin in the sample. These indices can be used to establish a criterion for unacceptable specimens. The indices are calculated from multiple wavelength readings of a patient sample diluted in buffer or saline. The calculated results are represented as an approximate hemoglobin concentration or as a semi-**quantitative** value. The same absorbance readings are also used to estimate relative **icterus** and **lipemia**.

Some analytes, such as potassium, can demonstrate an almost linear relationship between the amount of hemolysis and the increase in analyte. Table 2–1 shows such a relationship. This near-linear relationship has led to the suggestion that the indices should be used to correct results for the false increase (or decrease) in analyte concentration that is caused by the presence of hemoglobin. These calculations are not recommended because factors other than hemoglobin could also contribute to altered test values. For example, hemolyzed heel stick specimens from neonates can contain increased amount of colorless intracellular fluid with increased potassium. However, the indices can be used to apply appropriate modifying statements to those samples that the health-care staff chooses not to re-collect.

Chemicals leak from the cells in older specimens in which the serum was not separated from the clotted blood cells. Although the serum from old specimens may not appear hemolyzed, the effect may be the same as mild to moderate hemolysis. Old specimens should be rejected for patient initial reporting. Retesting older samples may be necessary for internal QA practices. The effect of hemolysis on sensitive results such as potassium, glucose, bicarbonate, and carbon dioxide and

phlebotomy - opening of a vein to withdraw blood

indices - plural of index; numbers used as indicators

quantitative - expressing test results by amount or concentration (a graded or proportional response)

icterus - yellowish pigmentation in the blood due to increased bilirubin

lipemia - fatty accumulation in the blood giving cloudy appearance

✓ **Common Sense Check**
Not only is it important to inform the clinician of the presence of hemolysis, it is also helpful, in cases of elevated potassium, to remark on the absence of hemolysis.

TABLE 2-1

Effect of Hemolysis on Potassium

Hemolytic Index	Approximate Hemoglobin (mg/dL)	Approximate Increase in Serum or Plasma Potassium
1	50	Not significant
2	100	0.4
3	150	0.5
4	200	0.7
5	250	0.9
6	300	1.0
7	350	1.2
8	400	1.4
9	450	1.6
10	500	1.7

most serum enzymes must be considered. An alternative to clotted tubes that are held for later retesting is the use of serum separator tubes. These contain an inert polymer that moves between the clotted blood cells and the serum during centrifugation. This gel barrier can prevent release of intracellular constituents for several hours. However, gel barriers can't be used for therapeutic drug monitoring since they can interfere with specimen testing. Separated blood, serum, or plasma is commonly held for up to 12 hours at room temperature or for 1 week in a refrigerator for repeat testing. This type of repeat testing, or internal QA practice, will be discussed more thoroughly in later portions of this chapter.

Case Scenario 2-1 Hemolysis: Why Is the Potassium Level So High Today?

Follow-Up

When the physician called the laboratory to inquiry about a 5.9-mmol/L plasma potassium concentration (reference range 3.5 to 4.5 mmol/L), he was concerned that sample hemolysis had falsely elevated the potassium result. Hemolysis can have a predictable false-positive relationship with serum potassium. The technologist checked the sample and determined that, in this case, there was no visible hemolysis, the age of the specimen was not excessive, and the result was likely an acceptable one. No earlier potassium results were reported on this patient, nor were there other electrolyte results to compare with this result as this was one of the early tests ordered. ●

CASE SCENARIO 2-2

The Contaminated Specimen: Unusual Electrolyte and Glucose Results

The paper printout from the chemistry instrument was marked with a flag next to the plasma glucose level. The glucose concentration was 48 mg/dL, critically lower than the reference range for fasting plasma glucose levels of

THE TEAM APPROACH
Because nonlaboratory staff such as nurses and physician assistants may collect blood specimens, it is important for the laboratory to adequately train and help maintain the phlebotomy skill level of these health care professionals. Job aids with pictures and simple directions can be provided in pocket guides and on computer pages when tests are ordered to help remind personnel of the specimen requirements for individual laboratory tests.

continued

Case Scenario 2-2 The Contaminated Specimen: Unusual Electrolyte
and Glucose Results *(continued)*

74 to 100 mg/dL. The technologist on duty was about to alert the clinician
about the critically low value when she noticed that the concentrations of
other tests for this specimen were only slightly higher than the critical range
lower limit and some results, such as chloride and sodium, were very elevated.

The technologist considered the reasons why so many results were abnormal, with many abnormally low. To solve the problem, the technologist considered what the tests have in common.

If the tests were all analyzed on the same chemistry instrument, it could indicate
a problem with a component of the instrument. An automated instrument receives
the sample of the specimen and performs the clinical chemistry test in a manner
similar to manual testing. In other words, a certain volume of patient sample is
mixed with reagent(s) and allowed to incubate until the chemical reaction forms a
measurable product, and then the product is measured. Calculations are then performed based on the measurements so that concentration of the substance can be
reported. Errors can occur in any of those steps and are termed *analytical errors*.
(Instrumentation is discussed in Chapter 3 in more detail.) In terms of this case,
glucose and several other analytes were analyzed and showed errors. Those analytes
were all measured by different methods involving a variety of chemical reactions, so
problems with all of the reagents, calibration, or calculations seem unlikely. Some
steps of automation that are common in all tests should be considered, including the
sample pipetting system. If this is plugged or partially plugged, erroneous results
could occur as a result of delivering the improper volume of sample into each test
cell. It may be unusual to observe some elevated results when the sampling system
is plugged, however.

Errors occurring with the sample have been already been discussed in regard to
hemolysis. Glucose is not as affected by hemolysis as potassium and other electrolytes. Other problems with specimen collection and handling will be discussed
further later in this chapter, including the effect of light or heat exposure and the
contamination of the specimen through the use of improper anticoagulants. Given
that many of the results in this situation are decreased and that the patient may be
receiving IV fluids, contamination of the blood specimen due to the dilutional
effect of IV solution should be considered.

Case Scenario 2-2 The Contaminated Specimen: Unusual Electrolyte
and Glucose Results

Follow-Up

The technologist contacted the patient's nurse to determine whether the
patient was receiving IV fluids. She also asked if it was possible that the specimen was contaminated with IV solution. The nurse confirmed that the patient
was receiving a saline (salt water solution) IV infusion and that the blood could
have been collected improperly from a vein above the IV line. A new employ-
ee had collected the specimen, and the proper procedure may not have been

continued

Case Scenario 2-2 **The Contaminated Specimen: Unusual Electrolyte and Glucose Results** (*continued*)

followed. The nurse drew a new sample, which gave improved results. A comparison of the results from both specimens is provided below.

Test	Reference Range	Critical Limit	Contaminated Sample	Re-collected Sample
Glucose (mg/dL)	74–100	≤40 or ≥450	48	72
BUN (mg/dL)	6–20	≥80	8	12
Creatinine (mg/dL)	0.9–1.3	≥5	0.5	0.8
Sodium (mmol/L)	136–145	≤120 or ≥160	148	142
Potassium (mmol/L)	3.5–5.1	≤2.8 or ≥6.2	3.1	4.5
Chloride (mmol/L)	98–107	≤80 or ≥120	122	106
CO_2 (mmol/L)	22–28	≤10 or ≥40	17	27

The glucose, blood urea nitrogen (BUN), and creatinine results in the initial sample, likely contaminated with IV solution, were approximately one-third lower than the values that were obtained from the redrawn sample. The sodium and chloride results were higher in the first sample due to saline contamination from the IV fluid. Total protein and albumin can also be considerably decreased when measured in specimens contaminated with IV fluid. The saline IV fluid used in this case has a higher sodium and chloride concentration than the patient plasma, so contaminating the blood specimen gave falsely increased sodium and chloride values while other analytes were diluted by the IV solution. ●

Specimen Contamination

The type of blood specimen contamination resulting from IV fluids would vary with the type of fluid being infused. A dextrose solution (sugar) IV infusion would yield extremely high glucose results in venous specimens collected above or near the infusion area. Total **parenteral** nutrition (TPN) fluid contains most of the required daily nutrients for a person who can't ingest food. TPN fluid contamination in a specimen creates gross **turbidity** along with elevated lipid and glucose values and potassium levels too high to be compatible with life.

In specimens from a patient receiving a saline IV infusion, potassium and protein results may be nearly one-third lower than in specimens not contaminated with saline IV solution. Sodium and chloride results will be falsely elevated due to contamination from saline IV fluid.

parenteral - bypassing the gastrointestinal system to provide nutrients directly to the bloodstream

turbidity - cloudiness of solution due to presence of light-blocking particles or molecules such as fats

Specimen Transport

in vitro - pertaining to laboratory conditions, such as specimens in a test tube

Many chemical compounds are stable within plasma or serum **in vitro** for only a short time. Levels of potassium, ammonia, lactate, bilirubin, glucose, CO_2, sodium, urea, and alkaline phosphatase, for example, are particularly affected by contact with blood cells, which can continue to undergo cellular metabolic processes after blood has been removed from the body.

Some chemicals, such as ammonia, lactate, bilirubin, and glucose, as well as the pH of a specimen, are unstable after removal of the specimen from the body unless held under specific conditions. For example, pH and ammonia can be preserved for an hour by placing the specimen in ice water if collected in the correct type of specimen tube and maintained covered with a stopper. Preservatives are often added along with anticoagulants to help maintain certain chemicals. Glucose will decrease as much as 12% per hour (5% to 7% in low-normal concentrations) if not separated from blood cells or preserved. In addition, within 4 hours, there can be as much as a 50% error in the results of tests such as carbon dioxide, sodium, urea, alkaline phosphatase, and other serum enzymes. Exposure to air and evaporation of water from the open specimen tube or in a patient sample can cause serious analytical errors for many routine clinical chemistry analytes such as enzymes and electrolytes, as well as errors in calculation of osmolality. Therefore, serum or plasma should only be used if received and separated from the cells within a few hours unless special conditions are met. Sodium fluoride is often used to preserve lactate and glucose levels by inhibiting glycolytic enzymes found in erythrocytes. Individual laboratories need to establish their own policies that maintain stability of the clinical chemistry analytes.

Additives to Blood

Using the wrong additives or the wrong amount of additive can cause adverse effects on blood specimens. For example, sodium oxalate, sodium fluoride, or sodium heparin cannot be used for samples needed for sodium analysis because they

TABLE 2-2

Common Clinical Chemistry Specimen Handling[6]

Analyte	Anticoagulant	Special Handling
Acetone	None (serum)	Stopper; freeze
Alcohol	None (serum)	Stopper
Bilirubin	None (serum)	Protect from light
Creatinine	None (serum)	Freeze
Glucose	None (serum)	Separate immediately; *or* Collect in NaF/oxalate (2 mg/mL)
Alkaline phosphatase	None (serum)	Stopper; avoid hemolysis; freeze
High-density lipoprotein cholesterol	Plasma in EDTA (2 mg/mL) tube	Freeze
Magnesium	Serum	Avoid hemolysis; separate immediately
Potassium	Serum or heparinized (0.2 mg/mL) plasma	Avoid hemolysis; separate immediately
Renin	Plasma in EDTA (2 mg/mL) tube	Chill during collection and centrifugation
Total proteins and electrophoretic fractions	Serum	Refrigerate (up to 1 month); freeze

increase the level of sodium. Similarly, ammonium heparin should not be used for specimens intended for plasma ammonia or urea testing because it adds to the chemical being measured. Sodium fluoride cannot be used for enzyme analysis samples because fluoride acts as an inhibitor to most enzyme activity. Ethylenediaminetetra-acetic acid (EDTA), sodium citrate, and sodium oxalate remove calcium and magnesium, so they cannot be used in samples that will be used for mineral analysis.[8] An increased anticoagulant-to-specimen ratio will dilute the specimen, causing a major impact on electrolytes, minerals, and pH. Table 2–2 lists common clinical chemistry specimens and the handling required for them to be accepted for analysis.

Sample Preparation

Sample preparation involves processing of the blood sample prior to and in preparation for analysis. Processing involves centrifugation, removal of protein (if applicable), and making an aliquot of the specimen in a test tube or sample cup so that the remaining specimen can be shared with other testing areas. Centrifugation is a common sample preparation technique since most clinical chemistry analyses are performed with serum or plasma. Keep in mind that clotted or whole blood cells can affect chemicals in the sample over a period of time, such that additional chemicals arise or some chemicals are consumed. Therefore, centrifugation should be timed to occur so that the testing can begin within an hour of collection. Some newer analyzers will perform this step as part of the automation, but for the most part, centrifugation is a separate and important step of sample preparation. Standards of practice in specimen handling and transport may be found in other resources such as publications by CLSI/NCCLS.

THE TEAM APPROACH

Communication is an important component of processing laboratory specimens and handling specimen problems. It is important to have clearly written policies for specimen rejection and to inform those who provide inadequate specimens of these policies. Delays in testing must also be communicated.

> **Case Scenario 2-3** Specimen Transport Delay: The Missing Glucose
>
> **Follow-Up**
>
> A physician had called to determine the morning glucose result for a patient who is diabetic. The technologist determined that the specimen was not in the laboratory but finally located it. The specimen had been left in the pocket of the nurse who had drawn the sample 4 hours prior to its discovery. The clotted blood sample was quickly transported to the laboratory and a glucose value of 136 mg/dL was obtained (reference range 74 to 100 mg/dL).
>
> Did the 4-hour delay in getting the sample to the laboratory have an impact on the glucose value? Yes. The 4-hour delay in separating serum from whole blood would most likely cause a preanalytical error in the glucose result because of in vitro cell glycolysis.
>
> If reported, the 136-mg/dL glucose result would likely have been considered within normal parameters for a random glucose test. The actual level was 210 mg/dL, which would likely have prompted intervention to lower the patient's plasma glucose. ●

Other Body Fluid Specimens

Measurements of chemicals in urine, cerebrospinal fluid, and other body fluids are also helpful in providing clinical laboratory information to aid in patient assessment. Each specimen tube must be properly labeled so that it can be traced back to the original patient sample and matched to the patient identification information and test requisition form. Barcode labels can be applied to specimen tubes that fit onto analyzers to make identification and pairing of the sample with the results easier.

Urine

Urine is a frequently requested specimen for renal function assessment and for assessment of metabolic conditions. The required type of urine specimen depends upon the analyte to be measured. For example, a timed 24-hour urine specimen is generally required for urinary protein. Accurate timing requires that the bladder be emptied just prior to beginning the timing sequence and then all of the urine voided must be saved during the following 24 hours in a large, properly labeled container. The urine container should be clean and contain no additives and should be retained at 2° to 4°C until collection is complete. If analysis is to be delayed following collection, the aliquot of the urine specimen can be retained at 2° to 4°C for up to a week or at –20°C if longer delay is needed.[4] Refer to Chapters 6 and 11 on renal function and endocrinology, respectively, for details of other types of urine specimens analyzed in clinical chemistry.

Cerebrospinal Fluid

Cerebrospinal fluid (CSF) is a commonly measured body fluid that provides valuable information to the health-care provider. Most CSF studies are performed on a specimen obtained by a physician or health-care provider through lumbar puncture (Fig. 2–1). Since only a small amount of CSF can be safely collected, it is imperative that it is handled carefully. If the CSF pressure is normal, at least 20 mL can be removed for testing without injury to the patient. The volume usually provided from an adult patient is about 20 mL. Due to the small volume, CSF must be

✓ Common Sense Check

It is important to open the specimen lids carefully with a gauze protector or in a special aerosol control box so that small droplets of serum or plasma are not sprayed around the room. These aerosols can allow entry of biohazardous bacteria and viruses into mucous membranes, such as into the eyes via spray, and into the nose or mouth via inhalation.

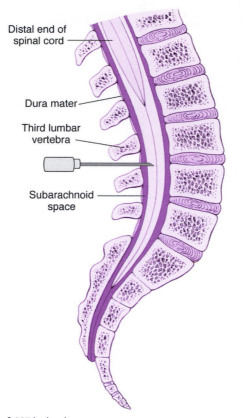

Distal end of
spinal cord

Dura mater

Third lumbar
vertebra

Subarachnoid
space

Figure 2–1. Collection of CSF by lumbar puncture. *(Adapted from Chabner DE: Medical Terminology: A Short Course. Philadelphia: WB Saunders, 1990.)*

shared between several testing areas, so it is necessary to conserve the sample and follow proper handling and transport requirements to avoid the need for recollection. Ideally, the specimens should be collected into three sterile tubes that are labeled sequentially.

The first tube should be used for chemical and immunologic studies, since it is most likely to be contaminated with dermal bacteria and therefore is not suitable for microbiological assays. The second tube is generally used for microbiological testing, and the third tube is used for total cell count, differential count, and cytological testing.

Due to the invasive nature of the collection process for CSF, analysis of the sample is generally requested in an urgent manner. Therefore, generally a short time frame is expected after collection for transport, analysis, and reporting. Many of the chemistry analytes can be preserved in a frozen aliquot of CSF if analysis is to be delayed. For hematology testing, cytological specimens, and microbiological testing, it is important to refer to specimen handling techniques for specific analytes within CSF to assure adequate preservation as recommendations may vary based on testing requirements.

Miscellaneous Body Fluids

For details about collection and handling of other body fluids such as amniotic fluid or sweat, please refer to specific details in chapters to follow. Table 2–3 lists typical requirements for other fluids and products.

> ✓ **Common Sense Check**
> If only one tube of CSF is obtained, it should be given to the clinical microbiology section first so that sterility can be maintained during their sampling. The tube is then delivered to areas requiring cell counting so that a well-mixed aliquot can be obtained. Clinical chemistry would receive the CSF specimen last since most of the testing would be performed on supernatant.

TABLE 2-3

Handling Requirements for Other Body Fluids and Samples[6]

Type	Collection and Handling Requirements
Amniotic fluid	Avoid light during routine testing; transport in ice may be necessary
Ascitic, pericardial, or pleural fluid	Sterile plain tube for culture. Liquid EDTA tube for cell counts and cell differentials.
CSF	Sterile tubes: the first for chemical and immunologic studies; the second for microbiological examination; and the third for microscopic and cytological studies.
Feces	Voided sample rather than examination glove residue; refrigeration prior to analysis; avoid contamination with urine or toilet bowl cleaners
Synovial fluid	Sterile plain tube for microbiological examination; heparinized or liquid EDTA tube for cell count and differential
Urine	Refrigeration of 24-hr specimen during collection; HCl to pH 3 is common for many analytes; NaOH to pH 8 for porphyrins, urobilinogen, and uric acid

ANALYTICAL VARIABLES AND QUALITY CONTROL

Quality control (QC) is an aspect of quality assessment (QA) that is used to assess the analytical phase of patient testing. QC samples are solutions or chemicals of known concentration that mimic a patient's specimen. They are tested along with patient specimens to monitor the validity of the analysis. Usually QC samples are collected, processed, and manufactured commercially. QC samples are often preserved and stored in a manner different than patient specimens, so they bypass the preanalytical phase of testing. QC results are not used to track the postanalytical phase of testing because they are not reported to physicians. They are very important, however, in helping to determine if current test results are validly measured in the testing phase.

Federal regulations require that two QC samples be analyzed at least once per day for each analyte using control procedures and rules that monitor the entire analytical process to detect immediate errors. The measurement of QC samples will detect problems of precision and accuracy over time.[9] Interpretation of control results is based on using specific rules for acceptance and rejection of QC results, documenting results and decisions, and having a process for resolving problems that result in rejection of results.

QC consists of various samples and procedures used to detect errors that occur due to test system failure, changes in environmental conditions, and differences in operator performance. Some instruments provide QC results from electronic detector output, known as "electronic QC" (EQC). These electronic performance indicators are acceptable to supplement analytical validity testing but cannot take the place of running QC samples along with patient samples to test all aspects of the analysis. QC rules should also monitor the accuracy and precision of the test performance over time.

Accuracy is the comparison of a result with the true value, while *precision* is the comparison of results with each other. A small amount of inaccuracy and imprecision is inevitable and accepted, but limits are set through federal regulations by the Clinical Laboratory Improvement Amendment (CLIA).

✓ **Common Sense Check**

Since the QC samples will be used to judge the reliability of analysis, it is important to handle the samples with care. It is imperative to check the expiration date and lot number, matching to the numbers in use. The QC samples must be well mixed, warmed up quickly to room temperature, and tested promptly. The QC sample container must then be capped and returned to the proper storage conditions, such as the refrigerator, as soon as possible to maintain freshness.

CASE SCENARIO 2-4

QC: More or Less Albumin?

The evening shift laboratory technologist was concerned when analysis of a patient sample reported an albumin concentration higher than its total protein. Since albumin is only one part of total protein, it would be impossible for albumin to be higher than total protein. The technologist checked the control results for both tests. The total protein controls were within limits of control, but both albumin controls were higher than 3 standard deviations (SD) above the expected mean.

QC Material	Observed Result	Expected Mean	1 SD
Level 1 (g/dL)	3.3	2.8	0.1
Level 2 (g/dL)	4.7	4.4	0.1

Quality Control Programs

The goal of a well-defined QC system is to detect immediate errors in an analytical run while minimizing the number of false rejections. The simplest type of QC procedure uses one rule to reject the analysis based on QC results falling outside of a range such as the 95% range. If this is used, 5% of the time, a result that falls just outside of the 95% range would be falsely rejected. Likewise, 5% of the results that are accepted within that range would also be a false rejection. These facts are based on probability that the correct decision was made 95% of the time when results that fall within this range are accepted. When testing is **qualitative**—that is, positive or negative—a simple one-rule policy is acceptable. Historically, manual testing was assessed with a one-rule rejection policy, tracking results over time to observe for errors.

False rejections are false alarms. They refer to the situation in which the testing process is actually acceptable but one QC result is occasionally and slightly outside of acceptable limits due to chance alone. Using multiple rules for acceptance and rejection, including some rules based on previous results, can lower the false rejection rate. This is especially important when automated testing is used, as in most clinical chemistry testing.

Adherence to a QC program with specific rules will help to achieve analytical goals during routine laboratory operation. As was mentioned earlier, QC samples may be purchased with known values for each analyte based on reported mean and SD. These are called assayed QC samples. QC samples may also be purchased without known values. Control materials should resemble as closely as possible the human material to be analyzed, with the same general makeup or specimen matrix. Controls may resemble calibrators provided by a vendor but are used differently. An assay should be calibrated with different material than the QC samples.[10] Control materials should be tested in the same manner as patient samples so all steps of the analytical process are checked. Two control levels for each analyte are recommended, and three are sometimes used. QC levels may be chosen based on the clinically useful limits of the analyte, **medical decision levels**, or an analytical measurement range. Additional controls should be utilized as necessary to challenge the entire analytical range. These samples are internally evaluated within the laboratory.

Internal QC is performed daily in the laboratory, whereas external QC or **proficiency testing** (PT) is performed only occasionally as a test of competency. An

qualitative - giving either positive or negative test results (a binary response)

medical decision level - the concentration or limit at which the test results are critically interpreted

proficiency testing - a means of verifying the accuracy of tests; can include participation in an external assessment program, splitting samples with another laboratory, or blind testing of materials with known values

outside agency provides samples and evaluates the results of testing. PT samples must be tested using the same procedures that are used for laboratory testing for routine QC and patient results. The results obtained from testing the PT samples are reported to the outside agency. The agency then provides a report of acceptance or rejection of the PT sample results for the participating laboratory based on the expected mean and SD testing results from all participating laboratories.

Both types of QC, internal and external, are an important part of TQM and are required by federal regulations and voluntary accreditation bodies such as the Joint Commission on Accreditation of Healthcare Organizations (JCAHO) and the College of American Pathologists (CAP).

A single lot number of control material should be purchased in quantities large enough to last 1 year. Adherence to manufacturer's storage requirements should increase the stability of most constituents. Most liquid controls are stored frozen at –10° to –20°C. Storage in a frost-free freezer, one that has repeated freeze-thaw cycles, should be avoided. Lyophilized material must be reconstituted according to the manufacturer's guidelines using the recommended diluent and a highly accurate (class A) volumetric pipette.

When a new lot number of control material is received, even when the mean and SD are provided by the manufacturer, each analyte should be assayed on 20 or more separate runs. A minimum of 20 data points is needed to establish a new mean and SD. These assays must be analyzed in parallel with the previous lot number control material.[11] A new mean and SD should be established if the control is unassayed or if it is different than the control data provided by the manufacturer. QC ranges can be set using several methods. Ranges can be set from the measured or provided SD so that statistically significant errors are detected, but they should comply with the federal guidelines for allowable SD. Federal guidelines also set fixed limits for precision, based on the SD and on total error.

Statistical analysis of control samples is based on the assumed gaussian distribution of the data. Figure 2–2 shows a typical gaussian, or bell-shaped, curve. With a gaussian curve of the population, 68% will be within 1 SD, 95% within 2 SD, and 99.7% within 3 SD of the mean. This means that 95% of acceptable QC results

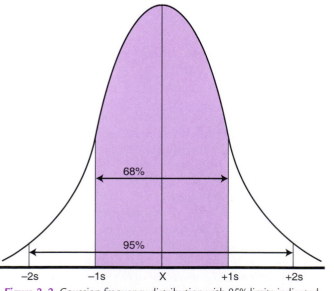

Figure 2–2. Gaussian frequency distribution with 95% limits indicated.

should fall within 2 SD of the mean. The following statistics are calculated from the collected data and applied to QC rules to judge for analysis acceptability.

Statistical Calculations

The *mean* ($\overline{X}$) is the sum of the control observations (x_1, x_2, ... x_i) divided by the number (n) of observations:

$$\Sigma\, x_i/n = \overline{X}$$

Practice calculating the mean of the following five results: 45, 44, 45, 48, 39 ($n = 5$).

$$(45 + 44 + 45 + 48 + 39)/5 = 221/5 = 44.2$$

The *standard deviation* (SD or *s*) is the measure of the dispersion of a group of values around the mean. It is derived from the curve of normal distribution. It is used to assess precision.

$$\text{SD}\,(s) = \sqrt{\frac{\Sigma(\overline{X} - x_i)^2}{n - 1}}$$

Practice calculating the SD of the following results: 45, 44, 45, 48, 39 ($n = 5$).

$$\text{SD}\,(s) = 3.3$$

Use a calculator or computer software to calculate this value. A statistical software package such as SPSS® or Microsoft Excel® or a programmable calculator should be used because generally 20 or more data points makes calculation by hand prone to error. Microsoft Windows® provides a simple statistical package with its calculator function to determine mean and SD.

The *coefficient of variation* (%CV) is the SD divided by the mean expressed as a percentage. This is another measure of percentage of imprecision.

$$\%\text{CV} = (\text{SD/mean}) \times 100$$

Practice calculating the %CV of the following results: 45, 44, 45, 48, 39 ($n = 5$).

$$\text{Mean} = 44.2$$
$$s = 3.3$$
$$\%\text{CV} = (3.3/44.2) \times 100 = 7.5\%$$

The *standard deviation index* (SDI) is the difference between an individual value subtracted from the group mean divided by the SD of the group; it is also known as the Z statistic:

$$\text{SDI} = (\overline{X} - x_i)/\text{SD}$$

Practice calculating the SDI of the following urea results: $\overline{X} = 44$, $x_i = 42$, $s = 2$

$$\text{SDI} = (44 - 42)/2 = 1.00$$

The *correlation coefficient* (*r*) is used to determine the consistency between two groups of samples or two testing methods. It is calculated using this formula:

$$r = \frac{\Sigma XY - \dfrac{\Sigma X \Sigma Y}{N}}{\sqrt{\left(\Sigma X^2 - \dfrac{(\Sigma X)^2}{N}\right)\left(\Sigma Y^2 - \dfrac{(\Sigma Y)^2}{N}\right)}}$$

Use a calculator or computer software to calculate this value. A statistical software package such as SPSS® or Microsoft Excel® or a programmable calculator should be used since this formula makes calculation by hand prone to error.

How Are These Values Used?

Mean and SD are calculations that assess the accuracy and precision of the analysis statistically. Errors of accuracy may be assessed by examining changes in the measured concentration of the control over time and comparing these concentration values to mean and SD ranges of the control. The deterioration of accuracy of the analytical system over time can be assessed by shifts and changes in the daily measurement of control concentration. By contrast, an imprecision problem will be demonstrated by an increase in the SD and %CV of results of the control concentration over time.

The SDI is a statistical calculation that is used for peer group comparisons. Participation in interlaboratory QC comparison programs provides peer group QC data based on the same methodology and the same instrument for the same lot number of control material. The SDI can be used to assess the validity of individual laboratory results as compared to a peer group QC result or proficiency sample by calculating the probability of the result obtained. It relates the bias, or difference from the true result, as compared with the SD expected. This calculation is used to assess PT results and other aspects of QA.

QC charts have historically been used to examine prior QC results within a particular range diagrammatically.[12,13] The most commonly used charts indicate day or run number on the abscissa and observed QC concentration, indicating mean, and SD ranges on the ordinate axis. One example of a QC chart is the Levey-Jennings control chart. A typical Levey-Jennings chart is depicted in Figure 2–3. By plotting the daily QC results, one can visualize the deviation of the results from the mean, typically noting when the results are greater than ±2 SD from the mean on a daily basis. Over time, watching for shifts and trends also helps to identify errors that become part of the system, or systematic.

$$\text{Mean} - 2\,s \text{ and Mean} + 2\,s = 95\% \text{ QC Range}$$

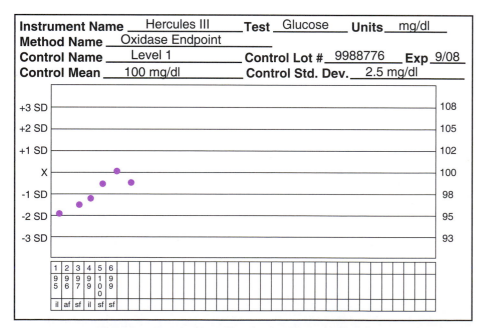

Figure 2–3. Levey-Jennings chart showing QC results for 6 days.

Practice calculating a common QC range (95% range) using a mean of 140 mmol/L and an SD of 2 mmol/L. The lower limit of the range is equal to the mean minus 2 times the SD, or $140 - (2 \times 2) = 136$ mmol/L. The upper limit of the range is equal to the mean plus 2 times the SD, or $140 + (2 \times 2) = 144$ mmol/L. In this example, the 95% QC range is 136 to 144 mmol/L.

The criteria used to determine acceptability of each control measurement are termed *control rules*, or QC rules. Westgard defined QC rules based on the earlier work of Shewhart, Levey, and Jennings.[14] Use of multiple control rules (commonly referred to as Westgard rules) can improve the performance of the control system. Individual rules have different capabilities for detecting different types of analytical error. A control rule or control decision is used to judge whether analysis is performing well. The QC ranges should take into consideration total error allowed by CLIA testing criteria.[12] Ranges can be tighter if clinical requirements are more demanding, but the SD limit should not be set so narrow that excessive time and resources are wasted checking false rejections.

As mentioned, the use of multiple rules improves the error detection and minimizes false rejections. There are six commonly used Westgard QC rules that can be used in whole or in part. Federal guidelines require that at least two rules should be selected to detect random and systematic error. Once a decision to reject the analysis is made based on QC sample results, the problem must be solved by taking corrective action for the system, with the ultimate consequence being accurate patient laboratory results. Problem-solving includes considering the quality of the QC sample, the accuracy of the calibration of the test, the reliability of equipment maintenance, and the reliability of the patient test. Many automated instruments provide clues to solving these problems with system monitors. Steps that are not automated should be retraced through the procedures and protocols to include sample expiration date, preparation, mixing, identification, and other steps involving the analysis phase, including maintenance and temperature stability checks.

A major requisite for multiple rule use is the stability of the control material over time. One must have a sufficient amount of the same lot number of control material and be able to store it to preserve the analytes so that deterioration from storage isn't the cause of analysis rejection. QC rules need to indicate the type of analytical error, that is, whether systematic inaccuracy or random error is causing imprecision, to aid in problem-solving. For example, an error due to imprecision may result from a pipetting problem as indicated by a random error in QC results. A systematic error may be caused by incorrect calibration, resulting in a problem with accuracy.[15]

QC Monitoring Rules

In the QC rule shorthand, the notation "subscript S" ($_S$) is designated for standard deviation. The first number is the number of the consecutive control observation. The number of standard deviations is placed before the $_S$, so that 2_{2S} means two consecutive controls greater than ±2 SD from expected mean. Control rules may be used when evaluating one control (within a control) or with two levels of control (across controls). The R_{4S} rule is used within one control only. Table 2–4 shows the QC monitoring rules commonly used in clinical chemistry. As was stated earlier, the goal of a QC system is to detect errors, including **random errors** and **systematic errors** such as **shifts** and **trends**. Figure 2–4 shows a flow chart for making decisions based on QC results.

A system is said to be "in control" when the control results fall within the QC limits and a rule isn't violated. If a rule is violated, the value falls outside the toler-

random error - error that occurs unpredictably due to poor precision

systematic error - error that occurs predictably once a pattern of recognition is established; predictable errors of the same sign and magnitude

shift - a sudden and sustained change in quality control results above the mean

trend - a gradual but steady change in quality control results moving up or down away from the mean

TABLE 2-4

Westgard QC Rules[14]

Abbreviation	Rule
1_{2S}	A single QC result falls outside the range, defined as ± 2 SD (use as a screening or warning rule that requires additional investigation of QC data). If this rule is used as the sole decision, it generates too many false rejections.
1_{3S}	A single QC result falls outside the range, defined as ± 3 SD (rejection of rule). This detects random error.
2_{2S}	Two consecutive QC results fall more than 2 SD on the same side of the mean (rejection of run). This detects systematic error.
R_{4S}	Two consecutive values differ by more than 4 SD (rejection of run). This detects random error.
4_{1S}	Four consecutive QC results are more than 1 SD away from the mean in the same direction. This indicates a shift in the control (warning or rejection rule). It detects systematic error. This rule may not be applicable for analytes with a narrow SD range.
10_{1S}	Ten consecutive QC results are more than 1 SD away from the mean in the same direction. This indicates a shift in the control (warning or rejection rule). This is the most sensitive check for systematic error. Because it can detect small shifts, a violation of this control rule may indicate an acceptable amount of error and serve as a warning rather than a rejection. A reagent or calibration problem should be suspected.

ance range, the series of analyses are considered "out of control," and measures to correct the problem must be taken. For example, when one control exceeds 3 SD from the mean, the 1_{3S} rule is violated. Figure 2–5 depicts this QC rule violation on a Levey-Jennings chart. Corrective actions depend on the method of analysis. You should consult the operating manual or procedure for causes of problems. When a control has been deemed to be "out of control," it is important to follow the corrective actions necessary to solve the problem and provide good patient results. If the problem resides with the control sample, analysis of patient results

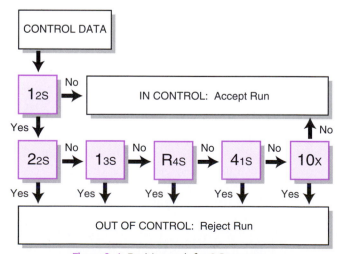

Figure 2–4. Decision path for QC program.

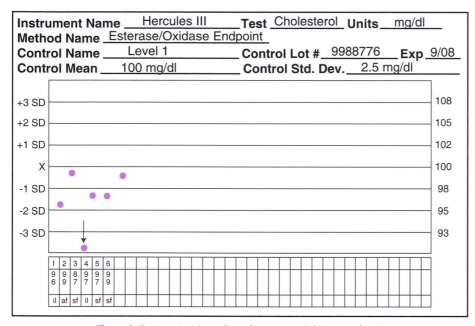

Figure 2–5. Levey-Jennings chart shows a 1_{3S} violation on day 3.

will not need to be repeated. It is imperative that analysis of the patients' samples be repeated if the corrective action involved the assay system.

Systems using three controls can make use of additional rules. When two of three QC measurements are outside limits, one should reject the result. This is known as the 2 of 3_{2S} rule. When six consecutive QC results are more than 1 SD away from the mean in the same direction, the results should be rejected based on a systematic error. This is the 6_{1S} rule. Finally, a 9_{1S} rule is when nine consecutive QC results are more than 1 SD away from the mean in the same direction. The analytical run should be rejected based on a systematic error.

Possible Solutions for Quality Control Problems

1. Repeat the control again after mixing.
2. Repeat the control using a fresh vial or another lot number.
3. Recalibrate the assay.
4. Replace the reagents.
5. Perform necessary maintenance.
6. Consult the trouble-shooting guide, supervisor, or service representative.[15]

Other QC rules that may be used include calculation of a moving average, delta checks, average of normals, and cumulative sum (cusum). A *moving average* is one that is recalculated periodically because the reference material varies over time. This control rule system is commonly used in hematology when a presumed healthy patient sample is repeated periodically throughout the day for precision and accuracy.

A *delta check* is generally performed by comparing an individual patient result throughout the day or week with computer detection of changes from earlier individual patient test results. This check is applied to certain analytes such as albumin and sodium that normally don't vary much throughout the day, but would not apply to those that vary significantly, such as glucose. The Greek letter delta generally refers to change. Bias is calculated from the previous result. This system has been effective in detecting specimen misidentification, which can be a serious problem in the clinical chemistry laboratory. Currently, when laboratory specimens or samples are misidentified, this is not detected by other methods of QC.[16]

A *Shewhart chart*, named after its inventor, was first used for studying the variation in output from a manufacturing process. These charts can distinguish unusual variations from common variations to help find local and sporadic problems with an instrument or transcription error. Shewhart charts can be used to monitor the testing process for the occurrence of future unusual variation and to measure and reduce the effects of common causes.[17]

Cumulative sum control charts, or *cusum charts*, are used to detecting a shift in results compared to the mean. They display cumulative sums of the deviations of measurements from the mean or target value. Cusum charts can be more sensitive to shifts in the process mean than Shewhart charts. Moving average charts are more sensitive to small shifts in the process average but may be difficult to interpret.[17]

Case Scenario 2-4 QC: More or Less Albumin?

Follow-Up

The technologist found that level 1 exceeded +3 SD from the mean for albumin and level 2 was exactly +3 SD from the mean. This indicates QC failure on both results. She checked the maintenance records and found the albumin channel cleaning procedure was 12 days overdue. After the necessary maintenance was performed and the channel recalibrated, the repeated results of both controls were on the mean. The technologist reanalyzed the patient samples in a reverse chronological order until the original values and the reanalyzed values matched. ●

CASE SCENARIO 2-5

QC: Shifting Lipase Results

The third-shift technologist found the lipase reagent bottle running low on the chemistry analyzer. He installed an additional bottle in order to be ready for the heavy workload from the intensive care units. The lipase reagent was a new lot number and required calibration before use. The two levels of control material analyzed following calibration showed an upward shift. The instrument flagged the QC with the following error statement: "QC recovery 2_{2S} across controls."

QC Material	Expected QC $\pm 2_S$	Observed QC
Control level 1 (U/L)	97 ± 2	102
Control level 2 (U/L)	45 ± 1	47

The technologist recalibrated the lipase reagent using a newly opened calibrator set. There was no improvement in the QC results. This time there were two QC error flags: "QC recovery 2_{2S} within controls;" and "QC recovery 2_{2S} across controls." *Recovery* in this context means "results obtained when compared to expected results."

Systematic and Random Errors

Systematic errors are always of the same sign and magnitude and produce biases (which can be positive or negative), while random errors are unpredictable. Systematic errors may be constant or proportional. Several may exist at the same time, and only the net bias will be evident. Systematic errors shift the mean of the distribution, while random errors widen the distribution. Shifts or trends are types of systematic errors.

A shift is defined as a change in QC results that happens abruptly and continues at the same level. This may be due to recent calibration, new shipment of control, or new lot number of calibrator. A trend is defined as a gradual change in one direction in QC recovery. This may be due to the aging of controls or reagents, or to needed maintenance.

Systematic error[18] may be due to

- aging reagents
- aging calibrators
- instrument components
- optical changes
- fluctuations in line voltage
- wear and tear of instrument
- reagent lot variability
- calibration differences
- technologist interactions

Trouble-shooting questions for a shift or trend include the following:

1. When was the reagent put on the instrument?
2. Did the trend start at that time?
3. Is it a new lot number?
4. Is it a reagent that requires operator intervention and preparation?
5. Was a new lot number of calibrator started?
6. Was the date of last calibration checked?
7. Was reagent prepared properly?
8. Was the correct calibrator lot number used?
9. Is there any maintenance that might need to be performed?
10. Has the manufacturer service engineer done recent repairs and maintenance?[18]

Random error[18] may be due to:

- reagent dispensing
- sample evaporation
- temperature of analyzer
- electro-optical mechanism
- calibrator reconstitution
- environmental conditions
- instability of instrument
- variation in handling techniques: pipetting, mixing, timing
- variation in operators

porcine - derived from swine (pigs)

Case Scenario 2-5 QC: Shifting Lipase Results

Follow-Up

The technologist was preparing to make a new bottle of reagent when he discovered a product information notice tucked in the bottom of the reagent box. This type of information comes with reagent kits to help in calibrating the instrument output with concentration. The information gave notice that the reagent was specific for human lipase but that control materials spiked with **porcine** lipase did not exhibit the same behavior as human lipase and lot-to-lot shifts could occur. The manufacturer recommended recalibrating the instrument with lipase standards when a new lot number of reagent is used and then analyzing human-based QC samples to check for analytical errors. It was also recommended that a few patient samples previously analyzed with the old lot of reagent be analyzed with the new lots to check for consistent patient results. Consistency of patient samples between the recently calibrated new lot number and the previously calibrated old lot number can be checked for correlation by calculating the correlation coefficient.

The technologist discovered that the QC material did contain porcine lipase, so recalibration was performed. The QC samples analyzed after this recalibration were found to not violate any QC rules. Previous and current QC results are shown below.

QC Material (Lipase)	Old Lot #	New Lot #
Control level 1 (U/L)	44	48
Control level 2 (U/L)	95	101

The patient samples were almost identical between the two lots, and the correlation coefficient (r) was determined with a statistical calculation to be +0.90. A strong positive correlation is $r = 0.90$ to 1.0, while a strong negative correlation is $r = -0.90$ to -1.0. Correlation values close or equal to zero show no correlation. In this case, since the values appear very close and the correlation coefficient verifies a strong correlation, you can assume that patient results were consistent between lot numbers after recalibration.

QC Material (Lipase)	Old Lot #	New Lot #
Sample A (U/L)	31	33
Sample B (U/L)	114	117
Sample C (U/L)	32	30
Sample D (U/L)	75	74
Sample E (U/L)	19	19
Sample F (U/L)	50	52
Sample G (U/L)	82	85
Sample H (U/L)	63	67 ●

> ## CASE SCENARIO 2-6
>
> **Introducing a New Test: Should We Offer hs-CRP?**
>
> The latest medical journals have been full of articles touting high-sensitivity C-reactive protein (hs-CRP) for cardiac risk assessment. Several physicians have approached the laboratory director about offering this test so that it doesn't have to be sent to a reference laboratory. The laboratory director has asked you to help investigate the new test. Where do you start?

Method Evaluation

New methods are generally proposed for improved laboratory service: expanding of the tests offered, decreasing turnaround time, improving precision and accuracy, reducing overall costs, or upgrading to an automated method. Methods should be selected and evaluated to assure that routine performance meets, at minimum, proficiency testing (PT) criteria. This includes issues of **sensitivity** and **specificity**. The following are factors that should be evaluated when considering whether or not to add a new test.

> Is there a sufficient need based on the number of potential patients for the test to be analyzed in-house?
> What are the intended goals for this test: screening, confirmation, or diagnosis?
> What degree of precision, accuracy, sensitivity, and specificity are required?
> What is the medical decision limit?
> What method should be selected?

There are practical considerations as well. You should consider what instrumentation is available in context with space and utilities for new instrumentation. In addition, increased workload, reagent storage and stability, hours of availability, special specimen requirements, handling of hazardous materials, and urgent or STAT applications should be considered.

If the test will be requested infrequently, it may be more cost effective to send it to a reference laboratory. Not only does the cost include the reagent and calibration material, but the expenditures for service contracts, instrument purchase or lease, labor costs, QC material, calibration verification, and PT must be taken into account. Extremely sensitive methods may require more intensive cleaning procedures as well as increased instrument preventive maintenance and service. The method with the smallest degree of error may not be suitable due to increased cost of short-lived reagents. A spectrophotometric assay may be the most cost effective but the enzyme-linked immunosorbent assay (ELISA) method for the same analyte may be more sensitive.

A review of new methods can be found with a technical and professional literature review, in manufacturer brochures, and by communicating with other clinical laboratory scientists or reading journal articles. The ideal method will have the properties that will give the best analytical performance. A method used as a **screening test** or initial test should detect everyone with the disease and have a high degree of sensitivity, whereas a method used as a **confirmatory test** needs a high degree of

sensitivity - the ability to detect small concentrations of the measured analyte

specificity - freedom from interference and cross reactivity, to determine solely the analyte purported to be measured

screening test - test to determine if patients have a disease before they present with symptoms; should be very sensitive

confirmatory test - using laboratory tests to verify that an initial test result is accurate; should be very specific

medical decision limit - the value for a test result that is used in making the diagnosis

specificity. Testing used to diagnose a disease state should detect all positives without giving any false positives. These tests require both high sensitivity and high specificity. Decisions have to be made as to the allowable precision, accuracy, and total error (the sum of random error and systematic error). Allowable error (E_A) is defined as the amount of error that can be tolerated without invalidating the medical usefulness of the analytical result. **Medical decision limits** can be determined by consultation with the medical staff.

The U.S. Food and Drug Administration (FDA) requires that manufacturers of equipment and reagents present evaluation data about the analytical performance of the method.[7] The laboratory's responsibility is to assess whether the manufacturer's claims are realistic and acceptable. Specifically, the new method needs to be checked for precision, reportable range (analytical measurement range), and accuracy. This is a federal mandate of CLIA '88, which specifies in the Final Rule that laboratories will need to perform validation studies for any new methods introduced after April 24, 2003. For procedures from FDA-approved commercially prepared kits, only precision, accuracy using patient comparison, and reportable range studies are required. For procedures developed or modified in-house, additional tests of validation must be performed, including interference studies and recovery studies.[9]

Precision estimates random analytical error of the method. The mean, SD, and %CV are calculated from the data obtained. The observed SD is judged against the allowable SD for acceptability. If the SD and %CV exceed the expected and allowable amounts, the remaining validation studies should not be performed until precision is improved or a more precise method is chosen. QC material may be used for this study and, in the process, QC ranges can be established. Test Methodology 2–1 details the precision procedure.

TEST METHODOLOGY 2-1.   TESTING PRECISION[19]

The Principle

Determining precision of a method is a test of random error. Samples should be chosen with analyte concentrations to include the medical decision level(s). Precision should be evaluated through 20 replicates of two to three different samples within one run of that test. It should also be tested over 20 days for between-day precision. Between-day replicates of the same samples should be done in duplicate. Results should be recorded on a form to be retained in the evaluation studies notebook. The date, time, and analyst are important to record, particularly for the between-day replication study. Mean, standard deviation (SD), and %CV should be calculated. SD and %CV that are equal to or less than the limits set by CLIA indicate an acceptable precision.

The Calculations

Data should be entered into a statistical computer program and mean, SD, and %CV should be calculated.

Example

Test: Glucose Method: Hexokinase with Hercules III
Materials: Acme control samples 1 and 2
Within-run replication study

continued

TEST METHODOLOGY 2-1. TESTING PRECISION[19] *(continued)*

Replicate	QC1	QC2	Sample 3	Date/Time	Analyst
1	126	200	NA	10/01/05 13:00	JEB
2	127	201	NA	10/01/05 13:00	JEB
3	127	198	NA	10/01/05 13:00	JEB
4	129	197	NA	10/01/05 13:00	JEB
5	126	202	NA	10/01/05 13:00	JEB
6	125	201	NA	10/01/05 13:00	JEB
7	127	200	NA	10/01/05 13:00	JEB
8	128	199	NA	10/01/05 13:00	JEB
9	127	202	NA	10/01/05 13:00	JEB
10	129	203	NA	10/01/05 13:00	JEB
11	127	197	NA	10/01/05 13:00	JEB
12	128	201	NA	10/01/05 13:00	JEB
13	127	202	NA	10/01/05 13:00	JEB
14	125	196	NA	10/01/05 13:00	JEB
15	126	200	NA	10/01/05 13:00	JEB
16	127	201	NA	10/01/05 13:00	JEB
17	128	199	NA	10/01/05 13:00	JEB
18	126	201	NA	10/01/05 13:00	JEB
19	127	199	NA	10/01/05 13:00	JEB
20	128	201	NA	10/01/05 13:00	JEB

QC1 Mean = 127
QC1 SD = 1.124
%CV = 1.124 × 100/127 = 0.89%

The *reportable range* is the range of specimen concentration over which the method may be used without dilution. It is also called the analytical measurement range (AMR). While checking the linear range, a check for a minimum detection limit can be made. The *minimum detection limit* is the smallest single result that can be distinguished from zero.[6] A preliminary evaluation or trial run can consist of within-run precision and linearity checks. If these two components do not meet the required goals, it is pointless to continue with the rest of the evaluation. Test Methodology 2–2 describes how to analyze the reportable range using standard solutions.

TEST METHODOLOGY 2-2. REPORTABLE RANGE[19]

The Principle

Reportable range is the lowest to highest concentration over which the method may be tested without sample dilution. The samples used in reportable range testing can be five or more accurate volumetric dilutions of an elevated patient sample, spiked patient samples pooled together, or commercially available linearity materials. The range should include most common clinical samples without need for dilution. The first check should be with aqueous material, such as a diluted standard since it has the ideal sample matrix. A subsequent check can be made with a matrix similar to patient samples. The evaluation range should match the claims of the manufacturer.

continued

TEST METHODOLOGY 2-2. REPORTABLE RANGE[19] *(continued)*

The Calculations

The average result for each of the six data points is compared with the assigned value using linear regression. Slope, *y*-intercept, and Pearson's correlation coefficient (*r*) are determined with a statistical program. The closer the slope is to 1.00, the *r* is to +1.00, and the *y*-intercept is to 0, the better the accuracy. A scatterplot of the data can also illustrate the highest point that remains close to the best fit line and the upper limit of linearity.

Example

Test: Glucose Method: Hexokinase with Hercules III
Materials: Acme standards 1–6
Reportable range study

Standard	Assigned Value "*x*"	Result #1	Result #2	Result #3	Average "*Y*"	Analyst	Date/Time
1	25	22	24	26	24	JEB	10/01/05
2	50	54	49	49	51	JEB	10/01/05
3	125	125	123	127	125	JEB	10/01/05
4	200	200	201	197	199	JEB	10/01/05
5	500	498	487	499	495	JEB	10/01/05
6	750	752	747	745	748	JEB	10/01/05

$$Y = bx + ar = 0.9xx$$
$$V = bx + a \; ; \; r = 0.9$$

reference method - a thoroughly investigated method with documented accuracy and precision

Patient comparison is a correlation of the new method with a comparative method. The comparison can be made between the new method and a **reference method** or the currently used methodology. Differences are interpreted as systematic analytical errors of the method. One method may have improved sensitivity due to better reaction conditions or improved specificity of the chemical reaction with less interferences. A patient comparison study is provided in Test Methodology 2–3.

TEST METHODOLOGY 2-3. PATIENT COMPARISON STUDY[19]

The Principle

A patient comparison study should encompass 40 to 200 patient samples, analyzed over several days, with values that range over the entire proposed reportable range. It is done to compare the results of the new method with a comparative method to test accuracy of the new method. It is recommended that the range of concentration should be 20% low, 50% normal, and 30% high. Fresh patient samples should be analyzed in duplicate, if possible, on two different runs. Testing should be completed within 4 hours to minimize effects of sample deterioration.

The patient data are calculated using linear regression analysis where the slope is the estimate of proportional analytical error and the *y*-intercept is an estimate of constant analytical error.

TEST METHODOLOGY 2-3.   PATIENT COMPARISON STUDY[19] *(continued)*

The Calculations

The data for the new method are compared with the data from the comparative method using linear regression. Slope, *y*-intercept, and Pearson's correlation coefficient (*r*) are determined with a statistical program. The closer slope is to 1.00, *r* is to +1.00, and *y*-intercept is to 0, the closer the results are in comparison with each other.

Example

Test: Glucose Method: Hexokinase with Hercules III
Materials: 40 patient samples
Comparison study

ID #	Average Test Result (Y)	Comparison Result (X)	Difference (Y − X)	Analyst	Date/Time
1	67	70	3	JEB	10/01/05 14:00
2	89	92	3	JEB	10/01/05 14:00
24	128	132	4	JEB	10/01/05 14:00
25	200	204	4	JEB	10/01/05 14:00
39	650	653	3	JEB	10/01/05 14:00
40	689	692	3	JEB	10/01/05 14:00

$$y = 0.99x + 3; r = +0.99.$$

Interference studies include common interference from hemoglobin, lipids, bilirubin, drugs, and anticoagulants. Samples can be checked against analytical methods known to be free from interference. The difference or bias can be judged against the allowable bias or total allowable error. Interference studies check for constant error.

Recovery studies involve adding a known volume of standard solution to a known volume of patient sample in one tube and, in a second tube, adding the same volume of diluent to the same volume of patient sample. The difference between the two is calculated and expressed as a percentage. The average recovery can be compared to the allowable bias or allowable total error to assess acceptability. Recovery studies estimate proportional systematic error.

Accuracy is further measured by comparison of test results with the new method to those with a reference or **gold standard method** for which accuracy has already been established. A gold standard method is the best available approximation of a true value, although not necessarily 100% accurate. A reference method is a thoroughly investigated method with documented accuracy and precision. This step may be necessary if there are significant variances in the patient comparison. If no reference method is available, the new method can be checked with PT material, assayed controls, calibrator material, or National Institute of Standards and Technology (NIST) samples. Accuracy checks for methodology bias.[20]

Other aspects of the analysis should be checked, including dilutions and calculations. If the instrumentation has an "auto dilute" function for the analyte, the automatic dilution should be checked against manual dilution for accuracy. The procedure is similar to the reportable range study in that results are compared with expected results and linear regression of the data can reveal helpful statistics. Automated analyzers should be checked for reagent and sample carryover.

Reference ranges should be established for a totally new methodology or confirmed for a method replacing one currently in use. Results of the method com-

gold standard method - test method that provides the best available approximation of a true value

parison study between the old method and new method should indicate, based on the correlation coefficient, whether the two methods are sufficiently correlated to allow using the same reference ranges with the new method.

Implementation of the new method should include personnel training, writing the procedure, and establishing QC procedures. Considerations for the Laboratory Information System would encompass interfaces, worksheets, load-lists, and automated processing systems as well as Charge Description Master (CDM) and Current Procedural Terminology (CPT) reimbursement codes. There should be communication with the clinical staff concerning the new method. Information should include specimen type, hours of availability, turnaround time, reference range, overall cost, and description of the clinical utility.

Minimization of preanalytical, analytical, and postanalytical errors is vital in providing reliable laboratory data. Specimen management is an important aspect of the preanalytical phase of testing. Specimen collection, transport, handling, referral, storage, and disposal are all aspects of specimen management. Care must be taken that the best policies for specimen management are written and carried out. This is necessary in order to assure that specimen integrity, analytical reliability, and accurate but timely reporting practices are maintained so that errors are minimized.

Case Scenario 2-6 Introducing a New Test: Should We Offer hs-CRP?

Follow-Up

The technologist determined that the frequency of hs-CRP requests for the previous 6 months averaged only three per day. Sending the samples to a reference laboratory was more cost effective than performing in-house testing.

Tests per year:	1095
Cost of reagent per test:	$ 3.75
Cost of calibrator per test:	$ 2.25
Cost of QC per test:	$ 4.33
Cost of PT participation per test:	$ 2.55
Cost of hardware modification per test:	$16.54
Total in-house cost:	$29.42
Reference laboratory cost:	$20.75

The technologist will review hs-CRP requests in 3 months to determine if they have increased in number. ●

Reliable laboratory results require commitment and care taken in the preanalytical, analytical, and postanalytical phases of testing. Proper collection, handling, and transport of the specimen prior to analysis is very important in order to assure the best sample for testing. In other words, the test result can only be as good as the specimen used in the test process. The analytical phase includes verification of instrument precision with a replication study, accuracy with a reportable range and patient comparison study, and overall reliability through the use of standard reference materials and calibrators, as well as QC samples. Following standardized procedures and using QC rules to make correct decisions about the tests performed are also critical aspects of the analytical phase.

POSTANALYTICAL FACTORS

Postanalytical factors are also important aspects of testing and primarily deal with reporting of results and other aspects that occur after the analysis phase. Just as the other two phases of testing have an effect upon the quality of laboratory test results, so does the report. If they are not delivered legibly and in a timely manner and are not positively identified with the patient sample, laboratory results are not valid no matter how carefully preanalytical and analytical errors were avoided.

Postanalytical factors include comparing the patient results to the correct reference ranges as well as taking into consideration abnormal results that correlate with critical situations. The latter involves the use of medical decision limits in which diagnostic decisions are based upon predictive values. Postanalysis includes verification that results are consistent with other laboratory results and do not reflect potential interferences. Finally, postanalysis includes reporting the results in a timely, accurate, legible manner to the appropriate health-care professionals while maintaining patient confidentiality.

CASE SCENARIO 2-7

Liver Function Tests: Elevated Alkaline Phosphatase Results

A clinical laboratory science student noticed an unusual enzyme pattern when reviewing a pediatric patient's test results, as shown below. Except for the elevated alkaline phosphatase (ALP), all the liver function tests were within the reference ranges and in agreement with results from a clinic visit 4 months earlier. She brought the results to the attention of the laboratory technologist supervising her training.

Test	Reference Range	Current Results	Prior Results
ALP (U/L)	40–360	395	75
ALT (U/L)	11–40	20	16
AST (U/L)	15–40	15	20
CK (U/L)	<144	103	89
LDH (U/L)	100–190	137	143
TBIL (mg/dL)	0.3–1.2	0.7	0.9

Reference Ranges

The reference range (or reference interval) for a laboratory test is a reference point to determine whether a disease is present or absent or if the patient is at risk for future disease states. This comparison may be used in monitoring the progression of a disease or therapeutic drug levels.[21]

Reference ranges may need to be established or confirmed when a new analyte is measured, a new or different analytical method is introduced, or there has been a significant reagent modification by the manufacturer. Laboratories are urged by manufacturers, as well as required by CLIA '88, to establish their own reference ranges. Range determinations can be a considerable investment in time, personnel, and resources.[22]

Large groups of suitable volunteers are difficult to assemble. Laboratories often rely on the employees and their spouses, blood donors, medical students, and healthy preoperative patients. This approach can limit the age range of the statistical population. The Clinical Laboratory Standards Institute (CLSI, formerly NCCLS) recommends a minimum of 120 subjects, while other researchers believe at least 200 are necessary for adequate statistical analysis. Publications by CLSI provide diagnostic laboratories with guidelines for determining reference ranges.[23]

In selecting volunteers for determining reference ranges, conditions in the preanalytical, analytical, and postanalytical phases of the study must be carefully controlled. Table 2–5 lists possible preanalytical factors that should be controlled. Analyte values from reference subjects must reflect all the preanalytical and analytical variables that can affect the results. Volunteer (reference subject) collections should occur over several days. Subjects should fill out a well-defined questionnaire that covers exclusion and partition criteria in addition to a written consent form.

In determining reference ranges, factors affecting the analytical phase that should be considered include instrument, reagent, calibration, calculations, lot-to-lot variables, technologists' variability, and instrument-to-instrument variations if analyzed on more than one system. QC should be included during the reference range determination in the same format as patient testing. Instruments should be in good control to prevent any bias in patient results.

Exclusion or partitioning criteria for determining reference ranges, as listed in Tables 2–6 and 2–7, can be used to select the reference population before specimen collection or can be applied during data review. Partitioning into subclasses such as age and sex should be done only if it is clinically useful and/or well grounded physiologically. The following are some partitioning examples:

1. Some age-related reference ranges are predictable, such as growth and sex hormones. Alkaline phosphatase is higher in young children than adults because of rapid bone growth. Estrogens are higher in sexually mature women than in young children. Bilirubin is higher in 2- to 4-day-old newborns than in older children or adults because of slower metabolic hepatic rates.
2. Creatinine is generally higher in males than females because males have larger muscle mass.
3. Race may play a factor in reference intervals. For example, alanine transaminase is higher in Hispanics than Caucasians, and blacks have higher creatine kinase values than Hispanics or Caucasians.
4. Socioeconomic status may determine quality of nutrition and hydration of a reference subject.
5. Hormone ranges can be partitioned by the time of the menstrual cycle: follicular, midcycle, luteal, or postmenopausal.

TABLE 2-5

Preanalytical Factors to Define for Reference Ranges

· Time of collection
· Body posture before collection
· Fasting or nonfasting state
· Type of sample: arterial, venous, capillary source
· Venous stasis
· Use of separator gel collection tubes

TABLE 2-6
Possible Reasons for Exclusion
· Illness, administration of blood products, hospitalization or surgery · Pharmacologically active agents—alcohol, tobacco, oral contraceptives, drug abuse (including vitamins), prescription drugs · Risk factors—obesity, high blood pressure · Genetic predisposition or carrier state · Risks from environment or occupation · Specific physiological states—stress, pregnancy and lactation, excessive exercise

6. People living at higher altitudes have higher hemoglobin and hematocrit values than those living at sea level.

Variations in analyte concentrations may be due to environmental conditions, including the air breathed and what is consumed. For example, geographic variations in analytes have been observed, such as with PO_2 values. This is due to changes in atmospheric conditions with higher altitudes and the amount of oxygen available. Compensation for environmental conditions by adaptations in oxygen-carrying capacity can maintain homeostasis in individuals acclimated to higher altitudes. There also has been a report of higher aminotransferase enzyme reference intervals in populations that have a greater degree of alcohol, and in particular beer, consumption. This is due to the fact that beer contains pyridoxal-5'-phosphate, a coenzyme in aminotransferase reactions.

Next in establishing reference ranges, the data are examined to determine if they have a gaussian distribution. Gaussian distribution of data is a probability curve that is bell-shaped and symmetric with equal values on each side of the mean. Outliers are removed and data are reviewed for exclusion criteria.

One statistical approach is to calculate the mean and SD and obtain a 95% confidence interval. This requires a gaussian distribution curve; however, the reference values of many analytes do not follow the gaussian form. Asymmetric curves can be "normalized" toward symmetry by adjusting the data with a square root or logarithmic transformation.

The nonparametric approach is easier to use. Nonparametric central limits encompassing 95% of the results are made by trimming off the lowest and highest 2.5% of observations accounting for the remaining 5%. This method is used for skewed and other non-normal data distributions.

TABLE 2-7
Possible Data Partition Criteria
· Age · Sex · Race · Human leukocyte antigen (HLA) type, ABO group · Physiological factors—stage of menstrual cycle, stage of pregnancy · Personal habits—exercise, alcohol use, tobacco use, diet

There is difficulty in getting ranges for all pediatric populations. Few samples are collected from children, especially infants. Published ranges can be found in the literature. When evaluating the possible adaptation of these ranges, care must be given to methodology used, how the sample was collected, and from whom it was drawn.

Mathematical transference can be used to adapt reference ranges from the literature or from other laboratories. Transference can be a complex issue and requires that certain conditions be fulfilled in order to be acceptable. The analyte should be tested on the same instrument system using the same methodology. Ideally, the reference range should be from the same geographic area on the same demographic population of test subjects. Preanalytical factors must also be comparable. The adapted reference range should be validated with a small number of reference subjects.[20]

Case Scenario 2-7 Liver Function Tests: Elevated Alkaline Phosphatase Results

Follow-Up

Alkaline phosphatase (ALP) comes from various locations, including liver, intestine, bone, placenta, and kidney. Physiological bone growth elevates ALP activity in serum to 1.5 to 2.5 times that of normal adult serum (reference range 30 to 90 U/L). Nonpathological ALP spikes are observed in actively growing children and are not necessarily a cause for concern. ●

Medical Decision Limits

Along with determining the reference ranges to correlate with absence of disease, it is also helpful for physicians to have a cutoff value to associate with specific diseases. In fact, that is the basic purpose of laboratory tests with the goal of detecting disease in its early stages. For example, a fasting plasma glucose of 126 mg/dL is used to classify diabetes. This is an example of a medical decision limit or cutoff. It helps to differentiate presence of a particular disease from absence of that disease. Medical decision limits are determined by quantifying the analyte of interest in a sampling of a patient population with the disease and a sampling of those without the disease. Next, with the results obtained from the analysis, the patients are classified based on disease presence and test result using a presumed medical decision limit. The four diagnostic categories are **true-positive**, **false-positive**, **true-negative**, and **false-negative**.

A true positive (TP) is a patient with the disease and a laboratory result at or above the medical decision limit. A true negative (TN) is a patient without the disease and a laboratory result below the medical decision limit. A false positive (FP) is a patient with a laboratory result above the medical decision limit but who is found not to actually have the disease, while a false negative (FN) is a patient with a laboratory result below the medical decision limit but who actually does have the disease. Good medical decision limits exhibit low diagnostic false positives and false negatives (such as 2% or less). Table 2–8 shows an example of the classification of patients based on fasting plasma glucose (FPG) and diagnosis of diabetes mellitus (DM). This information is then used to calculate the diagnos-

true positive - result at or above the decision limit in a patient who has the disease

false positive - result at or above the decision limit in a patient who does not have the disease

true negative - result below the decision limit in a patient who does not have the disease

false negative - result below the decision limit in a patient who has the disease

TABLE 2-8

Sensitivity and Specificy of Fasting Plasma Glucose

N = 200 DM; Classification	FPG ≥126 mg/dL	FPG <126 mg/dL
No, Negative for Disease	2, FP	99, TN
Yes, Positive for Disease	98, TP	1, FN

tic sensitivity and specificity of the medical decision limit for this analyte in predicting the disease.

The diagnostic sensitivity predicts the presence of a disease using a laboratory result such as elevated FPG for diabetes. Using the example above, the diagnostic sensitivity of FPG at the decision limit of 126 mg/dL predicts the likelihood of the patient having diabetes mellitus. **Diagnostic sensitivity** relates to the positive predictive value of a test, whereas **diagnostic specificity** relates to the negative predictive value. It is the percentage of patients with a positive result above the medical decision limit who actually have the disease. Diagnostic sensitivity also relates to the false-positive rate, which is equal to the percent specificity subtracted from 100%.

diagnostic sensitivity - the likelihood that, given the presence of disease, an abnormal test result predicts the disease

diagnostic specificity - the likelihood that, given the absence of disease, a normal test result excludes disease

$$\text{Predictive value of negative result} = \text{TN}/(\text{TN} + \text{FN}) \times 100\%$$
$$\text{Predictive value of positive result} = \text{TP}/(\text{TP} + \text{FP}) \times 100\%$$
$$\text{True-negative rate} = \text{diagnostic specificity} = \text{TN}/(\text{TN} + \text{FP}) \times 100\%$$
$$\text{True-positive rate} = \text{diagnostic sensitivity} = \text{TP}/(\text{TP} + \text{FN}) \times 100\%$$
$$\text{False-positive rate} = 100\% - \%\ \text{specificity}$$

Let us practice these formulas with the specific example of FPG at 126 mg/dL for the medical decision limit. In our example above, 200 patients had FPG levels determined by a recognized methodology. They were then diagnosed by their physicians as having diabetes by a second FPG level on another day and by history and physical examination. The test results were collated and classified as TP, TN, FP, and FN to determine the diagnostic value of the 126-mg/dL medical decision limit for classification of diabetes. Of the 200 results, 2 positive test results were false positives, 1 was a false negative, 98 were true positives, and 99 were true negatives.

$$\text{Predictive value of negative result} = \text{TN}/(\text{TN} + \text{FN}) \times 100\%$$
$$= 99/(99 + 1) \times 100\% = 99\%$$
$$\text{Predictive value of positive result} = \text{TP}/(\text{TP} + \text{FP}) \times 100\%$$
$$= 98/(98 + 2) \times 100\% = 98\%$$
$$\text{True-negative rate} = \text{diagnostic specificity} = \text{TN}/(\text{TN} + \text{FP}) \times 100\%$$
$$= 99/(99 + 2) \times 100\% = 98\%$$
$$\text{True-positive rate} = \text{diagnostic sensitivity} = \text{TP}/(\text{TP} + \text{FN}) \times 100\%$$
$$= 98/(98 + 1) \times 100\% = 99\%$$
$$\text{False-positive rate} = 100\% - \%\ \text{specificity} = 100 - 98\% = 2\%$$

Thus, this example shows that 126 mg/dL FPG is an excellent medical decision limit for the prediction of diabetes mellitus.

> ### CASE SCENARIO 2-8
>
> **Ionized Calcium: Falling Calcium Ions Postoperatively**
> The laboratory technologist was analyzing ionized calcium samples when she received a STAT sample from the postoperative recovery room. Analysis showed a very low ionized concentration of 2.5 mg/dL (reference range 4.6 to 5.1 mg/dL, critical value ≤3.0 mg/dL). The technologist immediately confirmed the results and called the postop unit. Concerned that the sample integrity may have been compromised, she questioned the nurse about the reliability of the sample. The nurse indicated that the critically low result was expected as the patient was beginning to show signs of **tetany**.

tetany - neuromotor irritability accompanied by muscular twitching and eventual convulsions

Critical Values

Critical values, otherwise referred to as panic or alert values, are medical decision level concentrations that would indicate a potentially or imminently life-threatening situation. Medical decision levels are the concentrations at which the test results are critically interpreted for purposes of diagnosis, monitoring, and therapeutic decisions. There may be several medical decision levels for a given analyte.

When a critical value is obtained, it is necessary to quickly notify the clinical team for immediate patient evaluation and treatment. Laboratories are mandated by CLIA '88 to establish a list of critical values as well as a written policy for notification and documentation. Critical values can be determined through the joint efforts of the medical staff, administration, risk managers, pathologists, and laboratory personnel. Medical and laboratory literature and information provided by the College of American Pathologists, such as the "Critical Value Q-Probes,"[24] can provide guidelines for list development. The list of critical values should encompass "point of care" tests as well.

The list should only include tests that are essential for the acute treatment of patients. Glucose, potassium, magnesium, sodium, total CO_2, inorganic phosphorus, calcium, and blood gases are examples of tests requiring critical value limits. There may be defined subsets of critical ranges, such as elevated total bilirubin for neonates or ammonia and iron in pediatric patients. The outpatient clinic may require a different critical cutoff than that established for the hospitalized patient. The overall goal of critical value selection is to enhance patient outcome while balancing resource and time constraints.

Laboratory personnel are responsible for screening results in a timely manner and evaluating a result before releasing it. Critical values warrant immediate notification of patient care personnel. CLIA regulations state to "alert the individual or entity requesting the test or the individual responsible for utilizing the test results."[25] This may include the physician, nurse, or other health-care giver. A reasonable attempt must be made to deliver results, exhausting all avenues of communication (e.g., telephone, beeper, answering service). It is not advisable to leave critical results on an answering machine, or send results through a fax machine or by e-mail. There is no guarantee of result retrieval in a suitable time frame.

The Joint Commission on Accreditation of Healthcare Organizations (JCAHO) has instituted a "read back" policy for critical values. This means that the individual receiving the critical results must write down the information and read back the patient's name, the analyte, and the critical result. Documentation of the individual's name and time of notification should be recorded.[26]

Case Scenario 2-8 Ionized Calcium: Falling Calcium Ions Postoperatively

Follow-Up

The hypocalcemia in this patient was due to many factors. Low calcium concentrations result from hypoalbuminemia caused by trauma, shock, and burns. The redistribution of plasma water during postburn edema further reduces the ionized calcium concentration because ionized calcium is freely diffusable. Ionized calcium homeostasis is regulated by vitamin D and parathyroid hormone. Researchers have found that both vitamin D and parathyroid hormone are affected by burns. Vitamin D metabolism is decreased due to failure to synthesize the active form of vitamin D (calcitriol). The calcium regulation is further affected by reduced secretion of parathyroid hormone.

An additional factor producing hypocalcemia was the presence of citrate in the transfused blood products, as the citrate complexed free calcium. Normally, ionized calcium concentration can return to reference values within 10 minutes of transfusion at a rate of 90 mL/kg/hr. In cases of trauma patients, rapidly transfused blood can overwhelm the regulatory mechanisms, resulting in a delayed return to reference concentrations.[27,28] During the course of the surgery, the patient was rapidly transfused with several units of blood. The patient required immediate calcium supplementation to forestall further tetany. ●

> **CLINICAL CORRELATION**
> Ionized calcium, approximately 45% of the total, is the physiologically active form. Adequate levels are necessary for the regulation of neuromuscular excitability, membrane permeability, and neurotransmitter release. Hypocalcemia can cause the heart to develop both contractile and electrical abnormalities. Hypotension or heart failure may occur.

SUMMARY

This chapter discussed the importance of assuring quality laboratory results through the use of a quality assurance system. The assurance of high-quality laboratory results relies on a commitment to all aspects of the testing system, including attention to preanalytical, analytical, and postanalytical factors. Maintenance of quality laboratory analysis includes the use of quality control materials and procedures that measure the validity of the analysis. Documentation and training are also key aspects of assessing and assuring quality laboratory results.

EXERCISES

As you consider the scenarios presented in this chapter, answer the following questions:

1. How is a shift different than a trend?

2. Compare and contrast systematic errors and random errors and provide an example of each.

3. Discuss three causes of hemolysis and three effects on common chemistry analytes.

4. Discuss two examples in which reference ranges may be different based on age or geographic variations.

5. Using calcium levels as an example and comparing with reference and critical values, discuss the importance of recognizing and quickly reporting a critically low calcium value.

6. Explain the effect of serum specimens contaminated with saline IV solution on common laboratory results, including electrolytes and protein levels.

References

1. Kazmierczak SC: Laboratory quality control: Using patient data to assess analytical performance. *Clin Chem Lab Med* 2003; 41:617–627.
2. Riebling N, Tria L: Six Sigma project reduces analytical errors in an automated lab. *MLO Med Lab Obs* 2005; 37(6):20, 22–23.
3. Montoya ID: Assessing the practice of laboratory medicine. *Clin Lab Sci* 2004; 17(2):66–67.
4. Seamark D, et al: Transport and temperature effects on measurement of serum and plasma potassium. *Scand J Clin Lab Invest Suppl* 1996; 224:275–280.
5. Stankovic AK: The laboratory is a key partner in assuring patient safety. *Clin Lab Med* 2004; 24:1023–1035.
6. Henry JB, Kurec AS: The clinical laboratory: Organization, purposes and practice. In Henry JB (ed): *Clinical Diagnosis and Management by Laboratory Methods*, ed 20. Philadelphia: WB Saunders, 2001.
7. Barrueto F Jr, et al: Cardioactive steroid poisoning from an herbal cleansing preparation. *Ann Emerg Med* 2003; 41:396–399.
8. Ritter C, Ghahramani M, Marsoner HJ: More on the measurement of ionized magnesium in whole blood. *MLO Med Lab Obs* 2004; 36(5):26–27.
9. U.S.Department of Health and Human Services: Medicare, Medicaid and CLIA programs: laboratory requirements relating to quality systems and certain personnel qualifications. Final rule. *Fed Regist* 2003; 68:3640–3714.
10. Westgard JO: Assuring analytical quality through process planning and quality control. *Arch Pathol Lab Med* 1992; 116:765–769.
11. Westgard JO (ed): Internal quality control testing: principles and definitions; approved guideline (NCCLS/CLSI Document C24-A). Wayne, PA: Clinical Laboratory Standards Institute, 1991.
12. Henry RJ, Segalove M: The running of standards in clinical chemistry and the use of the control chart. *J Clin Pathol* 1952; 5:305–311.
13. Levey S, Jennings ER: The use of control charts in the clinical laboratories. *Am J Clin Pathol* 1950; 20:1059–1066.
14. Westgard JO, Groth T: A multirule Shewhart chart for quality control in clinical chemistry. *Clin Chem* 1981; 27(3). Available at *www.Westgard.com/mltirule.htm*
15. Broome HE, et al: Implementation and use of manual multirule quality control procedures. *Lab Med* 1985; 19:533–537.
16. Ladenson J: Patients as their own controls: Use of the computer to identify "laboratory error." *Clin Chem* 1975; 21:1648–1653.
17. Parvin CA: Comparing the power of quality-control rules to detect persistent systematic error. *Clin Chem* 1992; 38:356–363.
18. Seehafer JJ: Corrective actions: What to do when control results are out of control. *MLO Med Lab Obs* 1997; 29(3):34–40.
19. Westgard JO: A method evaluation decision chart (MEDx): Chart for judging method performance. *Clin Lab Sci* 1995; 8:277–283.
20. Hartmann AE: Validation protocol for new method or instruments in the clinical laboratory. *Lab Med* 1983; 14:411–416.
21. Follas WD: Strategies for developing reference ranges. Advance for Medical Laboratory Managers, July 1, 1998. Available at *http://laboratory-manager.advanceweb.com*
22. Wachtel M, Paulson R, Plese C: Creation and verification of reference intervals. *Lab Med* 1995; 26:593–598.
23. Doumas BT (ed): How to define and determine reference intervals in the clinical laboratory; approved guideline, ed 2 (NCCLS/CLSI Document C28-A2). Wayne, PA: Clinical Laboratory Standards Institute, 2000.

24. Howanitz PJ: Errors in laboratory medicine: Practical lessons to improve patient safety. *Arch Pathol Lab Med* 2005; 129:1252–1261.

25. CLIA Sub Part K: Quality System for Non-waived Tests 493.1291. Available at *http://www.phppo.cdc.gov/clia/pdf/CMS-2226-F.pdf*

26. Joint Commission on Accreditation of Healthcare Organizations: 2006 National Patient Safety Goal 2 Laboratory Program. Available at *http://www.jcaho.org/accredited+organi-zations/patient+safety/06_npsg/06_npsg_lab.htm*

27. Toffaletti J: Physiology and regulation: Ionized calcium, magnesium and lactate measurements in critical care settings. *Am J Clin Pathol* 1995; 104(4 Suppl 1):S88–S94.

28. Toffaletti J: *Review Micrograph: Ionized Calcium Through Its First Decade*. Waltham, MA: Nova Biomedical, 2002.

Instrumentation is the tool of the clinical chemistry.

3

Laboratory Techniques and Instrumentation

Wendy Arneson and Jean Brickell

automation - ability of an instrument to perform a laboratory test with minimal human involvement

electrode - a terminal that detects changes in current or voltage in response to changes in the environment

spectrophotometer - instrument that uses a photodetector to measure the amount of a specific wavelength of light transmitted through a test solution to determine concentration

Instrumentation is the mainstay of clinical chemistry. Of all departments in the clinical laboratory, clinical chemistry is the most automated and dependent upon large-volume automated instrumentation. Automated instrumentation employs the same chemistry reactions used in manual biochemistry and general chemistry laboratories. **Automation** is able to achieve more precise and accurate results than manual methods due to more reliable control of volumes, timing, and analysis. Automation incorporates aspects of simpler laboratory equipment, including pipettes, **electrodes**, and **spectrophotometers**. The results gained from automated clinical chemistry analysis are dependent on calculations performed by the instrument relating to dilutions and conversions of photometer output to concentration. Knowledge of basic laboratory equipment, calculations, function of components within instruments, and chemical reactions will be discussed further in this chapter through the eyes of a student. This chapter describes the student's first experience in the clinical chemistry section of the laboratory. As this student works his way through measurement and analysis, the chapter will introduce the principles of basic clinical chemistry analysis.

OBJECTIVES

Upon completion of this chapter, the student will have the ability to

▪ Calculate dilutions with and without specific volumes and conversions of concentrations for commonly used clinical chemistry solutions.

▪ Describe the appropriate use of laboratory glassware, pipettes, and grades of water in the clinical chemistry laboratory.

▪ Discuss the proper use of a centrifuge, analytical balance, and glassware for diluting concentrated acid, including safe practices.

▪ Explain the principles of clinical chemistry testing instrumentation, including spectrophotometry, potentiometry, polarography, electrophoresis, osmometry, **immunoassay**, and chromatography.

▪ Differentiate methods of automating clinical chemistry instrumentation in terms of advantages, challenges, and applications.

immunoassay - test that measures the protein or protein-bound molecules concerned with the reaction of an antigen with its specific antibody

quantitative - expressing test results by amount or concentration (a graded or proportional response)

electrolytes - substances that ionize in solution and conduct electricity

HISTORY OF MEASUREMENT IN THE LABORATORY

The application of biochemical testing for medical testing began about 100 years ago. One of the first clinical chemists, Dr. Otto Folin, developed **quantitative** analytical methods for urine analytes of urea, ammonia, creatinine, uric acid, **electrolytes**, and acidity. He also developed early blood tests, including those for ammonia and creatinine, using the Jaffe method. Dr. Folin helped to establish the clinical significance of renal function and metabolic tests and published the first reference ranges for uric acid, nonprotein nitrogen (NPN), and protein in blood. He helped to develop methods for testing glucose and total serum protein in body fluids.

CASE SCENARIO 3-1

Teaching Applications of Laboratory Mathematics: How Do I Prepare This Solution?

A clinical laboratory science instructor will be teaching her students how to prepare reagents for a spectrophotometry exercise to be practiced later. They have in their work area a working analytical balance, glassware, cobalt chloride salt, deionized water, and 32% HCl **solution**. They need 500 mL of 1% HCl solution. This is the diluent needed to make 250 mL of a 22-g/L solution of cobalt chloride solution. How can 500 mL of 1% HCl be made using 32% HCl solution and deionized water?

solution - a mixture of two or more substances

MAKING THE DILUTION

When diluting a specific amount of solution, the following formula is used:

$$C_1V_1 = C_2V_2$$

The components of this formula are C_1, the starting concentration; V_1, the amount needed; C_2, the final, diluted concentration; and V_2, the total volume needed of the dilution solution. The concentration units and volume units must be the same to apply this formula. Converting units and volumes may be necessary.

For the problem in the case above: $C_1 = 32\%$, $V_1 =$ unknown, $C_2 = 1\%$, and $V_2 = 500$ mL. Since all units match, no conversions are necessary.

$$C_1V_1 = C_2V_2$$
$$32\% \times V_1 = 1\% \times 500 \text{ mL}$$
$$V_1 = 1/32 \times 500 \text{ mL}$$
$$V_1 = 15.625 \text{ mL or } 15.6 \text{ mL}$$

Case Scenario 3-1 **Teaching Applications of Laboratory Mathematics: How Do I Prepare This Solution?**

Follow-Up

With the calculation complete, the instructor will now teach the students how to use these calculations to prepare the solution. Fifteen point six milliliters (15.6 mL) of the concentrated acid will be diluted with enough water to make 500 mL of 1% HCl. Specifically, 15.6 mL of 32% HCl will be added to a 500-mL flask containing at least 200 mL of deionized water in a chemical fume hood. The solution is swirled gently and then enough deionized water is added to complete the total volume to 500 mL. This is sometimes abbreviated as QS (quantity sufficient) 500 mL.

The next step in reagent preparation, once the diluting solution is prepared, is to measure out the cobalt chloride salt. How can 250 mL of 22-g/L cobalt chloride solution be made using the 1% HCl? ●

✓ **Common Sense Check**
It is important to follow good laboratory safety practices. When using concentrated acids, bases, or volatile liquids, you should open the containers and measure volumes in a chemical fume hood so that harmful vapors are not inhaled by you or those around you. It is also important to add concentrated acids and bases to the diluting water to prevent a strong chemical reaction and possible spattering that could occur if water is instead added to the concentrated acid or base.

TABLE 3-1

Metric Units and Conversions

Metric Unit Prefix	Number Conversion
Kilo	1000
Deca	10
Deci	1/10
Centi	1/100
Milli	1/1000
Micro	1×10^{-6}
Nano	1×10^{-9}
Pico	1×10^{-12}

Preparation of Solutions

solute - the substance that is dissolved in the solution

solvent - the substance that is used to dissolve the solute

inert - chemically nonreactive

Solutions are composed of a **solute** within a **solvent** in a homogeneous mixture. The solute is the mass of the ingredient of interest while the solvent is the liquid that is considered **inert**, and not reactive. Concentrations of a solution generally involve a mass of solute dissolved in a certain volume of solvent.

Volumes and masses need to be in the same units in order to perform the conversion calculations. In other words, liters (L) needs to be converted to milliliters (mL) when determining how to make the cobalt chloride solution. Table 3–1 shows the metric prefix relationships and Table 3–2 the relationships between different volumes.

Conversions of Volumes

It is often necessary to convert volume amounts from one metric unit to another. For example, a common conversion is liters to deciliters (dL). A deciliter contains 100 mL and a liter contains 1000 mL.

Let us practice converting 0.3 liters to deciliters.

$$1 \text{ deciliter} = 0.1 \text{ L}$$

$$\frac{1 \text{ dL}}{x \text{ dL}} = \frac{0.1 \text{ L}}{0.3 \text{ L}}$$

$$\frac{1 \text{ dL}}{0.1 \text{ L}} = \frac{x \text{ dL}}{0.3 \text{ L}}$$

TABLE 3-2

Relationship of Volumes

1 kiloliter (kL)	1000 L	1,000,000 mL
1 liter (L)	1000 mL	1,000,000 μL
1 deciliter (dL)	100 mL	100,000 μL
1 milliliter (mL)	1000 μL	1,000,000 nL
1 microliter (μL)	1000 nL	1,000,000 pL

$$1 \text{ dL} \times 0.3 \text{ L} = 0.1 \text{ L} \times x \text{ dL}$$

$$\frac{1 \text{ dL} \times 0.3 \text{ L}}{0.1 \text{ L}} = x \text{ dL}$$

$$\frac{1 \times 0.3}{0.1} = x \text{ dL} = 3 \text{ dL}$$

$$3 \text{ dL} = 0.3 \text{ L}$$

Another quick way to perform this calculation is to multiply the number of liters by 10 to convert to deciliters or to divide by 10 to convert deciliters to liters. For example, using the previous problem, convert 0.3 L to deciliters.

$$0.3 \text{ L} \times 10 = 3 \text{ dL}$$

To convert 3 dL to L:

$$3 \text{ dL}/10 = 0.3 \text{ L}$$

Let us practice converting 0.7 mL to microliters (μL).

$$1 \text{ mL} = 1000 \ \mu\text{L}$$
$$1 \text{ mL}/1000 \ \mu\text{L} = 0.7 \text{ mL}/x \ \mu\text{L}$$
$$x \ \mu\text{L} = (1000 \ \mu\text{L} \times 0.7 \text{ mL})/1 \text{ mL} = 700 \ \mu\text{L}$$

Conversion between masses is calculated similarly. Table 3–3 depicts the relationships between different masses. Let us practice converting 0.55 grams (g) to milligrams (mg).

$$1 \text{ g} = 1000 \text{ mg}$$
$$1 \text{ g}/1000 \text{ mg} = 0.55 \text{ g}/x \text{ mg}$$
$$x \text{ mg} = (1000 \text{ mg} \times 0.55 \text{ g})/1 \text{ g}$$
$$x = 550 \text{ mg}$$

Another quick way to perform this calculation is to multiply grams by 1000 to convert to milligrams, or to divide by 1000 to convert milligrams to grams.

Calculations for Preparation of Solution Concentrations

Percentage (%) is the number of parts per 100 parts. Several common types of percentage concentrations are used in the clinical laboratory, including percentage weight per volume (**% w/v**) and percentage volume per volume (**% v/v**). Percentage volume per volume is the number of milliliters per 100 mL. This is common-

% w/v - number of grams per 100 mL

% v/v - number of milliliters per 100 mL

TABLE 3-3		
Relationship of Masses		
1 kilogram (kg)	1000 g	1,000,000 mg
1 gram (g)	1000 mg	1,000,000 μg
1 decigram (dg)	100 mg	100,000 μg
1 milligram (mg)	1000 μg	1,000,000 ng
1 microgram (μg)	1000 ng	1,000,000 pg

ly used when describing the strength of alcohol, such as 10% v/v ethanol. Percentage weight per volume is the number of grams per 100 mL. This is commonly used to describe a salt solution, such as 0.9% w/v NaCl. Rarely, a percentage is described using the mass of the solute and mass of the solvent. For example, percentage weight per weight (**% w/w**) is the number of grams per 100 g. Finally, **purity** is often used to describe a concentrated solution. It is a simple percentage such as parts per 100 parts.

The International System of Units (SI) is used so that values are understood from laboratory to laboratory and from country to country. Common SI units include micromoles per liter (μmol/L) and moles per liter (mol/L). *Molarity* is the number of moles expressed as molecular mass in grams per liter of solvent. The abbreviated unit name is mol/L. In order to determine the molecular mass (M.M.), you need to refer to the molecular formula and add the atomic masses of each atom in the molecule. For example, HCl has 1 hydrogen atom and 1 chloride atom. The atomic mass (A.M.) of hydrogen is 1.0 and that of chloride is 35.0, so the molecular mass in grams is 36 g. Therefore, 1 molar HCl contains 36 g HCl in 1 liter of H_2O.

> A.M. of H = 1.0
> A.M. of Cl = 35.5, rounded to 35
> M.M. of HCl = 36
> 1 mol/L HCl has 36 g HCl/liter H_2O

Other commonly used solution concentrations include molality and normality. *Molality* is the number of moles expressed as molecular mass in grams per kilogram of solvent. The abbreviated name is mol/kg. The number of moles is determined the same way for molality as for molarity. The only difference is that the mass of the solvent is used instead of volume in liters. For example, 1 molal HCl solution still contains 36 g of HCl in 1 kg of H_2O. *Normality* is the number of gram equivalent weights per 1 liter of solution. Equivalent weight takes into consideration the valence of the molecule as it dissociates into ionic groups in solution. It is often expressed as N or as Eq/L. For example, 1 N H_2SO_4 contains 49 g in 1 L of H_2O. This is determined from the molecular mass of 98.0 g, the sum of the atomic masses of each atom: A.M. H = 1.0×2, A.M. S = 32, and A.M. O = $16.0 \times 4 = 64$.

$$2 + 32 + 64 = 98$$

In normality, the valence of sulfuric acid needs to be considered as the ions dissociate into 1 sulfate ion (2−) and 2 hydrogen ions (2 × 1+) . The valence is the absolute value of either ion group, so in sulfuric acid it is 2 . Therefore, the equivalent weight of sulfuric acid is the molecular mass of 98 divided by the valence of 2 or 98/2 = 49. Thus 1 N H_2SO_4 is 1 Eq/L and contains 49 g in 1 L H_2O.

Conversions of Solutions

Sometimes solution units need to be converted prior to dilution or further use. For example, to convert a solution expressed as g/dL to molarity, you need to convert deciliters to liters and grams to molarity. To proceed, you should multiply the g/dL by 10 since there are 10 deciliters per 1 liter. Then you should divide by molecular mass since 1 mole is the molecular mass in grams. If you look at this in a formula, you will see how the units cancel in this equation with only mol/L remaining:

$$\frac{g \times 10 \text{ dL} \times 1 \text{ mol}}{dL \times 1 \text{ L} \times g \text{ M.M.}}$$

% w/w - number of grams per 100g (mass/mass)

purity - number of parts per 100 parts

Practice converting 44 g/dL HCl to mol/L. (Recall that HCl = 36 g M.M.)

$$44 \text{ g/dL} \times 10/36 = \text{mol/L} = 12.2 \text{ mol/L}$$

When converting molarity to g/dL, the reverse equation is applied. Multiply by the molecular mass in grams and divide by 10 to convert liters to deciliters.

$$\frac{\text{mol} \times 1 \text{ L} \times \text{g}}{\text{L} \times 10 \text{ dL} \times 1 \text{ mol}}$$

Practice converting 1.8 mol/L sulfuric acid to g/dL. (Recall that H_2SO_4 = 98 g M.M.)

$$1.8 \text{ mol/L} \times 98/10 = \text{g/dL} = 17.6 \text{ g/dL}$$

When converting molarity to normality, one needs to mainly consider the valence as the molecular mass in grams is common in both. The simple equation is molarity × valence = normality. The explanation for this simplistic formula is as follows and, when units are canceled, all that remains are multiplying valence by molarity to get Eq/L or normality:

$$\frac{\text{mol} \times \text{g (M.M.)} \times 1 \text{ Eq}}{\text{L} \times 1 \text{ mol} \times \text{g (M.M./Val)}}$$

Convert 3.0 mol/L H_2SO_4 to normality in Eq/L. (Remember the valence of sulfuric acid is 2.)

$$3 \text{ mol/L} \times 2 = 6.0 \text{ mol/L}$$

Some solutions are described in terms of density and purity (or percent assay) when purchased. It may be necessary to convert these units to normality to use the solution in reagent preparation. *Density* is the concentration of a solution expressed in grams per milliliter (g/mL). Density is often the designation for a concentrated acid or base. However, purity is often expressed along with density. *Purity* is a simple % w/w of the weight of the pure substance of interest in a chemical compound that contains chemicals other than the substance of interest. The following formula can be used to convert density and purity to molarity in mol/L: g/mL × purity × 1000/M.M./valence. This conversion may be better understood by seeing the entire formula.

$$\frac{\text{g} \times \text{assay purity (decimal form)} \times 1 \text{ mol} \times 1000 \text{ mL}}{\text{mL} \times \text{M.M.} \times 1 \text{ L}}$$

Convert concentrated HCl solution (37% assay purity, 1.19 g/mL density) to molarity. (The M.M. of HCl = 36.)

$$1.19 \times 0.37 \times 1000/36 = 12.2 \text{ mol/L}$$

pH and pOH Calculations

Concentration of a strong acid can also be presented in a way that represents the ionization of the hydrogen ions in solution, or the **potential**. Thus, pH is the potential of H^+ as it relates to the negative, or inverse, log of the hydrogen ion concentration, expressed as $[H^+]$, in mol/L. Mathematically, the pH of a strong acid is equal to the inverse log of the hydrogen ion molar concentration since it completely dissociates to hydrogen ions when in solution.

potential - force of electrical activity (in volts)

$$\text{pH} = \log (1/H^+) \text{ in mol/L}$$
$$\text{pH} = -\log [H^+]$$

What is the pH of 0.01 mol/L HCl?

$$pH \text{ of } 1 \times 10^{-2} \text{ mol/L}$$
$$pH = \log (1/1 \times 10^{-2})$$
$$pH = \log 100$$
$$pH = 2$$

What is the mol/L of HNO_3 of pH 7.0?

$$pH = \log (1/H^+)$$
$$7.0 = \log (1/H^+ \text{ mol/L})$$
$$\text{inv } \log 7.0 = 1/H^+ \text{ mol/L}$$
$$10{,}000{,}000 = 1/H^+$$
$$H^+ = 1 \times 10^{-7} \text{ mol/L}$$

Concentration of a strong alkaline solution can also be presented in a way that represents the ionization of the hydroxyl ions in solution. The potential of OH^-, or pOH, relates to the log of the **reciprocal** of the hydroxyl ion concentration in mol/L. Mathematically, the pOH of a strong alkaline solution is equal to the reciprocal of the log of the hydroxyl ion molar concentration since it completely dissociates to hydroxyl ions when in solution. Also, pOH is equal to 14 – pH of the solution.

reciprocal - opposite relationship

$$pOH = \log 1/[OH^-] \text{ in mol/L}$$
$$pOH = -\log [OH^-]$$
$$pH + pOH = 14$$

What is the pH of 0.01 mol/L NaOH?

$$pOH = \log 1/[OH^-] \text{ in mol/L}$$
$$pOH = \log (1/0.01)$$
$$pOH = \log 100$$
$$pOH = 2$$
$$pH = 14 - 2$$
$$pH = 12$$

Concentrations of weak acids or bases can also be presented in a way that represents the ionization of the hydrogen ions in solution, or the potential. However, the acid does not completely dissociate to hydrogen ion but also forms some weak salt. The proportion of hydrogen ions and salt formed when a weak acid dissociates in solution depends on its dissociation constant. pH is the potential of the dissociation constant added to the log of the ratio of salt concentration in mol/L to weak acid concentration in mol/L. This becomes most useful when predicting acid-base status of a patient's plasma based on the bicarbonate ion and carbonic acid concentrations. This will be discussed in more detail in Chapters 6 and 9. pK_a is the negative log of K_a, the dissociation constant.

$$pH = pK_a + \log (\text{salt conc./weak acid conc.})$$
$$pH = pK_a + \log (HCO_3^-/H_2CO_3)$$

What is the pH of the patient's plasma with HCO_3^- of 22 mol/L and H_2CO_3 of 1.1 mol/L given the pK_a of 6.1?

$$pH = 6.1 + \log (22/1.1)$$
$$pH = 6.1 + 1.26$$
$$pH = 7.36$$

Sample Dilutions

Patient **samples** may require dilution in order to be analyzed correctly. Most procedures are set up with a limited concentration range. Some procedures start with a set dilution such as 1/10. As was discussed earlier with reagent dilutions, dilutions are composed of a certain amount of concentrated sample and a certain amount of diluent mixed together to make a diluted sample. These types of dilutions are usually expressed as a fraction or ratio rather than with units of concentrations. A dilution is a fraction of the sample that can be represented for example, as x/y, where x is the sample volume and y is the sum of the sample volume and the diluent volume. A 1/4 dilution has 1 volume of sample and 3 volumes of diluent mixed together. Any volume can be used to create this dilution, but in order to get the correct fraction, the same unit of volume should be used for the sample and the diluent. For example, a 2/3 dilution could contain 2 mL of serum and 1 mL of pure water: $2/(2 + 1) = 2/3$. Another way that this dilution could be made is with 20 μL of serum and 10 μL of pure water or with 0.2 mL of serum and 0.1 mL of pure water.

What is the dilution that is created when 3 mL of saline is added to 2 mL of serum for a procedure?

$$\text{Dilution} = 2 \text{ mL}/(2 + 3 \text{ mL}) = 2/5$$

Large dilutions may be difficult to make because of the amount of diluent that needs to be added. For example a 1/1000 dilution may be difficult to create accurately even with 0.1 mL of serum and 99.9 mL of diluent. A series of dilutions, also called serial dilutions, may be a better way to make the dilution. Using the example of 1/1000, you could consider numerical combinations that make up 1000, such as 100×10.

$$1/1000 = 1/100 \times 1/10$$

To make a 1/1000 dilution with a series of dilutions, you could take 0.1 mL of serum and add to 9.9 mL of diluent to make the 1/100 dilution.

$$0.1/(9.9 + 0.1) = 1/(99 + 1) = 1/100$$

After that portion is mixed well, 0.1 mL of the 1/100 dilution can be added to 0.9 mL of diluent to make a 1/10 dilution of the 1/100 or $1/10 \times 1/100 = 1/1000$.

sample - a portion of the specimen to be used in analysis

✓ **Common Sense Check**
It is important when making a dilution that the amount of total volume is large enough to provide for the procedure but not so excessive as to waste precious sample. Careful attention to the total volume and sample volume is helpful.

CASE SCENARIO 3-2

Lab Glassware and Pipettes: Use Them Correctly

The clinical laboratory science student made up the reagent by measuring out the tap water in an Erlenmeyer flask and the concentrated reagent in a beaker. "Don't do that!" said the teaching mentor. "You must use the correct glassware and diluent when making up reagents."

Flasks

A *volumetric flask* is used for preparing large amounts of standard solutions and reagents that require highly accurate concentrations. This flask is a vessel with a tall, slender neck and a pear-shaped body with a flat bottom and is designed for a single volume, as indicated by the etched line on the neck of the bottle. The most

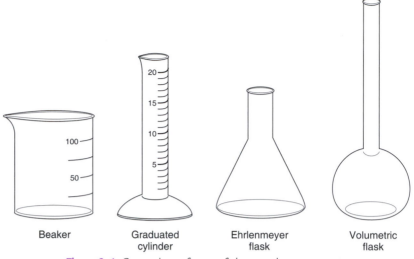

Figure 3–1. Comparison of types of glassware by appearance.

common volumes are 250, 500, 1000, and 2000 mL. However smaller volumes are available such as 100, 50, 25, and even 1, 2, and 5 mL. These flasks are "to contain" (TC) vessels, meaning that their accuracy is tested while it contains that volume. They are used for preparing a solution of known volume rather than determining the volume of an unknown fluid. Figure 3–1 shows a volumetric flask, Ehrlenmeyer flask, graduated cylinder, and beaker of similar sizes.

Ehrlenmeyer flasks are also used in solution preparation but are less accurate than volumetric flasks. This type of flask is a conical container with multiple volume markings that serve as estimates of volume and is available in a variety of sizes, such as 250, 500, and 1000 mL. The purpose of an Ehrlenmeyer flask is to help dissolve a solid solute into solution before transfer to a volumetric flask for final volume adjustment. The flask provides a larger surface area with its straight conical sides, so when a solution is swirled, it has maximum contact with the sides of the flask to help with dissolution. These flasks are also used in preparing a solution of known volume rather than determining the volume of an unknown fluid.

Beakers are simple flasks that are shaped like a drinking glass with a small pour spout. They also have volume markings and are available in a variety of total volume sizes. Beakers have the least accuracy of the three types of flasks. They would not be accurate in determining the total volume of an unknown fluid because the markings are not calibrated to a level of accuracy for that purpose. Beakers are used to hold stock solutions or diluents for short-term storage or during laboratory procedures.

Graduated Cylinders and Glass Pipettes

A graduated cylinder is a tall flask with multiple volume gradations. The purpose of this flask is to aliquot volumes of a fluid in making up a reagent dilution or to determine the volume of an unknown fluid. This type of glassware has a higher degree of accuracy than an Ehrlenmeyer flask since the volume markings are graduated to at least 5% of the total volume.

Glass pipettes are also used to deliver liquid of certain volumes and are calibrated at 20°C. There are two main types of glass pipettes: measuring and transfer. Glass pipettes are held vertically and need a device to provide suction to aspirate the fluid up to the volume markings. Safe practice requires the use of a suction bulb or device rather than sucking the fluid up with your mouth. Suction devices must be used even if you know the fluid to be distilled water since biohazards and toxins may become airborne and settle onto glassware. For the most accurate volumes, the pipette should be held vertically and the fluid adjusted to slightly above the intended volume and then adjusted down so that the lowest part of the fluid meniscus is at the intended volume.

Pipettes come in a variety of volumes and three main formats: to deliver drain out, to deliver blow out, and to contain. Pipettes that are calibrated "to deliver" (TD) but with no etched rings on the top should be allowed to drain out the fluid since the volume has been calibrated in this manner. This is typical of highly accurate pipettes such as transfer pipettes. Pipettes that are calibrated TD but with etched rings on the top should have the last drop blown out if the full volume is to be delivered. This type of pipette is typical of measuring pipettes in which the full volume or increments of volumes can be delivered. The final type of pipette, "to contain" (TC), is not used often in clinical chemistry. This type of pipette is used when diluting a highly viscous fluid such as whole blood. A TC pipette is calibrated to contain the designated volume so, in order to accurately dispense the full volume, the pipette must be rinsed out in the diluting fluid several times.

Two main types of glass pipettes are in common use in the clinical laboratory: measuring pipettes and transfer pipettes. Measuring pipettes deliver multiple volumes and are used when less accuracy of measurement is required, such as for delivering reagents or small amounts of solvent. This type of pipette should not to be used for making standard solutions or quality control materials. Examples of measuring pipettes are **serological** and Mohr pipettes. These pipettes will be discussed further below. Transfer pipettes deliver one volume and are used when a higher degree of accuracy required. A class A transfer pipette is accurate to within 0.1%.[1] This type of pipette is used for preparation of standard solutions to be used in calibration. Transfer pipettes resemble measuring pipettes except that only one measurement mark appears on the neck and there is a round or cylindrical bulb toward the middle or base of the pipette. Types of transfer pipettes include standard volumetric pipettes, Ostwald-Folin pipettes, and automated micropipettes. Test Methodology 3–1 describes the correct procedure for use of a glass pipette. Figure 3–2 depicts the correct technique for using a glass pipette.

serological - studying serum components of the blood; making a serum titer for clinical laboratory testing, such as an antibody titer

TEST METHODOLOGY 3-1. CORRECT OPERATION OF A GLASS PIPETTE

1. Place a mechanical suction bulb or device on the top of the glass pipette.
2. Insert the glass pipette into the fluid to a level that will aspirate fluid and not air bubbles.
3. Aspirate the fluid above the desired total volume by depressing the suction bulb, taking care not to aspirate it up into the bulb.
4. Remove the bulb, placing your finger over the top of the glass pipette.
5. Wipe off the outside of the pipette with gauze, taking care not to wipe the bottom, which could wick away fluid from inside the pipette.
6. Adjust the meniscus: read the meniscus at the bottom of the curve of the liquid.
7. Drain the liquid into the receiving vessel.
8. Place the suction bulb on the top of the pipette and blow out the last drop into the receiving vessel if this is a graduated pipette that calls for dispensing the last drop.

Serological measuring pipettes are graduated so that multiple volumes can be delivered. Typical serological pipette volumes range from a total volume of 0.2 ml to 10.0 mL and have gradations extending into the tip of the pipette. These are usually calibrated TD with a frosted or etched ring at the mouthpiece indicating the need to blow out the last drop as needed. They are termed *serological* because they are designed to easily make dilutions or titers of patient serum for serological procedures. These pipettes can also be used to make dilutions of serum or plasma for clinical chemistry procedures and are usually used for measuring out the diluent in a dilution. Figure 3–3 shows a typical serological measuring pipette.

Mohr pipettes are graduated, but the markings do not extend into the tip. Commonly these pipettes are available in total volumes of 2.0, 5.0, or 10.0 mL, but since there is no frosted ring at the mouthpiece, they are not blown out to deliver the full volume. If the full volume is to be delivered, the fluid is adjusted to a lower meniscus level. Due to the extra skill required with these pipettes, they are not common-

1. Use mechanical suction   2. Wipe off outside of pipette with gauze

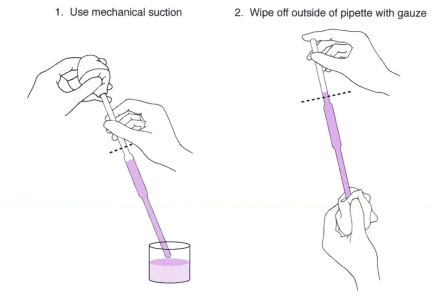

3. Adjust the meniscus; read meniscus at the bottom of the curved liquid

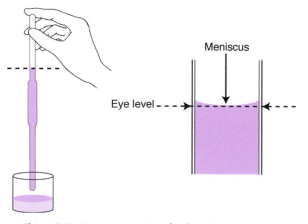

Figure 3–2. Correct operation of a glass pipette.

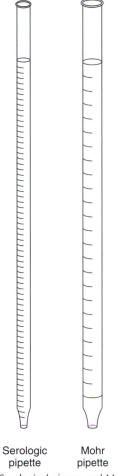

Serologic   Mohr
pipette   pipette

Figure 3–3. Serological pipette and Mohr pipette.

ly used in the clinical laboratory. Some pipette suction devices help to retain the fluid without the use of the fingertip, and they are recommended for this type of pipette. Figure 3–3 allows you to compare the serological and Mohr pipette.

Volumetric transfer pipettes are designed to indicate one volume. The volume calibration mark is etched into the neck of the pipette, but there is no etched ring at the mouthpiece. These markings indicate that these pipettes are TD drain out and the final volume should not be blown out for volume accuracy. The degree of accuracy is indicated on the pipette, and it is a higher degree of accuracy than in measuring pipettes. These pipettes have a cylindrical glass bulb near the center of the pipette that helps to distinguish them from other types of transfer pipettes. Figure 3–2 shows the typical appearance of a volumetric pipette.

Ostwald-Folin transfer pipettes are used for delivering small volumes of viscous solutions such as protein or whole blood standards. The mouthpiece has a frosted ring indicating that the last drop should be blow out in order to accurately deliver the full volume. To differentiate this type of pipette from a volumetric transfer pipette, there is a rounded bulb that is positioned closer to the delivery tip. *Sahli pipettes* are small transfer pipettes similar to Ostwald-Folin pipettes but are used for making dilutions of whole blood, typically for hematology procedures. These

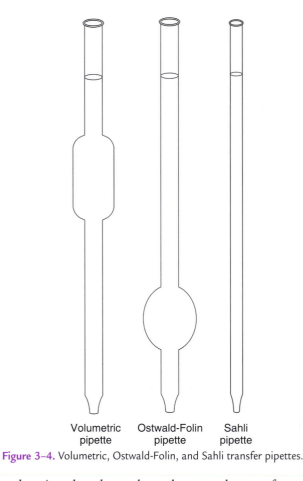

Volumetric   Ostwald-Folin   Sahli
pipette   pipette   pipette

Figure 3–4. Volumetric, Ostwald-Folin, and Sahli transfer pipettes.

pipettes are not class A and so do not have the same degree of accuracy as a volumetric pipette. However, they are considered accurate for performing manual cell counts from whole blood or viscous fluids. Figure 3–4 compares the appearance of a volumetric transfer pipette, Ostwald-Folin pipette, and Sahli pipette.

Case Scenario 3-2 Lab Glassware and Pipettes: Use Them Correctly

Follow-Up

To make up the 500 mL of 32% HCl solution correctly, the student should measure out 15.6 mL of 32% HCl with a 25-mL graduated cylinder. The concentrated HCl will be added to a 500-mL Ehrlenmeyer flask containing at least 200 mL of pure water in a chemical fume hood. The estimation volume markings on the Ehrlenmeyer flask are sufficient at this stage, but pure water must be used. The solution is swirled gently and then poured into a 500-mL or 1000-mL graduated cylinder. Then enough deionized water is added to complete the total volume to 500 mL, reading the bottom of the curved meniscus line as the volume. This action is sometimes abbreviated as QS (quantity sufficient) 500 mL. Since this solution is a diluent reagent rather than a standard solution, a volumetric flask is not necessary and using it may waste resources and risk breakage. It is suggested to use only one measuring device for each step to reduce the additions of inaccuracies. ●

✓ Common Sense Check

It is good safe practice to use a mechanical suction bulb to aspirate with a glass pipette rather than using your mouth to create suction. This would avoid accidentally aspirating harmful reagents, biohazards, or even soap.

Mechanical Micropipettes

Micropipettes can be easier to operate since they do not require switching between a suction bulb and the fingertip to control the volume held in the pipette. They deliver small volumes, usually less than 1.0 mL, with accuracy with the use of a suction button operated by moving your thumb. They are generally TC pipettes depending on the way they were initially calibrated.

The most commonly used pipettes have a piston with a button on top that, when depressed, creates a suction for aspirating and dispensing the volume. These pipettes are used with disposable pipette tips. They are manufactured with a one-stop or two-stop pipetting cycle. A one-stop pipette is the simplest type to use in that depressing the button will push out the air from the pipette tip. A two-stop air displacement pipette is similar except that there are two positions to depress the suction button. The upper position should be used to aspirate the fluid and the lower position is used to dispense the fluid and blow out the last drop. Figure 3–5 and Test Methodology 3–2 show the operation of a two-stop air displacement pipette. When determining at which stop the button was last left, it is recommended to put a fresh tip on and depress the button several times, observing the placement of the suction button.

> ✓ **Common Sense Check**
> Wear gloves when aspirating chemical reagents or biohazardous fluids to prevent skin damage or pathogens entering into minute cuts in your skin.

TEST METHODOLOGY 3-2. CORRECT OPERATION OF A MICROPIPETTE

Always follow the procedure provided by the vendor for the proper use of a micropipette. It is important to follow the recommendation for removing excess fluid from the outside of the pipette tip. For example, for positive displacement pipettes, the manufacturer often recommends dipping the filled syringe in distilled water to remove excess fluid clinging to the outside. For air displacement pipettes, as shown in Figure 3-5, the manufacturer recommends carefully wiping the outside of the pipette with a disposable tissue, taking care not to touch the bottom of the pipette tip.

It is also important to fully deliver the fluid according to the manufacturer's recommendations. For positive displacement pipettes, the syringe is rinsed into the receiving or diluting fluid so that the sample will be fully dispensed. For air displacement pipettes, there is a separate step in the dispense cycle that blows the final drop of fluid into the receiving container. In those cases, it is important to dispense the fluid toward the bottom of the receiving container so as to minimize loss by aerosolization or splashes.

1. If a disposable pipette tip is required, position the tip on the pipette.
2. Depress the plunger or suction button. If this is a two-stop pipette, the button is depressed to the upper position, which is generally around the halfway point.
3. While keeping the suction button depressed, place the pipette tip into the fluid to a level that will aspirate fluid and not air bubbles.
4. Slowly release the suction button up so that the fluid is aspirated, without air bubbles, into the pipette tip.
5. Remove the excess fluid from the outside of the pipette tip according to directions.
6. Dispense the fluid into the vessel by pushing the suction button down. If this is a two-stop pipette, the button is depressed all the way to the bottom.
7. For a one-stop pipette, the process is the same except that the button has only one position for aspirating and dispensing the fluid.

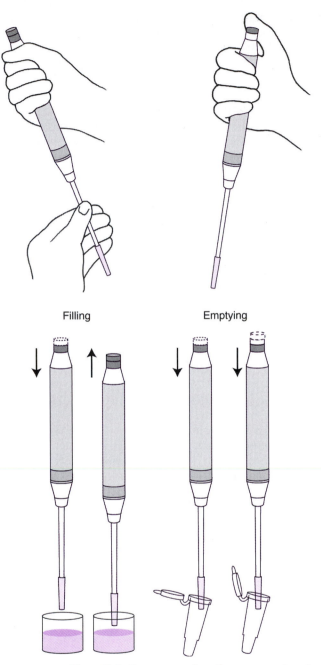

Filling   Emptying

Figure 3–5. Correct operation of a two-stop micropipette.

For delivering larger volumes of reagent repeatedly with a high degree of accuracy, a dispenser called a re-pipetter can be used. A re-pipetter is composed of a jar and a manual pump, and resembles a condiment dispenser. The volume can be adjusted by a screw, and this is necessary when calibrating to the volume desired. Volume accuracy can be checked with a graduated cylinder. An automated dilutor is also available and is typically accurate for even small volumes. The volume is usually measured by a syringe with a piston, and suction is created by a mechanical pump. Volume again can be checked with a graduated cylinder and calibrations made according to manufacturers' recommendations.

Pipette Validity

Pipette accuracy and precision must be checked periodically so that only valid pipettes are used. The most accurate method of validation is **gravimetric**. Gravimetric analysis of a pipette involves determining the mass of highly pure distilled water delivered by pipette using room-temperature water. The resulting mass is converted to volume using a density conversion factor for pure water adjusted to the temperature. Test Methodology 3–3 describes the gravimetric method for pipette calibration. There are also procedures for checking the validity of a pipette using a spectrophotometer. These procedures involve testing colored reagents such as potassium dichromate or p-nitrophenol with known **absorbance** at certain wavelengths. Since concentration relates to absorbance, volume can be determined from this procedure.[1] A screening method to check for validity of pipette operation is available using titrimetric verification. Since this method is not as sensitive in detecting pipette errors, it is expected by most accrediting agencies that gravimetric or spectrophotometric methods are used at least annually.

gravimetric - measuring mass to relate to density or other concentration

absorbance - the amount of light retained by a substance

TEST METHODOLOGY 3-3. GRAVIMETRIC PIPETTE CALIBRATION

1. Record the barometric pressure and temperature in °C of pure water (type 1), since these factors affect weight of substances.
2. Weigh a clean weighing vessel and adjust the scale to tare (zero mass).
3. Adjust the pipette to the desired volume and dispense according to the manufacturer's procedure into a previously weighed and tared vessel.
4. Use the following calculation:

$$(W_2 - W_1) \times Ft = \text{actual capacity in mL}$$
W_2 = weighing vessel after volume is pipetted into it (cover on)
W_1 = empty weighing vessel with cover (to 0.1 mg)
Ft = factor to adjust mass to volume based on temperature
(At 4°C, 1.0 g pure H_2O is 1.0 mL)

5. Repeat 10 times and determine the mean volume and standard deviation.
6. Perform calculations for % accuracy and precision. Use the manufacturer's specifications to determine accuracy and precision of the micropipette and to adjust the pipette accordingly. For example, a valid glass pipette has an accuracy >99.5 % and precision <0.5%.

% Accuracy = (actual volume from pipette/expected or nominal volume) × 100
% Precision = (standard deviation/mean volume) × 100

For an example calculation of pipette precision, let's use these data: $n = 10$, pipette expected volume = 100 μL, standard deviation = 4, pipette actual or mean volume = 98.

% Accuracy = (98/100) × 100 = 98%
% Precision = (4/98) × 100 = 4.1%

TABLE 3-4

Pipette Calibration Form

Pipette Serial #: _____

Date	Tech.	Pipette Volume	1st Sample	2nd Sample	3rd Sample	4th Sample	5th Sample	Mean	Standard Deviation	%CV	% Accuracy

Pipette calibration results should be recorded for long-term monitoring and to track changes over time with a particular pipette. This is an important aspect of quality assurance. The accuracy and precision of a pipette used in sample or standard solution dilution is critical to avoid analytical errors. Table 3–4 is an example of a pipette calibration form. Furthermore, pipette calibration should be verified as described in Test Methodology 3–4.

TEST METHODOLOGY 3-4.   VERIFICATION OF PIPETTE CALIBRATION

The following spectrophotometric procedure is used to verify calibration of "to deliver" transfer or measuring micropipettes that deliver volumes up to 1000 μL. This is an example of the use of *p*-nitrophenol in spectrophotometric verification of the calibration of a 10-μL pipette.

1. All glassware should be cleaned, rinsed with distilled water, and dried.
2. Reagents required: around 1.0 L of 0.01-mol/L NaOH and 100 mL of 105-mg/dL *p*-nitrophenol (PNP). Dissolve 105 mg of high-purity PNP in deionized water in a 100-mL volumetric flask. Fill to the mark, mixing thoroughly. Prepare dilutions of the stock PNP. Fill three 250-mL volumetric flasks with 250 mL 0.01-mol/L NaOH so that it reaches the volume mark. Add 1.0 mL of stock PNP to each flask using a different volumetric pipette each time. Mix well.
3. Make test solutions by adding 2.5 mL of 0.01-mol/L NaOH to each of 5 cuvettes. To each cuvette, using the test micropipette and following the manufacturer's direction for operation, add 10 μL of PNP solution. The manufacturer's directions should specify whether this pipette is to be dipped into rinse fluid or wiped with tissue prior to dispensing. Instructions may specify that the pipette is to be rinsed out into the receiving fluid, or to have the remaining drop blown out with the dispensing button followed by a tip discard. These are important aspects to follow consistently as they impact upon accuracy and precision of the pipette. In this example, 2500 μL + 10 μL, or 2510 μL, is the presumed total volume of each cuvette. Note that this volume would change depending on the size of the micropipette used.
4. Cover each cuvette and mix by inversion 8 to 10 times.
5. Using distilled water in the reference cuvette, adjust to zero absorbance at 401 nm in a previously warmed up spectrophotometer.

continued

TEST METHODOLOGY 3-4.   VERIFICATION OF PIPETTE CALIBRATION *(continued)*

6. Read the absorbance of each cuvette and record the absorbance readings on the attached chart. The presumed correct absorbance (Abs.) reading is 0.550.
7. Calculate the volume in microliters (µL) delivered by the pipette for each of the 5 tests using the following formula:

   (Abs. obtained/0.550) × 0.003984 × 2510 = volume delivered by pipette in µL

   The dilution of PNP is 1/251 = 0.003984, and 2510 is the total volume of each cuvette.
8. Determine the mean, standard deviation, and coefficient of variation (%CV) from the 5 volumes delivered by the pipette.
9. %CV is the measure of precision. Accuracy error is determined as:

   ([Expected volume – Obtained volume] × 100%)/Expected volume

   Accuracy should meet the manufacturer's guidelines or be <1.0 %, whichever is smaller.

CASE SCENARIO 3-3

Weighing Out Mass

The clinical laboratory science students need to measure out cobalt chloride salt using an analytical balance to make 250 mL of the 22-g/L solution. First they needed to determine how much cobalt chloride needs to be weighed out to make the solution.

$$\text{Concentration} = \text{mass/volume}$$

For example:

$$22 \text{ g/L} = 22 \text{ g/1000 mL}$$
$$22 \text{ g/1000 mL} = x \text{ g/250 mL}$$
$$250 \text{ mL} \times (22 \text{ g/1000 mL}) = x \text{ g}$$
$$5500 \text{ g/1000} = x \text{ g}$$
$$5.5 = x \text{ g}$$

So, 5.5 g of cobalt chloride must be obtained.

DETERMINING MASS

Weight is a function of mass and gravity, and its common English unit is the pound. Mass is a physical property of matter, and the common unit used to represent mass is the gram. Mass is typically determined with a balance. Balances are used in laboratories of all types, including teaching and clinical laboratories.

Balancing Act

Balances or scales are used in the clinical laboratory to weigh out chemicals in making media or reagents. Balances can also be used to check the function of a pipette using the gravimetric method, relating the mass of liquid dispensed by the pipette to its volume. There are two main types of balances: mechanical and electronic. Mechanical scales work by a fulcrum mechanism, with a more delicate fulcrum for measuring small mass to a high degree of accuracy. Double-pan, single-pan, and analytical mechanical balances are used in laboratory situations. Electronic balances are available that use electromagnetic force to balance the weight by restoring the balance arm back to null position.

The simplest mechanical scale is a double-pan balance. Currently, this type of balance is used in teaching situations but not used very often in the clinical laboratory. It has two pans, and the unknown mass is place in the left pan and standard weights are placed on right pan. It is the least accurate of all balances, since the mass is determined by placing standard weights on the right pan until the center balance needle rests on the zero or mid-point on the analog scale.

Single-pan scales are available in a mechanical format comprising a short arm with a weighing pan and external weights that can be slid onto the long arm to reach a balance. Electronic top-loading balances use a platform on which to place the item to be weighed; the platform is balanced via electromagnetic force. The output is visible on a light-emitting diode (LED) or liquid crystal diode (LCD) readout. Single-pan scales are employed in the clinical laboratory for measuring out nutrients when preparing bacteriologic growth media, for measuring out reagents for making histological stains, or for other uses. Although they have a moderate level of accuracy, they are easy to use and versatile and have large capacities of up to 20 kg.

Analytical balances are the most accurate type of balances. Mechanical versions have a single pan with internal weights to balance the unknown mass in the measuring pan. The mechanical analytical balance works by balancing on a very delicate fulcrum. This type of balance is very precise and accurate to 01 mg, but has a smaller capacity than single-pan top-loading balances. The electronic analytical balance works by an electromagnetic coil restoring the balance beam to a balanced position. It has the capability to determine the mass of the weighing vessel and reset to zero. This feature is called **tare** capability.

In order for balances to maintain proper function, periodic maintenance and functional checks must be performed. The balance must be installed on a sturdy counter or table free from vibrations. Prior to each use, the balance should be assessed as level. There is generally a liquid with a bubble within a level marker that can indicate if the balance is level. If the bubble is off-level, leveling screws may be used to adjust the length of each leg of the balance so that the balance can be properly leveled. The balance is level when the bubble is in the center of the level ring. After every use, the weighing pan should be placed in an arrest position so that it won't be attempting to measure mass, and any spilled chemical should be brushed off.

The accuracy of a single-pan balance is then checked with standard weights such as class S for larger masses and class J for smaller masses as determined by the National Institute of Standards and Technology (NIST). For example, an analytical balance at 0.100 g should be accurate to 0.000025 g when checking the class J standard weight.[1] The manufacturer's problem-solving guide should be consulted when inaccuracy is determined. Test Methodology 3–5 describes the procedure for maintaining and verification of balance function, and Table 3–5 provides a form for this purpose.

tared - adjusted a scale to zero, such as negating the mass of an empty vessel so that only the mass of an unknown is displayed

✓ **Common Sense Check**
Vibrations, air currents, extraneous dirt, and poor centering of the balance should be considered first as possible problems when a balance shows inaccurate or imprecise readings.

TEST METHODOLOGY 3-5. BALANCE MAINTENANCE PROCEDURE

With each use: Secure the weighing pan (arrested position), and use a clean camel hair brush to sweep away remnants of dust or chemicals into a dustpan. Verify that the weighing pan is free from dust and fingerprints prior to use. Verify placement on a vibration-free bench, in an area free from air drafts and direct sunlight. Adjust the lengths of the centering screw legs using the level bubble, as available. Zero the balance with an empty pan. Place a weighing vessel or paper on the pan and adjust the tare button to subtract out the mass of the vessel. Always secure the pan in standby mode before adding weight to the balance.

    Quarterly: Check the accuracy and precision of the balance by weighing NIST class S weights (50, 100, 200, 500, 2000, and 4000 mg) in triplicate, taking care to handle the standardized weights with clean cotton gloves or forceps in order to protect them.

TABLE 3-5

Balance Calibration Verification Worksheet

Laboratory _____ Month _____ Year _____
Balance Manufacturer and Model _____
Quarterly Verification

MASS OF NIST CLASS S

0.050 g	0.100 g	0.200 g
1.	1.	1.
2.	2.	2.
3.	3.	3.
4.	4.	4.
5.	5.	5.
Mean	Mean	Mean

MASS OF NIST CLASS S

0.500 g	2.00 g	4.00 g
1.	1.	1.
2.	2.	2.
3.	3.	3.
4.	4.	4.
5.	5.	5.
Mean	Mean	Mean

Accuracy of Balance: $\dfrac{(\text{Expected mass} - \text{Obtained mass} \times 100\%)}{\text{Expected mass}}$

0.050 g	0.100 g	0.200 g	0.500 g	2.00 g	4.00 g

Precision of Balance: $\dfrac{(\text{Standard deviation} \times 100\%)}{\text{Mean}}$

0.050 g	0.100 g	0.200 g	0.500 g	2.00 g	4.00 g

Documentation of validity acceptance based on manufacturer's specifications for accuracy and precision.
Date and signature of tech:

Case Scenario 3-3 Weighing Out Mass

Follow-Up

After determining that 5.5 g of cobalt chloride salt was needed, the CLS students used the analytical balance to weigh the cobalt chloride. This amount was placed into a 250-mL volumetric flask containing around 100 mL 1% HCl. This solution was swirled until totally dissolved and the remaining 1% HCl was added until the total volume of 250 mL was reached, swirling periodically to mix. When the final volume was reached, the flask was swirled and inverted 10 more times to get a mixed reagent before it was poured into a properly labeled brown glass container. ●

Centrifuges

The purpose of a centrifuge in the clinical laboratory is to separate substances of different mass or density. *Centrifugal force* is the outward force when a sample is spun at a high rate of speed. A centrifuge speeds up the natural separation that occurs by gravity over time. For example, centrifugation can separate serum quickly from clotted blood or plasma can be separated from anticoagulated blood cells. A centrifuge can also be used to separate precipitate from supernatant in a solution. The centrifugal speed is measured in revolutions per minute (rpm). Typical uses for the centrifuge include generating 1200 rpm for 10 to 12 minutes for serum from cells, 12,000 rpm for a microhematocrit, or 100,000 rpm for chylomicron separation. In addition, the force generated in centrifugation is important because it takes into account the effects of gravity (*g*) during centrifugation. For example, one typically needs to generate 14,000 *g* for a microhematocrit or 178,000 *g* for chylomicron separation. This force is called relative centrifugal force (RCF) and is also known as gravitational force. RCF, in units of *g*, for gravitational force, relates to revolutions per minute based on the size of the centrifuge radius in centimeters. The radius, or r, is determined by measuring the radius of the centrifuge arm from the center to the tip of centrifuge arm. The formula is

$$RCF = 1.12 \times 10^{-5} \times r \times rpm^2$$

RCF is calculated when comparing two different centrifuges used for the same purpose. This factor is helpful for calibrating revolutions per minute between the two centrifuges so that the correct revolutions per minute can be determined for each centrifuge.

There are three main types of centrifuges: horizontal-head, angle-head, and ultracentrifuges. *Horizontal-head centrifuges* are the swinging bucket type in which the centrifuge tubes are held in a vertical position when not moving but are horizontal when the centrifuge is fully in motion. They generate low speeds only but can produce a tight pellet of precipitate or clotted cells in the bottom of the tube. This type of centrifuge is recommended for serum separator devices. An *angle-head centrifuge* has a fixed 25- to 40-degree angle at which the tubes are held during centrifugation. The sediment packs at an angle but not as tightly as with a horizontal-head centrifuge. This type of centrifuge is adequate for cell packing, but since the sediment is at formed at an angle and not tightly packed, decantation is not recommended. The third type of centrifuge is an *ultracentrifuge*. This centrifuge generates the highest speeds. The centrifuge head is held at a fixed angle but generates tight sediment buttons due to the high speed generated. In order to reduce the heat produced by the friction generated by high centrifugal speeds, ultracentrifuges are refrigerated.[1] This type of centrifuge is especially useful for lipoprotein separations since refrigeration enhances the separation. Ultracentrifugation is also used in drug-binding assays, such as separating free drug from protein-bound drug, since ultracentrifugation is successful at sedimentation of proteins.[1]

Safety Considerations in Centrifugation

There are some important safety considerations regarding the operation of centrifuges. One of the most important considerations is to balance the load. If the centrifuge is allowed to generate speed when the load is imbalanced, it can cause serious vibrations that can break the test tubes, spilling the contents within. If the imbalance generates enough force, the centrifuge can fall over and cause serious damage and endanger the people in its vicinity. Another less obvious but equally dangerous safety consideration is the generation of aerosols, or microdroplets of the samples. These microdroplets can be inhaled or enter into mucosal membranes of the mouth, eyes, or nose with possible toxic or infectious disease consequences. Aerosols can be generated during vigorous shaking, when a vacuum is released, and during centrifugation. However, aerosols can be prevented by keeping the samples covered during centrifugation and by keeping the centrifuge lid covered during operation until the head comes to a complete stop. That way, if a tube breaks during centrifugation, the droplets can be contained within the centrifuge and not sprayed around the room. Several layers of gloves and tweezers may be needed to safely remove broken glass and while wiping up spills in the centrifuge. When opening centrifuged evacuated tubes, it may be necessary to open them in an aerosol containment box or wrap several layers of gauze around the top when opening it to catch any aerosol released with the vacuum.[2]

Maintenance is also required to keep the centrifuge functioning properly. Keeping the centrifuge clean and checking the brakes are important aspects of maintaining safe operation of the centrifuge. The main aspects of function checked are speed generated and the timing device. The revolutions per minute can be checked with a **tachometer**, a small strobe light with a photodetector that determines how many revolutions per minute are generated by the centrifuge. Test Methodology 3–6 describes the centrifuge maintenance procedure. Table 3–6 is a form for recording the centrifuge maintenance.

tachometer - device that measures speed in revolutions per minute

---

TEST METHODOLOGY 3-6.   CENTRIFUGE MAINTENANCE PROCEDURE

Weekly or biweekly depending on usage: Clean interior components with soap and water followed by freshly made 10% v/v bleach solution, including sample buckets. Wearing protective gloves, wipe interior sides and bottom, taking care when removing broken pieces of glass.

continued

TEST METHODOLOGY 3-6.   CENTRIFUGE MAINTENANCE

PROCEDURE *(continued)*

Monthly: Place two equally balanced containers into the centrifuge, cover, and operate at the most commonly used speed, listening for unusual vibrations. Check the braking mechanism to ensure a smooth, gradual stop. Check the timer of the centrifuge at 15 minutes, 10 minutes, 5 minutes, and 1 minute for the time the centrifuge motor is spinning (reaches the desired rpm until the motor shuts off) using a stopwatch.

Quarterly: Inspect gasket and check for wear and defects, and inspect cover latch for appropriate seal. Inspect head, head shaft, and coupling for evidence of wear, cracks in fitting, corrosion, uneven wear, and signs of fatigue. Inspect brushes for wear and replace according to manufacturer's instructions. Check the revolutions per minute at several commonly used speeds, including 3000 and 1500 rpm, while centrifuging a balanced load (after it has reached stable speed) using a tachometer aimed at the reflective strip viewed through the top of the centrifuge. If the revolutions per minute vary by more than 5%, consult the manufacturer's instructions for solving the problem. If an analog scale is provided for speed, the scale can be relabeled to match the actual speed. Lubricate the centrifuge shaft according to manufacturer's instructions, if applicable.

INSTRUMENTATION

An individual who enters the clinical chemistry laboratory today will face a plethora of equipment and electronic noises. Each piece of equipment has a unique place in assessing biochemical markers.

Each chemical test within the equipment represents three principles of instrumentation:

substrate - reactant in an enzyme-catalyzed reaction that is converted to product

1. the chemical reaction of the **substrates**, enzymes, and cofactors
2. the methodology of detecting the endpoint of the reaction
3. automation that synchronizes all aspects of testing

In trying to organize care and maintenance of the equipment, the medical technology student will find that instrumentation is based on a few basic principles that can be applied to many types of instruments.

TABLE 3-6					
Centrifuge Maintenance Procedure Checklist					
Month_____ Year_____	Weekly:	Monthly:		Quarterly:	
	Clean Interior	*Check Balance and Brake Including Brushes*	*Timer Check for 1, 5, 10, and 15 Minutes (list times)*	*Check rpm for 1500 and 3000 (list rpms)*	*Lubrication (if Necessary)*
Week 1					
Week 2					
Week 3					
Week 4					

Date and sign each cell of the table when check is performed.

CASE SCENARIO 3-4

Spectrophotometry: How Does It Work?

The student walked into the clinical chemistry laboratory on his first day of his clinical rotation. He was faced with numerous machines and electronic noises. The instruments did not look like the instruments that he had used in his student laboratory.

The supervisor introduced him to the mentor for the week and then left. "This is the Hercules III," said the lab tech, "our high volume chemistry instrument. It does all routine chemistries." As the day progressed, the student learned to load samples, enter patient information, and view test results. The next morning the student came early to watch the daily maintenance. "Basically, the Hercules III uses spectrophotometric and **ion-selective electrode** (ISE) technology," the lab technologist said. The student had experience with spectrophotometers and ion-selective electrodes in the student laboratory. The components are automated by discrete sample automation. These terms were familiar to the student.

ion-selective electrode (ISE) - electrode that measures the activity of one ion better than others

SPECTROPHOTOMETRY

Spectrophotometry is the mainstay of the automated clinical chemistry laboratory. Spectrophotometry is based on two principles: (1) substances **absorb** light at unique wavelengths and (2) the amount of light absorbed is proportional to the amount of substance that is present. Absorbance is equal to an **absorptivity** constant that is unique to the substance or molecule times the length of the light path through the substance times the concentration of the substance. These principles are summarized into Beer's law:

$$A = a\,b\,c$$

where A = absorbance, a = absorptivity constant for the substance, b = length of the light path through the substance, and c = concentration of the substance

Absorbance may be related to **transmittance**, T, the amount of light that is transmitted through the substance where Is = transmitted light through the test solution and Io = total possible light to be transmitted from the incidence beam:

$$A = -\log Is/Io = -\log T$$
$$\text{Since } A = \log (1/T)$$
$$A = \log 100 - \log \%T$$
$$\text{Then, } A = 2 - \log \%T = a\,b\,c$$

By choosing a wavelength of light that is optimal for the absorbance of the substance, absorption units represent the light that is absorbed by that substance and no other substances. The increase or decrease of light that is absorbed is proportional to the concentration of the substance. Percentage transmittance (%T) versus concentration is a nonlinear function. When %T versus concentration is plotted on linear graph paper, a curvilinear response is obtained. Figure 3–6 illustrates this relationship. %T is used only when plotted on semi-log paper to obtain a straight line. The straight line obtained can be used to determine the concentration of unknown samples. Absorbance versus concentration is a linear function, as

absorb - to take in or receive by chemical or molecular action

absorptivity - the amount of absorbance specific for a certain substance

transmittance - the amount of light not retained but passed through a test solution

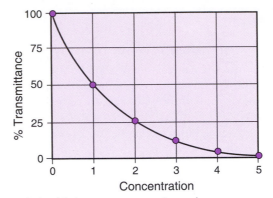

Figure 3–6. Relationship between concentration and percentage transmittance.

shown in Figure 3–7. The straight line obtained from this relationship can be used to determine the concentration of unknown samples.[3]

Simple spectrophotometry has been used for many years in clinical chemistry analysis. Specific types of chemical reactions measured by spectrophotometry will be discussed later in this chapter. There are several variations of spectrophotometric analysis that are based upon the principles defined by Beer's law. These types of spectrophotometry will be discussed in more detail starting with simpler spectrophotometric applications (endpoint, kinetic, and turbidimetry) and progressing to atomic absorption spectroscopy, nephelometry, chemiluminescence, and fluorometry.

Components of the Spectrophotometer

Since spectrophotometry is the process for measuring the amount of light absorbed by a substance, relating to the concentration of that substance, a spectrophotometer is an instrument that measures light of specific wavelengths. These are the components of a spectrophotometer: the light source, monochromator, sample holder, photodetector, readout device, and power source. Figure 3–8 illustrates the components of a simple spectrophotometer.

The lamp, or light source, provides wavelengths of light in the visible or ultraviolet (UV) range. A tungsten lamp is used for visible wavelengths (approxi-

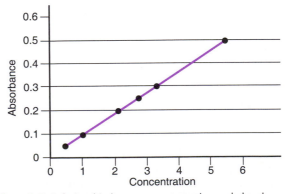

Figure 3–7. Relationship between concentration and absorbance.

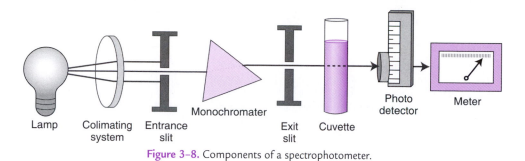

Figure 3–8. Components of a spectrophotometer.

mately 380 to 750 nm). Deuterium or mercury-arc lamps are used to produce UV light.

The monochromator, such as a filter, prism, or diffraction grating, is used to eliminate unwanted wavelengths of light and allow the desired light to reach the sample.

A sample holder holds the cuvette containing the test solution.

A photodetector detects light transmitted through the sample (because it was not absorbed) and converts the light energy to electrical energy.

The readout device indicates the absorbance or even concentration based on the calculations as shown above.

The power source provides stable energy for the components of the spectrophotometer.

A procedure for performing maintenance of a simple spectrophotometer is found in Test Methodology 3–7.

TEST METHODOLOGY 3-7. SPECTROPHOTOMETER MAINTENANCE PROCEDURE

1. Wavelength accuracy can be checked with a commercial filter, such as a didymium filter (peak at 585 nm), or with a prepared solution such as cobalt chloride (peak at 510 nm) or potassium dichromate (peaks at 350, 375, and 450 nm). Ultraviolet (UV) spectrophotometers are checked with a quartz mercury arc lamp or transmission standards. For example, didymium filters have 45%T at 610 nm. To correct for poor results, realign exciter lamp with wavelength selector.

2. Photometric linearity can be checked by running different concentrations of the same solution. Varying dilutions of a solution known to follow Beer's law are prepared and analyzed (examples of solutions to use: cobalt ammonium sulfate or cobalt chloride, copper sulfate, and alkaline potassium chromate). Absorbance versus concentration is plotted, and a linear plot indicates a linear response. Spectrophotometers that exhibit linearity inaccuracy should be tested for excess stray light (filter slit width is too wide) or a failing photocell.

3. Photometric accuracy can be checked with nickel sulfate solutions at 510 nm or special filters. Corrections for problems with photometric accuracy include realigning the excitor lamp or cleaning a dirty excitor lamp or photocell window. Corrections may be needed to the filter slit width or a damaged diffraction grating may need to be replaced.

continued

TEST METHODOLOGY 3-7.   SPECTROPHOTOMETER MAINTENANCE

PROCEDURE *(continued)*

4. Stray light can be checked with sodium nitrite solution, which should have <0.1%T at 355 nm. Correction for poor stray light results commonly involves cleaning dust off optical surfaces, including the mirrors, prisms, gratings, and lamp. Remove extraneous sources of light coming through the instrument cover. If these actions do not correct poor stray light results, it may be necessary to replace the excitor lamp.
5. Baseline stability detects excess baseline drift. It should be observed by setting an arbitrary wavelength and observing %T changes over 1 minute. Drift of more than 2%T indicates that the excitor lamp is failing.

Three Types of Spectrophotometric Methods

The spectrophotometer measures the absorbance of light of one of the components of a chemical reaction. Three examples of common types of chemical reactions that are measured by the spectrophotometer are endpoint **colorimetric**, endpoint enzymatic, and kinetic reactions (Table 3–7). The Jaffe reaction for creatinine is an example of an endpoint colorimetric reaction. The hexokinase reaction with glucose is an example of an endpoint enzymatic reaction in which enzymes **catalyze** the reaction to measure the analyte. An example of a kinetic method, which employs substrates and coenzymes to measure the **activity** of the enzyme, is that of measurement of alanine transaminase (ALT) using alanine, alpha-ketoglutarate, and pyridoxyl-5'-phosphate.

Endpoint Colorimetric Spectrophotometry

The first of these three types of spectrophotometric chemical reactions is the simple endpoint spectrophotometric reaction. The Jaffe reaction for creatinine analysis is an example of this method. In an endpoint spectrophotometric method, a colored product or **chromogen** forms that is measured by its ability to absorb visible light. Its reaction sequence is described with the other two reaction sequences in Table 3–8.

Endpoint Enzymatic Spectrophotometry

Some endpoint methods also use an enzyme to catalyze the chemical reaction. The final product is often a coenzyme that absorbs light strongly at lower wavelengths

colorimetric - determining an analyte from visible light absorption of a colored product

catalyze - to accelerate the rate of a chemical reaction without being consumed

activity - ability to produce motion or energy; for example, enzyme activity is the ability of the enzyme to influence the rate of a reaction

chromogen - colored product formed in a colorimetric reaction

TABLE 3-7

Common Types of Chemical Reaction Measured With Spectrophotometry

Chemical Reaction Type	What Is Measured	How Absorbance Is Measured*
Endpoint colorimetric	Chromogen	One reading
Endpoint enzymatic	Colorless coenzyme	One reading
Kinetic	Colorless coenzyme	Multiple absorbance readings

*Spectrophotometer is first set to 100% T/zero absorbance with a reference solution.

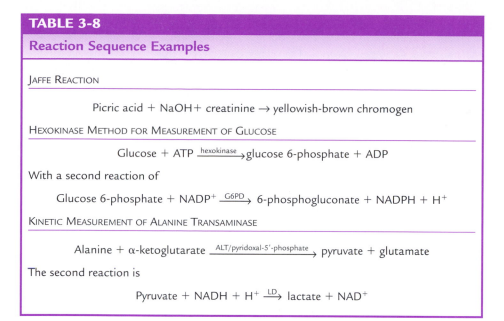

TABLE 3-8

Reaction Sequence Examples

JAFFE REACTION

$$\text{Picric acid} + \text{NaOH} + \text{creatinine} \rightarrow \text{yellowish-brown chromogen}$$

HEXOKINASE METHOD FOR MEASUREMENT OF GLUCOSE

$$\text{Glucose} + \text{ATP} \xrightarrow{\text{hexokinase}} \text{glucose 6-phosphate} + \text{ADP}$$

With a second reaction of

$$\text{Glucose 6-phosphate} + \text{NADP}^+ \xrightarrow{\text{G6PD}} \text{6-phosphogluconate} + \text{NADPH} + \text{H}^+$$

KINETIC MEASUREMENT OF ALANINE TRANSAMINASE

$$\text{Alanine} + \alpha\text{-ketoglutarate} \xrightarrow{\text{ALT/pyridoxal-5'-phosphate}} \text{pyruvate} + \text{glutamate}$$

The second reaction is

$$\text{Pyruvate} + \text{NADH} + \text{H}^+ \xrightarrow{\text{LD}} \text{lactate} + \text{NAD}^+$$

in the visible or near-UV spectrum. The hexokinase method for the measurement of glucose in body fluids is such a procedure; the analyte in this complex reaction is glucose. That is, glucose is the substance that is to be measured. Glucose absorbs light at many wavelengths. A test method aimed at directly measuring the absorbance of glucose would be subject to many types of interferences and would not be specific to glucose. Therefore, chemical reactions such as the hexokinase method have been developed in which a chemical reaction involving glucose, the enzyme, and other substances is used to produce **NADP**. NADP is the substance measured by the spectrophotometer because it absorbs light uniquely at 340 nm and is not subject to many types of interferences. The concentration of glucose is proportional to the consumption of the coenzyme in the reaction.

Kinetic Spectrophotometry

The last type of chemical reaction measured with spectrophotometry to be discussed is a kinetic reaction. As previously described, **coupled** sequential enzymatic reactions that produce **NAD** or NADP are commonly used for the measurement of other chemicals in the reaction since the change in absorbance at 340 nm is simple and relatively free from interference. Either the consumption of **NADH** or the production of ionized NAD (NAD$^+$) may be measured as a reflection of the concentration of other chemicals in the reaction. Measuring the catalytic properties of the enzyme is often accomplished by spectrophotometric analysis of the product that forms as change in absorbance of visible or UV light per minute. Coupled enzymatic reactions are chemical reactions that share a common intermediate. The product of reaction one is used as the substrate in reaction two. These may involve the analysis of NAD or NADP since change in absorbance at 340 nm during reaction of these molecules is simple and relatively free from interference. Enzyme activity is determined based on standardized reaction conditions.

Enzymes are proteins. They could easily be measured with immunoassay methods because of their antigenic properties. Quantification of enzymes in body fluids

NADP - nicotinamide adenine dinucleotide phosphate

coupled - chemical reactions that share a common intermediate

NAD - nicotinamide adenine dinucleotide

NADH - reduced nicotinamide adenine dinucleotide phosphate

is most clinically significant when the results closely relate to *recent* release from diseased or damaged tissues. Enzymes are often retained in circulation long after release from damaged tissues. Therefore, serum enzyme concentration, such as that reported in mmol/L, doesn't provide clinically useful information. Enzymes instead are reported in units of catalytic activity.

Methods of enzyme analysis involve measuring the ability of active enzyme to catalyze, or accelerate, the rate of a chemical reaction, converting substrate to product. The enzyme is not consumed in the reaction. Therefore, measuring enzyme levels by their ability to catalyze specific reactions in the test tube, or in vitro, provides the most clinically significant enzyme results and is the method of choice for enzyme testing. This method is known as kinetic spectrophotometry, in which the rate of product formation is determined by a change in absorbance per minute. Knowledge of quantification of an enzyme by its catalytic properties requires some understanding of kinetics as characterized by Michaelis and Menton. These principles are discussed in Chapter 1.

In kinetic analysis, multiple absorbance measurements are made. Average change in absorbance per minute is determined to assess that standardized reaction conditions were met during the time frame and provide increased accuracy for determining enzyme activity. **Zero-order kinetics** is the most accurate indication of enzyme activity because all active sites are filled with substrate. Substrate concentration is in excess and all other conditions in the reaction are optimal to allow the enzyme to work at its fastest speed. This condition is verified when change in absorbance per minute ($\Delta A/min$) is constant, despite a consistent linear increase or decrease in absorbance of product that is formed. If change in absorbance is not constant, then a variable other than enzyme activity is also present and results should not be calculated. This circumstance is often the case when enzyme activity is markedly elevated and substrate depletion occurs rapidly. Enzyme activity can be more accurately assessed when the sample containing the enzyme is diluted and the enzyme/substrate ratio is lower. Below is an example of absorbance results collected over time in order to determine $\Delta A/min$.

Absorbance	Time Elapsed (in reaction minutes)
0.230	1
0.250	2
0.270	3

$$\frac{\Delta A}{min} = \frac{(absorbance\ 2 - absorbance\ 1)}{min}$$

$$\frac{(0.250 - 0.230)}{(2 - 1)} = \frac{0.020}{min}$$

Endpoint activity is determined by taking an initial absorbance reading at the end of an incubation phase and a second absorbance reading at the end of a specific unit of time. If conditions remain constant during the time frame, change in absorbance per minute can be determined and related to enzyme activity. This method is less standardized than continuous monitoring of absorbance to determine enzyme activity but provides rapid and accurate results for many enzyme-catalyzed methods.

Multiple forms of enzymes exist, particularly when composed of two or more polypeptide chains or subunits. This unique composition of protein isomers, or **protomers**, can be associated with different distribution within tissues and with

---

CLINICAL CORRELATION

Serum enzyme activity is often a sensitive predictor of organ or tissue damage before the patient exhibits outward signs of disease. For example, levels of serum alanine transaminase (ALT) rise quickly in a patient with hepatitis or liver inflammation before other classic signs appear, such as jaundice or yellow-appearing skin or eyes.

zero-order kinetics - catalyzed reaction with all active sites of the enzyme filled with substrate so reaction occurs at its fastest rate; also called saturation kinetics

protomer - protein isomer in which the protein subunits have the same chemical formula but different spatial arrangements in the molecule

unique chemical and physical properties. Multiple forms of enzymes can also be produced as a result of postgenetic modification, such as from metabolism. The term **isoenzyme** refers to forms of the same enzyme that arise from unique gene sequences. Characterization of isoenzymes based on separation techniques can be used to indicate the tissue source of the enzyme activity and correlate with specific diseases. Separation and quantification techniques for isoenzymes and multiple forms of enzymes include **zone electrophoresis**, **ion-exchange chromatography**, **selective inactivation**, and **immunochemical** methods.[1]

Creating a Concentration (Calibration) Curve

Concentration of an analyte in a patient or quality control sample is determined after a series of standard solutions are analyzed and a graph of absorbance versus concentration is found to be a linear relationship. Solutions of unknown concentration are tested for absorbance; these absorbance results are read from the curve to determine concentration. Figure 3–9 presents a typical standard curve.

If this is a particularly stable test system, a standard curve does not need to be prepared each day. Instead, a constant proportionality can be used to calculate concentration from absorbance using Beer's law. This calculation is only valid if the absorbance readings and resulting concentrations fall within a specific range due to limits in **linearity**. The absorptivity constant and cuvette pathlength are held constant in the reaction and so do not appear in the calculation. The equation used for determining concentration of the patient or another unknown (unk) sample is as follows:

Concentration of unknown = (Concentration of standard/Absorbance of standard) × Absorbance of unknown

$$C_{unk} = (C_{std}/A_{std}) \times A_{unk}$$

For example, the absorbance results from a patient sample and an albumin standard in albumin analysis are shown below. Given these standard solution results, the concentration of the patient albumin can be determined.

Sample	Absorbance
2.5 g/dL albumin standard	0.250
Patient Jo Lin	0.500

Patient Jo Lin's albumin = (2.5 g/dL/0.250) × 0.500 = 5.0 g/dL

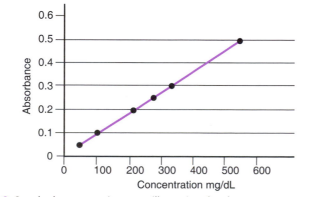

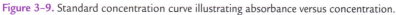
Figure 3–9. Standard concentration curve illustrating absorbance versus concentration.

isoenzymes - forms of enzymes with different amino acid sequences, giving unique properties, but having the ability to catalyze similar chemical reactions

zone electrophoresis - separating components of a mixture within a charged buffer solution by moving them through a porous filter based on electrical attractions

ion-exchange chromatography - separating components of a mixture based on different solubility characteristics and attraction to an electrically charged solid substance

selective inactivation - process of rendering some chemicals nonfunctional while keeping the function of other similar chemicals

immunochemical - chemical that is able to enter into an antibody-antigen reaction

linearity - relation of independent and dependent data points that produces a straight line

■■
CLINICAL CORRELATION
A patient's serum albumin level is compared with the reference range to determine if it appears to be abnormal. An elevated serum albumin level is indicative of dehydration, in which an insufficient amount of fluid in the blood causes some substances to appear relatively increased. Decreased serum albumin levels correlate with many types of diseases, including liver failure, extensive skin loss, and kidney diseases that cause loss of albumin via the urinary tract.

Common Clinical Chemistry Spectrophotometric Reactions

Table 3–9 summarizes the principles of common clinical chemistry test analysis, including rate versus endpoint spectrophotometric reactions.

OTHER PHOTOMETRIC TECHNIQUES

Nephelometry and Turbidimetry

In the clinical laboratory, turbidimetry and nephelometry are used to measure light scatter. Turbidity measures the decrease in the amount of light as it passes through a particulate solution. Nephelometry is used to measure the amount of light that is scattered as it passes through the particulate solution. Both methods can be used to determine the concentration of the particulate solution.

TABLE 3-9	
Chemical Reactions for Common Analytes	
Analyte	**Chemical Reaction**
Total Calcium	o-Cresolphthalein complex one + calcium $\xrightarrow{\text{alkaline pH}}$ chromophore (measured at 580 nm)
Glucose	Glucose + 2 H_2O + O_2 $\xrightarrow{\text{glucose oxidase}}$ gluconic acid + 2 H_2O_2 o-Dianisidine + H_2O_2 $\xrightarrow{\text{peroxidase}}$ oxidized o-dianisidine + H_2O
Urea	Diacetyl monoxime + urea $\rightarrow$ diazine (chromogen)
Urea	Urea $\xrightarrow{\text{urease}}$ carbonic acid + NH_4^+ NH_4^+ + a-ketoglutarate + NADH $\xrightarrow{\text{glutamic acid dehydrogenase}}$ NAD + NH_3 + glutamate
Bilirubin	Bilirubin glucuronide + diazotized sulfanilic acid $\rightarrow$ azobilirubin Azobilirubin + alkaline tartrate $\xrightarrow{\text{ascorbic acid, HCl}}$ reduced azobilirubin (measured at 600 nm)
Total Protein	Copper sulfate/sodium potassium tartrate/KI + protein peptide bonds $\rightarrow$ purple chromagen (measured at 540 nm)
AST	Aspartate + oxoglutarate $\xrightarrow{\text{AST/pyridoxal-5'-phosphate}}$ oxaloacetate + glutamate Oxaloacetate + NADH + H^+ $\xrightarrow{\text{MDH}}$ Malate + NAD^+
LD	Pyruvate + NADH + H^+ (pH 7.4) $\xrightarrow{\text{LD}}$ lactate + NAD^+
LD	Lactate + NAD^+ (pH 9.0) $\xrightarrow{\text{LD}}$ Pyruvate + NADH + H^+
ALP	4-Nitrophenyl phosphate + H_2O $\underset{\text{pH 10.3}}{\overset{\text{ALP Mg}^{+2}}{\rightleftharpoons}}$ p-nitrophenyl + phosphate ion p-nitrophenyl $\xrightarrow[\text{pH}]{\text{alkaline}}$ 4-nitrophenoxide
CK	Creatine phosphate + ADP $\xrightarrow{\text{CK/buffers (pH 6.7)}}$ creatine + ATP ATP + glucose $\xrightarrow{\text{HK}}$ glucose 6-phosphate + ADP Glucose 6-phosphate + $NADP^+$ $\xrightarrow{\text{G6PD}}$ 6-phosphogluconate + NADPH + H^+
Amylase	Starch $\xrightarrow{\text{amylase}}$ maltose + maltotriose + dextrins Maltose + maltotriose $\xrightarrow{\text{glucosidase}}$ glucose Glucose + ½ O_2 $\xrightarrow{\text{glucose oxidase}}$ H_2O_2 + gluconolactone

If the particle size is larger than the wavelength of the light source, then most of the light will be scattered in the forward direction at an angle of less than 90 degrees for the incident beam. This phenomenon is called **Mie scatter**. Particles that are smaller than the wavelength of the light source will scatter light in many directions and equally in the forward and backward direction. This phenomenon is known as **Raleigh scatter**.

Turbidimetry is used to measure small particles that reduce the amount of light that passes through the sample and scatter light in all directions. It can be measured with a simple spectrophotometer, using visible wavelengths of light. Beer's law applies to both turbidimetry and nepholometry in that concentration is proportional to the amount of light detected by the photodetector within upper-level limits of concentration. Turbidimetry is not as sensitive as nepholometry and must be timed precisely in order to get accurate results. When turbidimetry is part of an automated system, timing is controlled. Nephelometry is used to measure larger particles that deflect light forward. The intensity of light scatter is directly proportional to concentration of particles. Rate nephelometry may be used to measure the formation of precipitant complexes over time. Nephelometry is usually sensitive to low concentrations such as 1 to 10 mg/L. Nephelometry can also give precise results in an automated system. Sources of error may come from the sample itself. The matrix of the sample may affect the nephelometer reading. For example, lipemia of a serum sample may scatter light. Dilution of the serum reduces lipemia interference but also decreases sensitivity of the test measurement.

The position of the photodetector in nephelometry and turbidimetry depends on the direction of scattered light to be measured. Another difference in nephelometry when compared to simple spectrophotometry is the light source. The light source is usually a high-intensity light from a **laser** or a tungsten iodide lamp. Figure 3–10 shows the components of a nephelometer.

Mie scatter - large particles scattering light predominantly a in the forward direction

Raleigh scatter - small particles scattering light in all directions with maximum scatter forward and backward

laser - light amplification by stimulated emission of radiation; device using a high-energy beam of electromagnetic radiation

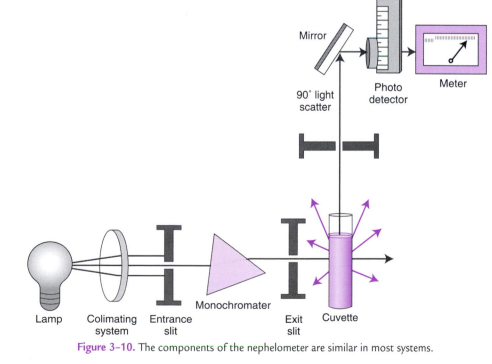

Mirror

90˚ light scatter

Photo detector

Meter

Lamp   Colimating system   Entrance slit   Monochromater   Exit slit   Cuvette

Figure 3–10. The components of the nephelometer are similar in most systems.

Atomic Absorption Spectrophotometry

Atomic absorption spectrophotometry (AAS), like simple spectrophotometry, measures light to determine the concentration of an analyte. However, this is a more complex type of spectrophotometry. Some unique features arise with the sample itself. Only metals such as divalent or some trivalent cations can be atomized easily, so this is a common method of analysis for metals such as lead. The element of interest is separated from the molecular state and placed in its unexcited, ground state. In the ground state, the element absorbs radiation at a narrow bandwidth of spectrum that is specific to the element. The excitation source emits the same wavelength of light that the atoms can easily absorb. Absorption of radiant energy follows Beer's law, such that concentration of the number of atoms present in the sample is proportional to the amount of absorption of the specific wavelength of radiation.

cathode - a negatively charged electrode that attracts cations (positive ions)

AAS uses a high-energy hollow **cathode** lamp (HCL) containing a filament of the same metal to be tested and a rare gas. Electrical discharge produced by the power source ionizes the rare gas atoms, causing collisions of the gas atoms with the metal atoms. The metal atoms emit radiant energy when they return to ground state. A rotating beam splitter, also known as a rotary chopper, generates a reference beam that bypasses the sample in the flame and, alternatively, a sample beam. The ratio between both paths is determined. Essentially, the decrease in radiant energy coming from the sample beam as compared to the reference beam is detected by the photodetector. The difference in energy between the two beams is due to the amount of energy absorbed.

The placement of the monochromator is after the cuvette, unlike in simple spectrophotometry. A monochromator between the flame and the photodetector eliminates extra wavelengths of light emitted by the flame before it reaches the photodetector. This helps to ensure that only light emitted by the lamp and not absorbed by the sample is detected. Figure 3–11 illustrates the components of the atomic absorption spectrophotometer.

AAS is highly sensitive for quantification of trace and toxic metals. It is not suitable for metals found in larger concentrations in plasma, such as sodium or potassium. Interferences in AAS include chemical, ionization, and matrix interference.

Fluorometry and Chemiluminescence

In the clinical laboratory, spectrofluorometry has been used for many years. It is most frequently found in highly automated immunoassay systems for measuring drugs, hormones, and other unique chemical analytes. **Fluorometers** measure

fluorometer - instrument that detects fluorescent emissions

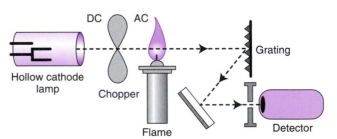

Figure 3–11. Components of the atomic absorption spectrophotometer.

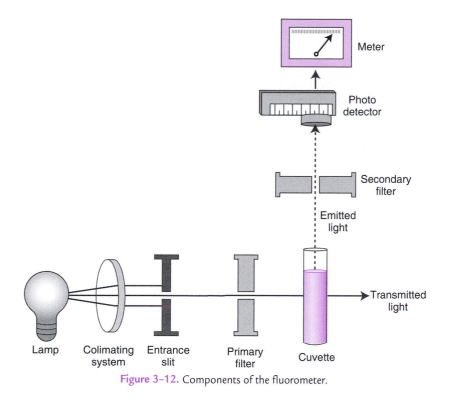

Figure 3–12. Components of the fluorometer.

fluorescence, a type of **luminescence** in which electrons within a chemical are induced to absorb light and become excited using high-energy radiation. The result is **emission** of low-energy light wavelengths very quickly (10^{-8} seconds). The arrangement of a fluorometer is similar to a simple spectrophotometer except that the excitor lamp is often a halogen, xenon, or laser lamp. Also, the spectrofluorometer contains a second set of monochromators, the emission filters, placed at a 90-degree angle to the excitor lamp but in line with the photodetector. This arrangement helps to ensure that only light emitted from the excited sample reaches the photodetector and not extraneous light from the lamp. Figure 3–12 shows the typical components of a fluorometer and the arrangement of the two sets of filters, the sample cuvette, and the photodetector.

Chemiluminescence is similar to fluorescence and is also used commonly with automated immunoassay methods. However, the cause of luminescence is due to a chemical reaction producing light emission rather than high-energy light absorption. A luminometer is the instrument that measures chemiluminescence. It is a simplified spectrophotometer that does *not* require a light source or monochromator since light is produced in the chemical reaction. The sample cuvette, photodetector, and readout device are the main components of a luminometer.

ANALYSIS WITH ELECTROCHEMISTRY

Electrochemistry is a type of analytical technique that measures ions in solution, by their electrical properties. These ions are called electrolytes and include ionized sodium (Na^+), potassium (K^+), chloride (Cl^-), bicarbonate (HCO_3^-), and calcium (Ca^{2+}). Electrochemistry also involves producing electrons or ions in a chemical

fluorescence - emission of low-energy light quickly after absorbing high-energy light; a type of luminescence

luminescence - production of light without the production of heat

emission - giving off or sending out

electrochemistry - measuring potential, current, or resistance to determine the activity of an analyte

resistance - opposing force to flow of electrons (in ohms)

current - electrical charge (in coulombs/second); measured in units of amperes

potentiometry - measuring electrical potential in voltage

coulometry - measuring aspects of current, including rate of electron flow; often used in titration of ions

amperometry - measuring current in amperes, including coulometric methods

voltammetry - measuring the current at an electrode using a specific voltage generated at another electrode

polarography - measurement of current flowing as electrons are formed in an oxidation-reduction system

osmometry - measurement of osmotic pressure from dissolved particles in a solution

reaction from nonionic analytes such as oxygen or urea nitrogen. Electrochemical reactions employ the relationship of electrical potential (E) to **resistance** (R) and **current** (I) so that, if two of these components are held constant, the third is measured and relates to the activity of the ion. The relationship is termed Ohm's law, in which $E = I \times R$. **Potentiometry, coulometry/amperometry, voltammetry, polarography,** and **osmometry** all operate upon these principles. Potentiometry is a system of measuring electrical potential, while amperometry measures current in amperes. Voltammetry is measuring the current at an electrode using a specific voltage generated at another electrode, while polarography, a type of voltammetry, measures current while controlling an increase in voltage. Osmometry is the process of measuring dissolved particles in a solution using a series of variable resisters. These methods will all be explored in more detail with specific procedures.

Potentiometry

Potentiometry is an electrical system of measuring change in electrical potential between a detecting electrode and a standard reference electrode in which current is kept constant. Ion-selective electrodes (ISEs) are used in potentiometry to measure the activity of one ion versus other ions. The electrodes are made of a unique material that is more selective for one ion compared to other similar ions. When the ion comes in contact with the electrode, there is a change in the potential compared to the reference electrode, measured as a voltage change, due to the ionic activity. ISEs are the most commonly employed methods of analysis for many electrolytes, including sodium and potassium, since spectrophotometric methods have proven to be less effective. Only free unbound ion is measured, which becomes significant when measuring such ions such as calcium and magnesium.

Clinical laboratories historically have used pH meters for many tasks, including adjusting the proper pH of reagents and determining the pH of clinically significant body fluids. Currently it is common practice to buy most reagents commercially prepared and pH balanced, so the pH meter is infrequently used for this task. Determining the pH of some body fluids has been simplified with the use of reagent pads or dipsticks. However, the pH electrode is still used in the clinical laboratory to measure the pH of arterial blood and to measure hydrogen ion concentration change in potentiometric reactions. The pH meter is used in student teaching laboratories and in some research and reference laboratory settings. Test Methodology 3–8 describes the typical calibration and maintenance of a pH meter prior to routine operation. Table 3–10 shows a pH meter maintenance checklist form.

TEST METHODOLOGY 3-8.   pH METER MAINTENANCE

1. With each use of the pH meter, record the temperature. Some meters require that temperature be dialed into the pH meter.
2. When measuring pH, set the cleaned probe in the fluid and set pH mode.
3. For a 3-point calibration, select a high pH buffer (such as 10.0), a low pH buffer (such as 3.0), and a neutral buffer solution (pH 7.0). All buffers must be fresh or properly stored and within the expiration period.

---

continued

TEST METHODOLOGY 3-8.   pH METER MAINTENANCE *(continued)*

4. The pH meter should be in the standby mode during rinsing and between measuring pH of samples or buffers. Rinse the pH probe thoroughly with deionized water. Allow to drip into a waste container and blot the probe gently.

5. Immerse the end of the probe completely in the high pH buffer solution, stirring the solution around the probe. Switch the meter from standby to read. Once a stable reading is obtained, after about 30 seconds, adjust the calibration to read 10.0 (or the value for whatever high pH buffer is used.)

6. Return the meter to standby, remove the probe from buffer, and rinse the probe thoroughly with deionized water, allowing water to drip off into a waste container, and blot gently.

7. Repeat calibration with the high pH buffer (steps 5 and 6) until the pH reading remains stable.

8. Immerse the end of the probe completely in the low pH buffer solution, stirring the solution around the probe. Once a stable reading is obtained, adjust the calibration (slope knob) to read 3.0 (or the value for watever low pH buffer is used.)

9. Repeat calibration with the low pH buffer until the pH reading remains stable.

10. Rinse the pH probe thoroughly with deionized water, allowing water to drip off into a waste container, and blot gently.

11. Immerse the end of the probe completely in the 7.0 buffer solution, stirring the solution around the probe. If pH 7.0 is obtained, the meter is calibrated. Record results on a form such as that shown in Table 3-10.

The pH meter is now ready to test pH of the unknown sample. Rinse with distilled water between each reading and place the pH meter in a standby setting in a neutral pH buffer solution between each reading.

The common laboratory method for many electrolytes is potentiometry using ISEs. An ISE contains a selective membrane or layer that interacts with one particular ion more than others, making it more specific to that ion. Electrical potential is set up with a reference electrode to which a standard voltage is applied and current is kept to zero. Change in potential is due to the presence of ions in the solution. For example, the ISE for Na^+ is composed of a unique glass or liquid membrane containing an organic **ionophore**, such as **monensin**. The ionophore for Cl^- is a unique liquid membrane or solid state indicator made of chloride salts, and that for K^+ is a valinomycin liquid membrane. Valinomycin forms a cagelike structure around chloride ions, retaining them in the liquid membrane when a constant current is applied.

Another major ion found in plasma is bicarbonate, HCO_3^-. It is measured as total carbon dioxide (tCO_2) by an ISE with a semipermeable membrane. The CO_2

ionophore - substance that attracts charged molecules (ions)

monensin - sodium ionophore used for ISEs; made from *Streptomyces* species

TABLE 3-10				
pH Meter Maintenance Checklist				
Recorded Temperature	Wiped Off Exterior With Damp Cloth	Checked Expiration Date and Proper Storage of Buffers	Replaced Probe in Fresh Storage Buffer	Date and Signature of Tech.

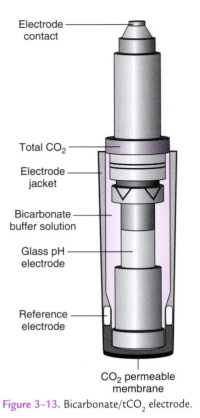

Figure 3–13. Bicarbonate/tCO₂ electrode.

in the serum or plasma is converted to gas and passes through the semipermeable membrane, where it reacts with a bicarbonate/carbonic acid buffer solution. This produces H⁺ in proportion with the amount of CO₂ gas due to the following chemical reaction:

$$H_2O + CO_2 \leftrightarrow H_2CO_3 \leftrightarrow HCO_3^- + H^+$$

ISE measures potentiometry due to change in pH produced. Figure 3–13 depicts this special type of ISE. This is the most common method for measuring bicarbonate ion in serum or plasma and gives results similar to the historical method, a colorimetric method that measures the change in pH in the buffer solution with a pH indicator. A recently emerging methodology for total carbon dioxide measurement is through use of a spectrophotometric enzymic method and **conductivity**. The enzyme urea amidolyase catalyzes the reaction of bicarbonate with urea to form several products, including ammonium ion. After first measuring endogenous ammonium ion, ammonium ion is catalyzed using glutamate dehydrogenase to produce ionized NADP (NADP⁺) from **NADPH** and change in absorbance at 340 nm is measured. Conductivity of ammonium will be addressed later. Test Methodology 3–9 describes analysis of electrolytes.

conductivity - the combined ability of ions to carry a charge

NADPH - reduced nicotinamide adenine dinucleotide phosphate

Coulometry/Amperometry

Chloride can be measured by coulometric-amperometric titration. Coulometry is a method employing measurement of coulombs, the flow of electrons per unit of time where titration is a process of determining an unknown concentration of a

TEST METHODOLOGY 3-9.   METHODOLOGY OF ELECTROLYTE ANALYSIS

The Reaction Principle

When the ion contacts the electrode, there is a change in potential compared to the reference electrode due to the ionic activity. An indirect ISE system dilutes the sample with diluent prior to analysis with the electrode. A direct ISE system measures the electrolytes in undiluted samples and will not be subject to falsely lowered sodium or chloride levels due to volume replacement by large amounts of chylomicrons or para-proteins.

Interferences

Hemolysis, release from muscle activity in fist clenching, or leakage from erythrocytes in older samples falsely increases potassium. Refrigeration of whole blood may enhance intracellular potassium release from erythrocytes. Indirect ISE systems cause false decrease of sodium and chloride due to dilutional effect by hyperlipidemia (>350 mg/dL) or hyperproteinemia (>10 g/dL) as those large lipid or protein molecules in unusually high amounts displace some of the volume of the plasma within the dilution. If a non-fasting specimen isn't available, chylomicrons may be removed by ultracentrifugation, wherein they collect into a device that allows separation of these fatty molecules from the rest of the serum or plasma. Another alternative is to use an instrument that measures sodium and other electrolytes by a direct ion-selective electrode.

The Specimen

Venous serum or lithium-heparinized whole blood or plasma, or heparinized arterial whole blood should be collected using a method to avoid hemolysis. Heparinized plasma is the specimen of choice and contains 0.3 to 0.7 mmol/L less potassium than serum due to platelet release during coagulation. Electrolytes may also be analyzed in body fluids such as urine, sweat, cerebrospinal fluid, and gastric fluids, and samples are stable if maintained in closed containers and analyzed promptly.

Reference Range (Adults)

Plasma Na	136–145 mmol/L
K	3.5–5.1 mmol/L
Cl	98–107 mmol/L
CO_2	22–28 mmol/L

substance by reacting it with an equivalent concentration of a known substance. For example, in an electrochemical titration, an anion can be titrated with a known quantity of cation. Amperometry is a specific type of electrochemical titration. It employs two electrodes charged with a constant electrical potential. Test Methodology 3–10 describes chloride analysis using coulometry.

Conductivity and Polarography

Conductivity is the combined ability of all ions in a solution to conduct or carry an electrical charge. Ammonium ions (NH_4^+) can be measured by conductivity. NH_4^+ generated from urea hydrolysis with urease or in the secondary reaction from carbon dioxide as mentioned earlier can be measured with conductivity. Alternating current is applied to the electrodes to generate electrical potential in order to prevent polarization of the electrodes. This allows for conductivity and resistance to be the reciprocal of each other.

TEST METHODOLOGY 3-10.   CHLORIDE ANALYSIS BY COULOMETRY

The Reaction Principle

Coulometry operates on the principle of Faraday's law. This method employs a silver anode that releases silver ions at a constant rate due to constant electrical potential. These ions react with chloride ions, forming insoluble silver chloride. When all of the chloride ions are reacted with the generated silver ions, there is a sharp increase in current conducted. Since current relates to electrical charge per unit of time, the time of titration is proportional to the chloride activity in the sample. This method is commonly used for sweat chloride analysis.

The Calculations

Calculations are performed by the instrument.

$$Eq.\ titrant = amperes \times time/F$$

where F = 96,487 $\times$ coulombs/Eq. wt.
For example:

$$Activity\ of\ Cl^- = amperes \times time/96,487 \times coulombs/35.5$$

Reference Range

serum Cl	98–107 mmol/L
sweat Cl	5–35 mmol/L

anode - a positively charged electrode that attracts anions (negative ions)

reduction - production of electrons and a positively charged ion; reaction at the cathode

oxidation - loss of electrons in a reaction; attraction of electrons produced in a reduction process at the anode

THE TEAM APPROACH

The partial pressure of oxygen is measured along with partial pressure of carbon dioxide and pH in arterial blood gas analysis. The analyzer may be located in a centralized laboratory, surgical suite, intensive care unit, respiratory care department or other areas of a health care facility. Although respiratory care therapists, nurses, or other allied health care professionals may be collecting the arterial blood specimen and analyzing for oxygen partial pressure, laboratory personnel are responsible for oversight of the instrument and quality assurance of the results.

Polarography is an electrochemical technique for measuring the concentration of reducible elements by means an cathode and measurement of the current flowing through an electrochemical cell to the **anode**. The electrical potential between the two electrodes is increased at a constant rate by an external voltage source, and **reduction** of the test substance occurs at the cathode. As the voltage reaches the standard electrode potential of the test substance, there is a sharp increase in electron flow as a result of reduction. The indicator electrode is usually a Ag/AgCl electrode in which **oxidation** occurs and the electron flow (current) is measured. The partial pressure of oxygen (PO_2) can be measured with a polarographic electrode, as described in Test Methodology 3–11. Figure 3–14 depicts the PO_2 electrode.

TEST METHODOLOGY 3-11. PO_2 MEASUREMENT BY POLAROGRAPHY/AMPEROMETRY

The Reaction Principle

PO_2 is measured by a polarographic electrode that is filled with buffer and covered with a semipermeable membrane. Dissolved oxygen diffuses through the membrane, reacts with the buffer, and is reduced at the platinum cathode charged with a direct current (DC) voltage. The resulting flow of electrons is measured by a meter versus the reference electrode maintained with a constant potential.

Reference Ranges

Adult arterial	83–108 mm Hg

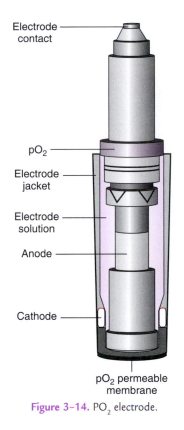

Figure 3–14. PO_2 electrode.

Voltammetry

Voltammetry is an electrochemical technique similar to polarography except that electrical potential is varied over time. There is typically a working reference electrode and direct current is applied to it initially as a large negative potential is generated. Metal ions are reduced at the surface of the reference electrode. This causes them to be strongly attracted to the surface of the electrode. In the next step, the direct current is applied as a large linear positive potential, causing the metal ions to be gradually re-oxidized and stripped from the electrode in order of their characteristic potentials. A microammeter records current versus applied potential to quantify individual metals.

Osmometry

Osmolality is defined as the concentration of solutes dissolved in a solvent, usually expressed as milliosmoles (mOsm) per kilogram of pure water. In plasma, all dissolved particles, including electrolytes, carbohydrates, waste products, vitamins, drugs, hormones, and the like, contribute to osmolality. However, the major osmotic substances are sodium, chloride, glucose, urea, proteins, and ethyl alcohol (when present). Sodium makes up roughly half of the plasma osmolality.

Plasma or serum osmolality can be estimated with the following formula:

1.86 (Na [mmol/L]) + (glucose [mg/dL]/18) + (urea N [mg/dL]/2.8) + 9

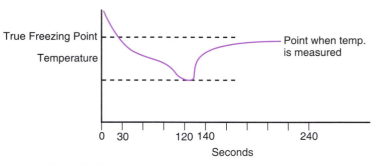

Figure 3–15. Freezing point osmometry: temperature versus time.

Glucose and urea nitrogen are converted to mmol/L by the factors listed, and 9 represents the typical contribution of ionized proteins, potassium, chloride, and calcium. Urine osmolality is also very useful in comparison to plasma osmolality in assessment of water regulation in regard to hormonal control and renal function.

Osmometry is the general term for analysis of osmolality. Dissolved particles affect a solution by altering the solution's colligative properties, such as lowering the vapor pressure or lowering the freezing point. These are the properties that can be measured in an osmometer to determine the osmolality of body fluids such as serum or urine. Figure 3–15 illustrates the relationship of temperature versus time in a freezing point osmometer in which the sample is rapidly supercooled below freezing point and then stirred, and the temperature rises as heat is generated. This procedure is described in Test Methodology 3–12.

TEST METHODOLOGY 3-12.   FREEZING POINT METHODOLOGY FOR OSMOLALITY MEASUREMENT

The Reaction Principle

A thermistor probe and stirring mechanism come in contact with the sample, which is supercooled to approximately –10°C, which should be below its freezing point. The stirring wire vibrates to initiate freezing to a slush stage and the heat of fusion warms the solution, causing equilibrium in temperature between freezing and thawing states. Variable resistance is measured, representing freezing point depression. At the end of this equilibrium, the sample freezes.

Osmolality in mOsm/kg H_2O is determined as the observed freezing point compared to the molal freezing point depression of pure water, –1.86°C. Figure 3-15 presents a diagrammatic representation of temperature of the solution over time.

The Specimen

Serum that is free from cells or gross hemolysis is the specimen of choice. Plasma is generally not allowed because of contributions to osmolality due to anticoagulants. Osmolality may also be analyzed in body fluids such as urine and gastric fluids, and samples are stable if maintained in closed containers and analyzed promptly or refrigerated at 2° to 8°C for up to 24 hours.

Reference Range (Adults)

Serum   275–298 mOsm/Kg

Sodium contributes nearly half of the osmolality in normal circumstances, but other solutes, such as urea, glucose, and alcohols, can contribute significantly to osmolality when they are present in excess. Alcohols cannot be detected by vapor depression osmometers but can be detected in freezing point depression (FDP) osmometers.[1]

Case Scenario 3-4 Spectrophotometry: How Does It Work?

Follow-Up

The student spent his week in high-volume clinical chemistry learning to apply the principles of spectrophotometry and electrochemistry. Along with learning how to organize work flow with the automated instrument, during less busy times the student was given a chance to practice calculations that explain the underlying theory. Many of those calculations, such as Beer's law for spectrophotometry and Ohm's law for electrochemistry, were familiar from general chemistry and physics classes he took as a first-year student. The student would be spending more time with automation later in his rotations, getting the chance to prepare calibration curves and sample dilutions and checking for linearity of reactions. ●

CASE SCENARIO 3-5

Separation: How Does It Work?

After his week in high-volume chemistry, the student went to special chemistry. "This is more like it. I have seen these instruments." His mentor explained that he would spend a week in **electrophoresis** and **chromatography**. "This is your week in the separation laboratory," the mentor said.

electrophoresis - a separation technique of different charged molecules in solution in an electrical field of varying potential

chromatography - a technique for separating similar molecules based on differential adsorption and elution

Electrophoresis

Electrophoresis is defined as the movement of charged particles when placed into an electrical field of varying electrical potential. Separation of charged particles during electrophoresis occurs when different molecules move at different rates. Electrophoresis is a tool that is used by clinical laboratory scientists/medical technologists to separate molecules prior to molecule identification. For example, serum proteins, when placed in a buffer of pH 8.6, become negatively charged and migrate to an anode, while the buffer particles migrate to a cathode.

Several forces affect the charged molecule during electrophoresis. The molecule will move in the direction of its opposite charge. Negatively charged molecules (anions) will move toward the positively charged electrode, the anode. Likewise, positively charged molecules (cations) will move toward the cathode, the negatively charged electrode. Electrical potential, or voltage, of the field, is directly related to the force on the charged molecules. The molecule is also affected by friction based on its shape. A larger and more asymmetric molecule will have a slower rate of movement in the electrical field due to friction. The forces that affect the charged molecule can be partially controlled through choice of voltage of the electrical field, viscosity and pH of the buffer solution in which electrophoresis takes place, and properties of the support medium for the sample.

During electrophoresis, current is carried between the cathode and anode by ions in the buffer solution. The voltage applied to the electrophoresis system is chosen to minimize heat and buffer evaporation, while maximizing molecule resolution. The charged molecules move through the pores of the support medium toward an opposite charge. The movement of large molecules may be restricted by pore size of the support medium. An ideal support medium does not interact with the charged molecule chemically or electrically, but acts as a filter to retard movement on the basis of size and shape. Cellulose acetate and agarose are two of the substances that can be used as a support medium for protein electrophoresis.

Movement is also due to buffer flowing across the support medium. The buffer moves in the opposite direction to the flow of negatively charged sample molecules. Buffer flow affects molecules having a small magnitude of charge more so than molecules having a greater charge. Gamma globulin proteins with pI of 7.2 actually flow from the application point toward the cathode. Although gamma globulins are negatively charged at buffer pH 8.6, the buffer flow is strong enough to carry these molecules against the electrical force. This process in which a solution moves relative to an adjacent stationary substance when placed in an electrical field is called electro-osmosis, or endosmosis. Figure 3–16 provides a simple illustration of electrophoresis.

Following electrophoresis, the protein fractions must be fixed in the support medium to prevent their loss during the staining process. The medium can be soaked in dilute acetic acid or trichloroacetic acid, or can be heated to denature the proteins. Proteins within an agarose medium can be precipitated out in a saline solution. This process fixes the fractions in the matrix of the support medium.

The fixed medium is ready for staining. Although many charged substances that were present in the sample have undergone electrophoresis through the medium, clinical laboratory scientists/medical technologists generally examine specific categories of substances during one test. The staining procedure allows the clinical laboratory scientist the opportunity to visualize one set of substances with specificity. Proteins may be stained with ninhydrin, which will visualize amino groups; ponceau S, which will nonspecifically help to visualize proteins on a cellulose acetate medium; Coomassie brilliant blue or amido black, which are specific for proteins; or Sudan black or oil red O, which can be used to visualize lipoproteins. After staining, excess stain is removed and the background of the support medium is cleared with a solvent. The medium is then dried and ready for analysis.

Once the medium has been stained and the background of the medium support has been cleared, the electrophoretic pattern can be scanned through a den-

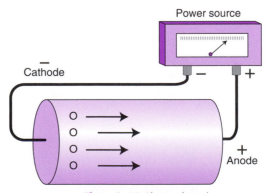

Figure 3–16. Electrophoresis.

sitometer. Densitometry works much the same way as a spectrophotometer; the stained electrophoretic pattern is scanned with a specific wavelength of light. The specific wavelength is chosen based on optimal absorbance by the stained protein. Depending on the density of the protein fraction, light is transmitted through to a photodetector that senses differences of light transmittance. Following Beer's law, the amount of light absorbance is proportional to the concentration of the protein in the fraction. As the densitometer scans the electrophoretic pattern at a specific wavelength, it produces a tracing, or graph, of the relative amounts of the protein fractions present. The densitometer will also print the percentage of the total that is detected for each protein fraction by a process called *integration*.

The process of densitometry is standardized. A gel that contains standard bands is scanned through the densitometer. The bands are standardized to transmit 10%, 20%, 40%, 60%, 80%, and 100% of the light source. As the light passes through the calibration standard, the operator adjusts electrical gain to correct transmittance to the standard percentage. As the densitometer scans the electrophoretic pattern, a tracing of the relative amounts of each protein band is produced. The densitometry report includes the electrophoretic tracing and calculation of the percentage of total protein that is detected for each protein fraction. If the concentration of total protein in the **specimen** is given, the absolute values of each protein fraction can be computed. Test Methodology 3–13 is a procedure for protein electrophoresis.

specimen - aliquot of body fluid or tissue from a patient

TEST METHODOLOGY 3-13.   PROTEIN ELECTROPHORESIS

The Reaction Principle

The patient's serum is placed into a sample trough within agarose gel, then placed in an alkaline buffer solution, and a standardized voltage is applied to allow separation of the major protein groups by electrophoresis. The result is six or more fractions of separated proteins, including the main fractions of albumin and alpha$_1$, alpha$_2$, beta$_1$, beta$_2$, and gamma globulins, from anode to cathode. Following electrophoresis, the agarose gel is processed in acetic acid and alcohol washes to fix the proteins. After a wash step, the protein fractions are stainined with Coumassie brilliant blue protein stain. After a second wash, fixed protein bands can be visualized and quantified with densitometry, in which light passes through the fixed medium and is absorbed by fixed stained protein bands.

The Calculations

% Protein fraction $\times$ total protein (g/dL) = protein fraction (g/dL)

For example, if the densitometer scans and measures relative amounts of protein fractions in an electrophoretic pattern for a specimen and the absolute amount of total protein is 8.0 g/dL, then the absolute concentration of each protein fraction can be computed as shown below.

Protein Fraction	Relative %	Absolute Concentration (g/dL)
Albumin	62.5	$0.625 \times 8.0 = 5.0$
Alpha$_1$ globulin	3.75	$0.0375 \times 8.0 = 0.3$
Alpha$_2$ globulin	8.75	$0.0875 \times 8.0 = 0.7$
Beta globuin	10.0	$0.1 \times 8.0 = 0.8$
Gamma globulin	15.0	$0.15 \times 8.0 = 1.2$
Total	100	8.0

CHROMATOGRAPHY

Chromatography is a technique for separating molecules based on their relative distribution between two different phases.[4] Separation takes place on a stationary or nonmoving phase under the influence of a mobile or moving phase. Molecules are separated based on their **solubility** and their interaction with these two phases. There are two general types of chromatography: plane and column.

solubility - the ability of a solute to dissolve in a solvent

Plane Chromatography

Plane chromatography is a separation technique that takes place on a flat surface or plane. The separation of substances in a solution occurs based upon differences in the solubility of molecules within two phases, a stationary and a mobile phase. The mobile phase, often a liquid, is the moving phase. The stationary phase is nonmoving and may be minute beads, polymer gel, or paper, for example. There are several types of plane chromatography, including paper and thin-layer chromatography. These will be described further.

Paper chromatography uses paper as the stationary phase and a solvent as the mobile phase. The solvent moves through the paper by capillary action. Separation depends on the solubility of solutes in the solvent, the polarity of solvent, and the polarity of solutes in the sample. In order to see the separated chemicals, a development step is needed. Visualization of the separated sample occurs by chemical reaction, which produces a color change. Density of the colored bands may then be measured by visible or fluorescent densitometry as a gauge of concentration. Introducing chemicals to react with the separated sample will help to develop the separated fractions, producing color changes that can be quantified with visible or fluorescent densitometry.

Thin-Layer Chromatography

Thin-layer chromatography (TLC) uses a thin layer of silica gel, alumina gel, polyacrylamide gel, or starch gel attached to a glass plate as stationary phase. The mobile phase is a liquid solvent. The fractions in the sample are generally quite soluble in the solvent and move with it up the stationary phase by capillary action. Separation of the solute fractions depends on their solubility in the solvent, the polarity of the solvent, the rate of diffusion, and the polarity of solutes in the sample. Separated fractions are also developed in TLC by applying a chemical to induce a chemical reaction with the separated fractions to produce color changes. Figure 3–17 shows a typical thin-layer **chromatogram**. Adaptations to TLC have been developed to include reverse-phase chromatography and high-pressure TLC. Reverse-phase chromatography uses a bonded silica thin-layer stationary phase that is more polar than the mobile phase. It is used for separating polar compounds.[4]

chromatogram - record of molecular separation taking place in chromatography

Column Chromatography

Chromatography can also take place within a column. Column chromatography involves the interaction of the sample mixture with a mobile phase, often a liquid or a gas, while the stationary phase is a medium in a column. Examples of station-

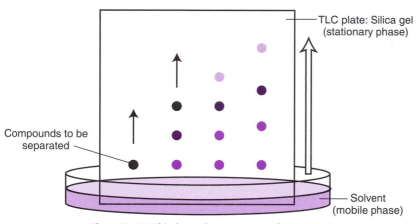

Figure 3–17. Thin-layer chromatogram of amino acid.

ary phase media include aluminum silicate gel and resin particles. The sample is injected into one end of the column, and then travels through the column medium via gravitational force or pressure from a liquid or gas carrier. Diverse substances within the sample will travel at different rates and **elute** from the column at different times. In column chromatography, the sample is placed into the column, and then flows down the column due to gravity or under the influence of pressure (gas or liquid), and separate fractions of solute are collected in reservoirs as **eluate**, the liquid coming through the column. Separated components can be detected by using different solvents that selectively elute certain compounds, which can then be quantified spectrophotometrically. Examples of column chromatography are described further. Typical laboratory analytes measured by this technique include glycosylated hemoglobin (Hb A_{1c}) nd Hb A_2 methods.[1]

Adsorption column chromatography employs a highly specific interaction of the solute by its attraction to the surface of solid particles of the stationary phase.[4] The adsorbant used is often silica gel with surface silanol and acidic groups that **adsorb** basic or alkaline charged substances. This has been used for separation of hemoglobin types such as glycosylated hemoglobin.[4]

In *partition column chromatography*, solutes within the sample interact with an inert, chemically unreactive solid support medium containing a thin film of liquid adsorbed onto its surface. Separation in this type of chromatography is based on **electrostatic** attractions or hydrogen bonding of the solutes to the liquid-coated stationary phase and is based on solubility differences of the solutes in the mobile and stationary phases. In *ion-exchange chromatography*, the sample is diluted with a buffer to give the solutes an electrical charge. These solutes interact reversibly with opposite-charged solid support molecules and mobile liquid phases. Varying the pH of the mobile phase allows elution at different times and can allow one to elute specifically charged solute particles. Thus, ion-exchange chromatography separates the solutes in the sample based on their solubility in the two phases as well as different electrical charges. This method has been used to separate hemoglobin S from other forms of hemoglobin in red blood cell lysed solutions.

In *steric exclusion column chromatography* (or size exclusion chromatography), the molecules are separated in the column based on size and hindrance by the pores in the gel medium. Size and molecular mass excludes certain molecules such that molecules with larger molecular mass elute faster from the column while molecules with smaller mass are retained in the gel medium longer.

elute - remove based on solubility

eluate - the liquid obtained from a column during separation; derived from washing

adsorb - attach to the surface of another material

electrostatic - producing electrical attractions within or between groups of molecules

steric - relating to the size of and distances between chemicals or side chains within the spatial arrangement of atoms in the chemical

Automated Chromatography

Various automated forms of column chromatography have been developed, to include high-pressure liquid chromatography (HPLC), gas chromatography (GC), and GC with mass spectrometry detection (GC-MS). Detector output from automated chromatography is plotted to display detector output versus time. Peaks are present in this chromatogram, with the peak area unique to the column characteristics and the detector. For example, the typical liquid chromatogram provides retention time, peak height ratio, and resolution for each detected compound. *Resolution* is the term that describes the separation and width of the peak, which takes into account conditions in the column. These automated methods of chromatography provide more specific and sensitive results than simple column chromatography, but they require more highly skilled and educated personnel. In addition, detailed protocols for collection, handling, and documentation must be followed when the testing is for clinical purposes. Automated column chromatography, in particular GC, is used for forensic testing of drug and alcohol levels.

HPLC is a type of column chromatography, but rather than relying on the force of gravity to move the samples and mobile phase through the column, it utilizes pressure to force sample through the column. The column can employ adsorption, ion-exchange, or other methods listed above. Fractions of separated solutes are commonly detected using UV spectrophotometers. Occasionally detection with HPLC is by thermal conductivity or use of electron capture detectors. Detector output is plotted on a graph, forming peaks of detector output (absorbance) versus time. HPLC can provide **qualitative** results in which the column retention time relates to the identity of the compound. Quantitative results may be calculated by relating the area under the curve of the unknown to the area under the curve of a known standard. Results are also quantitative in that the peak area can be determined, relating to the concentration of the compound when compared to a calibration curve of known standard solutions. Test Methodology 3–14 describes a drug analysis using HPLC.

qualitative - giving either positive or negative test results (a binary response)

TEST METHODOLOGY 3-14.   HIGH-PRESSURE (HIGH-PERFORMANCE) LIQUID CHROMATOGRAPHY METHOD OF SALICYLATE ANALYSIS

The Reaction Principle

Salicylate is the main ingredient of aspirin tablets. Excessive intake of salicylate results in toxicity. In the HPLC reaction, serum plasma is first precipitated with a reagent containing *o*-methoxybenzoic acid as an internal standard. Salicylate and other similar chemicals are then separated with an octadecylsilane reversed-phase chromatographic column and a solvent mobile phase. Quantification is performed by calculating the ratio of peak height absorbance at 313 nm of the analyte to that for the internal standard, then comparing this ratio with appropriate calibration standard ratios.

The Specimen

Heparinized plasma separated from cells promptly and stored at 4° to 6°C prior to analysis. Stability is enhanced for long-term storage at –20°C.

Therapeutic Range

150–300 mg/L

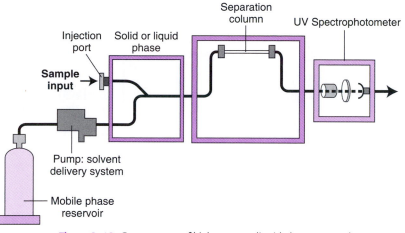

Figure 3–18. Components of high-pressure liquid chromatograph.

There are two main types of HPLC: reversed phase or normal phase. Normal-phase HPLC uses a solvent for the mobile phase, such as methanol, and a highly polar stationary phase such as silanol or nitrile groups bonded to silica packing. When a less-polar column packing such as octadecylsilane (C18) bonded to silica is used with a highly polar mobile phase such as distilled water or very dilute alcohol, the chromatography is termed reversed-phase HPLC.[4] Figure 3–18 illustrates the main components of a high-pressure liquid chromatograph, including the mobile phase pump, column, and detector.

Gas Chromatography

Gas chromatography utilizes an inert gas, often helium, as the mobile phase to move a sample through a column. The stationary phase in the column is a support medium surrounded by a thin liquid. The sample is rapidly heated to become vaporized, and flows with the carrier gas through the heated column, where separation occurs. In gas chromatography, an internal standard is added to all samples to account for fluctuations in the column and injection port temperature as well as changes in the carrier gas flow. The separated compounds are detected with flame ionization. In flame ionization detectors, an electronic signal is generated from each separated molecular component. Figure 3–19 illustrates the main components of a gas chromatograph, including the oven, column, gas tank, and detector. Other detection systems in gas chromatography include thermal ionic or electron capture detectors. The most accurate detector in gas chromatography is a mass spectrometer (GC-MS), which fractionates molecules into unique components that can then be separated electromagnetically to give a unique mass spectrum. Mass spectrometry provides improved specificity in detection of drugs of abuse or alcohol in patient samples.[1]

The information generated from the detector is in the form of peaks of measurable height and area of each separated chemical. By comparing the height and area of each peak from unknown samples to heights and areas of peaks of standards of known identity and concentration, the concentration of the unknown may be determined. Just as was described with HPLC, GC generates output that can be

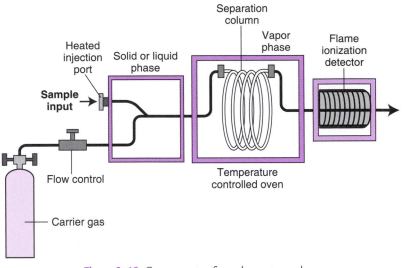

Figure 3–19. Components of gas chromatograph.

used to calculate retention time and peak area. The peak area is unique to the column characteristics and the detector. Column output is plotted versus distance measured as time. For example, the typical gas chromatogram provides retention time, peak height ratio, and resolution for each separate chemical fraction. Retention time, a peak at a certain time (t_R), is used to uniquely identify the chemical, while peak height ratio or peak area relates to concentration of the substance. *Resolution* is the term that describes the separation and width of the peak, which takes into account conditions in the column. The carrier gas moves through the column first and forms a peak on the graph as indicated by t_0 or t_m. This is sometimes called the dead time for the column. Figure 3–20 shows a simple gas chromatogram with t_0 and peaks t_1 and t_2. Test Methodology 3–15 describes a gas chromatographic method for alcohol quantification.

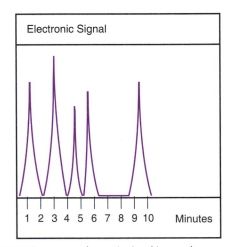

Figure 3–20. Time versus electronic signal in gas chromatogram.

TEST METHODOLOGY 3-15.   PRINCIPLE OF ALCOHOL TESTING BY GAS-LIQUID CHROMATOGRAPHY

The Reaction Principle

Specimens are diluted with *n*-propanol as an internal standard, and samples are then placed in sealed vials for headspace analysis. The headspace is the gaseous region just above the liquid level in the vial that contains the volatilized alcohol mixture. Vials are capped, sealed, and swirled to ensure complete mixing. The sealed vials are heated at 40°C for 30 minutes. Using a tuberculin syringe, a portion of the headspace is introduced into the gas chromatograph. The resolved components are detected using a flame ionization detector. The internal standard is used to mark the completion of the sample elution.

Interferences

Sources of error in gas chromatography include inadequate levels of carrier gas and incorrect column temperature, which can impede separation. Other sources of error include improperly identified or poorly preserved sample and improperly mixed or sealed test solution vials.

The Specimen

Sodium fluoride and potassium oxalated whole blood or serum kept in a sealed container with minimal airspace. Cleaning of the skin puncture site should be performed with a nonalcohol solution rather than the typical wipe. The sample must be collected in a closed system and may be arterial, venous, or capillary whole blood.

Reference Range

0 mg/dL (normal)

Figure 3–21 illustrates the typical output from gas-liquid chromatography of drugs from a patient sample. The separation pattern is highly dependent on the column contents and temperature conditions as well as the carrier gas. Often instrument output (the individual peaks) is a result of flame ionization detection. The adjusted retention times, used to qualitatively identity of the drug, are compared to purified standards, and peak height ratios can determine the concentration of the drugs.

Case Scenario 3-5 Separation: How Does It Work?

Follow-Up

The week in the separation laboratory was over. The student had an opportunity to learn about and practice electrophoresis and chromatography techniques. Some of the same principles learned about spectrophotometry were applied to electrophoresis when detecting and quantifying protein bands. A spectrophotometer using UV wavelengths was also used as the detector in HPLC. Principles of electrochemistry learned earlier were also helpful in understanding electrophoretic separation of charged particles and in electronic detectors of the gas chromatograph. It was time for the student to move onto the next week of clinical chemistry internship. ●

Serum Drug Screen

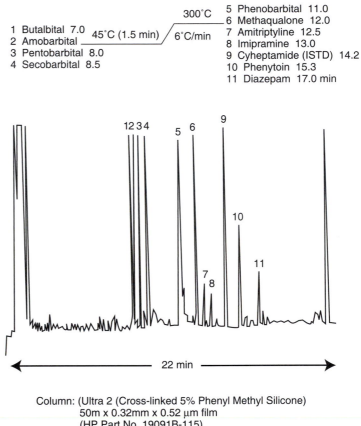

1 Butalbital 7.0
2 Amobarbital
3 Pentobarbital 8.0
4 Secobarbital 8.5

45°C (1.5 min)   6°C/min   300°C

5 Phenobarbital 11.0
6 Methaqualone 12.0
7 Amitriptyline 12.5
8 Imipramine 13.0
9 Cyheptamide (ISTD) 14.2
10 Phenytoin 15.3
11 Diazepam 17.0 min

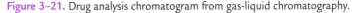

22 min

Column: (Ultra 2 (Cross-linked 5% Phenyl Methyl Silicone)
        50m x 0.32mm x 0.52 μm film
        (HP Part No. 19091B-115)
Carrier: μ(H$_2$) = 80cm/sec
Oven: Temperature program listed above
Injection 1μl, spitless
Detector: Flame ionization detector

Figure 3–21. Drug analysis chromatogram from gas-liquid chromatography.

CASE SCENARIO 3-6

Immunoassay: How Does It Work?

"This week you are in the immunoassay section," said the supervisor, "and you will get to know the Athena IV." The Athena IV was the new automated chemiluminescence analyzer. Thyroid-stimulating hormone, other hormones, and therapeutic drug levels were analyzed on the Athena. Although this instrument appeared quite different than the simple spectrophotometer that the student had used in the student laboratory, the supervisor reminded him that the Athena IV and other immunoassay analyzers measure the final product of the chemical reaction using the principles of spectrophotometry. In other words, although the reagents include new ingredients such as antibodies and luminescence-generating reactions, light was used to quantify the final product with a photometer similar to the simple spectrophotometer already used.

IMMUNOASSAY TECHNIQUES

An immunoassay is an analytical method that uses antibodies or **antigens** as reagents to measure specific chemicals, or analytes. The immunoassay has been in use for over 30 years. Results from immunoassays are the basis for many critical human health decisions involving detection of viruses and their antibodies, therapeutic drug monitoring, and screening for drugs of abuse. Over 70 clinical analytes are tested by immunoassay. The immunoassay technique is the basis for many home tests, and even home tests for pregnancy are based on this technology. Immunoassays are reliable and sensitive to very low concentration levels of analyte.

The key reagents in all immunoassays are antibodies or antigens. Most immunoassay tests that are performed in the clinical chemistry laboratory measure antigens, using antibodies as the reagent. Antibodies are proteins that are produced by the immune systems of higher animals. They are produced by specific white blood cells in response to "foreign" substances. Antibodies may be produced naturally, as a response to natural infections such as to mumps or chickenpox virus. They may also be produced as an acquired immunity in response to vaccinations. Antibodies physically bind to antigens. Immunoassays require minimum sample preparation since antibodies bind only to specific antigens. The strength of binding, or the affinity, determines the sensitivity of the method. Specificity allows detection of one antigen in the complex matrix of the sample.

The **antibody** consists of heavy and light chains of polypeptides that contain binding sites for an antigen. Figure 3–22 illustrates the basic structure of an antibody. Reagent antibodies are produced by injecting animals with the antigen or analytical target. The immune system responds only to high molecular weight **immunogens**, typically of molecular weight greater than 10,000. Many chemicals are smaller in molecular weight (**haptens**), and require preparation of a suitable immunogen in which the analyte is coupled to a carrier protein. Antibody and antigen reactions are subject to the **law of mass action**. The law of mass action simply states that free reactants will achieve equilibrium with bound reactants given time. Figure 3–23 depicts an antibody and immunogen.

Many different antibody-producing cells make **polyclonal** antibodies. Polyclonal antibodies may be made directly from animal blood and will bind with a variety

antigen - a protein or oligosaccharide that elicits an antibody response

antibody - an immunoglobulin produced by a B lymphocyte in response to a unique antigen

immunogen - high molecular weight molecule that stimulates antibody production; antigen

hapten - low molecular weight chemical coupled to a carrier protein to become a suitable immunogen

law of mass action - the rate of any given chemical reaction is proportional to the product of the activities (or concentrations) of the reactants

polyclonal - arising from many cell lines

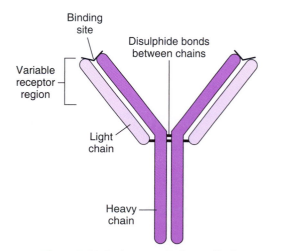

Figure 3–22. Basic structure of an antibody.

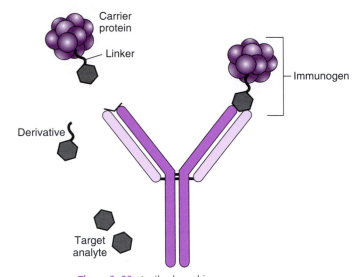

Figure 3–23. Antibody and immunogen.

monoclonal - arising from one cell line

hybridoma - a fused lymphocyte and myeloma cell used for making specific antibodies

clones - genetically identical cells

of antigens. **Monoclonal** antibodies are produced when mice are injected with the antigen, and antibody-producing lymphocyte cells are taken from the animals and fused with cells that grow continuously in culture to form **hybridomas**. A single hybridoma produces only one type of antibody by dividing to produce a large population of **clones** all making the same monoclonal antibody. Living hybridomas are frozen indefinitely in liquid nitrogen to produce an indefinite supply of uniform and consistent reagent antibodies of one type. Monoclonal antibodies have many advantages over polyclonal antibodies, including consistency between lots, indefinite supply, high specificity, and longer lead times, but have higher initial costs when compared with polyclonal antibodies.

Immunoassays are named by the acronym that describes the antibody-antigen response, such as ELISA (enzyme-linked immunosorbent assay). To organize the many methodologies that are used in immunoassay, assays are categorized by separation methodology, antibody-antigen reaction, or the label that is used to detect a reaction. Many formats have been used for immunoassay techniques. The choice of format is dependent upon the physical properties of the analyte, the need for quantitative versus qualitative result, the complexity of the sample matrix, sample preparation requirements, and simplicity of tests.

Types of Immunoassays

noncompetitive immunoassay - immunoassay that does not contain reagent antigen competing with patient antigen

tagged - labeled with some component that allows detection or visualization

epitopes - specific antibody binding sites found on an antigen

Type I is a single-site, **noncompetitive immunoassay**. In this format, an antibody of known antigenicity is **tagged** with label. The label is not part of the antigen-antibody reaction but is used to detect binding. Enzymes and fluorescent or chemiluminescent molecules are common labels for immunoassay reactions. Radioactive isotopes have historical significance in immunoassay, but are no longer routinely used to detect reactions. In type I immunoassays, the antibody is mixed with patient antigen. If the antigen contains specific **epitopes** for the antibody, binding will occur. Unbound antibody is then washed away and the label is measured. The amount of label present is directly proportional to the amount of the antigen.

A type II immunoassay, also known as a two-site immunoassay, is also noncompetitive but uses two antibody-binding reactions. Antibodies of known antigenicity are attached to a solid phase, such as plastic wells, tubes, capillaries, membranes, latex particles, or magnetic particles. Patient antigen is then added to the test system. Patient antigen with epitopes to the known antibody will bind to the fixed antibody. A second antibody that is tagged with a label is then introduced into the test system. If the patient antigen has an epitope for this second antibody, binding will occur. Excess labeled antibody is washed away. The remaining label is measured. The amount of label is directly proportional to the amount of antigen present in the patient sample.

Type III refers to an immunoassay that is both **competitive** and **homogeneous**. Patient antigen and reagent antigen that has been labeled are introduced to the testing system, which contains antibody in limited numbers. Patient and reagent antigen compete for the limited number of binding sites on antibody that are available. Based on the law of mass action, the ratio of antibody binding of patient to reagent antigen will be proportional to their concentrations. Binding of reagent antigen inactivates the label. Only free reagent antigen label will be measured. The amount of free reagent label measured is directly proportional to the amount of patient antigen that has bound to antibody. Figure 3–24 illustrates competitive immunoassays.

Type IV is a competitive **heterogeneous immunoassay**. This methodology is similar to type III methodology in that patient antigen and labeled reagent antigen compete for a limited number of antibody binding sites. However, the label is not inactivated by binding. Free and bound reagent antigen must be separated before the label is measured. Label may be measured on either the free or bound reagent antigen and is related to the amount of patient antigen in the sample.

competitive immunoassay - immunoassay in which patient antigen and labeled reagent antigen compete for the same binding site on the antibody

homogeneous assay - immunoassay in which bound and free antibody need not be separated before label is measured

heterogeneous immunoassay - immunoassay in which bound and free antibody must be separated before label is measured

Enzyme-Labeled Immunoassay

An enzyme is a common label that is used to detect an immunoassay reaction. After the antibody-antigen reaction has occurred, the product is determined by measuring the enzyme label. A procedure for measuring the product of the enzyme-catalyzed reaction must follow the immunoassay reaction. In most instances, substrate for the enzyme-activated reaction is added to the test system and the product of the reaction is measured by spectrophotometry. Examples of enzyme-labeled immunoassay include enzyme-linked (ELISA) and enzyme-multiplied immunoassays.

ELISAs are commonly used immunoassay techniques. An ELISA is a type II procedure. An antibody with known antigenicity is attached to a solid phase (usually a fiberglass membrane or multiwell plate). Patient antigen is then added to the test system. Antigen that is specific to the antibody will bind to the antibody. A second enzyme-labeled antibody that is specific to another site on the antigen is then added into the test system. Antigen that contains epitopes for both antibodies will be "sandwiched" between the antibodies. Free enzyme-labeled antibody is washed away. Substrate for the enzyme-catalyzed reaction is added and the product of the reaction is measured. The amount of enzyme activity is directly proportional to the amount of antigen present in the patient sample. Alkaline phosphatase and horseradish peroxidase enzymes are commonly used enzyme labels. Both enzymes catalyze reactions that produce colored compounds that can be measured on a spectrophotometer.

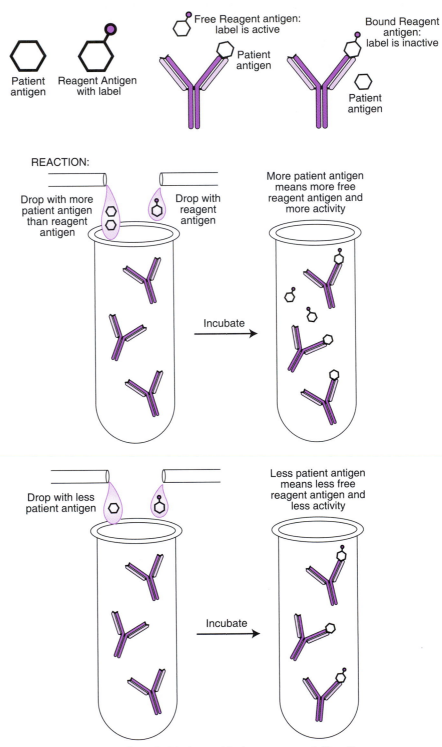

Figure 3–24. Competitive immunoassay. *A,* Type III.

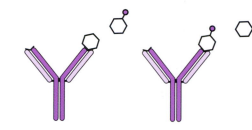

Free and bound reagent label
are both active

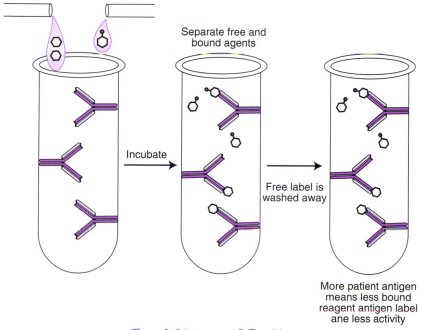

Figure 3–24. *(continued)* B, Type IV.

An enzyme-multiplied immunoassay technique (EMIT) is a type III procedure. Patient antigen and enzyme-labeled reagent antigen are mixed with a limited amount of antibody. Patient and reagent antigen compete for the limited number of binding sites that are available. Binding of reagent antigen inactivates the enzyme. Substrate is added to the test system, but only free reagent antigen will catalyze the enzyme reaction. Because more patient antigen will allow more enzyme-labeled reagent antigen to remain free and active, greater enzyme activity is an indication of increased patient antigen in the sample. Glucose-6-phosphate dehydrogenase (G6PD) is commonly used as enzyme label in EMIT procedures. When the antigen binds G6PD-labeled antibody, the active site of the enzyme is blocked. Substrate and a coenzyme (NAD) are added to the test system. The enzyme reaction is measured as change in absorbance as NAD is consumed.

Cloned enzyme donor immunoassays (CEDIAs) use a genetically altered enzyme as label. The enzyme exists in two sections; one section is bound as label to reagent antigen and the other section is introduced into the test system after antigen-antibody binding. The enzyme is active only when the two sections are intact. When reagent antigen is bound to antibody, the second section of the enzyme cannot bind to the first section and the enzyme remains inactive. The immunoassay procedure follows the type III format. Patient antigen and enzyme fragment–labeled reagent antigen compete for a limited number of binding sites on the antibody. The second section of the enzyme is added to the test system, and enzyme fragment–labeled reagent antigen binds to antibody, which results in inactivated enzyme. Increased amounts of patient antigen result in increased free reagent antigen and increased enzyme activity.

Microparticle-capture enzyme immunoassay (MEIA) employs a modified type II immunoassay format. The test cuvet contains antibody that is bound to latex microparticles. Patient antigen is allowed to bind to the antibody. A second antibody that is tagged with enzyme label is then added to the test system. Free labeled antibody is washed away and substrate is added to the test mixture. Enzyme activity is measured as an indication of the amount of antigen that is present in the patient sample. Alkaline phosphatase is commonly used as label, with 4-methylumbelliferyl phosphate as substrate. The fluorescent product of the reaction, methylumbelliferone, is measured.

Fluorescent-Labeled Immunoassay

The measurement of fluorescent compounds increases the sensitivity of the measurement of the label reaction. Methods that measure fluorescence must be carefully controlled for false-positive reactions from contaminating substances and false-negative reactions that can occur from fluorescence quenching. A fluorescence polarization immunoassay (FPIA) uses a type III immunoassay format with a fluorophore as label. Patient antigen and fluorescent-labeled reagent antigen compete for a limited number of antibody binding sites. Spectrophotometry, which uses polarized light, is used to excite the fluorophore, and the polarization of the emitted light is then measured. Small, unbound fluorophore-labeled reagent antigen will rotate quickly, emitting unpolarized light. Larger, bound fluorophore-labeled reagent will rotate more slowly, emitting **polarized light**. Increased patient antigen will result in greater amounts of unpolarized light.

polarized light- light which vibrates in one plane

Chemiluminescent-Labeled Immunoassay

Chemiluminescence is produced by compounds such as luminol and acridinium esters that have the ability to produce light energy by chemical reaction. The light may be seen as a flash or a glow. Immunoassay systems that measure chemiluminescence reactions often employ a type IV methodology. Patient antigen and chemiluminescent compound–labeled reagent antigen compete for a limited number of antibody binding sites. The label is not inactivated by binding. Upon separation of free and unbound reagent antigen, an enzyme (usually firefly luciferase) is used to produce chemiluminescence, which is measured with a luminometer. See the example of the use of chemiluminescent immunoassay in Test Methodology 3-16.

Particle Immunoassay

Particle immunoassays assess the formation or inhibition of a precipitation or aggregation event. Aggregation is measured by nephelometry or turbidimetry. Particle-enhanced turbidimetric immunoinhibition assay (PETINA) is a type IV immunoassay formatted procedure. Patient antigen and particle-labeled reagent antigen compete for a limited number of antibody binding sites. The binding of particle-labeled antigen to antibody produces aggregation and increased turbidity in the test solution, which can be measured by photometry.

TEST METHODOLOGY 3-16. CHEMILUMINESCENCE WITH THE ATHENA IV

The Reaction Principle

The Athena IV is a bench-top random-access immunoassay system that uses acridium ester as a chemiluminescent label capable of producing 150 tests per hour. Assay reagents are solid-phase paramagnetic particles that are mixed on the reagent tray so that they are maintained in solution. Sample and reagent are mixed and incubated for 7 minutes and stirred with the magnetic particles. Magnetic separation and wash steps follow to remove unbound antigen. A second reagent is added that enhances the reaction, followed by the last reagent, which oxidizes the acridium label. Chemiluminescence is measured at 430 nm by a photomultiplier tube.

Chemiluminescence is directly proportional to the amount of antigen from the sample.

The Calculations

Calibration curves of standard solutions over a range of concentrations are used to calculate the unknown results. Linear regression is performed by the microprocessor to determine linearity of the reaction, slope, and y-intercept.

Example Analytes

Hormones, drugs, and tumor markers are measured by this method.

Case Scenario 3-6 Immunoassay: How Does It Work?

Follow-Up

"This week you are doing immunoassays in the immunoassay section of the laboratory," the supervisor said to the student, "and you will get to know the Athena IV." The student learned that week that the Athena IV was the new automated chemiluminescence analyzer used to measure therapeutic drug and hormone levels. The basic lessons learned in biology classes, especially about the biochemistry of immunoglobulins and antigens, were helpful in understanding how substances could be assayed this way. The student learned that the detection system in the Athena IV immunoassay analyzer was a photodetector like a spectrophotometer. Also, he learned that chemiluminescence involves a chemical reaction that produces light, and it follows Beer's law in determining the unknown concentration of the analyte using measured light. ●

> **CASE SCENARIO 3-7**
>
> **Automation: How Does It Work?**
> The next week the student was back in high-volume chemistry. "You have seen many types of instrumentation," said the supervisor. "Automation is crucial to this laboratory. We report out over 300 chemistry laboratory results every day. We couldn't do that without automation because it is just too time-consuming to do this many tests by hand. Many of the chemical reactions must be carefully controlled by a computerized system." As the student loaded the Hercules III, he thought about the types of automation that he had seen. Later that day, the student was given time to read the analyzer's operating manual to understand how it works and further explore the calculations it uses to determine test results.

AUTOMATION

single-channel - able to perform only one test with a dedicated portion of the instrument

multichannel - able to perform a variety of tests at the same time with separate dedicated instrument components

discrete analysis - test reactions occur in separate compartments

continuous flow analysis - each sample passes through the same stream and reactions as all other samples, with only a brief washout phase between samples

random access - test reactions can be programmed to occur in a variety of sequences

batch analysis - a group of samples are analyzed at the same time for the same test

sequential analysis - performing a set of test reactions in a particular order on each sample in the order in which it is received

centrifugal analysis - using centrifugal force to achieve chemical reaction and analysis

Automation is the process of using a machine to perform steps in laboratory testing with only minimal involvement by the analyst. If one considers all of the steps needed to produce laboratory results from a given sample, at least nine separate steps can be identified. These include specimen identification, specimen volume measuring, sample pretreatment, reagent volume measuring, sample and reagent mixing, incubation, reaction timing and reaction analysis and calculations, and result presentation on a visual screen and/or in print. Automation can handle all or some of these steps. Automation may also involve specimen transport as well as reagent storage.

Many terms are to describe automated systems, including **single-channel** or **multichannel**, **discrete analysis**, **continuous flow analysis**, **random access**, **batch analysis**, **sequential analysis**, and **centrifugal analysis**. It is helpful to have an understanding of these terms as they are used in operating manuals and manufacturer's literature. *Discrete analysis* means that each test reaction takes place in a separate compartment that is either cleaned out or disposed of after use. Many general analyzers and immunoassay analyzers are discrete. *Random access* means that test reactions can be programmed to occur in a different order than the samples are placed on the instrument, and specific tests can be programmed for each sample. This is helpful when many samples are placed on an analyzer and are processing but an urgent test request must be added later. *Sequential analysis* means that all samples are processed in the order they are received, and multiple tests are performed in a certain order. These terms will be described further with examples.

Historically, the earliest automated instruments used either continuous flow or centrifugal analysis. In continuous flow analyzers, samples were aspirated into tubing to introduce samples into a sample holder, bring in reagent, create a chemical reaction, and then pump the chromagen solution into a flow-through cuvette for spectrophotometric analysis. Figure 3–25 depicts the flow-through process. The first analyzers were single channel, dedicated to only one test reaction. Sodium and potassium were measured in a multichannel analyzer by flame photometry, in which the sample was mixed with internal standard and then flowed into a flame.

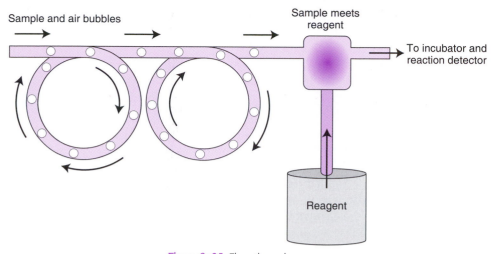

Figure 3–25. Flow-through process.

Emitted light was measured by a photometer. Sample **carryover** was a problem even when air bubbles or **washout** steps were used to clean out sample tubing and test reaction solutions between samples.

The flow-through process is currently utilized with instruments containing electrodes in which the sample is aspirated into tubing, pumped into electrode assemblies where electrochemical reactions occur, and finally rinsed into a waste container with a wash solution.

Centrifugal Analyzers

Centrifugal analyzers were developed as a result of space-aged technology and were one of the first types of discrete analyzers. Samples and reagents were mixed together, reacted, and flowed by centrifugal force into separate cuvettes in which spectrophotometric analysis could occur. These analyzers were capable of performing a batch of one type of test to completion. Then, after a washing out phase and setting up phase, a new batch of a different test could be performed. All patient test results were reported out at once for a particular batch.[5]

Continuous Flow Analyzers

Continuous flow analyzers are still used in some high-volume, multichannel analyzers that employ electrochemistry because the process is a rapid way of introducing samples to the ion-selective electrodes. Carryover is minimized since the products of electrochemistry are ions of low concentrations rather than a large amount of chromagen. However, air bubbles and wash fluids are used to remove remnants of sample before the next one flows in. Continuous flow is also used in some spectrophotometric instruments in which the chemical reaction occurs in one reaction channel and then is rinsed out and reused for the next sample, which may be an entirely different chemical reaction. Since disposable reaction cells are not used and liquid reagents are used, cost is low per test. Sample carryover is mini-

carryover - a sampling problem that occurs when remnants of a previous sample or test reaction product affect later samples

washout - water or wash solution flowing through a chamber after a sample has passed through it in order to clean it out and prevent carryover

mized by the use of air bubbles and an inert coating substance that forms a reaction capsule.[1]

Discrete Analyzers

Discrete analysis is also commonly used in many types of analyzers in clinical chemistry. Sample reactions are kept discrete through the use of separate reaction cuvettes, cells, slides, or wells that are disposed of following chemical analysis. This keeps sample and reaction carryover to a minimum but increases the cost per test due to disposable products. One system uses multiple layers of dry reagent embedded into gel layers compiled onto a plastic slide the size of a postage stamp. This dry slide system only introduces liquid from the patient sample and, although is more costly due to the disposable components, generates only dry waste. Some discrete systems reuse the reaction cuvette by thoroughly washing, rinsing with pure water, and drying it between patient samples. This technique helps to minimize cost by limiting disposable components as well as minimizing sample and test carryover.[1]

Specimen Identification

Automated instruments handle the stages of specimen testing in different ways. The sample container, whether it is a cup or the original tube, must be properly labeled so that it can be traced back to the original patient sample and matched to the patient identification information and test requisition form. Barcode labels can be applied to sample tubes that fit onto analyzers to make identification and pairing of the sample with the results easier. If sample cups or test tube samples are needed for the testing, it is important to properly label each sample cup with identifiers in order to trace back to the patient specimen and to match the identifier on test results. It is important to minimize the length of time that a sample tube or cup is open to the air since these conditions affect electrolyte and other test results. Some analyzers provide a lid that covers all patient samples during and after analysis. If the analyzer doesn't provide a sample cover, one must be place by laboratory personnel to maintain the stability of chemical analytes.

Sample Pretreatment

Proteins are present in large concentrations in serum (e.g., albumin at 35 g/L) and may interfere with some analyses. The effect of protein interference can be lessened by sample pretreatment. This is achieved usually by adding a large amount of diluent to dilute out interfering substances such as protein. Pretreatments may involve removal of protein with extraction reagents. Some therapeutic drugs, nonprotein hormones, and other analytes may be bound to protein in order to facilitate transport in blood. It may be necessary to remove protein for some assays to separate the free from protein-bound forms. This is often achieved with simple column chromatography incorporated into the automated method or by a precipitation and centrifugation step. Removal of proteins is often not needed with most basic chemistry tests. Diluting the sample prior to addition of reacting reagents can negate the effect of proteins. Instead of diluting the sample, one analyzer system has a top-spreading layer of film that traps proteins and prevents them from reaching the chemical reaction layer.

Reagent Handling and Pipetting

Reagents are stored by automated analyzers in room-temperature and refrigerated compartments. Small refrigeration compartments with computerized sensors monitoring the temperature and inventory of reagents are used to store labile reagents. Many systems use liquid reagents. Those that are flexible as to the source of their liquid reagents are called **open reagent systems**. Systems in which you can only purchase prepackaged reagents from the instrument manufacturer are called closed systems. These **closed reagent systems** may be more expensive due to lack of competition among vendors, but the quality of each reagent shipment should be more consistent. Reagent containers often contain barcode labels for ease of identification by the instrument and help in maintaining inventory.[6] Specimen volume and reagent measuring is usually done by positive displacement pipettes and tubing, with pumps generating suction to aspirate the sample and reagent volumes and deliver them to a reaction cell.

The Chemical Reaction

Sample and reagent mixing is performed by a variety of techniques, including centrifugal force, sound waves, vibration, stirring paddles, and a physical beater. Incubating in a carefully controlled heating block is necessary for enzyme-catalyzed reactions and is required by many testing methods. Reaction timing is carefully controlled by computerized timing devices that may control pumps or chains or other physical steps to move the reaction cell through the system.

Reaction Analysis

Reaction analysis is achieved at the end of the incubation phase by endpoint or continuous monitoring of light transmittance using spectrophotometry for most analytes. Ions are commonly measured by changes in potentiometry using ion-selective electrodes. A microprocessor performs calculations to convert absorbance or other measurements into units of concentration based on a standard curve. Test Methodology 3–17 describes a random-access automated method with a standard curve preparation for the calculation of unknown results.

Result Reporting

Patient and quality control results are then presented on a visual screen and printed on paper. Often, results can be sent to the electronic patient chart that is stored in the database of the hospital computer system. Sophisticated sensors send signals to the computer system to warn the operator of errors or problems of analysis. Warning sounds alert the operator to immediate technical problems; error flags on the laboratory report indicate results that must be verified. These cautionary activities provide continuous quality assurance of the technical process. For an example of the calculations in Test Methodology 3–17, see Table 3–11 and Figure 3–26.

open reagent system - analytical system that allows many sources for reagents

closed reagent system - analytical system for which the reagents, in a unique container or format, are provided only by the manufacturer

✓ **Common Sense Check**
Avoid loose clothing or dangling hair or jewelry that can get tangled in the moving parts of an analyzer, especially when it is opened up for maintenance. Gloves should be worn when handling all specimens and reagents to protect the skin. Protective eyewear may be necessary if aerosols are generated at the point of sampling.

TEST METHODOLOGY 3-17.   DISCRETE ANALYSIS WITH THE HERCULES III

The Reaction Principle

The Hercules is a random-access floor model system that uses disposable reaction cuvettes and concentrated liquid reagents that are automatically diluted prior to use. Instrumentation includes ion-selective electrodes for measurement of sodium, potassium, and chloride. The Hercules III can produce 400 results per hour (the test throughput). The test menu has 150 choices of analytes. Data entry can be with a keyboard and terminal or with a barcode and wand.

The sample wheel holds 50 patient samples in their original tubes with a piercing probe to enter through the tube stopper. Short samples can be placed in a labeled sample cup and are positioned in an alternate sample turntable, also used for quality control samples and STAT samples. Spectrophotometric readings are taken at 36-second intervals and used for both endpoint and kinetic reactions to ensure reaction stability. A second, bichromatic wavelength is also used to eliminate absorbance readings due to sample color or hemolysis. Results print on paper and can be transferred via computer interface to a hospital patient database. Online monitoring of all aspects of the system is achieved by electronic sensors, alarms, and troubleshooting codes that print in case of problems.

Calibration Steps

1. Following the kit manufacturer's instructions, four well-mixed fresh standards of various concentrations are analyzed to include the medical decision limits and upper limit of linearity of the procedure.
2. Absorbance of each standard is plotted on the ordinate (y axis), with its corresponding concentration on the abscissa (x axis), by the instrument microprocessor.
3. Linear regression is performed and a best-fit line is plotted through the 0,0 axis. Outliers are eliminated from the line.
4. The microprocessor calculates slope, y-intercept, and best-fit line using linear regression statistics and prints out results.
5. The operator must determine whether the curve meets the manufacturer's guidelines for intercept and slope. Intercept should always be close to 0, but unlike some linear regression results, slope will not always be 1.0.

The Calculations

The unknown concentrations are determined by the microprocessor as a reading from the best-fit line or by using the following regression formula: $y = bx + a$, where y is the measured absorbance of the unknown, "b" is the slope, x is the concentration to be determined, and "a" is the y-intercept. For example:

$$y = 0.044\,x + 0.0006$$

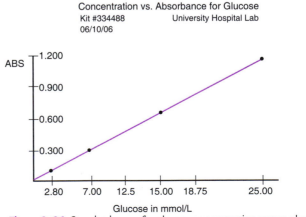

Concentration vs. Absorbance for Glucose

Kit #334488   University Hospital Lab
06/10/06

Figure 3–26. Standard curve for glucose concentration versus absorbance.

TABLE 3-11

Glucose Standards and Their Absorbance Using the Manual Glucose Method, Kit #334488

Concentration (mmol/L)	Abs.
2.8	0.125
7.0	0.310
15.0	0.665
25.0	1.101

Case Scenario 3-7 Automation: How Does It Work?

Follow-Up

The student arrived at the high-volume clinical chemistry laboratory with basic knowledge of principles of instrumentation. He left with understanding of the similarities and differences of large-volume automated instruments. ●

Total Laboratory Automation

As described previously, steps of the analytical and postanalytical phase of testing commonly can be performed by an automated clinical chemistry analyzer. The steps that must still be performed manually include those of the preanalytical phase, beginning with collection of the blood sample, labeling, transport, storage, and processing, including centrifugation. However, since the 1980s some preanalytical steps have been handled by automation. Many institutions have a robotic or mechanical transport mechanism from the patient's site to the laboratory. In addition, some laboratories also have a robotic system that centrifuges, de-caps, and splits sample aliquots, transports samples to the analyzer, and places them onto the instrument. Those specimens have been labeled with a barcode at the bedside that can be read by the robotic transport system as well as the analyzer identification station so that specimens can be tracked. Although these systems are available, they are usually only implemented in large reference laboratories since the need for total automation precludes their use for facilities that process low numbers of specimens.[5]

FUTURE INSTRUMENTATION PRINCIPLES IN CLINICAL CHEMISTRY

Miniaturization of analyzers has continued since automation was first introduced in the 1950s. Ion-selective electrodes have become smaller and can now be placed in hand-held devices. As memory capacity expands, microprocessors and computers are becoming smaller in size. Minute electronic components called *microchip devices* have been developed to carry out electrophoresis separation of proteins with immunoassay quantification.[6] Work is underway to create even smaller electronic devices that help to perform clinical diagnostic testing. The term *nanotechnology* is used to describe many types of devices in which the characteristic dimensions are very small (<1000 nm). Future trends in clinical chemistry testing will include the use of smaller and smaller diagnostic components.[7]

Instrumentation that can perform testing without requiring a blood sample from venipuncture or skin puncture is called *noninvasive*. Several noninvasive or minimally invasive instruments have been developed, including those for transcutaneous oxygen saturation, glucose, and bilirubin testing.[8] Limitations to miniaturization or noninvasive technology at this point seem to be based on the concentration of the analyte desired for testing compared to other chemicals present in that same body fluid.

SUMMARY

Much has happened in clinical chemistry testing since Dr. Folin helped to develop many of the basic biochemical reactions. Many aspects of clinical testing have become automated, including specimen labeling, transport, complex analysis, and result reporting. However, some elements have remained the same, including use of endpoint detection of chemical reactions with spectrophotometry and electrochemistry. The fundamental calculations and principles learned in general chemistry and physical science (physics) are foundations for these methods of testing. In this chapter, we joined a clinical laboratory science student as he learned about working in clinical chemistry, applying some of the biochemical principles and aspects of analysis learned in introductory chapters of this textbook. Table 3–12 reviews the general calculations most commonly used in clinical chemistry. Table 3–13 reviews the important safety practices described in this chapter.

TABLE 3-12

Summary of Calculations

Dilutions with specific volume specified	$C_1V_1 = C_2V_2$
Dilutions without specified volume	sample volume/(sample + diluent volume)
Simple conversions	1 deciliter = 0.1 L; 1 gram = 1000 mg; 1000 microliters = 1 mL
Concentrations	% w/v = number of g/100 mL
Concentrations	1-mol/L HCl has 36 g HCl/liter H_2O (A.M. H = 1.0, A.M. Cl = 35)
Conversion of concentrations	g/dL to mol/L = $\dfrac{g \times 10\ dL \times 1\ mol}{dL \times 1\ L \times g\ M.M.}$
Conversion of concentrations	mol/L to g/dL = $\dfrac{mol \times 1\ L \times g}{L \times 10\ dL \times 1\ mol}$
Conversion of concentrations	g/mL to molarity = $\dfrac{g \times assay\ purity\ (decimal\ form) \times mol \times 1000\ mL}{mL \times molecular\ mass \times 1\ L}$
Conversion of concentrations	pH = log $(1/H^+)$ in mol/L for strong acid

TABLE 3-12 (continued)

Summary of Calculations

Conversion of concentrations	$pH = pK_a + \log (HCO_3^-/H_2CO_3)$ for carbonic acid
% Accuracy	% accuracy $= \dfrac{\text{actual volume from pipette}}{\text{expected or nominal volume}} \times 100$
% Precision	% precision $= \dfrac{\text{standard deviation}}{\text{mean volume}} \times 100$
Centrifuge calibration	$RCF = 1.12 \times 10^{-5} \times r \times rpm^2$
Spectrophotometry	$A = a\,b\,c$
Spectrophotometry	$A = 2 - \log \%T$
Spectrophotometry	$C_{unk} = C_{std}/A_{std} \times A_{unk}$
Osmometry	1.86 (Na [mmol/L]) + (glucose [mg/dL]/18) + (urea N [mg/dL]/2.8) + 9
Protein densitometry	% protein fraction $\times$ total protein (g/dL) = protein fraction (g/dL)

TABLE 3-13

Summary of Safety Features

- When using concentrated acids, bases, or volatile liquids, you should open the containers and measure volumes in a chemical fume hood so that harmful vapors are not inhaled by you or those around you.
- Add concentrated acids and bases to the diluting water to prevent a strong chemical reaction and possible spattering that could occur if water is instead added to the concentrated acid or base.
- Use a mechanical suction bulb to aspirate with a glass pipette rather than using your mouth to create suction. This would avoid accidentally aspirating harmful reagents, biohazards, or even soap.
- Wear gloves when aspirating chemical reagents or biohazardous fluids to prevent skin damage or pathogens entering into minute cuts in your skin.
- Balance the load in a centrifuge to prevent serious vibrations that can break the test tubes, spilling the contents within. If the imbalance generates enough force, the centrifuge can fall over and cause serious damage and endanger the people in its vicinity.
- Avoid making aerosols. Aerosols can be generated during vigorous shaking, when a vacuum is released, and during centrifugation. Aerosols can be prevented by keeping the samples covered during centrifugation and by keeping the centrifuge lid covered during operation until the head comes to a complete stop.
- Avoid loose clothing or dangling hair or jewelry that can get tangled in moving parts of an analyzer, especially when it is opened up for maintenance. Gloves should be worn when handling all specimens and reagents to protect the skin. Protective eyewear may be necessary if aerosols may be generated at the point of sampling.

EXERCISES

As you consider the scenarios presented in this chapter, answer the following questions:

1. Calculate how much stock 10 molar acetic acid is needed to make 250 mL of 2.0 molar acetic acid.

2. Convert mg/dL to mmol/L for calcium.

3. Describe how to prepare a 1/10 dilution of patient serum using pure water for a procedure that requires 50 μL for a procedure. It is recommended to make slightly more that double the total volume needed in case the procedure must be repeated.

4. Explain how to make 500 mL of 0.3 molar NaOH from an available stock solution that has 1.50 g/mL with 59% purity.

5. Describe the appropriate use of a volumetric flask, a graduated cylinder, a volumetric pipette, and a mechanical one-stop micropipette for making up a glucose standard dilution, reagent preparation, stock standard solution, and patient sample dilution.

6. Discuss the proper use of a centrifuge for spinning down clotted blood specimens, including safe practices.

7. Differentiate potentiometry (ISE) from polarography using a simple description of the electrodes involved, what is measured as the endpoint, and an example analyte.

8. Differentiate chemiluminescent immunoassay from enzyme immunoassay in terms of the type of label on the antibody and how the chemical reaction proceeds and is measured.

9. What is the difference between continuous flow automation and discrete analysis?

10. Using as an example the Jaffe reaction for serum creatinine, what steps could be performed by automation?

References

1. Bermes EW, Kahn SE, Young DS: Introduction to principles of laboratory analyses and safety. In Ashwood ER, Burtis CA, Bruns DE (eds): *Tietz Textbook of Clinical Chemistry and Molecular Diagnostics*. Philadelphia: WB Saunders, 2006.

2. Uldall A, et al: International Federation of Clinical Chemistry (IFCC) Scientific Division, Committee on Analytical Systems: Guidelines (1990) for selection of safe laboratory centrifuges and for their safe use with general purpose appendices concerning centrifuge nomenclature, quantities and units, and calculation of centrifugal acceleration. *Clin Chim Acta* 1991; 202(1-2):S23–S40.

3. Freeman V: Spectrophotometry. In Haven M, Tetrault G, Schenken J (eds): *Laboratory Instrumentation*, ed 4. New York: Van Nostrand Reinhold, 1995.

4. Ettre LS: The centenary of the invention of chromatography. *J Chromatogr Sci* 2003; 41:225–226.

5. Tetrault G: Automated chemistry analyzers. In Haven M, Tetrault G, Schenken J (eds): *Laboratory Instrumentation*, ed 4. New York: Van Nostrand Reinhold, 1995

6. Boyd JA, Hawker C: Automation in the clinical laboratory. In Burtis CA, Ashwood ER (eds): *Tietz Textbook of Clinical Chemistry*, ed 2. Philadelphia: WB Saunders, 1994.

7. Wilding P, et al: Manipulation and flow of biological fluids in straight channels micromachined in silicon. *Clin Chem* 1994; 40:43–47.

8. Maisels MJ, Kring E: Transcutaneous bilirubinometry decreases the need for serum bilirubin measurements and saves money. *Pediatrics* 1997; 99:599–601.

4

Evidenced-based criteria for the diagnosis and assessment of carbohydrate disorders direct the choice of the laboratory testing that is provided for the health care team.

Diabetes and Other Carbohydrate Disorders

Jean Brickell, Vicki Freeman, and Wendy Arneson

This chapter describes the role of the laboratory in assessing and monitoring diseases of carbohydrate metabolism. The chapter emphasizes the role of laboratory in the most common disorder of carbohydrate metabolism, diabetes mellitus, with a focus on the measurement of glucose. The chapter also explores the assessment of the metabolism of **disaccharides**, **polysaccharides**, and **monosaccharides** other than glucose. Please refer to Chapter 1, The Biochemistry of Disease, for a discussion of the metabolic pathways of carbohydrates.

disaccharides - simple carbohydrates composed of two monosaccharides

polysaccharides - complex carbohydrates composed of more than 20 monosaccharides

monosaccharides - simple carbohydrates that cannot be broken down to further sugars by hydrolysis

etiology - the cause of disease

sulfonylurea - one of a class of oral drugs used to control hyperglycemia in type 2 diabetes mellitus

benzoic acid analog - a compound that is structurally similar to $C_7H_6O_2$ and used for control of type 2 diabetes

alpha-glucosidase inhibitor - blocks hydrolysis of an alpha glucoside for control of type 2 diabetes

glycemic - pertaining to control of blood glucose levels

infiltration - deposition and accumulation of an external substance within a cell, tissue, or organ

glycogenesis - formation of glycogen

lipogenesis - formation of fats

gluconeogenesis - formation of glucose from excess amino acids, fats, or other noncarbohydrate sources

glycogenolysis - glycogen stored in the liver and muscles is converted to glucose 1-phosphate and then to glucose 6-phosphate

OBJECTIVES

Upon completion of this chapter, the student will have the ability to

▰ Describe the Clinical Practice Guidelines of the American Diabetes Association for classification, diagnosis, and assessment of diabetes mellitus.

▰ List common preanalytical errors resulting from improper specimen collection and handling for glucose, ketones, lactate, and glycated hemoglobin.

▰ Describe the principles of glucose, ketone, and glycated hemoglobin analyses, including commonly encountered sources of analytical interferences.

▰ Compare results of carbohydrate and ketone testing with expected and previous findings and correlate results with pathology.

▰ Suggest appropriate course of action that is needed when encountering common sources of discrepancies in patient test results.

DIABETES MELLITUS

Diabetes is a family of disorders that is characterized by hyperglycemia. The disorders of diabetes differ in their **etiology** and symptoms and in the consequences of disease. The American Diabetes Association (ADA) estimates that approximately 7% of the population of America suffers from diabetes. Therefore, it is a serious public health threat and economic burden on health care funds.[1–3]

Timely, specific therapeutic intervention may reduce the serious consequences of diabetes. To aid the physician in choosing appropriate therapy, the laboratory plays a role in diagnosis of the disease, identification of the type of the disorder, and assessment of progression of the tissue damage. Insulin replacement, diet management, and exercise have been shown to reduce the consequences of type 1 diabetes mellitus. Type 2 diabetes mellitus is best controlled by weight loss, diet management, and drug therapy, such as **sulfonylureas**, **benzoic acid analogs**, metformin, thiazolidinediones, and **alpha glucosidase inhibitors**. Insulin may be prescribed for type 2 diabetics who fail to achieve **glycemic** control with other measures. The therapeutic goal for both type 1 and type 2 diabetics is glycemic control, that is, maintaining blood glucose at or near normal concentration levels.

The current criteria for diagnosis of diabetes rely on the etiology of disease. Four forms of diabetes have been classified. These four forms are type 1, type 2, gestational diabetes, and other specific causes of diabetes. The etiologies of these four forms of diabetes are described in detail in Table 4–1.

Type 1 diabetes is characterized by lack of insulin production and secretion by the beta cells of the pancreas. One cause of the hyperglycemia of type 1 diabetes mellitus is an autoimmune destruction of the beta cells of the pancreas. The cell-mediated response causes **infiltration** of the pancreas and reduction in the volume of beta cells. As a protein hormone, insulin acts through chemical responses to receptors on the cells of target tissues. In the muscle, insulin stimulates glucose uptake into cells and enhances **glycogenesis**. In adipose tissue, insulin stimulates glucose uptake into cells and enhances **lipogenesis**. In the liver, insulin has a negative effect, inhibiting **gluconeogenesis** and **glycogenolysis**. Autoantibodies are present in the circulation of many individuals with type 1 diabetes. There appears to be a genetic susceptibility to development of autoantibodies, with certain histocompatibility antigens predominant in the type 1 diabetes population. However, the development of disease is complex; triggering factors, such as rubella, mumps,

TABLE 4-1

Etiologic Classification of Diabetes Mellitus

Type 1 diabetes (beta cell destruction, usually leading to absolute insulin deficiency)
  Immune mediated
  Idiopathic
Type 2 diabetes (may range from predominantly insulin resistance with relative insulin
  deficiency to a predominantly secretory defect with insulin resistance)
Gestational diabetes mellitus (GDM)
Other specific types
  Genetic defects of beta cell function
  Genetic defects in insulin action
  Diseases of the exocrine pancreas
  Endocrinopathies
  Drug- or chemical-induced
  Infections
  Uncommon forms of immune-mediated diabetes

Source: American Diabetes Association: Diagnosis and classification of diabetes mellitus. *Diabetes Care* 2006; 29(Suppl 1); reprinted with permission.

and other viral infection, and chemical contact may be necessary for progression of disease.[4]

Type 2 diabetes is characterized by decline in insulin action due to the resistance of tissue cells to the action of insulin. The problem is intensified by the inability of the beta cells of the pancreas to produce enough insulin to counteract the resistance. Thus, type 2 diabetes is a disorder of both insulin resistance and relative deficiency of insulin. Insulin resistance syndrome, also known as metabolic syndrome and syndrome X, affects the metabolism of many nutrients, including glucose, triglycerides, and high-density lipoprotein (HDL) cholesterol. Individuals who are diagnosed with metabolic syndrome may show abdominal **obesity** and high blood pressure. Such individuals are at increased risk for cardiovascular disease. Metabolic syndrome is explored further in Chapter 10 (Assessment of Nutrition and Digestive Function). The etiology of type 2 diabetes is complex and multifaceted. There is evidence to show that there is an association of obesity with the development of type 2 diabetes. Other factors, such as family history of type 2 diabetes and lack of physical activity, have also been associated with the disorder. Previous diagnosis of gestational diabetes is a risk factor for type 2 diabetes, as are increasing age, hypertension, and dyslipidemia. Increased risk for developing the disease is also associated with membership in certain racial and ethnic groups, such as African-Americans, Hispanic-Americans, Native Americans, Asian-Americans, and Pacific Islanders.[5]

Gestational diabetes is similar in etiology to type 2 diabetes; however, it is defined as diabetes that is diagnosed in pregnancy. Pregnancy is associated with increased tissue cell resistance to insulin. Most pregnant women will compensate with increased secretion of insulin; those individuals who are unable to compensate may develop gestational diabetes. The hyperglycemia of gestational diabetes diminishes after delivery; however, the individual who has developed gestational diabetes is at higher risk for the development of type 2 diabetes thereafter.

The fourth form of diabetes is termed *other specific causes of diabetes*, and was previously called secondary diabetes. This form of hyperglycemia may be the

obesity - body mass index ≥ 30 kg/m^2

protease inhibitor - a medication that inhibits the action of enzymes

glucocorticoids - adrenal cortical hormones primarily active in protecting against stress and affecting protein and carbohydrate metabolism

ketoacidosis - the accumulation of keto acids in the blood causing metabolic acidosis

CLINICAL CORRELATION
Type 1 and type 2 diabetes mellitus differ in their clinical presentation as well as their etiology. Type 1 diabetics are usually younger and thinner than type 2 diabetics. Type 1 diabetics present with acute symptoms, while type 2 diabetes develops more slowly over time. Type 1 diabetics are more prone to develop ketoacidosis than type 2 diabetics.

secondary result of non–insulin-related events. Blood glucose levels are increased in endocrine disorders, such as Cushing's syndrome; in exocrine disorders, such as cystic fibrosis; and as a response to specific drugs, such as **protease inhibitors** and **glucocorticoids**. Other causes of this form of diabetes are the result of genetic defects that affect pancreatic beta cells or the action of insulin.

The disorders of diabetes differ in their presentation as well as their etiology. Approximately 10% of diabetics are of the type 1 variety. The type 1 disease state usually occurs as acute illness, while type 2 diabetes progresses slowly over time. Type 1 glucose blood levels are usually more severe than type 2. Type 1 diabetics are more likely to develop **ketoacidosis** than are type 2 diabetics. Due to the etiology of disease, type 1 diabetics are insulin dependent, while most type 2 diabetics are not. Type 1 diabetics are younger (<18 years old when diagnosed) and thinner; type 2 diabetics are usually older (>40 years old when diagnosed) and more likely to be obese. However, these characteristics of presentation are not uniform to all type 1 and type 2 diabetics. Type 1 diabetes may be diagnosed after the age of 18 years. Type 2 diabetes may develop in obese children. Type 2 diabetics may need insulin if glycemia cannot be controlled by other measures.

Carbohydrate metabolism, including glucose metabolism, is regulated by the action and counteraction of the endocrine system. Two hormones, insulin and glucagon, have predominant influence on the pathways of carbohydrate metabolism. The actions of these two hormones counteract each other. Insulin is released in response to increased blood glucose. Insulin acts upon the membrane-bound receptors of tissue cells to allow the movement of glucose in the cell. Insulin also stimulates glycogenesis, lipogenesis, and glycolysis and inhibits glycogenolysis. Glucagon is released in response to a need for increased blood glucose. Glucagon stimulates glycogenolysis and gluconeogenesis. Insulin and glucagons are both produced in the pancreas, insulin in the beta cells and glucagons in alpha cells of the islets of Langerhans.

Other hormones also affect carbohydrate metabolism. Epinephrine, a hormone that is released by the adrenal medulla at times of stress, inhibits insulin secretion and stimulates glycogenolysis and lipolysis. Glucocorticoids, such as cortisol, are released from the adrenal cortex to reduce blood glucose concentration by inhibiting gluconeogenesis the absorption of dietary glucose. Thyroxine, a thyroid hormone, increases glycogenolysis and gluconeogenesis and inhibits absorption of dietary glucose through the intestine.

Glucose Challenge Test and Other Diagnostic Tests

The hallmarks of the laboratory's role in diagnosis of type 1 and type 2 diabetes are the fasting glucose test and the glucose challenge test. For 3 days before the challenge test, the patient should consume at least the minimum daily requirement of carbohydrates and exercise normally. An overnight fast of 10 to 16 hours is required the night before the test. The patient should not smoke or take medications on the morning of the test. Only water is allowed during the testing period. Blood is drawn before the ingestion of glucose liquid and at 2 hours after ingestion. The time period starts when the patient begins to drink the glucose liquid; all the liquid should be consumed within 5 minutes. Seventy-five grams of glucose are given to adults; children are given 1.75 g/kg of weight, but not more than 75 g. If testing will occur within 1 hour of the draw, blood is collected without anticoagulant and serum is tested. Blood may be collected into a gray-top vacuum tube, which contains sodium fluoride and sodium or potassium oxalate, if there will be

TABLE 4-2

Reference Ranges for Blood Glucose Levels

	Normal	Impaired	Indication of Diabetes
Fasting blood glucose (mg/dL)	70–99	100–125	≥126
2-Hour postprandial blood glucose (mg/dL)	<140	140–200	≥200

delay in testing. The preservative sodium fluoride will reduce glycolysis for up to 24 hours at room temperature. Several methods for testing for blood glucose are available. Reference ranges for interpretation of blood glucose results for the glucose challenge are provided in Table 4–2.

Another test for glucose, the random (or casual) blood glucose test, may also be measured to aid in the diagnosis of diabetes. A random blood glucose of greater than or equal to 200 mg/dL in an individual with symptoms of diabetes, such as **polyuria**, **polyphagia**, and **polydipsia**, is also indicative of diabetes. Table 4–3 lists the ADA criteria for diagnosis of diabetes mellitus.

Diabetes cannot be diagnosed by testing urine for glucose. The renal threshold, or the blood level at which a substance will appear in the urine, for glucose is approximately 175 mg/dL. At that level, urine testing would not identify an individual at the diagnostic level for fasting blood glucose, 126 mg/dL, and would not distinguish between diabetic and nondiabetic individuals adequately.

Patients who are at risk for gestational diabetes are given a one-step or two-step glucose challenge. As the first step in the two-step challenge, the patient is given a 50-g glucose load. The patient need not be fasting for the test. Blood is drawn for glucose testing at 1 hour after ingestion of the glucose solution. A 1-hour glucose level of less than 140 mg/dL rules out a frank diagnosis of gestational diabetes. Patients who have 1-hour levels of greater than or equal to 140 mg/dL are challenged with a 3-hour glucose tolerance test. The glucose load for a 3-hour toler-

THE TEAM APPROACH
The administration of a glucose challenge test is a team effort. Laboratory staff rely on nursing staff to provide fasting instructions. The integrity of the test result depends upon the reliability of patient preparation.

polyuria - excessive secretion and discharge of urine

polyphagia - excessive hunger

polydipsia - excessive thirst

✓ **Common Sense Check**
A positive test for glucose in urine suggests that the blood glucose level is above 175 mg/dL.

TABLE 4-3

Criteria for the Diagnosis of Diabetes Mellitus*

1. Symptoms of diabetes plus random (casual) plasma glucose concentration ≥200 mg/dL (11.1 mmol/L). *Random* is defined as any time of day without regard to time since last meal. The classic symptoms of diabetes include polyuria, polydipsia, polyphagia, and unexplained weight loss.

OR

2. Fasting plasma glucose (FPG) ≥126 mg/dL (7.0 mmol/L). *Fasting* is defined as no caloric intake for at least 8 hours.

OR

3. 2-Hour postload glucose ≥200 mg/dL (11.1 mmol/L) during an oral glucose tolerance test, using a glucose load containing the equivalent of 75 g anhydrous glucose dissolved in water.

*These criteria should be confirmed by repeat testing on a different day. The 3-hour oral glucose tolerance test (OGTT) is not recommended for routine clinical use.

Source: American Diabetes Association: Diagnosis and classification of diabetes mellitus. *Diabetes Care* 2006; 29(Suppl 1); reprinted with permission.

ance test is 100 g. Blood is drawn at fasting, and at 1, 2, and 3 hours postingestion. Diagnosis of gestational diabetes is made if any two of the following results are observed:

Fasting blood glucose: ≥95 mg/dL
1 hour blood glucose: ≥180 mg/dL
2 hour blood glucose: ≥155 mg/dL
3 hour blood glucose: ≥140 mg/dL

Alternatively, the patient may be given 75g of glucose for the tolerance test. Criteria for fasting, 1-hour, and 2-hour glucose levels are the same as the 100-g glucose tolerance test; however, a 3-hour blood test is not drawn.

For the one-step approach, the glucose tolerance test is performed directly without the 50-g glucose screening test. This approach is best used for women who are at high risk for development of gestational diabetes based on personal and family history and examination findings. Test Methodology 4–1 presents the specifics of glucose testing.

TEST METHODOLOGY 4-1.   GLUCOSE

Current procedures that measure glucose use enzymatic methodology.

The Reaction: Enzymatic Method

Three enzymatic approaches to the measurement of glucose have been explored. Enzymatic methods are specific for glucose.

The *hexokinase method* is the reference method for glucose. The method involves two coupled reactions:

$$\text{Glucose} + \text{ATP} \xrightarrow{\text{hexokinase, Mg}^{2+}} \text{G6PO}_4 + \text{ADP}$$

$$\text{G6PO}_4 + \text{NADP}^+ \xrightarrow{\text{G6PD}} \text{6-phosphogluconate} + \text{NADPH} + \text{H}^+$$

The increase in absorbance of NADPH at 340 nm is measured as directly proportional to glucose. The hexokinase reaction may also be coupled to an indicator reaction and measured through the development of a colored product.

The *glucose oxidase method* is specific for beta-D-glucose. The initial reaction:

$$\beta\text{-D-Glucose} + \text{O}_2 \xrightarrow{\text{glucose oxidase}} \text{gluconic acid} + \text{H}_2\text{O}_2$$

may be coupled with a peroxidase indicator reaction:

$$\text{H}_2\text{O}_2 + \text{reduced chromagen} \xrightarrow{\text{peroxidase}} \text{oxidized chromogen} + \text{H}_2\text{O}$$

or may be assessed by measuring oxygen consumption, using an oxygen electrode. The *glucose dehydrogenase method* involves the measurement of NADH production:

$$\text{Glucose} + \text{NAD}^+ \xrightarrow{\text{glucose dehydrogenase}} \text{D-gluconolactone} + \text{NADH} + \text{H}^+$$

The Specimen

Glucose in serum, plasma, and cerebrospinal fluid (CSF) may be measured by these methods. Glucose levels in serum or plasma are 10% to 15% higher than those in whole blood. Serum or plasma must be separated within 1 hour to prevent degradation by glycolysis. Glucose is stable for 24 hours in whole blood when preserved with sodium fluoride.

Reference Ranges

Serum or plasma (fasting)	74–100 mg/dL
CSF	60% of serum or plasma level

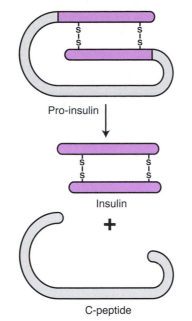

Figure 4–1. Proinsulin, insulin, and C-peptide.

Since type 1 diabetes is characterized by low levels of insulin and type 2 diabetes is usually characterized by normal or high levels of insulin, it might appear that the results of blood insulin tests would be the means for distinguishing between type 1 and type 2 diabetes. However, the difficulty in measuring this hormone accurately diminishes its usefulness for diagnosis. Large differences in results have been noted between laboratories using the same analytical methods to measure insulin.[6] In addition, the specimen that is tested may contain exogenous insulin that the patient is receiving as insulin treatment, or antibodies to insulin that can interfere with measurement.

Concentration of C-peptide reflects the production of endogenous insulin by the pancreas. Insulin is stored in the pancreas as the biologically inactive protein proinsulin. Proinsulin is cleaved into the active hormone, insulin, and an inactive peptide, C-peptide. Figure 4–1 illustrates this molecule. Therefore, the concentration of C-peptide represents the concentration of the endogenous insulin that is produced in the pancreas and is not affected by insulin antibody interference. However, because of the lack of analysis standardization, the ADA does not recommend the use of either insulin or C-peptide measurement for diagnosis of type 1 diabetes.[5]

The presence of autoantibodies to pancreatic islet markers confirms a diagnosis of type 1 diabetes. Islet cell cytoplasmic autoantibodies are seen at the onset of 70% to 80% of type 1 diabetes cases. Glutamic acid decarboxylase autoantibodies are also found at the onset of 70% to 80% of type 1 diabetes cases, and insulinoma-2–associated autoantibodies are found with about 60% of such cases.

Tests of Diabetes Control and Disease Progression

Laboratory testing for diabetes after diagnosis of the disease is directed toward the assessment of the progression of disease. The laboratory offers analysis that helps the physician determine the extent of glycemic control and the risk for the severe consequences of hyperglycemia. While the biochemical processes that cause the

microvascular - pertaining to small blood vessels

CLINICAL CORRELATION

Hyperglycemia is associated with pathological changes in both diabetic and nondiabetic patients, such as impaired immunity, blindness, renal disease, and neuropathy. Hyperglycemia of diabetes is associated with cardiovascular disorders, stroke, and limb amputation.

CLINICAL CORRELATION

Research shows that maintaining control of blood glucose concentration over time will reduce the consequences of diabetes. The laboratory provides evaluation of glycemic control through measurement of glycated hemoglobin.

microalbuminuria - small amounts of albumin found in the urine, also called dipstick-negative increase in the excretion of albumin in urine

physiological damage have not been fully determined, it is clear that hyperglycemia is associated with a wide variety of pathological changes in both diabetic and nondiabetic patients. In both diabetic and nondiabetic critically ill patients, hyperglycemia is associated with impaired immunity that results in increased susceptibility to infection. The **microvascular** pathologies in the retina, renal glomerulus, and nervous system, which occur as chronic complications of diabetes in many patients, may produce blindness, renal disease, and neuropathy, respectively. Hyperglycemia of diabetes is associated with cardiovascular disorders, stroke, and limb amputation. Controlling hyperglycemia reduces the risk of such consequences and improves patient outcome.[7,8]

The results of the Diabetes Control and Complications Trial (DCCT) and the United Kingdom Prospective Diabetes Study (UKPDS) show that glycemic control impacts many aspects of the possible sequelae of diabetes. The DCCT followed over 1000 type 1 diabetics over a 9-year period. Two groups were studied, those who received the standard care of the time and those who received intervention to maintain glycemic control. Control of glucose over time was measured by testing for hemoglobin A_{1c} (Hb A_{1c}). The mean Hb A_{1c} for the group that received standard care was 9%. The mean Hb A_{1c} for the group that received special treatment to control glycemia was 7%. This group exhibited a 76% reduction in retinopathy, 69% reduction of neuropathy, and 44% reduction in nephropathy as compared to the group that received standard care.[9,10]

The UKPDS investigated treatment outcomes of type 2 diabetic patients over approximately a decade. As in the DCCT, two groups were studied. One group received treatment to keep blood glucose less than 250 mg/dL, while the second group received treatment to keep blood glucose at the 110-mg/dL level. The study showed that, as with type 1 diabetes, aggressively controlling blood glucose reduces risk for kidney failure and microvascular complications that lead to blindness. These studies and others illustrate the importance of glycemic control: that by carefully monitoring blood glucose, the risk for systemic complications may be reduced.[11,12]

In addition to diagnostic analysis and assessment of glycemic control, the laboratory provides information that will help the physician detect onset of specific pathology that may result from hyperglycemia, through analysis of ketones, creatinine, **microalbuminuria**, acid-base status, lipids, and other measurements. Table 4–4 lists clinical practice guidelines for monitoring diabetes mellitus with laboratory tests.

TABLE 4-4
Clinical Practice Guidelines for Monitoring Diabetes Mellitus[13,14]
RECOMMENDATIONS FOR GLYCEMIC CONTROLS

Glycated hemoglobin
    Normal: <6%
    Goal: <7%

TESTING GUIDELINES

Glycated hemoglobin
    If unstable: quarterly
    If stable: 2 times per year
Lipid profile: yearly
Microalbumin: yearly

CASE SCENARIO 4-1

Diabetes Mellitus Type 1: The Emergency Department

Brandon is a 15-year-old with a 7-year history of type 1 diabetes. He presented to the emergency department with the following laboratory test results:

Test	Brandon	Reference Range
Plasma		
Na (mEq/L)	136	136–145
K (mEq/L)	4.6	3.5–5.1
Cl (mEq/L)	90	98–107
CO_2 (mEq/L)	10	23–29
Anion gap	41	10–20
Glucose (mg/dL)	315	74–100 (fasting)
Serum		
Ketones	30 mg/dL (positive)	Negative
Urine		
Glucose	2+	Negative
Protein	1+	Negative
Ketones	3+	Negative

Brandon appeared confused and disoriented; his blood pressure was 132/90 mm Hg. Within the past year, Brandon showed poor glucose control and was admitted to the hospital for treatment of frank hypertension (144/90 mm Hg). His parents were having a difficult time helping him comply with his treatment plan, which included daily home monitoring of capillary glucose, insulin therapy, and dietary recommendations.

LABORATORY RESULTS IN TYPE 1 DIABETES

A brief examination of the laboratory results in this case suggests an individual with poor glucose control over a long period of time who was experiencing an acid-base imbalance. The increased plasma glucose, serum ketones, whole plasma lactate, urine glucose, and urine ketones were typical of uncontrolled type 1 diabetes.

The decreased CO_2 suggested an acid-base disturbance, most likely metabolic acidosis. The increased anion gap suggested the existence of unmeasured anions, most likely keto acids, in Brandon's blood. The laboratory results for serum and urine ketones also suggested an acid-base imbalance. Ketoacidosis is one form of metabolic acidosis that occurs in response to a patient's inability to metabolize glucose for energy.[15] The enzymes that metabolize glucose are present in most cells, but not in the extracellular fluid. Without the action of insulin, glucose cannot enter the cell. In the absence of cellular glucose, fatty acids are oxidized for production of energy. Ketones are by-products of excessive beta-oxidation of fatty acids.[16] The ketones beta-hydroxybutyric acid, acetoacetate, and acetone are products of this process. The ketones produced from the degradation of fatty acids to acetylcoenzyme A (acetyl-CoA) are related by the following formula:

$$\text{Acetyl-CoA} \rightarrow \rightarrow$$
$$\text{Acetoacetate} + \text{NADH} + \text{H}^+ \rightarrow \text{NAD} + \beta\text{-Hydroxybutyrate} +$$
$$\text{H}^+ \rightarrow CO_2 + \text{acetone}$$

Beta-hydroxybutyric acid is present in the largest amount: 78% of the ketones that are present in blood are beta-hydroxybutyric acid. Acetoacetate represents 20% and acetone is present as 2% of the measured ketones. The extent of ketosis correlates well with the degree of acidosis. Methods of testing for ketones are presented in Test Methodology 4–2.

TEST METHODOLOGY 4-2.   KETONES

The Reaction: Sodium Nitroprusside

This method uses a sodium nitroprusside reagent that also contains glycerine, disodium phosphate, and lactose.

$$\text{Sodium nitroprusside} + \text{acetoacetic acid} + \text{acetone} \rightarrow \text{lavender color}$$

False-positive reactions are due to medications such as L-dopa, methyldopa, 8-hydroxyquinoline, and phenolphthaleins. False-negative reactions can occur due to exceeding linearity of reaction. Dilutions of suspected highly positive results are required to verify actual reaction. False-negative reactions are also due to decreased reaction of the reagent with the serum ketone bodies and can be eliminated by crushing the reagent tab prior to addition of serum. Another cause of a false-negative reaction is use of an older serum or urine sample. Fresh serum or urine is required since the volatile component, acetone, will evaporate and some conversion of acetoacetate to the more volatile acetone can also occur over time.

The Reaction: Enzymatic (β-Hydroxybutryate Dehydrogenase [BHDH]/ Diaphorase) Method

$$\beta\text{-Hydroxybutyrate} + \text{NAD}^+ \xrightarrow{\text{BHDH}} \text{acetoacetate} + \text{NADH} + \text{H}^+$$
$$\text{NBT} + \text{NADH} \xrightarrow{\text{diaphorase}} \text{NBT (colored)} + \text{NAD}^+$$

Negative interference (up to 60%) is due to excess acetoacetate, which reverses the chemical reaction, and dilution of the sample is required to get more accurate β-hydroxybutyrate levels in those cases. Generally there is better correlation of β-hydroxybutyric acid (BHBA) with diabetic ketoacidosis except in early response to treatment. Just as in measuring acetoacetic acid during early stages of insulin therapy, there is increased conversion of BHBA to acetoacetate despite lessening of acidosis.[16]

The Specimen

Serum, plasma, and urine may all be measured for ketones. Sample must be fresh or kept covered to prevent evaporation of the volatile forms.

Reference Ranges

Sodium nitroprusside method for acetoacetic acid and acetone:
  Serum and urine   Negative or <10 mg/dL
Beta-hydroxybutyrate dehydrogenase method for beta-hydroxybutrate:
  Serum   0.02–0.27 mmol/L

Case Scenario 4-1 Diabetes Mellitus Type 1: The Emergency Department

Additional Laboratory Results

In addition to the immediate concern of ketoacidosis, the physician was also concerned about development of nephropathy. Brandon's urea and creatinine were analyzed a few hours later with the following results:

Test	Brandon	Reference Range (Adolescent)
BUN (mg/dL)	25	6–20
Creatinine (mg/dL)	1.1	0.5–1.0

The blood urea nitrogen (BUN)/creatinine ratio was 25/1.1 or 23/1. An increased ratio with a normal or near-normal creatinine is typical of prerenal disorders. Brandon's creatinine was within normal limits, suggesting a prerenal **uremia**, such as dehydration.

uremia - a toxic condition associated with renal insufficiency produced by the retention in the blood of nitrogenous substances normally excreted by the kidney

Dehydration is a common occurrence in the ketoacidosis of diabetes. Hyperglycemia produces hyperosmolarity. The hyperosmolar state initiates multiple physiological responses, including increased renal excretion of glucose and ketones, resulting in polyuria and fluid oncotic shifts. Eventually polydipsia, or excessive thirst, is triggered and, if fluid replacement occurs, the dehydration is minimized. Fluid replacement therapy along with restoring normoglycemia is often an aspect of restoring normal conditions to the patient in diabetic ketoacidosis.[15]

Case Scenario 4-1 Diabetes Mellitus Type 1: The Emergency Department

Brandon's History

Brandon's mother noticed his first symptoms when he was 8 years old, following an uneventful chickenpox infection. His symptoms appeared suddenly. His mother noted that he urinated more frequently than usual, he had increased thirst and appetite, and he had been losing weight. At the office of his pediatrician, Brandon was tested for glucose with a random blood glucose concentration result of 560 mg/dL. Laboratory testing of his urine revealed increased glucose and ketones. The pediatrician diagnosed type 1 diabetes mellitus based on the glucose level of the **random (or casual) blood draw**, which was above 200 mg/dL, and his classic symptoms of type 1 diabetes: polydipsia, polyuria, and rapid weight loss. The diagnosis was confirmed with a fasting glucose test of 255 mg/dL from blood drawn on another day. His physician placed him on a strict course of therapy, including diet change. Brandon's mother monitored his blood glucose at home to maintain it as close to normal as possible. Brandon was seen periodically by the pediatrician to determine the control of his glycemia. He was placed on carefully monitored insulin therapy.

Brandon has shown poor glycemic control with episodes of postprandial hyperglycemia and early-morning hypoglycemia by self-monitoring blood glucose technique. His parents reported early difficulties in motivating Brandon to comply with daily home monitoring of blood glucose and his treatment

random (or casual) blood draw - blood collected at any time of day without regard to duration since last meal

continued

Case Scenario 4-1 Diabetes Mellitus Type 1: The Emergency Department *(continued)*

regimen. During Brandon's admission for treatment of hypertension in the previous year, the following additional lab results were obtained:

Test	Brandon	Reference Range
Serum creatinine (mg/dL)	0.5	0.5–1.0
Creatinine clearance (mL/min/1.73 m^2)	183	93–131
Urine albumin excretion rate (μg/min)	240	<20
Hb A$_{1c}$ (%)	11.6	4–6
Blood pressure (mm Hg)	132/90	120/80

Hypertension and Microalbuminuria

Hypertension, defined as blood pressure greater than or equal to 140/90 mm Hg, is a common complication of diabetes. Hypertension is associated with other microvascular complications of the disease and is risk factor for the development of cardiovascular disease. Cardiovascular disease is the major cause of death in diabetics.

Renal disease is a serious complication of diabetes, occurring in 20% to 40% of patients with diabetes. Microalbuminuria is an early marker of diabetic nephropathy. *Microalbuminuria* is a term that is used to describe albumin in the urine in amounts that are slightly above normal. Since many urine dipsticks are not sensitive to these small amounts, microalbuminuria is sometimes described as "dipstick-negative albuminuria." Other methods of testing for microalbuminuria are described in Test Methodology 4–3.

TEST METHODOLOGY 4-3.   MICROALBUMINEMIA

The Reaction Principle

Quantitative tests for urine albumin use nephelometry or immunoassay methodology. Nephelometry measures the complexes that are formed with antibodies to albumin. Immunoassay measures the radioactive or enzyme labels that change when albumin binds an antibody.

Latex agglutination tests measures immune complexes that are formed with latex-attached antibodies. Agglutination is reported as a semiquantitative measure of albumin present in the urine.

The Specimen

A timed urine collection is recommended; 24-hour, 8- to 12-hour, or 1- to 2-hour timed specimens are acceptable. A first morning, random urine specimen may be tested; the result is reported as an albumin/creatinine ratio. Urine should be stored at 4°C or preserved with sodium azide.

Reference Ranges

Condition	Albumin (μg/min)	Albumin/Creatinine (mg/24 hr)	(mg/g)
Normal	<20	<30	<20
Microalbuminuria	20–200	30–300	20–30
Overt albuminuria	>200	>300	>30

Yearly testing for microalbuminuria is recommended by the ADA Clinical Practice Guidelines for monitoring diabetics. Patients with microalbuminuria who progress to macroalbuminuria are likely to progress to renal disease over a period of years.[17,18]

In the early stages of nephropathy, microalbuminuria reveals increased glomerular permeability of the renal nephron. At this stage, the progression to end-stage renal disease may be slowed or prevented by treatment and glycemic control. The ADA recommends testing for microalbuminuria in all postpubescent patients who have had diabetes for at least 5 years.

Case Scenario 4-1 Diabetes Mellitus Type 1: The Emergency Department

Follow-Up

During Brandon's next two routine clinic visits, his physician noted hypertension and 2+ proteinuria. Brandon's physician is concerned that Brandon is not compliant with his home monitoring schedule and treatment regimen. The physician referred Brandon for diabetic education. Brandon was also referred to a kidney specialist for assessment of the renal complication of his disease. ●

CASE SCENARIO 4-2

Diabetes Mellitus Type 2: Mrs. Powtee and the Diabetes Center

Mrs. Nancy Powtee is an obese, 47-year-old, African-American woman who lives a sedentary life. She had been experiencing fatigue, unusual thirst, and frequent urination for the past few months. She got up several times during the night to urinate and was thirsty at these times also. Lately, she noticed tingling and numbness in her fingers and feet and noticed that she dropped items frequently. She also reported that she lost weight recently, although she was not dieting. On the advice of family members, she scheduled an appointment with Dr. Tom Johnson, a family practice physician. On the basis of her history, he ordered laboratory tests, which returned the following results:

Test	Mrs. Powtee	Reference Range
Serum (Fasting)		
Glucose (mg/dL)	365	74–100
Total cholesterol (mg/dL)	243	148–268
HDL cholesterol (mg/dL)	20	34–87
Triglycerides (mg/dL)	416	44–223
Whole Blood		
Hb A_{1c} (%)	10.4	4–6

continued

Case Scenario 4-2 Diabetes Mellitus Type 2: Mrs. Powtee
and the Diabetes Center *(continued)*

Urine

Glucose	4+	Negative
Ketones	Negative	Negative
Protein	Negative	Negative

When Dr. Johnson showed the laboratory results to Mrs. Powtee, he
explained that he believed that she has type 2 diabetes. The physician
explained that she had an insulin problem; her body was making enough
insulin but her body cells could not use the insulin properly. Although
she had plenty of glucose in her blood, her body could not use the glucose
for energy because glucose could not enter her body cells. Instead, her
blood glucose was eliminated in her urine.

Dr. Johnson explained that the disease was more frequent in women of
her age, sedentary lifestyle, and race. He stated that many diabetics had family
members with diabetes, but Mrs. Powtee could not recall family members
who had diabetes. The physician explained that diabetes increases the risk for
developing kidney disease, cardiovascular disease, and blindness. Mrs. Powtee
was understandably upset. Her physician told her that type 2 diabetes is usually much more easily managed than type 1 diabetes. She may be able to control
the disease by exercise, diet change, and weight loss. Dr. Johnson performed a
foot examination to check for microvascular and neuropathic problems. The
examination was normal except for some callus formation.

Dr. Johnson asked the office staff to make appointments for Mrs. Powtee
at the diabetes center, where she could attend classes for self-monitoring her
blood glucose and receive nutritional counseling. He prescribed an oral diabetes agent to increase cellular sensitivity to insulin and decrease the release
of glucose by the liver. He also scheduled a second appointment for Mrs. Powtee to have a fasting blood glucose test to confirm his diagnosis. There are
many identified risk factors for the development of type 2 diabetes mellitus.

Dr. Johnson made his diagnosis on the basis of her elevated random glucose
above 200 mg/dL and the presence of symptoms. Mrs. Powtee had some of
the classic symptoms of diabetes: polyuria, polydipsia, and unexplained weight
loss; symptoms of fatigue, blurred vision, and numbness and tingling in the
extremities are also common symptoms of diabetes. The criteria that are used
to diagnose type 1 diabetes are also used to diagnose type 2 diabetes. ADA
Clinical Practice Guidelines for monitoring type 1 diabetes mellitus are also
recommended for type 2 diabetes. In contrast to type 1 diabetes, type 2 diabetes is not usually controlled through insulin treatment. However, insulin
treatment in the later stages of the disease may be prescribed. Although long-
term complications are associated with type 2 diabetes, ketoacidosis is seldom
seen.

Mrs. Powtee was seen at the diabetes center a few days after her visit to
the doctor. Such facilities focus on preventive care and offer programs that
help the patient slow or stop progression of disease. At the center, she saw

continued

Case Scenario 4-2 Diabetes Mellitus Type 2: Mrs. Powtee and the Diabetes Center *(continued)*

the diabetes educator, who was a registered nurse, and the dietitian. The diabetes educator taught her how to use her glucose monitor. (Test Methodology 4–4 describes the use of self-monitoring glucose meters.) She learned to wash her hands before the procedure, take a capillary blood sample, use the glucose monitor, and record her glucose levels. The diabetes educator suggested that Mrs. Powtee test her blood every morning to monitor her fasting level, and before and after a meal to monitor her response to glucose. Her target levels were set at 80 to 120 mg/dL for her fasting level and below 140 mg/dl 2 hours after a meal. Her goal was to meet her target levels for at least 50% of her tests.[19]

TEST METHODOLOGY 4-4.   SELF-MONITORING GLUCOSE METERS

At-home or near-patient monitoring by POCT with glucose meters provides information so that therapeutic intervention may be initiated immediately.

The Reaction Principle

Glucose meters use the same chemical reactions that are used in glucose analysis in the laboratory: glucose oxidase, hexokinase, and dehydrogenase. Most systems use dehydrated reagents embedded in pads on plastic strips. The strip is inserted in the meter, where the reaction is measured. The reaction may be a color change that is measured by reflectance spectrophotometry, or the reaction may produce a change in current that can be measured by electrochemistry.

The Specimen

Capillary or anticoagulated whole blood is measured. The sample is placed directly on the test pad.

Calibration may be performed automatically on some instruments or performed with code test strips. Some instruments are calibrated to report the estimated glucose levels in plasma or serum.

Reportable range varies widely from instrument to instrument. Readings beyond the reportable range of the instrument should be measured on different equipment.

Reference Range

Whole blood glucose is approximately 10% to 15% lower than serum or plasma glucose levels.

The educator also provided written information to Mrs. Powtee about her Hb A_{1c} result of 10.4%. ●

Glycated Hemoglobin

Hb A_{1c}, a glycated hemoglobin, is an indicator of long-term glycemic control. In adults, hemoglobin is a mixture of three forms: Hb A_1, Hg A_2, and Hb F, with Hb A_1 predominating. Hemoglobin A_1 consists of three subforms: Hb A_{1a}, Hb A_{1b}, and

THE TEAM APPROACH

Since it is important for diabetic patients to eat meals on a regular basis and balance their food intake with activity versus their blood glucose level, it is not practical or necessary for them to fast for 8 to 10 hours prior to a visit to a diabetes center or physician's office for follow-up. Glycated hemoglobin levels do not require a fasting specimen and can be used in conjunction with the patient's self-monitored blood glucose records to determine glycemic control over the past few months. Laboratory personnel may need to communicate this information with nursing or clinic staff when initially setting up services for those patients.

Hb A_{1c}, with Hb A_{1c} predominating. The term *glycated hemoglobin* describes a chemically stable conjugate of any of the forms of hemoglobin with glucose. Glycated forms of hemoglobin are formed slowly, nonenzymatically, and irreversibly at a rate that is proportional to the concentration of glucose in the blood. The level of glycated hemoglobin in a blood sample provides a glycemic history of hemoglobin glycation over the life span of the erythrocyte, the cell that contains the hemoglobin. The average lifespan of the erythrocyte is 120 days, and glycated hemoglobin describes the average glucose levels in the blood over that life span. Clinically, glycated hemoglobin is used to reflect glycemic control over the previous 90 to 120 days. Glycated hemoglobin measurements are unaffected by daily variation of glucose from diet and exercise. Glycated hemoglobin measurements are, however, influenced by conditions that affect the life span of the hemoglobin molecule, such as sickle cell disease and hemolytic disease, which can falsely decrease glycated hemoglobin results.

To approximate the study of the Diabetes Control and Complications Trial, methodology for testing glycated hemoglobin has been standardized to measure hemoglobin A_{1c}, as described in Test Methodology 4–5. The National Glycohemoglobin Standardization Program helps standardize Hb A_{1c} determinations to DCCT values. Hb A_{1c} test methods may be awarded a "certificate of traceability to the DCCT reference method" if the method meets criteria for precision and accuracy of the Standardization Program. Hb A_{1c} is that form of glycated hemoglobin formed by condensation of glucose with the amino-terminal valine residue of each beta chain of hemoglobin A. Hb A_{1c} is the preferred standard for assessing glycemic control.[20]

TEST METHODOLOGY 4-5.   HEMOGLOBIN A$_{1c}$

The American Diabetes Association Clinical Practice Guidelines recommend Hb A_{1c} testing for patients with diabetes.[21] Because Hb A_{1c} estimates the average blood glucose over the preceding 2 to 3 months, the guidelines recommend measurement of Hb A_{1c} every 3 months for the patient for whom glycemic control has not been established and twice a year for patients who have glycemic control. The goal of therapy is an Hb A_{1c} result of less that 7%. Results that are above the goal may signal the need for a change in therapy.

Glycated hemoglobin may be separated and identified on the basis of charge and structure differences. Methods of analysis include ion-exchange or affinity **chromatography**, electrophoresis, isoelectric focusing, and immunoassay.

The Reaction Principle

Ion-Exchange Chromatography

Hemoglobin molecules are separated on the basis of charge. A hemolysate of the specimen is applied to a cation (negatively charged) exchange resin column. A buffer is applied, and the column elute is collected in aliquots. The pH of the buffer is chosen so that glycated hemoglobin molecules are less positively charged than Hb A. At this charge, glycolated hemoglobin does not bind as well to the column and is eluted first. A second buffer elutes Hb A. Hemoglobin aliquots are measured spectrophotometrically, and glycated hemoglobin is calculated as a percentage of the total hemoglobin. This method is not specific for Hb A_{1c} and will report false increases of Hb A_{1c} in blood that contains increased amounts of labile pre-A_1 and Hb F. False decreases are reported in blood that

continued

TEST METHODOLOGY 4-5.   HEMOGLOBIN A$_{1c}$ *(continued)*

contains Hb S and Hb C. Hb A$_{1c}$ levels of patients with disorders in which red blood cell (RBC) survival is decreased may be falsely decreased.

Electrophoresis

Hemoglobin varieties are separating on the basis of charge. Hemolysate of the specimen is applied to an agar gel support. Electrical potential is applied across the support, andhemoglobin components within the specimen are separated on the basis of the differences of the charges. The method is not specific for Hb A$_{1c}$. Because Hb A$_1$ migrates faster than Hb A, Hb A$_1$ is referred to as fast hemoglobin. Hb A$_{1c}$ may be falsely increased with specimens containing labile pre-A$_1$ or Hb F. False decreases in Hb A$_{1c}$ level may be reported in patients with disorders in which RBC survival is decreased.

Isoelectric Focusing

Hemoglobin varieties are separated on the basis of their migration patterns in a pH gradient. Isoelectric focusing is a method of electrophoresis in which components are separated according to their isoelectric points. The isoelectric point is the pH at which the protein is neutral; electrophoresis takes place in a pH gradient. The method is specific for Hb A$_{1c}$. This method is not in common clinical use in the United States, but is used more commonly in Europe.

Affinity Chromatography

This method is based on differences in structure. The hemolysate passes through an affinity column that consists of inert cellulose or agarose matrix covalently bound to a ligand such as *m*-amino-phenylboronic acid. Glycated hemoglobin reacts to the boronic acid reversibly. Nonglycated hemoglobin elutes first. A second buffer dissociates glycated hemoglobin from the resin column. Glycated hemoglobin is calculated as a percentage of total hemoglobin.

Immunoassay

This method is based on differences in structure. Enzyme immunoassay uses monoclonal antibodies that are directed specifically to Hb A$_{1c}$. This methodology has been developed for the use of capillary specimens.

The Specimen

The preferred specimen is whole blood that has been collected in EDTA, heparin, or fluoride anticoagulant. Capillary blood may be used for some procedures such as immunoassay. A hemolysate of washed RBCs is tested. Whole blood may be stored for 1 week at 4°C. Hemolystate may be stored for 4 to 7 days at 4°C or 30 days at –70°C.

Interference

Falsely increased Hb A$_{1c}$ may be reported for blood with increased Hb A$_{1a}$ levels. Falsely decreased Hb A$_{1c}$ may be reported in individuals with disorders in which RBC survival is decreased.

Reference Range for Glycated Hemoglobin

Hb A$_{1c}$ is reported as a percentage of the total hemoglobin:

    Hb A$_{1c}$ 4.0%–6.0%

Case Scenario 4-2 Diabetes Mellitus Type 2: Mrs. Powtee and the Diabetes Center

The diabetes educator explained to Mrs. Powtee that her Hb A_{1c} would be tested at the diabetes Center at least every 6 months to determine the average of her blood glucose levels over the previous 3- to 4-month period. Studies have shown a correlation between mean plasma glucose concentration and Hb A_{1c} (Table 4–5).

TABLE 4-5

Correlation Between Hb A_{1c} Level and Mean Plasma Glucose Levels on Multiple Testing Over 2–3 Months[22]

Hb A_{1c} (%)	Mean Plasma Glucose	
	mg/dL	*mmol/L*
6	135	7.5
7	170	9.5
8	205	11.5
9	240	13.5
10	275	15.5

Mrs. Powtee also attended a nutrition class. She and the dietician discussed changes in eating habits that would help Mrs. Powtee meet her blood glucose goals. She learned to record her meals so that she and the dietician could continue to monitor her carbohydrate intake. Finally, Mrs. Powtee joined the exercise group and planned activities that she could do at home.

point-of-care testing (POCT) - testing that does not require specimen preparation and provides rapid results at or near the patient's location

THE TEAM APPROACH
Management of diabetes is accomplished through a physician-coordinated team. The team may include physicians, nurse practitioners, physician's assistants, nurses, dietitians, pharmacists, and laboratory personnel. The team prepares and implements an individual therapeutic plan that centers on patient self-management.

Diabetes centers provide **point-of-care testing (POCT)** for consistent and regular management of glycemia and monitor markers that predict the development of hyperglycemia-related pathology. At diabetes centers and other facilities that provide preventive care for patients with chronic diseases, patients are helped to take responsibility to monitor their illness and plan activities to improve long-term outcome of the pathological consequences of the disease process. Such facilities help to reduce the progression of disease toward secondary complications and mortality. Patients receive education and support to make appropriate lifestyle changes. Medical personnel are available to monitor risk factors on a regular basis. POCT provides rapid biochemical analysis in a timely manner, allowing necessary changes to therapy during the patient visit.

Case Scenario 4-2 Diabetes Mellitus Type 2: Mrs. Powtee and the Diabetes Center

Follow-Up

Six months after her first visit to the diabetes center, Mrs. Powtee had met her goals. Seventy percent of her home blood glucose tests were in the target range. Her symptoms were diminishing and her Hb A_{1c} was 8.0%. She continued to attend nutrition sessions and exercise regularly. ●

CASE SCENARIO 4-3

Gestational Diabetes Mellitus: The Prenatal Clinic

Jan Brown is a 32-year-old Native American woman who is in her 26th week of pregnancy. During her first prenatal visit, Mrs. Brown's urine was tested for glucose and protein; both tests were negative. At her last prenatal visit, the results of her urine test for protein and glucose were

Test	Mrs. Brown	Reference Range
Protein	Negative	Negative
Glucose	Positive	Negative

Mrs. Brown is overweight and has a family history of diabetes. Her age, ethnicity, family history, and weight put her at risk for gestational diabetes mellitus. Mrs. Brown's physician uses the recommendations of the National Diabetes Association for laboratory testing for diagnosis of gestational diabetes. The criteria for diagnosing gestational diabetes are based on the original research of O'Sullivan and Mahan[23] and modified by Carpenter and Coustan.[24] The National Diabetes Group protocol for diagnosis of gestational diabetes is outlined in Table 4–6. In this protocol, the physician first orders a 50-g glucose challenge to screen for diabetes. For this screening test, the patient need not be fasting. Blood is drawn 1 hour after the glucose solution is consumed. Mrs. Brown's results are shown below:

Test	Mrs. Brown	Reference Range
1-hour glucose (50 g)	210 mg/dL	<140 mg/dL

Because the screening test is positive, the physician asks Mrs. Brown to return to the laboratory after an 8-hour fast. Mrs. Brown is instructed to refrain

TABLE 4-6

The National Diabetes Group Recommended Screening and Diagnosis Testing for Gestational Diabetes Mellitus

SCREENING

Pregnant women over 25 years of age should be screened between 24 and 28 weeks of gestation. A 50-g glucose load should be administered. Glucose level should be tested at 1 hour. A glucose level of 140 mg/dL or greater should be followed by a glucose tolerance test.

DIAGNOSIS

The test should be administered after an overnight fast. A 100-g glucose load is administered. Blood is drawn at fasting, 1-, 2-, and 3-hour levels. Two or more levels that exceed the following criteria indicate gestational diabetes mellitus.

Fasting	95 mg/dL
1 hour	180 mg/dL
2 hour	155 mg/dL
3 hour	140 mg/dL

continued

Case Scenario 4-3 Gestational Diabetes Mellitus: The Prenatal Clinic *(continued)*

from eating or drinking fluids, other than water, overnight for 10 to 16 hours before the test. She is cautioned not to smoke or take medications on the morning of the test. During the testing period, she will be allowed only water. A fasting sample is drawn and she is given a 100-g glucose solution. Mrs. Brown's blood is drawn every hour for 3 hours with the following results:

Test	Mrs. Brown	Reference Range
Fasting	144 mg/dL	≥95 mg/dL
1 hour	155 mg/dL	≥180 mg/dL
2 hour	210 mg/dL	≥155 mg/dL
3 hour	152 mg/dL	≥140 mg/dL

Gestational diabetes mellitus is defined as glucose intolerance that develops during pregnancy.[25] Between 1% and 14% of all pregnant women, depending on the population studied, will develop gestational diabetes. Women with risk factors for developing gestational diabetes should be screened for gestational diabetes between the 24th and 28th week of gestation. Women who are at low risk for developing gestational diabetes need not be screened. Table 4–7 lists character-istics that define low risk for gestational diabetes. Table 4–5 depicts the National Diabetes Group recommendations for screening and diagnostic testing for gestational diabetes mellitus. The measurement of urine glucose is detailed in Test Methodology 4–6.

TEST METHODOLOGY 4-6.   URINE GLUCOSE

Urine glucose may be measured either qualitatively or quantitatively.

The Reaction: Qualitative Measurement

Glucose may be measured as a reducing substance using the Benedict's copper reduction reaction. Glucose reduces cupric ions to cuprous ions to produce a yellow or red cuprous compound. All reducing sugars will produce a positive result. Other reducing substances, such as ascorbic acid, may also produce positive reactions.

Urine test strips use the glucose oxidase reaction. The test strip is impregnated with glucose oxidase, peroxidase, and a chromogen. The reaction is specific for glucose. Ascorbic acid and urates may inhibit the reaction and cause false-negative results. Contamination of urine with hydrogen peroxide or an oxidizing agent such as bleach may cause a false-positive reaction.

The Reaction: Quantitative Measurement

Urine glucose may be measure quantitatively using chemical methods (hexokinase method or glucose oxidase method). Uric acid in urine may cause falsely lowered results in glucose oxidase methods, which use hydrogen peroxide and peroxidase indicator reactions.

The Specimen

Random or 24-hour specimens may be analyzed. Glucose must be measured promptly or preserved with glacial acetic acid or sodium benzoate.

Reference Range

Urine (random)	<30 mg/dL

TABLE 4-7

Characteristics That Define Low Risk for Development of Gestational Diabetes Mellitus[5]

Age <25 years
Weight normal before pregnancy
Not a member of an ethnic group with a high prevalence of diabetes, such as Hispanic-American, Native American, Asian-American, African-American or Pacific Islander
No known diabetes in first-degree relatives
No history of abnormal glucose tolerance
No history of poor obstetric outcome

Case Scenario 4-3 Gestational Diabetes Mellitus: The Prenatal Clinic

The results of Mrs. Brown's laboratory tests confirmed her physician's diagnosis of gestational. Since gestational diabetes increases the risk to both mother and child for harm, the physician referred her for diabetes education immediately. The goal of treatment for gestational diabetes is the goal of all diabetics, glycemic control. Mrs. Brown was taught to monitor her blood glucose and was given nutritional counseling to include caloric reduction for weight loss and moderate physical exercise. Her physician asked her to schedule regular appointments to verify blood glucose levels. If she is not able to control her glycemia through self-monitoring, diet change, and exercise, insulin therapy will be considered.

The growth and maturation of the fetus is dependent upon nutrients that cross the placenta from the mother. Although insulin is not able to cross the placenta, glucose does cross from the mother's blood to the fetus. Increased fetal glycemia causes the fetal pancreas to increase secretion of insulin. The extra glucose is stored, leading to fetal **macrosomia** and increased difficulty at delivery. At birth, the newborn's pancreas continues to secrete insulin, producing severe neonatal hypoglycemia.

macrosomia - increased size and weight of the fetus

Case Scenario 4-3 Gestational Diabetes Mellitus: The Prenatal Clinic

Mrs. Brown is also at risk for developing hypertension and **pre-eclampsia** and may require a cesarean delivery. The fact that she has developed gestational diabetes mellitus puts her at risk for developing other types of diabetes mellitus, usually type 2, in the future.

pre-eclampsia - a complication of pregnancy characterized by increasing hypertension, proteinuria, and edema

Early diagnosis and treatment of gestational diabetes is beneficial in delaying the development of type 2 diabetes and reducing severe consequences. While screening the whole population for the disease may not be effective, screening may be effective for those individuals who are at risk for the development of type 2 diabetes. Lifestyle change, glycemic control through self-monitoring of blood glucose, and pharmacological treatment of glycemia improve insulin resistance.

Case Scenario 4-3 Gestational Diabetes Mellitus: The Prenatal Clinic

Follow-Up

Mrs. Brown delivered a healthy, normal-sized infant. She continued her diet and exercise plan and lost weight. These basic lifestyle changes will help her avoid developing gestational diabetes with future pregnancies and other types of diabetes after pregnancy. ●

CASE SCENARIO 4-4

Transient Neonatal Hypoglycemia: The Big Baby

"He is a big baby, isn't he?" his mother asked. Baby Morgan was delivered at Riverside Medical Center to a 33-year-old mother who had no prenatal history. Baby Morgan was indeed larger than normal. The nurses in the nursery noticed that Baby Morgan seemed lethargic and unresponsive. A whole blood glucose done in the nursery was 23 mg/dL. Although neonatal blood glucose levels are usually lower than adult blood glucose levels, Baby Morgan's glucose level worried the nurses. Hypoglycemia in neonates may be caused by prematurity, maternal diabetes, and maternal toxemia.

Upon questioning the mother, the physician learned that Mrs. Morgan had a history of delivering big babies and having sugar problems during pregnancy. Mrs. Morgan probably had developed gestational diabetes. The fetus of a mother with gestational diabetes oversecretes insulin. When the neonate is born, fetal hyperglycemia is ended. Since the fetal pancreas is accustomed to oversecretion of insulin, the neonate goes into severe hypoglycemia. This hypoglycemia is usually transient.

Hypoglycemia

Hypoglycemia is characterized by blood glucose levels that are less than normal. Exact definition of the glucose level in hypoglycemia is under debate; symptoms of hypoglycemia usually occur when blood glucose has fallen below 50 mg/dL. Two types of hypoglycemia occur, reactive (postprandial, or after meals) and fasting (postabsorptive). Hypoglycemia that is caused by a stimulus such as excessive insulin administration, ethanol ingestion, or over-regulation of diabetes is termed *reactive hypoglycemia*. Reactive hypoglycemia is not usually related to any underlying disease; fasting hypoglycemia often is. Reactive hypoglycemia may be diagnosed with Whipple's triad: low blood glucose with classic symptoms of hypoglycemia, which are alleviated by glucose administration.

Hypoglycemia that occurs after fasting is rare. *Fasting hypoglycemia* may occur as a response to insulin-producing tumors of the pancreas (insulinomas) or other tissues, hepatic dysfunction, glucocorticoid deficiency, sepsis, or low glycogen stores. Fasting hypoglycemia may be diagnosed with differentiation of the etiology by a 72-hour fast that is conducted in a hospital.[26] During the fast, blood specimens are drawn for glucose, insulin, and C-peptide determination. Most patients with true fasting hypoglycemia show low glucose blood levels within 12 hours after the fast begins. Insulin and C-peptide levels help differentiate among the causes of the hypoglycemia. The ADA discourages the use of the 5-hour glucose tolerance test for the diagnosis of hypoglycemia.

Case Scenario 4-4 Transient Neonatal Hypoglycemia: The Big Baby

Follow-Up

Baby Morgan's hypoglycemia was indeed transient. As revealed by capillary blood glucose monitoring several times a day for 3 days, his glucose levels returned to the normal reference range for his age group. As the effects of maternal hyperglycemia dissipated, the neonatal pancreas responded properly to Baby Morgan's first nutrients. Mrs. Morgan was referred to the diabetes educator for nutritional counseling and exercise classes to control her weight. She also received information about gestational diabetes, which included warnings about the dangers of hyperglycemia during pregnancy for both mother and child. ●

CASE SCENARIO 4-5

Galactosemia: Double the Work or Worth the Price?

The technologist working at the body fluids bench in the clinical laboratory was supervising John, the medical technology student. John noticed that it was the policy to test the urine samples of neonates with a glucose dipstick by a specific method and also with a reducing substance method. John commented to the technologist that, although all of the babies had negative glucose dipstick results, the laboratory was still required to test by the alternative method.

GALACTOSEMIA

The glucose method found in urinalysis testing with chemical test strips is specific for glucose due to the specificity of the glucose oxidase enzyme involved. The principle of the urine test strip method is discussed in Test Methodology 4–6 earlier in this chapter. This qualitative or semiquantitative method is more sensitive and specific for glucose than copper reduction methods. The lower limit of sensitivity for urinary glucose by the glucose oxidase method is 100 mg/dL, while the sensitivity in copper reduction method is 250 mg/dL. When inhibitors are present, the lower limit of sensitivity for urinary glucose by the enzymatic test strip method is limited somewhat. False-positive results in the glucose oxidase method are due to contamination of urine with strong oxidizing substances such as bleach/hypochlorite or hydrogen peroxide. False-negative reactions are due to ascorbic acid, urates or salicylates, or high amounts of ketones.[16]

The reducing substance method will react with glucose, galactose, lactose, fructose, and other reducing substances such as ascorbic acid but not with sucrose, a nonreducing sugar. This method is clearly not specific for galactose, but when used in conjunction with the specific methods for glucose, it can at least rule in or out the presence of glucose and indicate need for more specific testing to determine whether another reducing substance is present, such as galactose. Test Methodology 4–7 gives the details of urine reducing substance testing.

TEST METHODOLOGY 4-7.   URINE REDUCING SUBSTANCE (GALACTOSE SCREENING)

The principle reagent in the copper reduction method contains copper sulfate, sodium hydroxide, sodium carbonate, and sodium citrate.

The Reaction

$$\text{Reducing substance} + \text{copper sulfate } (Cu^{3+}) \longrightarrow \text{cuprous oxide/}$$
$$\text{cuprous hydroxide } (Cu^{2+})$$

The result is measured qualitatively as a colored product ranging from green (moderate amount of reducing substance) to orange (high amount of reducing substance).

Interference

Interference due to air oxidation is minimized by the bubbles that form in the process. Ascorbic acid, uric acid, salicylates, and many other substances can also act as reducing substances, giving false-positive results. False-negative result can occur with amounts of > 2000 mg/dL glucose, which will cause a "pass-through" phenomenon in which the end color is closer to green than orange. Diluting samples suspected of containing a high amount of reducing sugar is recommended.[16]

The Specimen

Fresh urine

Reference Range

Negative

Chromatography can be used to separate the sugars found in a urine sample. Sugars can be separated using a specific type of filter paper and an organic solvent. The sugars, when allowed to interact with the paper and solvent over a specified period of time, will migrate different distances on the paper. They can then be visualized by spraying with a developing solution. The migration ratio of the distance in centimeters (cm) traveled by the sugar when compared with the distance traveled by the solvent is known as the retention factor (Rf). This Rf characterizes the type of sugar. For example, a typical Rf for galactose by this method is 0.45.[27]

Galactose is present in urine of patients with neonatal **galactosemia**.[28] Neonatal galactosemia is an **inborn error of metabolism** for galactose due to deficiency of one of three possible enzymes. The most common defect is that of galactose-1-phosphate uridyl transferase, causing an accumulation of galactose. Some aspects of glucose metabolism are affected, such as a decrease in glycogenolysis, as conversion to glucose is inhibited by galactose accumulation. Since galactose is primarily supplied from lactose in dairy products, this inborn error of metabolism becomes evident early in life. Initial symptoms of galactosemia are diarrhea and vomiting after the ingestion of milk. Continued accumulation of galactose results in more serious conditions such as mental retardation, cataracts, and possibly liver disease.

galactosemia - an inherited disorder marked by the inability to metabolize galactose due to a congenital absence of the enzyme galactose-1-phosphate uridyl transferase

inborn error of metabolism - an inherited metabolic disease that often causes deficiency of an enzyme

Prevention of permanent damage to the developing brain, eyes, and liver involves removal of sources of galactose from the diet, especially milk products.[28]

Case Scenario 4-5 Galactosemia: Double the Work or Worth the Price?

Follow-Up

The medical technology student, John, commented to the teaching technologist that all of the babies had negative glucose dipstick results but the laboratory was still required to test by the alternative method. After further discussion, it became clear that a nonspecific test such as the copper reduction method would screen for galactose, fructose, and other reducing substances in the urine. Reducing sugars usually do not accumulate in the urine of newborns, but may be present due to inborn errors of metabolism. If a positive test result is found with the copper reduction method, more specific tests would be necessary to determine the amount and type of sugar present. ●

OTHER CARBOHYDRATE METABOLIC DISORDERS

There are other disorders that affect glucose and carbohydrate metabolism. Glycogen storage diseases often result in hypoglycemia, lactic acidosis, and ketosis. There are several types of glycogen storage diseases. Fructosuria is associated with lactic acidosis, ketosis, and the presence of reducing substances in excess. The laboratory plays a role in assessing these rare, but important, carbohydrate metabolic disorders.

Glycogen Storage Disorders

Glycogen storage diseases such as type I (von Gierke's disease) are rare disorders due to enzyme defects and accumulation of glycogen in liver and skeletal muscle.

- Glycogen storage disease type I is due to glucose-6-phosphatase deficiency causing ineffective glycogenolysis, hypoglycemia during fasting states, growth retardation, ketosis, lactic acidosis, and pronounced hepatomegaly due to accumulation of glycogen in liver and, to some degree, muscle. Determining insulin and glucagon levels as well as measuring glucose response after administration of epinephrine (the epinephrine tolerance test) may be helpful in obtaining a diagnosis.
- Types II, V, and VII are due to other enzyme defects and tend to cause milder symptoms and accumulation of glycogen primarily in skeletal muscle.
- Types III and VI, like type I, are also liver forms of glycogen storage disease but are rarer in occurrence.
- Type IV is a severe liver form of glycogen storage disease with cardiac and skeletal muscle disease.

Fructosuria

Fructosuria can be due to enzyme defects in fructokinase, fructose-1-phosphate aldolase, or fructose-1,6-diphosphatase. These are rare autosomal recessive inherited diseases, with only fructokinase deficiency causing a harmless presence of fructosuria. Serious consequences occur when fructose is provided by dietary intake of fruits, honey, and syrup (such as corn syrup), resulting in ketosis, lactic acidosis, and liver failure. Chromatography can be used to separate and measure individual carbohydrates.

Additional Testing to Aid Interpretation of Carbohydrate Disorders

Lactate

The measurement of lactate has been associated with several carbohydrate disorders in this chapter, including diabetes mellitus and glycogen storage diseases. Lactic acid is a by-product of glucose metabolism in the Embden-Myerhof pathway resulting directly from the conversion of pyruvate and NADH in the presence of lactate dehydrogenase (LD).

$$Lactate + NAD^+ \xleftarrow{LD} pyruvate + NADH$$

Equilibrium favors the right side of the reaction at a pH of approximately 7.5 and the left side at a pH of approximately 9.0 to 9.6.

Lactate formation is most prevalent in erythrocytes, the brain, liver, kidneys, and skeletal muscle in association with decreased uptake of pyruvate by the citric acid cycle. Blood levels accumulate when the liver is saturated with lactate during strenuous exercise, decreased tissue oxygenation, toxin accumulation, or diseases. Tissue oxygenation problems are associated with **hypovolemia**, shock, and heart failure, particularly of the left ventricle. Diseases such as diabetes mellitus, liver disease, and malignancies or accumulation of toxins from methanol, ethanol, or salicylate metabolism can result in impaired oxygen use by mitochondria and increased production of lactate.[16] Testing for lactate is described in Test Methodology 4–8.

hypovolemia - decreased blood volume; may be caused by fluid losses or inadequate fluid intake

■■ **CLINICAL CORRELATION**

Two types of lactic acidosis occur. Type A is associated with hypoxia, or decreased tissue oxygenation. Type A lactic acidosis may be caused by blood loss or heart diseases in which hemoglobin delivery to tissue is reduced. Type B lactic acidosis is caused by metabolic disorders, such as diabetes mellitus.

TEST METHODOLOGY 4-8.   LACTATE

The Reaction Principle

Enzymatic spectrophotometric methods are available for measuring lactate in which the hydrogen peroxide generated from lactate conversion to pyruvate in the presence of lactate oxidase reacts with a chromogen to form a color.

$$L\text{-Lactate} + O_2 \xrightarrow{\text{lactate oxidase}} pyruvate + H_2O_2$$
$$H_2O_2 + noncolored\ chromogen \xrightarrow{\text{peroxidase}} colored\ dye$$

This has been incorporated into dry film technology, and reflectance of a red dye at 540 nm is measured in proportion to the patient's lactate.[16]

Lactic acid can be measured by an amperometric biosensor electrode containing lactate oxidase. The lactate from the patient sample diffuses into the enzyme layer within the membrane, where lactate is dehydrogenated and hydrogen peroxide is formed. The hydrogen peroxide forms in proportion to the patient's lactate and generate a current.[16]

The Specimen

Heparinized venous plasma or either venous or arterial whole blood is measured. CSF may also be measured. Any exercise or interference with blood flow may affect accurate results. Tourniquet use is not recommended. Care should be taken to reduce RBC glycolysis after collection by use of fluoride preservative in the collecting tube, delivering the specimen on ice and immediately separating the plasma from the cells.

TEST METHODOLOGY 4-8. **LACTATE** *(continued)*

Lactate accumulation causes depletion of bicarbonate, elevated anion gap, and metabolic acidosis in a process similarly to ketoacidosis. Lactic acidosis is relatively common in chronically ill patients, particularly with circulatory problems, and further complicates their recovery. It is associated with diabetic patients as well as those with congestive heart failure and is associated with a very high mortality rate when present for more than a short time.

Reference Range (Adult)

Whole blood, venous   5–12 mg/dL

QUALITY ASSURANCE

CASE SCENARIO 4-6

Does the Result Reflect the Physiology? Capillary Glucose: To Wipe or Not to Wipe

Ms. Garcia, the clinical laboratory point-of-care testing (POCT) supervisor, was checking on quality assurance issues in the diabetes clinic and noticed that nurses were instructing new patients to collect the first drop of blood from the finger-stick sample to analyze in the glucose device rather than wiping away the first drop. She considered this practice as a deviation from the usual standard of practice and wanted to clarify this to avoid preanalytical variations in glucose. Ms. Garcia decided to check with the manufacturer's information as well as other sources.

Standard practice for collecting capillary samples, like all patient samples, involves uniform steps in an attempt to provide an ideal capillary sample. For example, the disinfectant is allowed to evaporate for a short time in order to avoid hemolyzing or diluting the sample. Squeezing of the skin is avoided to prevent outflow of debris and tissue fluid. Likewise, wiping away the first drop of blood to eliminate the impact of tissue fluid and debris is considered standard practice in capillary collection.

Case Scenario 4-6 Does the Result Reflect the Physiology? Capillary Glucose: To Wipe or Not to Wipe

Follow-Up

With the advent of newer methodology in glucose monitoring devices, there is a trend by manufacturers to develop less invasive techniques and smaller blood samples for glucose testing. Based on the results of extensive studies, many of the training materials provided by manufacturers of these new glucose-monitoring devices for patients and health care professionals no longer recommend wiping away the first drop of blood.[29–32] They continue to recommend proper cleansing and drying of the site and often warn to avoid squeezing or massage prior to and during capillary collection. ●

CASE SCENARIO 4-7

Comparing Results: POCT vs. Laboratory Results

Ms. Morris was hospitalized with congestive heart failure and type 2 diabetes mellitus that currently requires insulin therapy. Her blood glucose was below 50 mg/dL when the nurse tested it using a point-of-care (POC) device. Since it was the policy of the hospital to verify all POC glucose results below 50 mg/dL and above 450 mg/dL, a venous sample was obtained. Surprisingly, the venous plasma glucose was 129 mg/dL. This situation occurred again the next day in that the capillary glucose was abnormal and required a venous sample for verification. The venous sample obtained at the same time was close to 100 mg/dL higher than the capillary glucose.

Some of the questions considered by the technologist in charge of POC testing were as follows:

1. Is there a difference between whole blood and plasma glucose values?
2. Is there a difference between the accuracy and precision of the POC glucose device and the laboratory instrument?
3. How could the patient's condition affect the capillary and venous glucose result?

There is evidence that differences exist in whole blood capillary glucose results compared to venous plasma or serum glucose results. Fasting whole blood has about 10% to 15% less glucose when compared to fasting venous plasma due primarily to the amount of packed red cells and water within the cells present in the whole blood sample. When hematocrit is above or below the expected reference range, or when the patient is dehydrated and whole blood becomes more viscous, this may be more of a concern.[16,33] Some whole blood glucose analyzers are calibrated to plasma results.[31] In other words, the analyzer performs a calculation so that the glucose result is adjusted up by 10% to 15% and reported in values comparable to plasma. This makes comparison between POC glucose values and venous serum or plasma easier, particularly when an institution is using both methods for evaluating the patient's glycemic state for therapy.

There is generally not a significant difference between fasting venous and fasting capillary glucose levels. However, a big variation may exist between random (or nonfasting) capillary and venous blood glucose levels due to intracellular transport. The storage of blood prior to glucose analysis can affect the results considerably. Heparinized or clotted whole blood allows cell glycolysis to continue, causing a significant loss in plasma glucose. The rate can typically be 7% decline in glucose per hour, and if the patient has elevated numbers of white blood cells, the rate can be 10% or more. This is equivalent to about a 5- to 10-mg/dL glucose decline each hour in normal fasting levels of glucose. This can be eliminated by separating the serum from clotted cells using centrifugation and gel barriers or separation devices. If separation of serum or plasma is not possible or the methodology requires whole blood and delayed analysis, the preferred preservative for the sample is sodium fluoride.[34] This is found in conjunction with sodium oxalate in the standard gray-top blood collection container. However, some newer methods of POC using glucose dehydrogenase have interference with this anticoagulant, so prompt analysis using capillary blood is the only option.[35] Moderate to gross hemolysis will cause inter-

TABLE 4-8

Analytical Interferences in Glucose Analysis

Method	Interfering Substance
Glucose oxidase	Ascorbic acid, uric acid, bilirubin, hemoglobin, tetracycline, glutathione, galactose, D-xylose
Hexokinase	RBC phosphate esters, bilirubin, triglycerides (>500 mg/dL), drugs, fructose

ferences in some methods as well, so care should be taken in collection and handling of the blood sample prior to glucose analysis.[16]

Accuracy and precision of POC glucose devices have been reported to compare well with glucose analyses performed by laboratory-based instrumentation. For example, in method comparison studies provided by the manufacturer, the Bayer Glucometer Elite® whole blood glucose values compared favorably (bias of 4% to 6%) with laboratory instruments utilizing both glucose oxidase and hexokinase methods. The same POC instrument exhibited precisions of 3% to 6% coefficient of variation. The method comparison process is described further below. Accuracy can also be affected by analytical variations, such as interference from commonly occurring chemicals within the whole blood or plasma. Ascorbic acid, uric acid, salicylate, hemoglobin, and other reducing substances can falsely decrease the reaction of glucose oxidase with glucose due to inhibition of the chromagen. This is minimized by dilution of the sample.[16] Table 4–8 lists interferences in glucose methods.

Case Scenario 4-7 Comparing Results: POCT vs. Laboratory Results

Follow-Up

In this situation, Ms. Morris, a patient with congestive heart failure and type 2 diabetes mellitus, had significantly different capillary blood glucose values than venous plasma glucose on several occasions. She died a few days later as a result of her congestive heart failure. ●

Heart failure is the inability of the heart to circulate blood effectively enough to meet the body's metabolic needs. This inadequacy will potentially cause a difference in analytes in venous blood compared to capillary blood. Microvascular disorders can also cause poor circulation, affecting the capillary circulation more so than venous circulation, and are indicated by cold and/or pale fingertips. In those circumstances, venous blood glucose is more likely accurate than capillary glucose values.

CLINICAL CORRELATION
Heart failure may affect the left ventricle, right ventricle, or both. Forward-failing heart failure causes the forward flow of blood to the tissues to be inadequate because the left ventricle is unable to pump blood to the systemic circulation with enough force. This inadequacy will decrease circulation to the capillaries.

Comparing Methods: Evaluating the New Method

Method comparisons are necessary when introducing a new method of analysis so that clinical decision-making is not affected adversely. For example, when a POC glucose device was used to guide insulin therapy changes, results obtained with the new device were compared with the results provided by the analyzer. A study[31] was carried out in a hospital laboratory comparing the arterial whole blood glucose results from 123 patients with the Bayer Glucometer Elite XL® device and with the Nova-SP-9®. Both instruments use glucose oxidase methods. Partial pressure of O_2 was analyzed to consider variation due to innate oxygen within the samples. The following data were obtained:

Range = 24–476 mg/dL, n = 123, bias = –4.8%, r = 0.986, y = 1.11x – 20.96

The bias from the POC device was –4.8% compared with the Nova analyzer. The correlation coefficient was 0.986, with 1.000 considered a perfect correlation between the two instruments. Linear regression was performed on the data to obtain slope and y-intercept. The slope of 1.11 represents a slight proportional error when compared to 1.00. The y-intercept of –20.96 represents an approximately 21-mg/dL constant error in which the POC device will consistently provide lower arterial whole blood glucose values than the laboratory instrument. Similar results have been obtained with the Accu-Chek, with an even lower bias and but a constant error of +8.4 mg/dL.[29] Overall, the data point to reasonable correlation and moderate constant errors between the two instruments.

One aspect that may introduce a significant difference in capillary versus venous blood is the impact of the patient's circulation. Due to normal circulation, typically capillary blood compares more closely to arterial blood than to venous blood. Glucose within venous blood is as much as 1.3% (7 mg/dL) lower than capillary blood glucose due to tissue utilization and impact on circulation. Patients with peripheral microvascular disease, congestive heart failure, or other circulatory problems may have diminished circulation to the fingertips causing an impact on analytes measured in finger-stick samples.[35,36] Samples obtained from earlobes may also be different than venous samples due to the effect of circulatory problems. Warming the site prior to collection may help to normalize this effect.[16]

How Are POC Glucose Values To Be Used According to ADA Guidelines?

POC glucose devices are not to be used for diagnosis but rather for monitoring daily glycemic control relative to diet, activity, and therapy. (Refer to the earlier discussion of the ADA criteria for diagnosis of diabetes.) Newer, more precise POC instruments may be used to closely target insulin therapy to glucose results. The current insulin dosage target is to achieve a fasting plasma glucose of 100 mg/dL.[9] Glucose monitors must be able to report results calibrated to plasma results and be highly accurate and precise methodologies to achieve this goal. Frequent analysis of glucose quality control samples can help to assess the reliability of the instrument and reagent strips in providing patient results.

SUMMARY

The clinical laboratory provides information for health care providers to diagnose diabetes and other carbohydrate disorders. The laboratory also provides information to help monitor the progression of disease and manage it with changes in therapy as needed. Laboratory results contribute to health promotion and disease prevention by identifying individuals who are at high risk for developing future carbohydrate disease. The clinical laboratory scientist must have a thorough understanding of the disease process and the ability to produce laboratory results that accurately represent the physiological concentration of carbohydrates in the body.

EXERCISES

As you consider the scenarios presented in this chapter, answer the following questions:

1. Describe the Clinical Practice Guidelines of the American Diabetes Association for the diagnosis of type 1 diabetes, type 2 diabetes, and gestational diabetes.

2. Discuss test specificity for the common methods for analyzing blood glucose.

3. Describe the evidence that indicates that control of blood glucose levels will reduce the severe consequences of diabetes.

4. Explain the use of the measurement of Hb A_{1c} levels in the diagnosis and treatment of diabetes.

5. Compare glucose levels of whole blood and serum.

6. Explain the etiology of neonatal hypoglycemia.

7. When is a less specific method for sugar, such as a reducing sugar method, clinically significant?

8. What specimen collection and handling considerations should be made for ketone testing?

9. In what situations should one attempt to correlate the glucose results with the ketone results?

10. What are some abnormal forms of hemoglobin that may interfere with glycated hemoglobin analysis?

References

1. American Diabetes Association: Diabetes statistics. Available at *http://www.diabetes.org/diabetes-statistics.jsp* (accessed Feb 13, 2006).
2. *Diabetes Surveillance.* Bethesda, MD: U.S. Department of Health and Human Services, 1999.
3. National Center for Health Statistics: *National Hospital Discharge Survey.* Atlanta: Centers for Disease Control and Prevention, 1998.
4. Dokhee TM: An epidemic of childhood diabetes in the United States? Evidence from Allegheny County, Pennsylvania. Pittsburgh Diabetes Epidemiology Research Group. *Diabetes Care* 1993; 16:1606–1611.
5. American Diabetes Association: Diagnosis and classification of diabetes mellitus. *Diabetes Care*, 2006; 29(Suppl 1).
6. Clark PM: Assays for insulin, proinsulin(s) and C-peptide. *Ann Clin Biochem* 1999; 36:541–564.
7. Van den Berghe G, et al: Intensive insulin therapy in critically ill patients. *N Engl J Med* 2001; 345:1359–1367.
8. Krinsley JS: Effect of an intensive glucose management protocol on the mortality of critically ill adult patients. *Mayo Clin Proc* 2004; 79:992–1000.
9. The Diabetes Control and Complications Trial Research Group: The effect of intensive treatment of diabetes on the development and progression of long-term complications in insulin-dependent diabetes mellitus. *N Engl J Med* 1993; 329:977–986.

10. The DCCT/EDIC Research Group: Retinopathy and nephropathy in patients with type 1 diabetes four years after a trial of intensive therapy. *N Engl J Med* 2000; 342:381–389.

11. The UK Prospective Diabetes Study Group: Intensive blood-glucose control with sulphonylureas or insulin compared with conventional treatment and risk of complications in patients with type 2 diabetes (UKPDS 33). *Lancet* 1998; 352:837–853.

12. The UK Prospective Diabetes Study Group: Effect of intensive blood-glucose control with metformin on complications in overweight patients with type 2 diabetes (UKPDS 34). *Lancet* 1998; 352:854–865.

13. Goldstein DE, et al: Tests of glycemia in diabetes (Technical Review). *Diabetes Care* 1995; 18:896–909.

14. Sacks DS, et al: Guidelines and recommendations for laboratory analyses in the diagnosis and management of diabetes mellitus. *Diabetes Care* 2002; 25:750–786.

15. Beers M, Berkow R: *The Merck Manual of Diagnosis and Therapy*, ed 17. Rahway, NJ: Merck & Co., 1999.

16. Cohen HT, Spiegel DM: Air-exposed urine dipsticks give false positive results for glucose and false-negative results for blood. *Am J Clin Pathol* 1991; 96:398–400.

17. Gall MA, et al: Risk factors for development of incipient and overt diabetic nephropathy in patients with non-insulin dependent diabetes mellitus: Prospective, observational study. *BMJ* 1997; 314:783–788.

18. Ravid M, et al: Long-term renoprotective effect of angiotensin-converting enzyme inhibition in non-insulin-dependent diabetes mellitus: A 7-year follow-up study. *Arch Intern Med* 1996; 156:286–289.

19. American Diabetes Association: Self-monitoring of blood glucose (Consensus Statement). *Diabetes Care* 1987; 10:93–99.

20. Little RR, et al: The National Glycohemoglobin Standardization Program (NGSP): A five-year progress report. *Clin Chem* 2001; 47:1985–1992.

21. Goldstein DE, et al: Glycated hemoglobin: Methodologies and clinical applications. *Clin Chem* 1986; 32:B64–B70.

22. Rohlfing CL, et al: Defining the relationship between plasma glucose and HbA_{1c}: Analysis of glucose profiles and HbA_{1c} in the Diabetes Control and Complications Trial. *Diabetes Care* 2002; 25:275–278.

23. O'Sullivan JB, Mahan CM: Criteria for the oral glucose tolerance test in pregnancy. *Diabetes* 1964; 13:278.

24. Carpenter MW, Coustan DR: Criteria for screening tests for gestational diabetes. *Am J Obstet Gynecol* 1982; 144:768–773.

25. Metzger BE, Coustan DR (eds): Proceedings of the Fourth International Workshop-Conference on Gestational Diabetes Mellitus. *Diabetes Care* 1998; 21(Suppl 2): B1–B167.

26. Service FJ: Hypoglycemic disorders. *N Engl J Med* 1995; 332:1144–1152.

27. Young DS, Jackson AJ: Thin-layer chromatography of urinary carbohydrates: A comparative evaluation of procedures. *Clin Chem* 1970; 16:954.

28. Davis B, Mass D, Bishop M: *Principles of Clinical Laboratory Utilization and Consultation*. Philadelphia: WB Saunders, 1999.

29. *Accu-Chek Comfort Curve, 2003 Operator's Manual*. Indianapolis, IN: Roche Diagnostics Corp., 2003.

30. *Accu-Chek Instant Plus 1996 User's Manual*. Indianapolis, IN: Boehringer Mannheim Corp., 1996.

31. *Miles Glucometer 3 Blood Glucose Meter 1999 User's Manual*. Elkhart, IN: Bayer Inc. Diagnostics Division, 1999.

32. *One Touch II Blood Glucose Monitoring System 1992 User's Manual*. New Brunswick, NY: Johnson & Johnson, 1992.

33. Barreau PB, Buttery JI: The effect of the haematocrit value on the determination of glucose levels by reagent strip methods. *Med J Aust* 1987; 147:286–288.

34. Chen AV, et al: Effectiveness of sodium fluoride as a preservative of glucose in blood. *Clin Chem* 1989; 35:315–317.

35. Thomas SH, et al: Accuracy of fingerstick glucose determination in patients receiving CPR. *South Med J* 1994; 87:1072–1075.

36. Atkin SH, et al: Fingerstick glucose determination in shock. *Ann Intern Med* 1991; 114:1020–1024.

5

Hemoglobin synthesis is a vital process that can be affected by many aspects, including environmental ones, and often provides clinical clues, including changes in laboratory results.

Hemoglobin Production Disorders and Testing

Vicki Freeman and Wendy Arneson

In this chapter, we will discuss hemoglobin synthesis, conditions that affect the normal formation of hemoglobin, and how these conditions are detected through laboratory testing. There are four scenarios in this chapter illustrating correlation of laboratory values with disorders including iron-deficiency anemia, lead poisoning, and hereditary porphyrias. By working through the problems as they are presented, the student will learn about iron, ferritin, lead, porphyrin, porphobilinogen, and glycated hemoglobin testing based on preanalytical and analytical situations. The side boxes in this chapter provide common sense tips, definitions of terms, and brief descriptions of clinical correlations as well as reminders of the team approach in health care. Text boxes within the chapter outline methodology for laboratory assessment of hemoglobin production disorders.

OBJECTIVES

Upon completion of this chapter, the student will have the ability to

- List three (3) physiologic functions of iron in the body.
- Discuss the common methods of analysis, endpoint detection, specimen collection and handling requirements, and sources of error for iron, TIBC, whole blood lead, and glycated hemoglobin.
- Evaluate serum iron, TIBC, transferrin, and % saturation results compared to reference ranges and correlate with iron-deficiency anemia, anemia of chronic diseases, and hemosiderosis.
- Identify the structures of uroporphyrin I and III, coproporphyrin I and III, protoporphyin III (IX), and delta-aminolevulinic acid.
- Describe the effect of lead in heme synthesis.
- Evaluate whole blood lead level and possible sources of toxicity.
- Describe the enzyme defects in acute intermittent porphyria and hereditary coproporphyria.
- Describe the principle, specimen collection and handling requirements, and interferences in the Watson-Swartz test and the porphyrin tests.

CASE SCENARIO 5-1

Case of Iron-Deficiency Anemia: Iron-Poor Blood

The laboratory performed a routine CBC on a 40-year-old female who was schedule to have elective surgery. The following test values were obtained:

Test	Result	Reference Range
Hemoglobin (g/dL)	10	11.7–15.5
Hematocrit (%)	29.9	35–45
MCV (fL)	75	80–100
MCHC (g/dL)	30	32–34
WBC ($\times 10^9$/L)	6.0	4.0–11.0
Platelet count ($\times 10^9$/L)	200	150–400

The morphology showed a few pencil forms and occasional target cells. The physician then ordered serum iron and ferritin levels and a TIBC.

HEME SYNTHESIS

A series of enzymatic reactions that begin with coenzyme A and glycine pyridoxal phosphate lead to the formation of heme (Fig. 5–1).

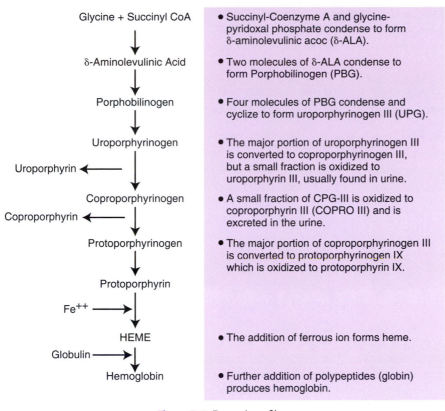

Figure 5–1. Formation of heme.

ABSORPTION, TRANSPORT, AND STORAGE OF IRON

As shown in the heme synthesis model in Figure 5–1, iron is an essential element of heme and hemoglobin. Iron is also a constituent of methemoglobin, myoglobin, and several enzymes. Iron is used by the body, in conjunction with the hemoglobin molecule, to transport oxygen to the cells, where it participates in oxidative mechanisms.

How Is Iron Absorbed in the Body?

Iron, ingested in the ferric $(3+)$ state, must be converted to the ferrous $(2+)$ state to be absorbed. This conversion takes place in the stomach, where the gastric HCl provides the acidity to reduce the iron. This absorption mechanism is the body's method of regulating the amount of iron in the body. Iron that is not absorbed is excreted through the feces.

How Is Iron Stored in the Body?

Approximately 25% of the iron in the body is stored in the liver, spleen, and bone marrow as **ferritin**, or ferric iron (Fe^{3+}) bound to an **apoferritin** protein molecule.

ferritin - the storage form of iron found in the liver, spleen, and bone marrow

apoferritin - the protein portion of ferritin, the storage form of iron

transferrin - a beta$_1$ globulin transport protein for carrying iron in blood plasma

When the body needs iron for synthesis of heme, myoglobin, or other molecules, it is released from the ferritin and is then bound to the beta$_1$ globulin molecule, **transferrin**, to circulate in the body, primarily to the hematopoietic tissue to be used in heme synthesis.

How Is Iron Transported in the Body?

The majority of the iron in the body is found bound to transferrin. The cellular uptake of iron is mediated by a cell-surface transferrin receptor (TfR). The amount of transferrin receptor expressed on a cell is proportional to a cell's need for iron. A proteolytic product of the transferrin receptor (called soluble transferrin receptor [sTfR]) circulates in plasma, and its concentration is proportional to the total concentration of cellular TfR. In the case of a deficiency of apoferritin, excess iron is deposited as small iron oxide granules, called **hemosiderin**. Figure 5–2 depicts the physiologic processes affecting iron, including absorption, transport, and storage.

hemosiderin - granular iron oxide found in the bone marrow or other cells

ASSESSING IRON LEVELS AND FORMS

In order to understand how iron testing is performed, it is important that the mechanisms controlling the absorption, transportation, and storage of iron are comprehended. Iron, transferrin, and ferritin can be measured directly by laboratory techniques. Additionally, an indirect method of measuring transferrin concentration and the saturation of the transferrin molecule can be performed. The total iron-binding capacity (TIBC) is an indirect measurement of the transferrin concentration. This test measures the total amount of iron that apotransferrin has the capacity to bind. Alternatively, the unsaturated iron-binding capacity (UIBC), the

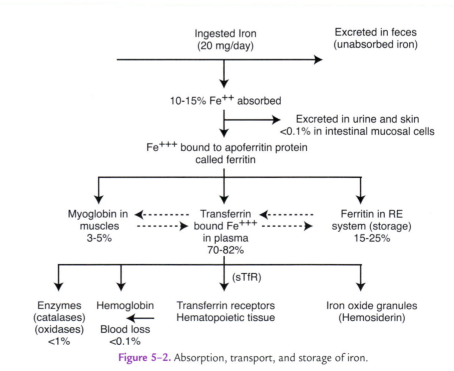

Figure 5–2. Absorption, transport, and storage of iron.

amount of protein (apotransferrin) still available to bind iron, can be measured. TIBC can also be expressed in terms of percentage of the saturation of the transferrin molecule (called % *saturation*). One less commonly utilized laboratory test to assess iron status is sTfR. This can be measured to determine the cellular requirement of iron. Since most cellular iron utilization is by erythroid precursor cells, the circulating sTfR is proportional to the rate of erythropoiesis and becomes elevated in iron deficiency, when cells become more competitive for the iron.[1]

TIBC measures the total amount of iron that apotransferrin has the capacity to bind. TIBC is measured by incubating serum containing transferrin with ferric ammonium citrate so that all free sites are saturated with iron. Excess unbound iron is removed and the remaining fully saturated transferrin is measured by an iron method.

Serum ferritin is the best diagnostic test for iron deficiency because it is a measurement of the iron stores in the body. Iron deficiency is indicated by a decreased ferritin concentration in adults of below 15 µg/L compared to a reference range of 20 to 250 µg/L, in children of lower than 6 µg/L (7 to 140 µg/L), and in babies of lower than 12 µg/L (50 to 200 µg/L). These cutoffs detect most cases of iron deficiency; however, deficiencies can occur in the low-normal range.[2] It is also important to be aware that serum ferritin is an acute-phase reactant, and its concentration may be increased in the presence of infections, systemic inflammations, malignancies, liver diseases, and chronic renal failure. Oral contraceptives can cause increases in serum transferrin levels, and serum iron levels can become transiently increased after oral iron ingestion, which results in low transferrin saturation levels when taking oral contraceptives and iron supplements. So, while a low serum ferritin is diagnostic of iron deficiency, normal serum ferritin values do not exclude a deficiency state, and other tests such as serum iron and % transferrin saturation may be needed. Additionally, the ratio of sTfR to serum ferritin (R/F ratio) may be used to provide an estimate of iron stores. sTfR is not affected by oral contraceptives or iron intake. The R/F ratio is affected by inflammatory processes.[3]

Case Scenario 5-1 Case of Iron-Deficiency Anemia: Iron-Poor Blood

Additional Test Results

Initial results from a complete blood count (CBC) on a 40-year-old woman led the physician to order serum iron and ferritin levels and a TIBC. The results of the follow-up tests on this patient with suspected iron-deficiency anemia (IDA) were as follows:

Test	Result	Reference Range
Serum iron (µg/dL)	20	50–170
Serum ferritin (µg/L)	5	20–200
TIBC (µg/dL)	550	250–400

In adults, a serum ferritin level less than 12 µg/L is the most common cutoff value used to denote absence of iron stores. In the past, a combination of serum ferritin less than 12 µg/L and % saturation of transferrin less than 16% was used to identify iron deficiency. However, with newer methods of analysis that remove the interference of copper, the cutoff value for transferrin saturation has been lowered

---

✓ **Common Sense Check**
The amount of TIBC should be larger than serum iron concentration since TIBC includes serum iron. If an analytical error occurs or the numbers are accidentally reversed, TIBC concentration could possibly appear smaller than serum iron. This indicates a need to check for analytical or transcription errors.

■■ **CLINICAL CORRELATION**
Hemolytic anemia is associated with decreased to normal serum iron levels resulting from red blood cell (RBC) destruction, while pernicious anemia is associated with decreased to normal serum iron and TIBC levels due to defective iron storage.

■■ **CLINICAL CORRELATION**
Hemochromatosis is associated with increased serum iron, normal to increased TIBC, and decreased serum ferritin levels due to increased rate of absorption and less ferritin production.

■■ **CLINICAL CORRELATION**
Hepatitis is correlated with increased serum iron and TIBC levels due to increased release of iron and ferritin from storage forms.

■■ **CLINICAL CORRELATION**
In cirrhosis, serum iron, TIBC, and ferritin levels are all decreased due to decreased production of protein.

CLINICAL CORRELATION
In nephritic syndrome, serum iron and TIBC levels are decreased due to increased loss of protein and iron.

CLINICAL CORRELATION
In lead poisoning, serum iron is decreased due to decreased RBC formation.

CLINICAL CORRELATION
In malignancies, serum iron is decreased due to impaired release from stores, while in pregnancy the increased demand on iron stores causes potential for decreased serum iron if iron supplements are not taken.

CLINICAL CORRELATION
The laboratory features in patients with hemoglobinopathies or thalassemia include microcytic, hypochromic red blood cells with anisocytosis, poikilocytosis, and mild thrombocytosis. There is usually increased serum ferritin and % transferrin saturation and normal to decreased levels of transferrin and TIBC.

microcytic - of smaller than normal size (red blood cells)

hypochromic - having a large pale central area due to less hemoglobin (red blood cells)

anisocytosis - variation in sizes of red blood cells: smaller, larger or both

poikilocytosis - unusual shape of red blood cells

hemoglobinopathies - diseases that result in structural abnormalities of globin chains

thalassemias - diseases resulting from decreased synthesis of globin chains

to 10% to 12%.[4] Identification of iron deficiency in the elderly is usually based on the same criteria as for adults. However, age-specific criteria should be applied to this population as the sensitivity of serum ferritin in detecting iron deficiency is reduced (due to elevated serum ferritin levels during inflammation) and hemoglobin levels in elderly men may be lower than in 18- to 44-year-old males.

Case Scenario 5-1 Case of Iron-Deficiency Anemia: Iron-Poor Blood

Follow-Up

The hematologic results and serum iron and ferritin levels in the iron deficiency case study are low, while the TIBC is increased. These results are indicative of IDA as they demonstrate a low level of iron in storage and in the bloodstream, but an increased capacity to bind more iron on the transferrin protein molecule. ●

Iron Deficiency

The laboratory features of iron deficiency include a constellation of findings in the hematology profile. Iron deficiency causes red blood cells that are small (**microcytic**) with **hypochromia**, of varying sizes (**anisocytosis**), and of odd shapes (**poikilocytosis**). It may possibly cause mild thrombocytosis as well. IDA is also associated with reduced ferritin, iron, and % transferrin saturation levels and increased levels of transferrin and TIBC. Test Methodology 5–1 provides details on the various types of iron measurement. Similar findings, except for low iron levels, may be present in patients with **hemoglobinopathies** or **thalassemia**, which should be excluded when clinically appropriate.

TEST METHODOLOGY 5-1.   IRON MEASUREMENT

The Reaction

Colorimetric Iron Procedures

Method 1:

$$Fe^{+++}:Transferrin \xrightarrow{acid} Fe^{+++} + apoferritin$$
$$Fe^{+++}: \xrightarrow{Reducing\ Agents^*} transferrin + 2Fe^{++}$$
$$Fe^{++} + complexing\ chromogen^{**} \rightarrow colored\ complex$$

Method 2:

$$Fe^{+++}:transferrin \rightarrow Fe^{+++} + apoferritin$$
$$Fe^{3+} + hydroxyamine \rightarrow Fe^{++}$$
$$Fe^{++} + bathophenanthroline^{**} \rightarrow decrease\ in\ absorbance$$

Other methods of iron measurement include:
Electrochemical coulometry (sums up electron transition)
Atomic absorption spectroscopy

continued

> **TEST METHODOLOGY 5-1.   IRON MEASUREMENT** *(continued)*
>
> *Method of TIBC Measurement*
>
> Saturate all binding sites with excess Fe (ferric ammonium citrate or ferric chloride). Remove excess unbound iron (using ion-exchange resin or chelation by $MgCO_3$, followed by centrifugation and decanting the supernatant containing saturated transferrin). Run as per iron method above.
>
> **The Specimen**
>
> Serum, free from visible hemolysis. Patient should be fasting as iron levels can become transiently increased by iron ingestion. Morning specimen is best as iron has a diurnal variation with higher concentrations later in the day.
>
> **The Calculations**
>
> UIBC = TIBC – serum iron.
> % Saturation of iron = serum iron × 100/TIBC
>
> **Reference Ranges for Iron**
>
> | | |
> |---|---|
> | Adult male | 65–170 µg/dL |
> | Adult female | 50–170 µg/dL |
> | Infants or children | Age-specific |
>
> **Reference Ranges for TIBC**
>
> | | |
> |---|---|
> | Adult | 250–450 µg/dL |
> | Infant | 100–400 µg/dL |
>
> These reference ranges are highly method dependent and should be established by each laboratory based on their patient population and method of analysis.
>
> ---
> *Potential reducing agents include ascorbic acid, hydrazine, thioglycollic acid, or hydroxylamine.
> **Potential chromogens include bathophenanthroline sulfate, diphenylphenanthroline, ferrozine, or tripyridyltriazine.

When an increase in hemoglobin of 10 to 20 g/L (1 to 2 g/dL) in 2 to 4 weeks is seen following a trial of iron therapy, then the diagnosis of iron deficiency is supported. Other tests may be ordered, including free erythrocyte protoporphyrin and serum free transferrin receptors, which are not affected by concurrent diseases. However, they are not available in most diagnostic facilities.[5]

Practice Calculation: UIBC and % Saturation of Iron

A 45-year-old male had the following test results for serum iron, TIBC, and % saturation of iron: iron was 70 µg/dL (reference range, 65 to 170 µg/dL) and TIBC was 210 µg/dL (250 to 450 µg/dL). Use the following formulas to determine UIBC and % saturation of iron:

UIBC = TIBC – serum iron
% saturation of iron = serum iron × 100/TIBC

For this patient:

UIBC = 210 – 70 = 140 µg/dL
% saturation of iron = 70 × 100/210 = 33.3%

TABLE 5-1

Correlation of Iron Studies with Conditions

	Iron	TIBC	Ferritin
Iron-deficiency anemia	↓	↓	↓
Cirrhosis	↓	↓	↓
Pernicious anemia	↓ to Normal	↓	
Hemochromatosis	↑	Normal to ↑	
Hepatitis	↑	↑	
Nephrosis and bleeding	↓	↓	
Hemolytic anemia	↓ to Normal		
Lead poisoning	↓		
Pregnancy	↓		
Malignancies	↓		
Infections	↓		

Interpretation of Iron Results

There are several causes of excessive serum iron, including hemosiderosis and hemochromatosis. Hemosiderosis is a condition of maintaining excessive levels of iron in storage. Hemochromatosis causes excessive iron deposition in organs and is characterized by the development of bronze color in the tissues. Both of these conditions are associated with excessive levels of serum iron and % saturation of the transferrin with iron.

Causes of decreased iron include anemia of chronic disease and iron deficiency. Iron deficiency can be due to a variety of situations, including increased demand for iron, blood loss, and lack of dietary intake of iron. Table 5–1 shows the typical pattern of iron study results, including serum iron, TIBC, and ferritin levels found in conditions of iron excess and iron deficiency.

CASE SCENARIO 5-2

Low Hemoglobin of Unknown Cause: Lead Poisoning from Paint in an Old House

A mother brings her active 2-year-old son to the pediatrician for a routine visit. The physician orders a CBC. When the laboratory returns the test results, she notices that the child's hemoglobin is 10.2 g/dL, a slight decrease from the normal range of 11 to 14 g/dL. The mother reports her son has been healthy for the most part, but has had some constipation and what appears to be abdominal pain. He does eat well, and she gives him a vitamin supplement that includes iron. Upon further questioning, the mother discloses that they live in an older home that hasn't been repainted in a long time, and the woodwork especially is not in good shape.

The physician orders further testing, including serum iron and ferritin levels, a blood lead level, and an erythrocyte protoporphyrin level. Given the tests just mentioned, what disorders does the physician suspect her patient has?

continued

Case Scenario 5-2 Low Hemoglobin of Unknown Cause: Lead Poisoning from Paint in an Old House (*continued*)

Additionally, she orders urine delta-aminolevulinic acid and coproporphyrin levels. The child and mother are sent to the laboratory for blood to be drawn and for instructions on the urine collection. What is the physician trying to either rule out or in?

MEASURING LEAD LEVELS

Lead is measured in whole blood by a variety of methods, as described in Test Methodology 5–2. Principle methods for lead testing include atomic absorption spectrophotometry and anodic stripping voltammetry.

TEST METHODOLOGY 5-2.   LEAD TESTING

The Reaction Principle

The specimens are diluted and aspirated into a calibrated atomic absorption spectrometer that has a good-quality graphite furnace programmed to dry the sample, char the sample at 700°C, and atomize at 2500°C, holding at 5 seconds. The absorbance peaks and peak area of duplicate samples are recorded. Concentration is determined from the calibration curve.

The Specimen

Whole blood collected with a lead-free needle, collecting tube (the royal blue–top tube is metal free), and stopper. The anticoagulant used will depend on the method of measurement; EDTA is common. Capillary blood is not recommended due to the increased possibility of contamination.

Urine should be collected directly into a plastic container from which the surface lead has been removed with an acid wash.

Since the difference between a normal and an elevated level is very small, any contamination must be avoided.

Reference Ranges

Infant	<10 μg/dL
Adult	<25 μg/dL

Lead Poisoning Effect on Heme Synthesis

It is now timely to take a look at the effect of lead on heme synthesis. Figure 5–3 shows the same heme synthesis pathway that was presented in Figure 5–1; however, Figure 5–3 shows the points in the pathway where lead inhibits the enzymes, causing a disruption in heme synthesis. Lead poisoning inhibits delta-aminolevulinic acid (δ-ALA) dehydrase, coproporphyrinogen oxidase, and ferrochelatase enzymes, causing a buildup of the substances earlier in the pathway. Increased δ-ALA, coproporphyrin, and protoporphyrin are commonly found in urine.

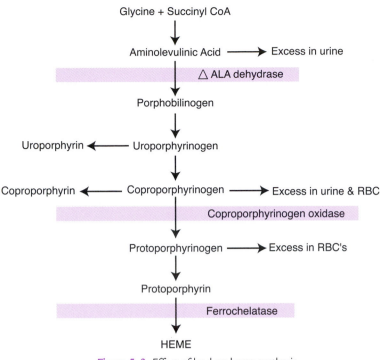

Figure 5–3. Effect of lead on heme synthesis.

Tests of Lead Inhibition of the Heme Pathway

Increased levels of urinary δ-ALA and urinary porphyrins are sometimes used as diagnostic tests of lead poisoning in adults. Erythrocyte protoporphyrin (EPP) levels in whole blood samples have been used as a screening test for lead poisoning. Another potential test is the zinc protoporphyrin (ZPP) test. ZPP forms from excess protoporphyrin IX combining with Zn when Fe is not available. Free protoporphyrin and zinc protoporphyrin are not measured routinely but are available from reference laboratories and can also be measured fluorometrically.

What Is the Best Test for Determining Lead Toxicity in Children?

The single best test for detection of toxic lead exposure is the measurement of whole blood lead. In 1991, the Centers for Disease Control and Prevention (CDC) established the whole blood analysis of lead as the recommended test and set lower lead levels to indicate lead toxicity. The current diagnostic level is greater than 10 μg/dL for children.[6] In adults, lead levels of greater than 30 μg/dL indicate significant exposure. According to the CDC, EPP levels are not sensitive indicators of low-level lead; they are sensitive only for high-level exposures. ZPP is considered a supplemental lead test but is not used extensively because of poor diagnostic sensitivity in cases of iron deficiency and anemia of chronic disease and due to poor diagnostic sensitivity limits of 25 μg/dL. Current guidelines recommend that all children up to age 6 be screened yearly using whole blood lead testing, with the highest priority going to children ages 1 to 3 years.[7]

In Case Scenario 5-2, the physician ordered serum iron and ferritin levels. How do these tests fit into the differential diagnostic criteria? What is the physician trying to either rule out or in?

Earlier, it was discussed that ferritin was the best diagnostic test for iron deficiency but that deficiencies can occur in the low-normal range of ferritin. In order to identify iron deficiency in children, age-specific reference ranges should be employed. A serum ferritin level of less than 10 to 12 μg/L is indicative of iron deficiency in children and is often used as a sole measure of iron status or used in combination with another parameter. The physician ordered ferritin and iron to determine if the child was suffering from iron-deficiency anemia.

Additionally, the physician ordered a blood lead level, erythrocyte protoporphyrin level, and urinary delta-aminolevulinic acid and coproporphyrin in addition to the ferritin and iron levels. Low levels of hemoglobin may be present in iron-deficiency anemia or in disorders other than iron-deficiency anemia. In this case, it appears that the physician is considering lead poisoning as a potential cause of the anemia due to the home environment, since lead often comes from older paint or glazes of walls, furniture, or ceramic pottery.

Causes of Elevated Lead Levels in Adults and Children

Lead poisoning historically was a common problem with children. The CDC periodically surveys children on health and nutritional parameters and has reported that only about 4.4% of children currently have elevated blood levels compared with 88% of children in the 1970s. This is due to many factors, including the fact that lead is no longer a component of paint found in homes or furniture or a component of gasoline. Children in the past were frequently exposed by ingesting or inhaling lead from paint chips or by ground contamination from leaded gasoline.[8] Lead poisoning still occurs in part due to children exposed to lead in older homes that contain lead in paint and varnish, especially when released during home remodeling. Lead poisoning of children and adults is also a result of mining and industrial exposure.

THE TEAM APPROACH
Whole blood and urine lead levels may be tested in adults. Special lead-free collection containers need to be provided to the blood collection staff. Since urine should be collected in a lead-free container, an acid-washed plastic container needs to be provided to the patient.

Case Scenario 5-2 Low Hemoglobin of Unknown Cause: Lead Poisoning from Paint in an Old House

Additional Test Results

In our lead poisoning case, the laboratory results on the child were as follows:

Test	Child	Reference Range
Serum iron level (μg/dL)	120	50–100
Serum ferritin level (μg/L)	150	7–140
Whole blood lead (μg/dL)	60	≤10
Erythrocyte protoporphyrin (μg/dL)	150	17–77
Urine δ-aminolevulinic acid (mg/dL)	12.2	1.5–7.5
Urine coproporphyrin (μg/dL)	220	13–179

continued

Case Scenario 5-2 Low Hemoglobin of Unknown Cause:
Lead Poisoning from Paint in an Old House *(continued)*

The whole blood lead level was well above the medical decision limit, indicating lead poisoning. Iron deficiency was ruled out based on the serum iron and ferritin levels. The mother was instructed to have the paint and varnish in her home tested for lead and to remove the sources of lead from her home to which her son had access. The boy was started on chelation therapy, which helps remove the lead from his body. Lead levels will be checked periodically, as the redistribution of lead from tissue and bone stores can result in the return of elevated blood lead levels. ●

CASE SCENARIO 5-3

Acute Variegate Porphyria: Darkening Urine Samples in the Laboratory

The young South African woman's urine, sent to the laboratory for routine urinalysis, became dark upon standing. The laboratory performed a porphyrin screen and a brilliant pink fluorescence was visible when illuminated with ultraviolet light. The history of the woman revealed that she had became emotionally disturbed and appeared to be hysterical a few days after a laparotomy. Prior to her operation she had taken, over a period of a week, prescribed medication to help her sleep that contained barbiturates. When first seen by her physician, the patient had complained of severe abdominal and muscle pain and general weakness. Her tendon reflexes were absent, and she had frequent episodes of vomiting and was constipated.

What was the cause of the urine changing color? What specimen handling procedures should have been followed on the urine specimen? Whatfollow-up testing should be performed on the urine specimen and on a blood sample?

PORPHYRINS

porphyrins - cyclic compounds called tetrapyrroles that are formed by the linkage of four pyrrole rings

porphyrinogen - tetrapyrrole that is a precursor of heme

Porphyrins are cyclic compounds called tetrapyrroles that are formed by the linkage of four pyrrole rings through methylene (methane) bridges,[9] as depicted in Figure 5–4. Heme precursors are called **porphyrinogens**. In biological liquids, particularly at acidic pH, porphyrinogens oxidize into porphyrins, which are found in body fluids. Porphyrins are derivatives from porphin, composed of a four-pyrrole nucleus. Only three porphyrins are of clinical significance: uroporphyrin, coproporphyrin, and protoporphyrin (Fig. 5–5).

The chemical properties of the porphyrin molecules play an important role in the pathogenesis of the porphyrias. Conjugated double bonds give coloration (maximum of absorbance around 405 nm) and fluorescence (around 620 nm). Nuclear substitution of the pyrroles by carboxyl groups alters the solubility of each different molecule. Carboxyl groups make the porphyrin more soluble in water. Porphyrins with less than 4 carboxyl groups are not found in appreciable amounts in urine and are excreted mostly in bile and feces. Porphyrins deposit in the skin, which causes an inflammatory reaction when exposed to ultraviolet (UV) light. Protoporphyrin with 2 carboxyl groups is soluble in lipids and insoluble in water. These solubility properties cause protoporphyrin to concentrate more in the cellu-

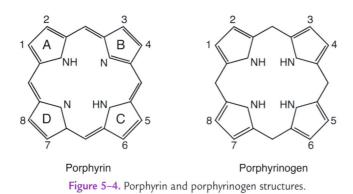

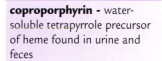

Figure 5-4. Porphyrin and porphyrinogen structures.

lar membranes and cause inflammatory reactions with burning sensations soon after exposure to the sunlight.

Coproporphyrin, containing 4 carboxyl groups, is excreted by both urinary and fecal routes. Uro- and coproporphyrins are soluble in water; **uroporphyrin**, with 8 carboxyl groups, is more highly soluble than coproporphyrin. They concentrate in intra- and extracellular fluids and cause bulbous skin lesions late in the disease course. The porphyrins' solubility also determines their elimination profile: uroporphyrin is eliminated through urine while protopophyrin is essentially eliminated in feces. Coproporphyrins are eliminated through both methods. Porphyrin

coproporphyrin - water-soluble tetrapyrrole precursor of heme found in urine and feces

uroporphyrin - highly water-soluble precursor of heme found in urine

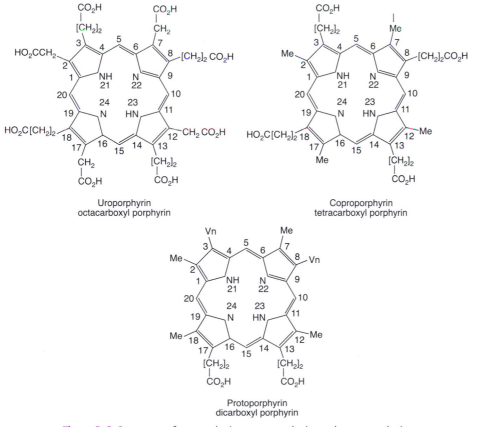

Figure 5-5. Structures of uroporphyrin, coproporphyrin, and protoporphyrin.

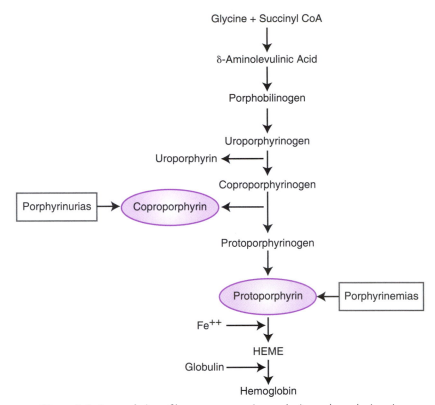

Figure 5–6. Accumulation of heme precursors in porphyrias and porphyrinemias.

precursors (δ-ALA and porphobilinogen [PBG]) are freely eliminated by the kidneys, and their blood levels are always quite low.

Porphyrin Conditions

The three common porphyrin conditions are based on the accumulation of porphyrin metabolites in the urine, the red blood cells, or in the entire body. **Porphyrinurias** and **porphyrinemias** are secondary conditions. In porphyrinuria there is a moderate increase in urine coproporphyrin production, while in porphyrinemia there is an increase in erythrocytic protoporphyrin concentration, as depicted in Figure 5–6. Lead intoxication can cause both of these conditions. Additional causes of porphyrinuria include liver damage, accelerated erythropoiesis, and infection. Other causes of porphyrinemia include iron deficiency, impaired iron absorption, and chronic infection.

The third condition, porphyria, may be either inherited or acquired. The common feature in all porphyrias is the excess accumulation in the body of porphyrins and porphyrin precursors. These are natural chemicals that normally do not accumulate in the body. Precisely which one of these porphyrin chemicals builds up depends upon the type of porphyria. The inherited type is a result of a deficiency in one of the enzymes in the heme synthesis pathway, as depicted in Figure 5–7. The classification is based upon the organ involved (i.e., liver or bone marrow; Table 5–2). For example, x-linked sideroblastic anemia is caused by a defect in δ-aminolevulinic acid synthase and results in impaired heme synthesis.

porphyrinuria - condition in which the urine contains excess coproporphyrin

porphyrinemia - condition in which the red blood cells contain excess protoporphyrin

■■ CLINICAL CORRELATION

In the hepatic type of inherited porphyria, the defect in porphyrin metabolism is within the liver. In hepatic porphyria, porphyrins and related substances are produced in excessive amounts from the liver.

■■ CLINICAL CORRELATION

The inherited erythropoietic type of porphyria is a defect of porphyrin metabolism within the blood-producing tissues, such as the bone marrow.

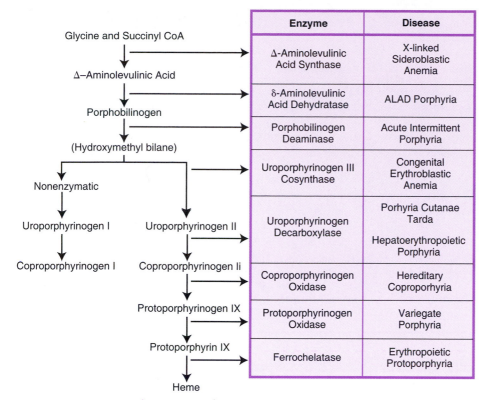

Figure 5-7. Porphyrias and their enzyme defects.

	Enzyme	Disease
	Δ-Aminolevulinic Acid Synthase	X-linked Sideroblastic Anemia
	δ-Aminolevulinic Acid Dehydratase	ALAD Porphyria
	Porphobilinogen Deaminase	Acute Intermittent Porphyria
	Uroporphyrinogen III Cosynthase	Congenital Erythroblastic Anemia
	Uroporphyrinogen Decarboxylase	Porhyria Cutanae Tarda / Hepatoerythropoietic Porphyria
	Coproporphyrinogen Oxidase	Hereditary Coproporhyria
	Protoporphyrinogen Oxidase	Variegate Porphyria
	Ferrochelatase	Erythropoietic Protoporphyria

TABLE 5-2

Porphyrias

Type	Enzyme Involved	Major Symptoms	Laboratory Tests
X-linked sideroblastic anemia (XLSA)	δ-Aminolevulinic acid synthase		Bone marrow exam
ALAD porphyria	δ-Aminolevulinic acid dehydratase (ALAD)	Abdominal pain	CBC with differential Increased urinary δ-aminolevulinic acid (δ-ALA)
Acute intermittent porphyria	Porphobilinogen deaminase	Abdominal pain Neuropsychiatric symptoms	Increased urinary porphobilinogen
Congenital erythropoietic porphyria	Uroporphyrinogen III cosynthase	Photosensitivity	Increased urinary uroporphyrin No change in porphobilinogen
Porphyria cutanea tarda	Uroporphyrinogen decarboxylase	Photosensitivity	Increased urinary uroporphyrin No change in δ-aminolevulinic acid and porphobilinogen

continued

TABLE 5-2 (continued)

Porphyrias

Type	Enzyme Involved	Major Symptoms	Laboratory Tests
Hepatoerythro-poietic porphyria	Uroporphyrinogen decarboxylase	Photosensitivity	Same as in PCT plus increased protoporphyrins in RBCs
Hereditary copro-porphyria	Coproporphyrino-gen oxidase	Photosensitivity	Decreased activity of copro-porphyrinogen oxidase
		Neurological symptoms	Increased coproporphyrin in feces & urine
Variegate porphyria	Protoporphyrino-gen oxidase	Photosensitivity	Increased urinary uroporphyrin, fecal coproporphyrin, and protoporphyrin
		Abdominal pain Neuropsychiatric symptoms	
Erythropoietic protoporphyria	Ferrochelatase	Photosensitivity	Increased fecal and RBC protoporphyrin

hepatic - pertaining to the liver

erythropoietic - pertaining to blood cell production

■■ **CLINICAL CORRELATION**
The acquired type of porphyria is caused by liver disease or occurs in response to toxic metals or drugs. Other biomarkers for liver disease are often present, including elevated serum bilirubin and liver enzymes.

■■ **CLINICAL CORRELATION**
Accumulation of porphyrinogens in the skin can cause photosensitivity, an inflammatory reaction worsened by sunlight. Patients may also have abdominal pain, constipation, and vomiting or more severe complications.

The group of eight[10] inherited disorders involves a defect in the heme biosynthetic pathways (conversion of glycine to heme) and results in abnormal porphyrin metabolism and an overproduction or accumulation of heme precursors (see Table 5–2). These conditions can be further divided into two groups: **hepatic** or **erythropoietic**.

The symptoms and treatments of the different types of porphyrias are not the same. Cutaneous porphyrias are porphyrias with skin manifestations. The acute porphyrias are characterized by sudden attacks of pain and other neurological symptoms that can be both rapidly appearing and severe. If an individual has the characteristic enzyme deficiency but has never developed symptoms, the condition is considered latent. There can be a wide spectrum of severity between the latent and active cases of any particular type of porphyria. However, in all cases there is an identifiable abnormality of the enzymes that synthesize heme that leads to accumulation of intermediates of the pathway and a deficiency of heme.

Porphyrins absorb visible light strongly, causing itchy skin, fluid accumulation, swelling, and the like. The most damaging wavelength is 405 nm, which is the peak of the absorption spectra of porphyrins, and this wavelength is not blocked by window glass. This sensitivity leads to skin blisters, fluid accumulation, and severe inflammation of the skin (called *photodermatitis*) on exposure to sunlight, with possible disfigurement. An acquired form of porphyria due to lead poisoning, which inhibits delta-aminolevulinic acid dehydrase, ferrochelatase, and copro-oxidase, causes a buildup of delta-aminolevulinic acid and porphyrins in the urine. This was discussed in an earlier section of this chapter.

Porphyrinogens, such as porphobilinogen, can undergo oxidation to their corresponding porphyrins through a light-catalyzed reaction. The porphyrin compounds, when accumulating in urine, cause it to become a dark red or purple color (red-violet at acid pH, red-brown at alkaline pH). The metabolites are irreversibly oxidized by light, and the urine will darken upon standing if it contains porphyrinogen. Urine containing excessive amounts of porphyrin, when organic solutions are added, will fluoresce when exposed to UV light (400 nm). This property is used in the laboratory detection of porphyrin. Random urine can be used for laboratory measurement, but must be protected from light since these chemicals will degrade when exposed to light. Total fecal porphyrins may also be measured and can be separated and quantified individually by high-pressure liquid chromatography (HPLC). Additionally, using nonhemolyzed plasma, porphyrins can be measured directly by fluorescence scanning. Normally there are only trace amounts of porphyrins in plasma. Therefore, a marked increase in the amount of fluorescent porphyrins would be indicative of a cutaneous porphyria. If the total plasma porphyrins are increased, HPLC can be used to determine which type of porphyrins predominate.

Case Scenario 5-3 Acute Variegate Porphyria: Darkening Urine Samples in the Laboratory

Follow-Up

In the case of acute variegate porphyria in a South African young woman, the urine sample sent to the laboratory for routine urinalysis became dark upon standing. The laboratory performed a porphyrin screen, in which a brilliant pink fluorescence was seen under ultraviolet light. When first seen by her physician, the patient had complained of severe abdominal and muscle pain and general weakness. Her tendon reflexes were absent and she was vomiting and constipated. Within 24 hours she was totally paralyzed and within 2 days she died.

The questions posed earlier can now be answered. The cause of the darkening urine was the presence of porphyrinogens that, when exposed to light, were oxidized to the porphyrin derivative. In cases in which porphyria is suspected, the urine sample should be protected from light as soon as it is collected.

Follow-up testing for porphyrinogens might include the Watson and Schwartz test (Fig. 5–8).[12] The physical and chemical properties of porphyrins are detected and measured by a UV test, as described in Test Methodology 5–3.

> **THE TEAM APPROACH**
> Routine urine handling requires properly labeled and covered containers but usually doesn't require protection from light. If porphyrinogens or porphyrins are suspected, the specimen should also be protected from light, and communication with nursing staff may be necessary to get a light-protected urine sample.

TEST METHODOLOGY 5-3.   URINE PORPHYRIN, PORPHYRINOGEN, AND PORPHOBILINOGEN

The Reaction: Porphyrin

A qualitative screening test[11] is based on the principle that porphyrins fluoresce in an organic solution when exposed to UV light. A mixture of amyl alcohol, ethyl ether, and glacial acetic acid is shaken with a urine aliquot and allowed to separate. The upper organic phase is irradiated with a long UV wavelength light and observed for pink fluorescence in comparison to a porphyrin standard. The upper, organic layer will exhibit pink fluorescence if porphyrins are present.

Interference

Drugs and metabolites may cause interfering fluorescence in the organic layer.

continued

Case Scenario 5-3 Acute Variegate Porphyria: Darkening Urine
Samples in the Laboratory *(continued)*

**TEST METHODOLOGY 5-3.   URINE PORPHYRIN, PORPHYRINOGEN,
AND PORPHOBILINOGEN** *(continued)*

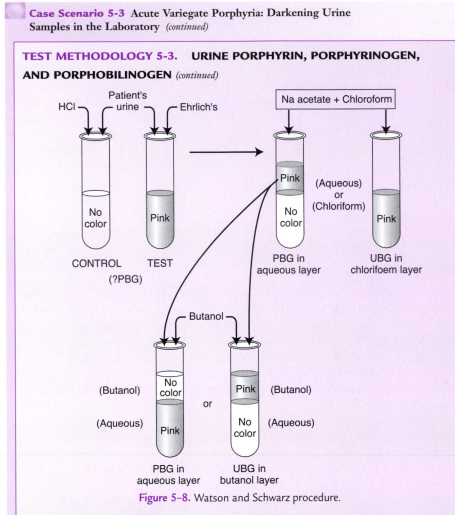

Figure 5–8. Watson and Schwarz procedure.

The Reaction: Porphyrinogen

Watson and Schwartz developed a qualitative test used in the detection of porphyrinogen. It uses Ehrlich's reagent, consisting of *p*-dimethylaminobenzaldehyde. Red color remaining in the aqueous supernatant (upper layer) is usually due to porphobilinogen. To increase specificity, the upper layer is further extracted with butanol. Porphobilinogen is then found in the lower aqueous layer. Any red color in that layer is due to porphobilinogen.

Porphobilinogen + Ehrlich's aldehyde reagent → red color

Interferences

Urobilinogen, indole, and indicane can all react pinkish-red. Further extractions can remove compounds such as chloroform, which extracts urobilinogen (UBG) to the lower level, or *n*-butanol, which extracts UBG to the upper level. Variations to improve specificity and minimize interferences include the addition of sodium acetate to increase pH, buffer, and enhance color. In the primary extraction, chloroform is added to extract UBG to the lower organic layer while porphobilinogen (PBG) stays in the upper aqueous layer. Confirmatory extraction with *n*-butanol extracts UBG into the upper (*n*-butanol) layer and PBG stays in the lower (urine) layer. For verification, HCl is added to a fresh urine aliquot. If color develops, interfering substances are present.

Case Scenario 5-3 Acute Variegate Porphyria: Darkening Urine
Samples in the Laboratory *(continued)*

TEST METHODOLOGY 5-3.   URINE PORPHYRIN, PORPHYRINOGEN,

AND PORPHOBILINOGEN *(continued)*

The Reaction: Porphobilinogen

A new semiquantitative screening test for urinary PBG is available. In this test, the urine is pretreated with ion-exchange resin and the color of the Ehrlich-PBG reaction is matched against a color chart for semiquantitative estimation of concentrations greater than 6 mg/L.[13] This test is recommended as a replacement for the Watson and Schwartz test. If positive, more specific tests should then be performed.[14]

THE SPECIMEN

Random urine; protect the specimen from light until analysis.
   Reference Ranges
   Negative is the normal result.

Hemoglobin Synthesis in the Context of Porphyrins

As mentioned at the beginning of this chapter, hemoglobin is synthesized from heme and globin. There are four subunits of the hemoglobin molecule: two identical pairs of polypeptide chains (the globins) each with a cleft on the exterior, which contains the heme (iron-porphyrin) group.[7] The types of polypeptides are named alpha, beta, delta, gamma, or epsilon.

Normally, the adult has more than 96% of total hemoglobin (Hb) as Hb A. This is composed of four polypeptides that are made of two alpha and two beta chains. There also may be a small percentage of Hb F, composed of two alpha chains and two gamma chains, and a small percentage of Hb A_2, composed of two alpha chains and two delta chains. *Hemoglobinopathies* are diseases that result in structural abnormalities of globin chains, while *thalassemias* are diseases resulting from decreased synthesis of globin chains. Both types of disorders affect the proportion of normal hemoglobins. A clinical hematology textbook can provide more details about those disorders.

CASE SCENARIO 5-4

**Problems With Glycated Hemoglobin Analysis:
Is the Hemoglobin A_{1c} Acceptable?**

Mr. Washington is an African American newly diagnosed type 2 diabetic. He has been referred to the diabetes clinic for his first 3-month check-up. Records show that, when he was diagnosed as a diabetic, his two fasting plasma glucose values were 132 mg/dL and 129 mg/dL (compared with the reference range of 74 to 100 mg/dL) and his glycated hemoglobin was 6.9% (4% to 6%). He also had a mild microcytosis noted on his CBC but normal hemoglobin and hematocrit. His current fasting plasma glucose is 115 mg/dL (74 to 100 mg/dL), and records show only two occasions during the past 3 months in which the fasting whole blood glucose exceeded 126 mg/dL (74 to 100 mg/dL). His current glycated hemoglobin is 7.8% (4% to 6%). The technologist in charge of the

continued

Case Scenario 5-4 CST:Problems With Glycated Hemoglobin Analysis: Is the Hemoglobin A$_{1c}$ Acceptable? *(continued)*

diabetes center is questioning the glycated hemoglobin result since it seems to be higher than expected given the previous results. He will consult the manufacturer's information and other resources to learn what may cause false-positive interferences in glycated hemoglobin.

GLYCATED HEMOGLOBIN

As discussed in Chapter 4 (Diabetes and Other Carbohydrate Disorders), glycated hemoglobin, of which hemoglobin A$_{1c}$ is the most stable, reflects sustained average plasma glucose over the life span of the erythrocytes. Since the average erythrocyte life span is 120 days, glycated hemoglobin, especially Hb A$_{1c}$, is an indication of long-term glucose control. It should not be used for diagnosis of diabetes but correlates well with risk of micro- and macrovascular complications such as retinopathy, neuropathy, microangiopathy, and cardiovascular disease.

There are several methods for determining glycated hemoglobin, including ion-exchange and affinity or high-performance liquid column chromatography. These methods all separate hemoglobin forms by their interaction with a mobile and stationary phase within a column. Quantitation of the glycated versus total hemoglobin can then be achieved spectrophotometrically. Some of these methods do experience analytical interferences due to temperature, altered forms of hemoglobin due to disease states such as uremia or alcoholism, or the presence of abnormal forms of hemoglobin such as S, C, or F.[15]

CLINICAL CORRELATION

Decreased levels of hemoglobin and poikilocytosis, including sickle-shaped red blood cells, are associated with hemoglobin S disease or sickle cell anemia.

How Can Electrophoresis Be Used to Analyze Hemoglobin A$_{1c}$?

Agar gel electrophoresis at pH 6.3 is also a method used to separate hemoglobin forms. This method relies on separation of the hemoglobin types based on differences in charge, molecular mass, and other aspects that affect migration in an electrical field. Electrophoretic separation is primarily of Hb A$_1$ from Hb A, followed by densitometry at 415 nm, which will help to quantify the amounts. This method has become highly automated and common for processing large volumes of tests. Although this method has less variation due to temperature or pH fluctuations, interference does exist due to Hb F and labile forms.[2]

Immunoassay methods are also used to quantify glycated hemoglobin using specific antibody to Hb A$_{1c}$. The antibody is specific due to structural differences in glycated hemoglobin when compared with other forms of hemoglobin. This method is also becoming widely available in clinical laboratories, including an application in a small point-of-care device available for testing in clinics where quick turnaround time is essential. This method is less precise and accurate than chromatography, but interference due to unusual forms of hemoglobin is less common than with some types of chromatography.

Case Scenario 5-4 Problems With Glycated Hemoglobin Analysis:
Is the Hemoglobin A$_{1c}$ Acceptable? *(continued)*

Follow-Up

Mr. Washington's Hb A$_{1c}$ was analyzed in the diabetes clinic by the electrophoretic method. It was suspected that Mr. Washington suffered from a hereditary persistence of hemoglobin F, which often manifests itself with up to 30% Hb F and slight microcytosis but no clinical evidence of anemia. Since electrophoresis does suffer from interference due to hemoglobin F, the sample was sent to a reference laboratory that performed glycated hemoglobin testing by HPLC. The Hb A$_{1c}$ value obtained by HPLC was 6.0% (reference range 4% to 6%), which seemed to correlate better with the average glucose values obtained over the past 3 months. Affinity chromatography is an alternative method that also does not suffer from interference due to variant forms or nonglycated forms of hemoglobin. However, it is not used as extensively due to manual steps involved. It has been replaced by more automated methods such as electrophoresis or HPLC. For more details on the principles of electrophoresis and chromatography, please refer to Chapter 3. ●

SUMMARY

Conditions that affect the normal formation of heme, such as iron deficiency, lead poisoning, and enzyme defects in the heme synthetic pathway, are relatively common events. These diseases can be detected through laboratory testing of iron, ferritin, lead, porphyrin, and porphobilinogen along with other hematologic and clinical data. Glycated hemoglobin is a normal form of hemoglobin A$_1$ but, in increased amounts, it indicates long-term hyperglycemia. Some methods of glycated hemoglobin analysis have interference from the presence of unusual or abnormal amounts of hemoglobin, such as hemoglobin F. The case scenarios in this chapter illustrated correlation of laboratory values with disorders including iron-deficiency anemia, lead poisoning, and hereditary porphyrias. Specimen collection and handling as well as a type of interference in glycated hemoglobin testing were also emphasized.

EXERCISES

As you consider the scenarios presented in this chapter, answer the following questions:

1. Define the following terms important to the measurement of various forms of iron: ferritin, transferrin, apoferritin, hemosiderin, TIBC, UIBC, % saturation, and serum transferrin receptors.

2. Discuss the absorption, transport, and storage of iron in the body.

3. Discuss the determination of TIBC and the calculation of UIBC and % saturation.

4. Identify the causes of increased and decreased iron and TIBC in the blood.

5. Explain a source of lead poisoning in children and the medical decision limit used.

6. Describe the basic structure and solubility of porphyrins and porphyrinogens.

7. Explain the effect of lead in heme synthesis.

8. Discuss the analysis of hemoglobin A_{1c} by an electrophoresis method.

References

1. Looker AC, Loyevsky M, Gordeuk VR: Increased serum transferrin saturation is associated with lower serum transferrin receptor concentration. *Clin Chem* 1999; 45:2191–2199.
2. Tietz NW: *Clinical Guide to Laboratory Tests*, ed 3. Philadelphia: WB Saunders, 1995.
3. Thomas C, Thomas L: Biochemical markers and hematologic indices in the diagnosis of functional iron deficiency. *Clin Chem* 2002; 48:1066–1076.
4. Looker AC, et al: Prevalence of iron deficiency in the United States. *JAMA* 1997; 277:973–976.
5. Guidelines and Protocols Advisory Committee: Investigation and management of iron deficiency (G&P2004-085), 2004. Available at *http://www.hlth.gov.bc.ca/msp/protoguides/gps/irondef.pdf*
6. National Center for Environmental Health: Preventing lead poisoning in young children, 2005. Available at *www.cdc.gov/nceh/lead/Publications/PrevLeadPoisoning.pdf*
7. National Center for Environmental Health: Managing elevated blood lead levels among young children: recommendations from the Advisory Committee on Childhood Lead Poisoning Prevention, 2002. Available at *www.cdc.gov/nceh/lead/CaseManagement/caseManage_main.htm*
8. National Center for Environmental Health: Available at *www.cdc.gov/nceh/lead/about/fedstrategy2000.pdf*
9. Nelson DL, Cox MM: *Lehninger Principles of Biochemistry*, ed 4. New York: WH Freeman, 2004.
10. American Porphyria Foundation: Porphyria types, 2006. Available at *www.porphyriafoundation.com/*
11. Zaider E, Bickers DR: Clinical laboratory methods for diagnosis of the porphyrias. *Clin Dermatol* 1998; 16:284.
12. Watson CJ, Schwartz S: A simple test for urinary porphobilinogen. *Proc Soc Exp Biol Med* 1941; 47:393.
13. Deacon AC, Peters TJ: Identification of acute porphyria: evaluation of a commercial screening test for urinary porphobilinogen. *Ann Clin Biochem* 1998; 35(Pt 6):726–732.
14. Anderson KE, et al: Recommendations for the diagnosis and treatment of the acute porphyrias. *Ann Intern Med* 2005; 142:439–450.
15. Goldstein DE, et al: Glycated hemoglobin: methodologies and clinical applications. *Clin Chem* 1986; 32:B64–B70.

The clinical laboratory provides objective information for the assessment of renal disorders.

6

Assessment of Renal Function

Wendy Arneson and Jean Brickell

electrolyte - substances that ionize in solution and conduct electricity

nonprotein nitrogen - catabolites of protein and nucleic acid metabolism, including urea, ammonia, creatinine, creatine, and uric acid

This chapter presents nine laboratory situations that are pertinent to the role of the clinical laboratory in assessment of renal function. By working through the scenarios as they are presented, the student will gain knowledge about the physiological impact of **electrolytes**, **nonprotein nitrogen** waste products, and other kidney function tests on renal health and pathology. Each scenario allows you to examine the laboratory assessment process, including the impact of preanalytical factors, such as specimen collection and handling; the effects of variation on the analytical procedure; and the importance of postanalytical factors, such as communication of results. In this chapter, you will explore your role in providing the laboratory results that aid in diagnosis and monitoring of renal disorders. The side boxes in this chapter provide common sense tips, definitions of terms, brief descriptions of pathophysiology, and clinical correlation as well as reminders of the team approach in health care. Text boxes within the chapter outline methodology for laboratory assessment of renal function.

OBJECTIVES

Upon completion of this chapter, the student will have the ability to

▪ Evaluate patient sample collection and handling processes in terms of impact on their renal function and electrolyte analysis.

▪ Discuss commonly encountered sources of analytical interference in urea-nitrogen, creatinine, or other renal function testing analysis.

▪ Describe the principle of analysis of urea, creatinine and uric acid, in terms of key reagents, their role and endpoint detection.

▪ Discuss the principle of analysis of Na, K, Cl, and total CO_2 (HCO_3^-), in terms of electronic components, reagents, and endpoint detection.

▪ Provide appropriate criteria for interpreting renal function and electrolyte laboratory test results.

▪ Determine the appropriate course of action that is needed to resolve problems that occur during renal function and electrolyte testing.

◼ CASE SCENARIO 6-1

Glomerular Nephritis: Jennie

"Jennie's here," the phlebotomist announced to the laboratory technicians in the break room. Jennie was a favorite among laboratory personnel at River City Medical Clinic. Jennie, a bright 17-year-old, was recovering from acute glomerular **nephritis** and had been a regular visitor to the laboratory over the past few weeks. Jennie came to the clinic regularly to have her blood and urine tested to monitor the status of her disease.

Several months before, Jennie had a sore throat. She did not go to the doctor and recovered without medication. However, a few weeks later Jennie was still listless and nauseated. She noticed that her urine was very dark and tinged red; she was also not producing much urine. Jennie's mother took her to their primary care physician. At the physician's clinic, the laboratory results showed blood and protein in Jennie's urine. A few red blood cell casts were seen on

nephritis - inflammation of the kidney

Case Scenario 6-1 Glomerular Nephritis: Jennie *(continued)*

microscopic examination of the urine. From the preliminary laboratory results and the history of sore throat, the physician suspected a renal glomerular inflammation and ordered blood work to assess the findings further.

The initial blood work showed increased production of antibody to a streptococcal infection with a high **antistreptolysin-O (ASO) titer**. Her plasma creatinine, **blood urea nitrogen (BUN)**, and plasma sodium were high. Her other electrolytes—potassium, chloride, and carbon dioxide—were within the reference ranges. The pediatrician ordered a 24-hour urine for creatinine **clearance**.

antistreptolysin-O (ASO) titer - measure of antibodies to a protein component of group A *Streptococcus* bacteria

blood urea nitrogen (BUN) - urea concentration in the blood; historically, urea was measured as nitrogen remaining from a protein-free filtrate of the blood

clearance - the elimination of a substance, as related to its removal from the blood plasma by the kidneys

CREATININE METABOLISM

Creatine is synthesized in the liver, pancreas, and kidneys from the amino acids arginine, glycine, and methionine. Creatine is transported through the circulatory system to muscle, brain, and other organs, where it is converted to phosphocreatine and acts as an energy reservoir much like ATP. Creatinine is produced as a waste product of creatine and phosphocreatine. Because much of the creatinine is produced in muscle, the amount of creatinine that is measured in blood is proportional to the patient's lean muscle mass. The waste product, creatinine, enters the blood supply, where it is removed through the kidneys.

Creatinine clearance measures the ability of the glomerulus to filter chemicals from the blood. The best substance to use for glomerular clearance would be a chemical that is filtered completely through the glomerulus and not reabsorbed through the nephron tubule. Creatinine meets that criterion for clearance and is also an endogenous substance; that is, it is produced in the body. Other substances, such as inulin, may be used for evaluation of creatinine clearance; however, they are exogenous substances and must be introduced into the body. Creatinine clearance is measured as a rate; therefore, the test must be timed. The test measures the movement of the substance from blood to urine; therefore, both blood and urine concentrations of the chemical must be measured.

Test Methodologies 6–1 and 6–2 provide more information about measuring creatinine in blood and urine, and performing the 24-hour creatinine clearance test, respectively.[1-5]

TEST METHODOLOGY 6-1.   CREATININE

Creatinine may be measured by chemical or enzymatic methods.

Chemical Methodology

The Reaction

In the Jaffe reaction, creatinine reacts with picric acid in an alkaline environment to generate an orange-red product. The reaction is not specific for creatinine. The orange-red color may be generated by protein, glucose, ascorbic acid, acetone, acetoacetate, pyruvate, guanidine, and cephalosporins. The methodology is dependent upon picric acid concentration, alkaline pH, reaction temperature, reaction time, and wavelength at which the product is measured.

continued

TEST METHODOLOGY 6-1.   CREATININE (continued)

The Specimen

Serum, plasma, and urine may all be measured by the Jaffe reaction.

Reference Ranges

Male	0.9–1.3 mg/dL
Female	0.6–1.1 mg/dL
Children	0.3–0.7 mg/dL

Enzymatic Methodology

The Reaction

Enzymatic approaches to the measurement of creatinine have also been explored. Creatininase, creatinase, and creatinine deaminase have all been used to produce a measurable product that reflects creatinine concentration. Reactions are coupled with enzymatic reactions that can be measured spectrophotometrically, such as NADH to NAD^+ or H_2O_2 to H_2O.

The Specimen

Serum, plasma, and urine may be measured enzymatically. Fluoride and ammonium heparin should not be used as anticoagulants in enzymatic methods.

Reference Ranges

Reference ranges are specific to the method used. In general, enzymatic methods produce lower reference ranges than nonenzymatic methods.

TEST METHODOLOGY 6-2.   CREATININE CLEARANCE

Creatinine clearance is an imperfect measure of glomerular filtration rate. The use of creatinine to estimate glomerular filtration rate is based upon three assumptions: (1) creatinine is filtered through the glomerulus, (2) relatively low amounts of creatinine are reabsorbed through the nephron tubule, and (3) creatinine production is constant over time. Although creatinine can provide a rough estimate of glomerular filtration rate, error may be encountered. Such factors as increased tubular reabsorption of creatinine, reduced creatinine generation from muscle tissue, and dietary changes in nitrogenous compounds may affect creatinine clearance.

The Specimen

Properly collected specimens are essential for accuracy of the creatinine clearance test. Two specimens are collected, a 24-hour urine and a blood specimen that is drawn during the 24-hour urine collection or not more than 24 hours before or after the urine collection. The laboratory may add 6-mol/L HCl or boric acid to the container as preservative.
   The patient is instructed to collect the urine as follows:
1. Void and discard this urine.
2. Start timing the 24-hour period immediately after voiding
3. Collect all the urine voided for the next 24 hours. Keep the urine in a cool place.
4. At 24 hours, void and add this urine to the collection container.
5. Bring the urine to the laboratory as soon as possible.

continued

TEST METHODOLOGY 6-2. **CREATININE CLEARANCE** *(continued)*

The Calculation

At the laboratory, the specimen is well mixed, the volume is measured, and then an aliquot is taken for testing. The urine specimen is diluted 1:10 with distilled water and measured for creatinine. The urine creatinine is multiplied by 10 for the dilution. Creatinine clearance is calculated as follows:

$$\frac{\text{Urine creatinine (mg/dL)} \times \text{volume (mL)} \times \text{average surface area (m}^2)}{\text{Plasma creatinine (mg/dL)} \times \text{time (min)} \times \text{patient surface area (m}^2)}$$

Complete collection of the 24-hour urine is necessary in order to report the creatinine clearance accurately.

Several formulas are available to estimate creatinine clearance. The Schwarz formula estimates creatinine clearance from serum creatinine.[5] This formula is used for pediatric patients:

$$\text{Creatinine clearance} = (k \times \text{Ht})\text{Creat}$$

where $k = 0.45$ if age <1 year, $k = 0.55$ if age $= 1$ to 12 years, Ht = height in cm, and Creat = serum creatinine.

Reference Ranges

Male	95–130 mL/min
Female	80–120 mL/min

Case Scenario 6-1 Glomerular Nephritis: Jennie

Diagnosis of Jennie's Kidney Disorder

As a consequence of Jennie's streptococcal infection, a portion of the functional units in Jennie's kidney lost their ability to filter waste products from her blood. Jennie's sore throat was probably group A beta-hemolytic streptococcal infection, or "strep throat." The infection provoked an antibody response, which resulted in the formation of antigen-antibody complexes circulating in her blood, as indicated by her high ASO titer. The complexes caused inflammation of the renal glomeruli, which resulted in reduction of the **filtration** capability of the glomeruli and, consequently, the reduction of the flow of waste products from blood to urine.

GLOMERULAR NEPHRITIS

Glomerular nephritis may be caused by immunologic damage such as **systemic lupus erythematosus**, poststreptococcal damage, or hypersensitivities to drugs. The cause also may be nonimmunologic in origin, such glomerular nephritis that is produced by **diabetic nephropathy**. Chronic glomerular nephritis is a slower developing disease and may be **idiopathic**, and is characterized by gradual **uremia** and loss of functioning nephrons.

The kidney is a component of the urinary tract system, which consists of kidneys, ureters, urinary bladder, and urethra. The urinary tract functions as a pathway for the elimination of metabolic by-products and unessential chemicals. The kidney maintains the water, ionic, and chemical balance of blood by filtering chemicals

filtration - the process of removing particles from a solution by passing the solution through a membrane or other barrier

systemic lupus erythematosus - chronic autoimmune inflammatory disease involving multiple organ systems

diabetic nephropathy - disease of the kidney, including inflammatory, degenerative, and sclerotic conditions, caused by diabetes

idiopathic - diseases without recognizable cause

uremia - a toxic condition associated with renal insufficiency produced by the retention in the blood of nitrogenous substances normally excreted by the kidney

CLINICAL CORRELATION
Acute glomerular nephritis is characterized by a sudden onset of hematuria and proteinuria and a decrease in glomerular filtration rate characterized by a rise in plasma creatinine and a fall in creatinine clearance compared with reference ranges.

from the blood and conserving, or reabsorbing, those chemicals that are needed for adequate metabolism. The kidneys maintain the balance of plasma constituents, while excreting those substances that are no longer needed by the body.

The central portion of the kidney consists of tubules that drain the kidney cortex and medulla. The cortex, or outer portion of the kidney, appears red and contains the blood vessels, which bring blood to the kidney, and nephrons, the functional units that filter and maintain the chemical stasis of the blood. The medulla appears as a series of pyramids within the cortex and contains straight tubules and collecting ducts (Fig. 6–1).

There are about 1 million nephons in each kidney. In association with blood vessels that serve the kidney, the nephrons make up the cortex and medulla of the kidney. Each nephron contains a glomerulus, proximal tubule, loop of Henle, and distal tubule. The glomerulus filters blood plasma from arterioles into Bowman's space and hence in the proximal tubule of the nephron. The integrity of the glomerulus membrane, which consists of the endothelium, basement membrane, and epithelium, and renal blood flow determine the *glomerular filtration rate*. The glomerulus has multiple small pores through which chemicals are filtered from the blood. In a healthy kidney, the pores exclude any substance with a molecular radius more than 4 nm. The glomerulus also selects by charge. Substances that are neutral or have positive charge are more likely to pass through the pores of the glomerulus than substances that are negatively charged. For example, albumin, which has a molecular radius of less than 4 nm but is negatively charged, does not readily pass through the pores of the glomerulus. In a healthy kidney, cellular blood components should be excluded from the filtrate because of their size.

Once in the proximal tubule, the filtrate flows through the rest of the nephron: the proximal tubule, loop of Henle, distal tubule, and collecting tubule. Some tubule cells, especially those in the distal portion of the nephron, exchange sodium and water back into the blood supply. Sodium is exchanged in the presence of the hormone aldosterone and water is exchanged in the presence of antidiuretic hormone (ADH). The exchange of chemicals back into the blood supply is called **reabsorption**. Exchange may occur as active transport, which occurs against the concentration gradient of the chemical and uses energy, or as passive transport, which occurs with the gradient from high to low concentration of the chemical.

Because of the ability of the nephron to filter and reabsorb certain chemical from the blood, the measurement of the concentration of these chemical in the blood and urine serves as a functional evaluation of the kidney and specific areas of the nephron. The measurements of the concentrations of creatinine, blood urea nitrogen, and electrolytes all serve as functional evaluations of different areas of the kidney.

CLINICAL CORRELATION
In a patient with stable weight, glomerular filtration rate is inversely related to serum creatinine; as serum creatinine rises, glomerular filtration rate decreases. Most proteins are too large to filter through the glomerulus and into urine unless the glomerulus is damaged. While the predominant protein that appears in urine filtrate from damaged glomeruli is albumin, the type of proteins found in urine filtrate indicates the severity of damage.

reabsorption - to absorb again, as related to the movement of particles through the nephron, the movement of particles from the renal filtrate back into blood

CLINICAL CORRELATION
The evaluation of blood urea nitrogen (BUN) is a gross indicator of renal function. Damaged nephrons are unable to clear urea from the bloodstream, resulting in an increased BUN. The level of BUN is also affected by patient hydration, protein diet, and gastrointestinal bleeding.

Case Scenario 6-1 Glomerular Nephritis: Jennie

Follow-Up

At the laboratory, the clinical laboratory scientist (CLS) directs Jennie to void and discards this urine. The CLS writes down this time and gives it to Jennie as the starting time of the 24-hour collection. The CLS draws blood for a plasma creatinine measurement. The CLS gives Jennie basins in which she will void and directs Jennie to place all the urine that is voided in the urine

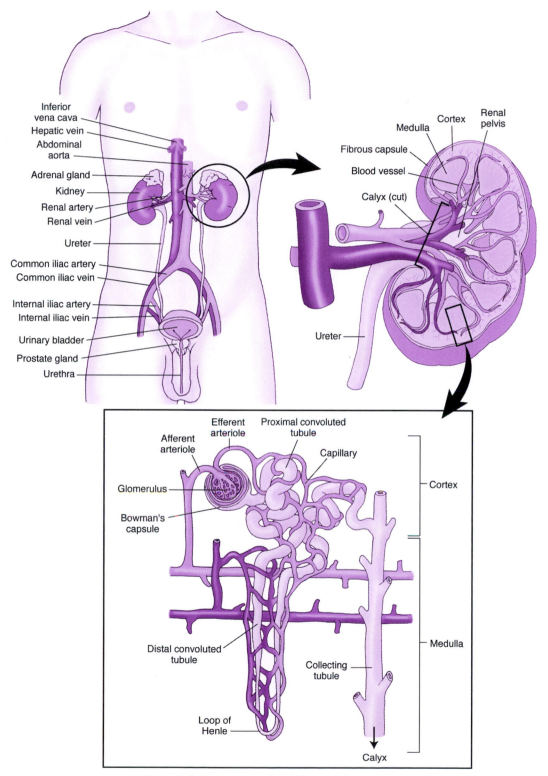

Figure 6–1. The anatomy of the kidney and the nephron.

Case Scenario 6-1 Glomerular Nephritis: Jennie *(continued)*

container and place it in a cool place. Jennie follows the directions and returns the completed 24-hour urine collection to the laboratory on the following day.

Urine creatinine	96 mg/dL
Plasma creatinine	2.1 mg/dL
24-Hour urine volume	950 mL
Height	5 ft 2 in.
Weight	105 lb

The nomogram in Figure 6–2, where the average surface area is given as 1.73 m², can be used to calculate the surface area of Jennie's body. With the values from the 24-hour urine collection, Jennie's creatinine clearance is calculated to be 42 mL/min. The test result confirms the pediatrician's suspicion that Jennie has acute glomerulonephritis.

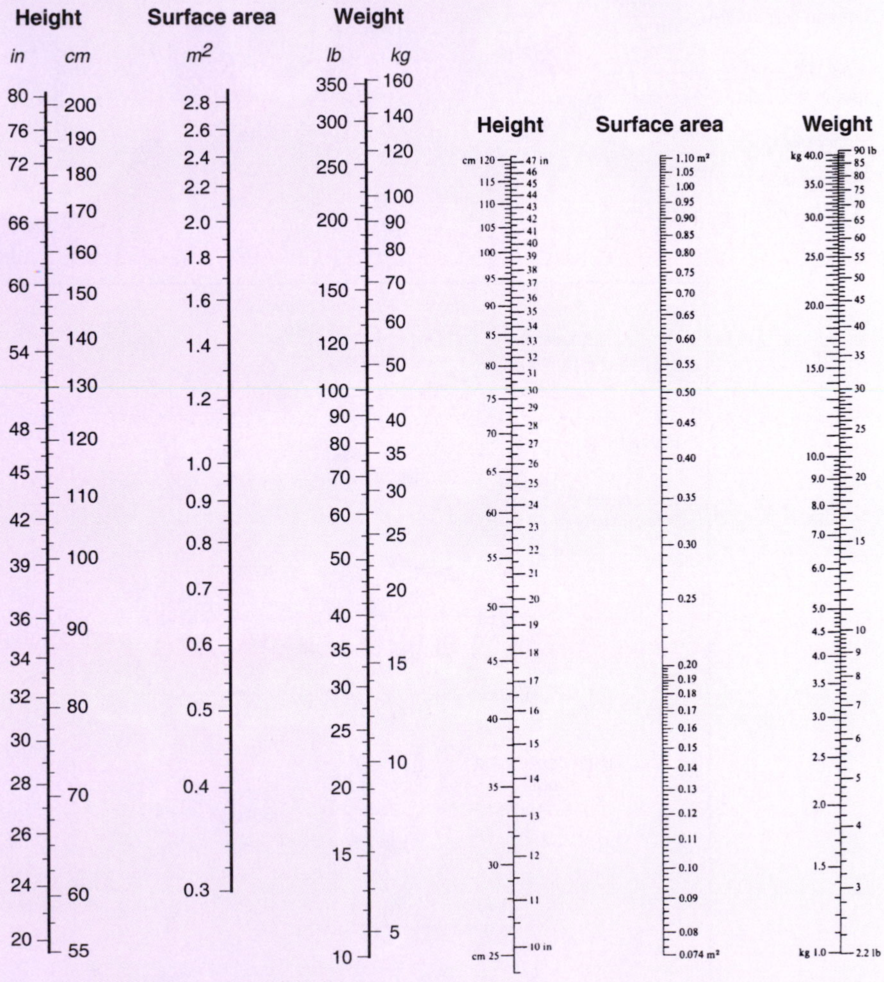

Figure 6–2. Adult and pediatric nomograms for the calculation of body surface area. *Source: From the formula of Du Bois and Du Bois. Arch Intern Med 1916; 17:863. Copyright 1916. American Medical Association. Reprinted by permission.*

Case Scenario 6-1 Glomerular Nephritis: Jennie *(continued)*

Jennie had a full recovery. Since a small percentage of individuals who have acute glomerulonephritis develop progressive glomerulonephritis or chronic renal failure, her physician will watch for changes in her creatinine and electrolytes in her serum and for protein and blood in her urine for the next several months. ●

CASE SCENARIO 6-2

Nephrotic Syndrome Assessment: The Diabetic Patient

The CLS measured the volume of the 24-hour urine that had just been submitted by Emily, a 35-year-old woman with type 1 diabetes mellitus. The CLS knew from previous tests on Emily's urine that the urinary protein concentration would be high. The patient had diabetic nephropathy. One of the consequences of long-term diabetes is the glycosylation of tissue proteins and the increased incidence of vascular disease. Diabetic nephropathy is a secondary consequence of effect of diabetes on the glomerulus. The capillary walls of the glomeruli become more permeable to chemicals, allowing the passage of chemicals of increasing size. The charge selectivity mechanism of the glomeruli may also be lost. The glomeruli permit the passage of protein of increasing size. This disease and other diseases of nephrotic syndrome are characterized by heavy proteinuria of greater than 3.5 to 4.0 g/day.

NEPHROTIC SYNDROME

Diabetic nephropathy is one cause of nephrotic syndrome. The syndrome also may be caused by a primary defect of the kidney, or it may be secondary to diabetes, carcinomas, systemic lupus erythematosus, or drug therapies. The syndrome may result from autoimmune renal damage, such as from systemic lupus erythematosus or toxic reactions to bee stings; or from chronic glomerular nephritis or nonimmunologic disorders, such as renal vein thrombosis, serious infections, and toxic reactions to drugs or carcinomas. Nephrotic syndrome is characterized as a renal condition compromising the integrity of basement glomerular membrane and tubular epithelium, often resulting in large porous openings.[6]

Albumin is the major protein that is lost from the blood. Albumin concentration in the blood is usually less than 3 g/dL. Other proteins are lost also; transferrin, ceruloplasmin, immunoglobulins, and complement may be filtered from the blood, resulting in iron-deficiency anemia, copper deficiency, and immunodeficiency. In contrast, urine protein concentrations increase, especially albumin, transferrin, and lipoproteins. Determination of urinary protein and albumin is described in Test Methodologies 6–3 and 6–4, respectively. Lipids may be taken up by renal tubular epithelial and other cells in urine. When these cells appear in the urine, they produce characteristic oval fat bodies, which are highly refractile when examined under bright-light microscopy. Examination of the cells using polarized light results in the appearance of "Maltese cross" formations in cells containing cholesterol.

CLINICAL CORRELATION

Nephrotic syndrome is characterized by severe hypoproteinemia, massive proteinuria (>2.5 g/day), edema, hyperlipidemia, oval fat bodies, lipiduria, and hyponatremia. Hyperlipemia results from cholesterol accumulation in the blood because of the low concentration of cholesterol carrier proteins.

TEST METHODOLOGY 6-3.   URINARY PROTEIN

Because the concentration of protein in urine is less than the concentration in blood, more sensitive methodology must be performed to measure the concentration of urine proteins than of serum proteins.

The Reaction Principle

Several methods exist for the measurement of urinary protein.

Turbidometric

Protein may be precipitated with sulfosalicylic acid, trichloroacetic acid, or benzethonium chloride. The turbidity of the precipitate is measured photometrically.

Dye-Binding

Dye binds to amino groups; the resulting color change is measured colorimetrically.

The Calculation

(Urine protein concentration [mg/dL] × urine volume [dL])/day

Example (Refer to Case Scenario 6–2)

Emily's urine protein concentration was 120 mg/dL; her urine volume was 1000 mL. Her 24-hour urine protein is calculated as follows:

(120 mg/dL × 10 dL)/day = 1200 mg/day or 1.2 g/day

The Specimen

A 12- or 24-hour collection may be used. A 24-hour collection is preferred since some variation in excretion may occur over a 24-hour period. Urine should be collected as described for creatinine clearance. Urine should be kept cool.

Reference Range

Urine protein   <100 mg/day

TEST METHODOLOGY 6-4.   URINARY ALBUMIN

Tests for microalbuminuria must be sensitive to low concentrations of albumin. Urinalysis dipsticks measure protein through the effects of protein on pH; these techniques are not sensitive to low concentration of albumin in the urine. Semiquantitative immunologic methods screen for low concentrations of albumin. Positive semiquantitative results must be confirmed by a qualitative method.

The Reaction Principle

Dye binds to albumin and causes a shift in the maximum absorption. Methyl orange, bromcresol green, and bromcresol purple dyes have all been used.

The Calculation

(Urine albumin concentration [mg/dL] × urine volume [dL])/day

The Specimen

A 12- or 24-hour collection may be used. A 24-hour collection is preferred since some variation in excretion may occur over a 24-hour period. Urine should be collected as described for creatinine clearance. Urine should be kept cool.

Reference Range

The excretion of 30 to 300 mg of albumin per 24-hour period on two of three collections is indicative of microalbuminuria

Case Scenario 6-2 **Nephrotic Syndrome Assessment: The Diabetic Patient**

Additional Test Results and Follow-Up

Emily's blood work shows a normal creatinine concentration, low levels of protein and albumin, and high levels of cholesterol and triglycerides. Urinalysis results show 4+ proteinuria.

Emily's nephrotic syndrome was diagnosed in the early stages of the disease. As Emily's diabetes progressed, her physician screened her urine for **microalbuminuria**. The American Diabetes Association (ADA) recommends periodic testing for microalbuminuria in adult diabetics. Microalbuminuria has prognostic significance for the development of renal disease in diabetic patients, especially those patients with type 1 diabetes.[6,7] ●

microalbuminuria - small amounts of albumin found in the urine, also called dipstick-negative increase in the excretion of albumin in urine

CASE SCENARIO 6-3

Azotemia Assessment: Out of Proportion

The CLS made the usual "common sense check" of the laboratory results before sending them out to the physician. The electrolytes were in proper proportion, but the BUN-to-creatinine ratio was unusual. An examination of the laboratory request did not show an indication of renal disease. The patient's BUN was increased, the creatinine was normal, and the BUN-to-creatinine ratio was above 20;1. The patient clearly had **azotemia**, but the cause of the azotemia was not evident.

✓ **Common Sense Check**
Normally, the BUN-to-creatinine ratio in serum is 10:1 to 20:1.

azotemia - an elevated level of urea in the blood

AZOTEMIA

Urea is the waste product of the degradation of amino acids into CO_2 and ammonia. Urea is synthesized in the liver and transported through blood to the kidney, where it is filtered through the glomerulus. Almost half of the urea is reabsorbed back into the blood by passive transport in the nephron tubule. Azotemia may indicate renal disease or a nonrenal disorder that causes a secondary increase of blood urea as a consequence of disease. Test Methodology 6–5 shows methods of evaluating urea.

TEST METHODOLOGY 6-5.   UREA

Two methods for measuring the concentration of urea are commonly used, the urease method and the colorimetric method.

The Reaction

Urease Methods

$$Urea + H_2O \xrightarrow{urease} 2NH_4^+ + HCO_3^-$$

The ammonia that is liberated in the reaction above may be measured in a variety of ways:
1. The reaction may be coupled with a reaction that drives NADH to NAD^+.
2. The conductivity of the ammonium ion may be measured.

continued

TEST METHODOLOGY 6-5.   UREA *(continued)*

3. The Berthelot reaction may be used:

$$NH_4^+ + NaOCl + phenol \xrightarrow{\text{nitroprusside}} indophenol$$

4. An indicator dye may be used.
5. The reaction may be coupled with a reaction that produces H_2O_2.

Colorimetric Method

The diacetyl monoxime reaction is used to produce a color change:

$$Diacetyl\ monoxime + urea \xrightarrow{\text{acid}} diazine\ (yellow\ compound)$$

The Specimen

Serum or plasma may be tested. Anticoagulants containing fluoride or citrate should not be used.

Reference Range

Serum or plasma   6–20 mg/dL

✔ **Common Sense Check**
Laboratory results that commonly correlate should be compared before reporting. For example, BUN and serum creatinine are normally both elevated in kidney disease. BUN can also be elevated in other conditions. It is unusual, however, for serum creatinine to be elevated while BUN remains normal. In this case, a problem with the results may exist.

The reference range for the BUN-to-creatinine ratio is 10:1 to 20:1. Increases in the ratio may be caused by prerenal, renal, and postrenal factors. Prerenal changes include variation of protein intake and dehydration. Renal disorders that affect the BUN-to-creatinine ratio include renal failure and glomerular damage. Postrenal changes that affect this ratio include urinary tract infections. Table 6–1 lists causes of increases or decreases to this ratio.

Case Scenario 6-3 Azotemia Assessment: Out of Proportion

Follow-Up

Upon further investigation, the CLS found that Emily was on a high-protein diet. The azotemia was a result of the increase of urea that was produced from ammonia in the breakdown of the amino acids of the proteins. ●

TABLE 6-1

Interpretation of the BUN-to-Creatinine Ratio

BUN-to-Creatinine Ratio	Causes
Increased ratio with normal creatinine level	Prerenal uremia
	High protein intake
	Gastrointestinal bleeding
Increased ratio with increased creatinine level	Postrenal obstruction
Decreased ratio	Acute tubular necrosis
	Low protein intake
	Starvation
	Severe liver disease

CASE SCENARIO 6-4

A Case of Renal Failure: A Review of the Laboratory Results

The technologist, measuring the volume of 24-hour urine, noted that it was to be analyzed for creatinine clearance and for urinary sodium. The laboratory requisition indicated that a serum creatinine and sodium had been obtained during the 24-hour collection period, so an additional specimen was not required. She reviewed the results of the last 24 hours on this patient:

Test	Patient	Reference Range
Na (mmol/L)	126	136–145
K (mmol/L)	6.5	3.5–5.1
Cl (mmol/L)	100	98–107
CO_2 (mmol/L)	7	22–28
BUN (mg/dL)	45	6–20
Creatinine (mg/dL)	2.8	0.6–1.1

The serum creatinine and urea were increased, and three of the four electrolytes that were measured were abnormal. The technologist completed analysis of the urine creatinine and sodium, and then calculated creatinine clearance. The results were noted:

Test	Patient	Reference Range
Creatinine clearance (mL/min)	36	80–120
Urinary sodium (mmol/24 hr)	230	27–287

The technologist considered the connection between the creatinine clearance and urinary sodium results and also recognized that this patient had low urinary output, or **oliguria**. The patient had indications of renal failure.

renal failure - loss of renal function for control of water and electrolytes, decline in filtration and removal of wastes, and loss of nutrients

oliguria - decreased urine output, <400 mL of urine per day (a common sign of renal insufficiency)

TYPES AND ASPECTS OF RENAL FAILURE

Renal failure is classified as either acute or chronic. *Acute renal failure* occurs suddenly, often secondary to sudden acute illness or to therapy. Acute renal failure is characterized by loss of sodium in blood and increased fraction of sodium **excretion** in the urine (FE_{Na}), especially when compared to creatinine clearance. Loss of sodium is due primarily to decreased tubular function, which helps regulate sodium and other electrolyte levels as well as water balance. Glomerular filtration rate is usually less than 20 mL/min. *Chronic renal failure* occurs over a longer period of time, with renal insufficiency progressing through several clear-cut stages. Chronic renal failure may also be secondary to an underlying illness. Chronic renal failure is often caused by chronic illness with complications that affect the kidney, such as the immunologic damage of systemic lupus erythematosus or the nonimmunologic damage of diabetic nephropathy or **multiple myeloma**.

Acute renal failure may be classified as prerenal, renal, or postrenal in origin. Prerenal acute renal failure may be caused by decreased circulation, low blood volume, or decreased fluid volume reaching the kidney. Postrenal acute renal failure may occur as the result of urinary obstruction, which reduces the flow of urine from the kidney. Reduced glomerular filtration rate is often the indication of

excretion - the elimination of waste products from the body

multiple myeloma - a malignant disease characterized by the infiltration of bone and bone marrow by neoplastic plasma cells

STAT - immediately or at once

postrenal acute renal failure. Renal classifications of acute renal failure are usually secondary to acute tubular necrosis, however, glomerular function will eventually be lost as well.

CALCULATION OF FRACTIONAL EXCRETION OF SODIUM

Fractional excretion of sodium is defined as the fraction of sodium actually excreted by the body relative to the amount filtered by the kidney. FE_{Na} is not a test, but rather a calculation based on the concentrations of sodium and creatinine in blood and urine.

$$FE_{Na} = Na \text{ Clearance} \times 100\%/\text{creatinine clearance}$$

FE_{Na} of less than 1% indicates decreased blood flow to the kidney, while FE_{Na} of greater than 1% (and usually greater than 3%) suggests kidney damage.[8–11]

Case Scenario 6-4 A Case of Renal Failure: A Review of the Laboratory Results

Follow-Up

Urinary excretion of sodium in this patient was increased, along with slightly decreased creatinine clearance and declining urine output, indicating early stages of acute renal failure. The renal failure is most likely of renal origin as indicated by the urinary sodium and creatinine values. Loss of sodium and resulting electrolyte and mineral imbalance have serious consequences if not treated. This patient received dialysis and fluid and electrolyte therapy until the condition was reversed. ●

CASE SCENARIO 6-5

Renal Tubular Acidosis: A Matter of Balance

While analyzing basic chemistry profiles and urine in the **STAT** laboratory, the CLS noticed a pediatric patient who had repeated urinary results with 1+ proteinuria and alkaline pH. The demographics of the patient revealed a 13-month-old male patient with an admitting diagnosis of failure to thrive. The laboratory results from a blood sample revealed:

Test	Patient	Reference Range (Children)
Sodium (mmol/L)	128	138–145
Potassium (mmol/L)	3.2	3.4–4.7
Chloride (mmol/L)	98	98–107
Bicarbonate (mmol/L)	11	22–28
BUN (mg/dL)	24	5–18
Creatinine (mg/dL)	1.5	0.3–0.7
Calcium (total; mg/dL)	7.6	8.6–10.6
Glucose (mg/dL)	60	60–100
Phosphorus (mg/dL)	1.7	4.0–7.0
Anion gap (mmol/L)	22	10–20

Case Scenario 6-5 Renal Tubular Acidosis: A Matter of Balance *(continued)*

In addition to the abnormal urinalysis results, the nonprotein nitrogen waste products, BUN, and creatinine were elevated. The results for electrolytes and minerals were abnormal as well.

RENAL CONTROL OF ACID-BASE BALANCE

Refer to the earlier description of renal anatomy and physiology. The proximal convoluted tubules are responsible for reabsorption of electrolytes, glucose, amino acids, and other nutrients to their **renal threshold** levels via active transport. Water is reabsorbed via osmosis. The loop of Henle primarily reabsorbs water and sodium chloride. The distal convoluted tubules, under stimulation from aldosterone, further regulate sodium and chloride reabsorption in exchange for potassium secretion. These tubules also respond to parathyroid hormone for the reabsorption of calcium and magnesium in exchange for phosphorus. The collecting ducts further regulate water reabsorption under regulation of antidiuretic hormone.

The distal convoluted tubules secrete protons such as H^+ and NH_4^+, waste products from the normal process of metabolism. Thus, the kidneys are important in the regulation of acid-base balance. In addition, Na^+, HCO_3^-, and $H_2PO_4^-$ are secreted to combine with H^+ to **buffer** urinary filtrate and form the weak acid H_2CO_3. This chemical dissociates to form H_2O and CO_2 in the presence of carbonic anhydrase and then dissociates further to form HCO_3^- and H^+. The resulting bicarbonate is reabsorbed to help maintain acid-base balance in blood plasma. Bicarbonate is part of the bicarbonate/carbonic acid buffering system for blood pH in the body. The bicarbonate balance of this system is classified as the metabolic component of the buffer system.

Ammonium and phosphate buffering systems also contribute to buffering hydrogen ion concentration of the urinary filtrate. The secretion and reabsorption of H^+ and bicarbonate, as well as Na^+ and K^+, are under the influence of several hormones such as aldosterone and angiotensin II.[12]

The dissociation constant of carbonic acid is compatible with the normal blood pH of 7.40, and it can form bicarbonate to combine with H^+, producing H_2O and CO_2 for respiratory regulation and excretion. Thus, the bicarbonate system is the most significant buffer for human blood. Both renal control of bicarbonate and hydrogen ion excretion and respiratory control of carbonic acid, in the form of carbon dioxide gas, help to regulate and maintain normal pH. The normal ratio of 20:1 for bicarbonate ion (mmol/L) compared to carbonic acid (mmol/L) is sufficient to regulate blood pH to 7.40. This has been characterized by the following formula:

$$7.40 = 6.1 + \log (HCO_3^-/H_2CO_3)$$

where 6.1 is the pK_a and 7.40 is the normal blood pH. When the blood pH is outside of the normal reference range, and/or the bicarbonate or CO_2 values are abnormal, an acid-base disturbance exits. For more information about acid-base balance, please refer to Chapter 9 (Assessment of Respiratory Disorders). The following text summarizes acid-base disturbances due to metabolic or renal involvement.

The classification of *acid-base balance* in blood is based upon blood pH beyond the normal reference range. The cause of pH imbalance is linked to the metabolic (or renal) component, which is HCO_3^-, or the respiratory component, H_2CO_3.

renal threshold - plasma level at which the kidneys no longer reabsorb a substance so that it is excreted into urine as waste

buffer - a mixture of chemicals that resist changes in pH by combining with free H^+ (proton acceptor) and OH^-, generally a strong salt and weak acid or base; human buffer systems include anionic proteins, deoxyhemoglobin, phosphate buffers, and bicarbonate/carbonic acid buffers

TABLE 6-2

Causes and Clinical Signs of Metabolic Acidosis

Metabolic Acidosis

pH <7.35
HCO_3^- <22 mmol/L
Compensating PCO_2 <35 mm/Hg (H_2CO_3)

	Causes
Production of organic acids	
Ketosis	Carbohydrate deprivation, starvation, or diabetes mellitus
Lactic acidosis	Extreme muscle metabolism; circulatory problems with anaerobic conditions
Formic acid or acetic acid	Alcohol toxicities
Loss of bicarbonate	Diarrhea; severe intestinal, pancreatic, or biliary fistula
Loss of bicarbonate reabsorption and H^+ excretion	Renal tubular acidosis, renal failure

Reference ranges: whole blood arterial pH, 7.35–7.45; whole blood arterial PCO_2, 35–45 mm Hg; bicarbonate, 22–28 mmol/L.

alkalosis - increase in blood alkalinity due to an accumulation of alkaline substances or reduction of acids

acidosis - increase in the acidity of blood due to an accumulation of acids or an excessive loss of bicarbonate

metabolic acidosis - acidosis resulting from increase in acids other than carbonic acid

metabolic alkalosis - alkalosis in which plasma bicarbonate is increased with a proportionate rise in the plasma concentration of carbon dioxide

respiratory acidosis - acidosis caused by retention of carbon dioxide due to pulmonary insufficiency

respiratory alkalosis - alkalosis with an acute reduction of plasma bicarbonate and a proportionate reduction in plasma carbon dioxide

Alkalosis occurs when pH exceeds the upper limit of the reference range (7.45), while **acidosis** is associated with pH less than the lower limit of the reference range (7.35). Given the relationship of the buffer components to regulating pH, bicarbonate ion concentrations are directly related to pH and carbonic acid, as determined by the partial pressure of carbon dioxide (PCO_2), is inversely related. Thus, a situation that causes a decrease in bicarbonate ion will lower the ratio and cause a decrease in pH. This is termed **metabolic acidosis**[13] (Table 6–2). **Metabolic alkalosis** is a condition that will raise the bicarbonate ion concentration, increasing the bicarbonate/carbonic acid ratio and causing an increase in pH value (Table 6–3). Conditions of **respiratory acidosis** are caused by increased carbonic acid levels, in which the lungs are unable to properly excrete carbon dioxide gas. **Respiratory alkalosis** is caused by a deficit of carbonic acid and hyperventilation of carbon dioxide gas (Fig. 6–3).

TABLE 6-3

Causes and Clinical Signs of Metabolic Alkalosis

Metabolic Alkalosis

pH >7.45
HCO_3^- >28 mmol/L
Compensating PCO_2 >47 mm/Hg (H_2CO_3)

	Causes
Loss of H^+	Severe vomiting or nasogastric suction; certain diuretics
Excess bicarbonate	Treatment with sodium bicarbonate, sodium lactate, citrate, or acetate

Reference ranges: whole blood arterial pH, 7.35–7.45; whole blood arterial PCO_2, 35–48 mm Hg; bicarbonate, 22–28 mmol/L.

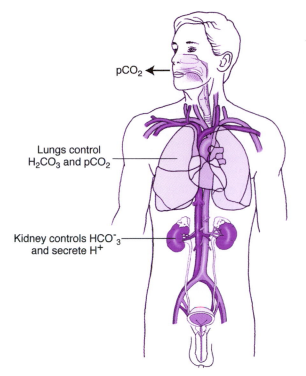

pCO₂ ←

Lungs control
H₂CO₃ and pCO₂

Kidney controls HCO⁻₃
and secrete H⁺

Figure 6–3. Metabolic control of pH.

THE ROLE OF ELECTROLYTES

The four major electrolytes are sodium (Na^+), potassium (K^+), chloride (Cl^-), and bicarbonate (HCO_3^-). Sodium and potassium are **cations**, with sodium in greater concentration extracellularly and potassium in greater concentration intracellularly. Chloride and bicarbonate are **anions**. Control of cation concentration is maintained by the *Na-K-ATPase pump*.

Sodium

Because of the high concentration of sodium in extracellular fluid, such as plasma water, sodium plays a major role in maintaining **osmotic pressure**. Sodium levels in body fluids are maintained by renal reabsorption in the proximal convoluted tubules, based on a sodium threshold. Sodium balance is also maintained by the influence of the hormone aldosterone on the distal convoluted tubules, as a consequence of changes in blood volume and blood pressure. Extremely high or low sodium concentrations in plasma will cause severe osmotic pressure changes that can induce serious consequences to several organs. The most immediate effect is swelling on the brain and potential coma.[14]

Potassium

Potassium, the major intracellular cation, is also controlled by the Na-K-ATPase pump. Potassium maintains cardiac rhythm and contributes to neuromuscular con-

cation - an ion carrying a positive charge

anion - an ion carrying a negative charge

osmotic pressure - pressure that develops when two solutions of different concentration are separated by a semipermeable membrane

duction. Imbalances in potassium level, as indicated by hyperkalemia or hypokalemia, will cause cardiac arrhythmias and neuromuscular weakness.

Chloride

Chloride is one of the major extracellular anions that helps maintain electrical neutrality with sodium. Chloride contributes to the maintenance of acid-base balance by participating in the *isohydric shift*. The isohydric shift describes the maintenance of hydrogen ion concentration as shifting of hydrogen ion occurs between fluid spaces. The shift refers to the buffering of H^+ with HCO_3^- and other buffers intracellularly and movement to extracellular fluid spaces. H^+ produced from dissolved CO_2 and carbonic acid is buffered in plasma by deoxyhemoglobin and plasma buffers. Thus, the H^+ and CO_2 concentrations are similar in venous and arterial blood due to their flow into and out of cells, including the capillary, venous, and arterial extracellular fluids. The chloride shift is the movement of Cl^- ions opposite to bicarbonate ions during acid-base compensation and, thus, maintains electrical neutrality as due to increased protonation of proteins and hemoglobin.

Bicarbonate

Bicarbonate ion is produced from carbon dioxide as it reacts with the water in the plasma. It forms from the reaction:

$$CO_2 + H_2O \leftrightarrow H_2CO_3 \leftrightarrow H^+ + HCO_3^-$$

Bicarbonate is the major component of the extracellular buffer system, and is controlled by renal tubular cells and erythrocytes, the previously described metabolic component of the buffer system.

While total CO_2 (tCO_2) includes many components, the majority of plasma CO_2 exists in the form of bicarbonate ion. Some bicarbonate is found in cells (intracellularly), where it maintains electrical neutrality in conjunction with potassium. Bicarbonate may move to extracellular fluid in order to buffer H^+, forming H_2CO_3. Carbonic acid is a weak acid that will act as a buffer and not contribute to the pH of the body fluids. Dissolved carbon dioxide gas is measured as PCO_2 by blood gas analyzers and contributes to H_2CO_3 levels. Dissolved CO_2 and PCO_2 make up a small percentage of carbon dioxide forms. A minute amount of carbon dioxide in plasma is bound to carrier proteins.[15]

RENAL TUBULAR ACIDOSIS

Renal tubular acidosis (RTA) is a tubular defect of acid-base regulation. This condition is characterized by alkaline pH of the urine with acidic blood plasma pH, which causes depletion of potassium and bicarbonate ions. Typically, secondary muscle and bone weakness occurs due to the profound electrolyte and mineral imbalance, especially from hypokalemia. Renal tubular acidosis can be classified as a primary disorder, such as a proximal tubular defect associated with Fanconi's syndrome or Wilson's disease, two genetic disorders.[16,17] Renal tubular acidosis can also be a distal tubular defect, occurring secondary to medullary cystic disease or as a complication of renal transplantation.[18]

Fanconi's syndrome is more common in young patients as a hereditary disorder and results in complications in development and strength of bones and muscles and in tissue repair due to mineral and protein deficiencies.[19] In adults, the syndrome may also be secondary to renal toxicity or complications from renal transplantation.

Case Scenario 6-5 Renal Tubular Acidosis: A Matter of Balance

Follow-Up

The patient's fixed alkaline pH, proteinuria, bicarbonate deficit, and electrolyte and mineral imbalances are typical of renal tubular acidosis. Given the age of the patient as well as the hypocalcemia, hypophosphatemia, and hypoglycemia, the scenario is typical of renal tubular acidosis resulting from Fanconi's syndrome. In this case, treatment with large doses of bicarbonate, electrolytes, and minerals was used to help restore and maintain acid-base balance. ●

CASE SCENARIO 6-6

Hyperkalemia Due to Hemolysis: The Difficult Venipuncture

The technologist had difficulty in obtaining blood from the 75-year-old female dialysis patient. After several attempts, the sample slowly filled a heparinized collection tube two-thirds full and then stopped filling. The needle was withdrawn, and the sample was gently but thoroughly mixed and labeled. This sample was injected into the bedside multianalyzer. The potassium was 6.1 mmol/L and creatinine was 3.8 mg/dL, but all other parameters were within normal values. The technologist decided to centrifuge the remaining portion of the heparinized whole blood sample to observe for **hemolysis** due to the difficulty in obtaining the venous sample. It appeared hemolyzed, and a second sample was obtained with the help of the nurse practitioner.

HEMOLYSIS

Consider the effect of hemolysis on electrolyte and renal function analyses. Recall that potassium, inorganic phosphates, and magnesium are classified as intracellular electrolytes due to their higher distribution inside cell fluids when compared to plasma and other extracellular spaces. Therefore, rupture of cellular membranes, such as those of erythrocytes, will release these intracellular electrolytes into plasma, falsely increasing the amount to be measured. Excessive squeezing of a finger during capillary puncture or prolonged tourniquet use for venipuncture will cause falsely increased plasma or serum potassium. Vigorously shaking a whole blood specimen or an unseparated sample older than a few hours will also disrupt erythrocyte membranes, causing false elevations of serum or plasma potassium levels.

Hemolysis affects the analysis of electrolytes and minerals found in plasma. Grossly hemolyzed specimens will affect analysis of sodium and chloride due to a dilutional effect. Variation will also occur due to the presence of interfering chemicals that absorb at wavelengths that are similar to the test analysis. Hemolysis should be avoided when plasma or serum samples for renal function tests, electrolytes, and minerals are analyzed.[7]

CLINICAL CORRELATION
Fanconi's syndrome is a complex group of disorders resulting from impaired renal reabsorption of glucose, amino acids, and phosphorus, potassium, sodium, and bicarbonate ions and often the inability to secrete hydrogen ions and regulate acid-base balance.

hemolysis - rupture of erythrocyte cell membrane causing release of intracellular contents

THE TEAM APPROACH
Hemolysis is usually not visible in a whole blood sample, which is often the sample of choice for point-of-care instrumentation in critical care, emergent care, or outpatient settings. Thus, it is important to have well-trained collection personnel who can recognize and avoid the typical conditions that cause hemolysis. Phlebotomy training must address mechanisms for successful routine and difficult venipuncture techniques, capillary sample collection, and strategies for obtaining blood specimens from a variety of patients. A discussion of specimen collection and handling conditions that could lead to hemolyzed or hemoconcentrated samples and the effect of these errors on laboratory results should be included in training sessions and procedure manuals for phlebotomy.

Avoidable causes of hemolysis include the following:

1. Failure to place the needle bevel in the center of the vein lumina or partial occlusion of a vein during venipuncture.
2. Squeezing or intense pressure on fingertips or heel during capillary collection.
3. Retaining tourniquet on arm for longer than 1 minute.
4. Failure to separate serum or plasma from cells within 1 hour of collection.
5. Shaking or vigorous inversion of the blood sample, especially prior to clotting.

Unavoidable/pathophysiological causes of hemolysis include the following:

1. Intravascular hemolysis, which can result from the patient's disorder, such as hemolytic anemia
2. Transient hemolysis, which may result from some surgeries such as open heart surgery or heart valve replacement

Case Scenario 6-6 Hyperkalemia Due to Hemolysis: The Difficult Venipuncture

Follow-Up

A second specimen was obtained using a special technique (butterfly infusion set needle), and it filled the smaller evacuated container quickly and completely. The results from this sample were closer to the reference ranges, appeared not to be hemolyzed, and correlated with successful dialysis treatment. The hemolyzed cells from first sample caused erroneous potassium and creatinine laboratory data and should not have been reported on the patient's chart.

CASE SCENARIO 6-7

Pseudohyponatremia? A Problem With Analysis

While analyzing samples in the STAT lab, the technologist noted a creamy tomato soup appearance of a heparinized whole blood specimen. The specimen was accompanied by a requisition for electrolyte analysis from the emergency department. The results of laboratory testing are listed below.

Test	Patient	Reference Ranges
Sodium (mmol/L)	135	136–145
Potassium (mmol/L)	3.6	3.5–5.1
Chloride (mmol/L)	99	98–107
Bicarbonate (mmol/L)	24	22–28
Anion gap (mmol/L)	16	10–20

The technologist considered the following question: When does lipemia, a relatively common occurrence in nonfasting patients, cause methodological interferences for electrolytes? The technologist recalled that lipemia may interfere with analysis of sodium by some methods. After consulting the operating procedure for the whole blood analyzer, the technologist learned that the method that was used to analyze sodium in this laboratory employed a direct ion-selective electrode (ISE). Lipemia does not affect this method.

ELECTROLYTE ANALYSIS

Ion-selective electrodes (ISEs) are the most commonly employed methods of analysis for many electrolytes, including sodium and potassium, although spectroscopic and spectrophotometric methods also exist. Only free unbound ion is measured by the ISE. This limitation becomes significant when measuring such ions such as calcium and magnesium. ISEs consist of or are covered by a unique material that is more selective for one ion than other ions. When the ion comes in contact with the electrode, there is a change in the potential compared to the reference electrode, measured as a voltage change, due to the ionic activity.[20] Test Methodology 6–6 describes the specific principles of ISEs.

TEST METHODOLOGY 6-6.   ELECTROLYTES

The ion-selective electrode (ISE) for sodium is often made of a lithium aluminum silicate or other composite silicon dioxide glass compound that selects for Na^+ more readily than K^+ or H^+. The ISE for potassium typically contains a selective membrane containing valinomycin. The valinomycin binds well with the potassium ions. The total plasma carbon dioxide (tCO_2) gas cell/electrode contains an acid to convert HCO_3^- to gas, which diffuses through a silicone membrane and reacts with a bicarbonate/carbonic acid buffer to produce H^+ in proportion to the amount of tCO_2 in the plasma. The H^+ ions are detected by an ISE made of silicon dioxide/lithium and calcium oxide glass that selects for H^+ in preference to Na^+ and registers a change in potential versus the silver chloride reference electrode. Chloride can also be measured by an ISE of unique composition. A silver chloride membrane solid state electrode measures the activity of Cl^- and is highly accurate.

The Reaction Principle

When the ion comes in contact with the electrode, there is a change in the potential compared to the reference electrode measured as a voltage change, due to the ionic activity.

The Specimen

Venous serum or lithium-heparinized whole blood or plasma, or heparinized arterial whole blood should be collected by a method to avoid hemolysis, release from muscle activity, or leakage from erythrocytes. Heparinized plasma is the specimen of choice and contains 0.3 to 0.7 mmol/L less potassium than serum due to platelet release during coagulation. Refrigeration may actually enhance intracellular potassium release from erythrocytes. Electrolytes may also be analyzed in body fluids such as urine, sweat, cerebrospinal fluid, and gastric fluids and are stable if maintained in closed containers and analyzed promptly.

Reference Ranges for Plasma (Adults)

Sodium	136–145 mmol/L
Potassium	3.5–5.1 mmol/L
Chloride	98–107 mmol/L
Bicarbonate	22–28 mmol/L

The ISE system that dilutes the sample with diluent prior to analysis with the electrode is termed *indirect*. It is compromised by hyperlipidemia or hyperproteinemia as those large lipid or protein molecules in unusually high amounts displace some of the volume of the plasma within the dilution. For example, if triglycerides are >350 mg/dL and/or total protein is >10 g/dL, interference may begin to be experienced. The effect of hyperlipidemia or hyperproteinemia is to falsely lower the measured sodium and sometimes chloride levels due to this dilutional effect.

Chloride also can be measured by coulometric-amperometric titration, with silver ions released at a constant rate and forming insoluble silver chloride. The time of titration is proportional to the chloride activity in the sample. This method is commonly used for sweat chloride analysis.

A recently emerging methodology for total carbon dioxide measurement employs an enzyme, urea amidolyase. The enzyme catalyzes the reaction of bicarbonate with urea to form several products, including ammonium. Ammonium is then measured using glutamate dehydrogenase (after first assessing the endogenous ammonium ion concentration) to produce $NADP^+$, and a change in absorbance at 340 nm is produced.[21]

Lipemia, or creamy appearance of blood plasma due to exogenous triglycerides, is generally at its most pronounced within 2 hours after ingestion of a meal but can persist for up to 8 hours. These exogenous triglycerides are also termed *chylomicrons*. The standard collection of routine laboratory tests of samples obtained in the early morning after an 8- to 10-hour fast avoids lipemia and its potential analytical interferences, and standardizes values that are affected by the diurnal variation of hormones. Electrolytes and renal function tests may be monitored at other times of the day as well and in emergent situations when an overnight fast is not possible. Chylomicrons may be removed from the sample by ultracentrifugation or blood collection into a device that allows separation of these fatty molecules from the serum or plasma specimen.

Direct ISE systems measure electrolytes in undiluted samples. This methodology will not be subject to falsely lowered sodium or chloride levels due to volume replacement by a large presence of chylomicrons or paraproteins.[20]

Calculation of Anion Gap

The anion gap is a calculation of the difference between anions and cations in blood. The gap represents chemical anions other than those used in the formulas (sodium, potassium, chloride, and bicarbonate) that might be present in blood. The gap is used to estimate acid-base and electrolyte disturbances.

There are two commonly used formulas for calculation of the anion gap, with or without the inclusion of potassium ions. The most commonly used formula is

$$(Na + K) - (Cl + HCO_3^-)$$

The formula

$$(Na) - (Cl + HCO_3^-)$$

can be used but is generally being replaced by the formula that includes potassium. The reference range is slightly different if both cations are included in the calculation (10 to 20 mmol/L), while it is 7 to 16 mmol/L if the calculation does not include potassium.

Use of Anion Gap

In normal situations, electrolytes exist in body fluids within a balance to provide electrolyte neutrality. In other words, the total sum of anions, including chloride, bicarbonate, and ionized proteins, equal the sum of all cations, such as potassium, sodium, and calcium (Fig. 6–4). The major electrolytes account for the majority of

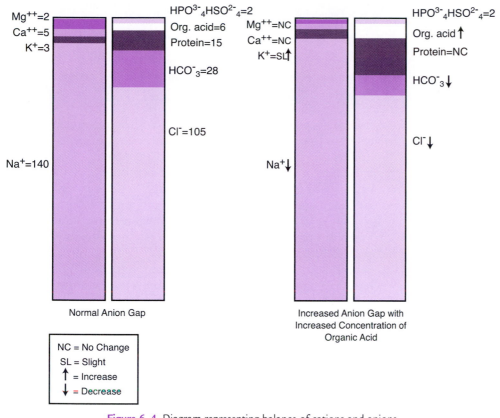

Figure 6–4. Diagram representing balance of cations and anions.

the ions with only about 15 mmol/L contributed by unmeasured anions. The anion gap represents those unmeasured anions that are present in body fluids providing electrolyte balance and neutrality, such as lactate, sulfates, phosphates, ketones, organic acids, and ionized proteins.

The use of an anion gap calculation can be helpful for classification of acid-base status, for recognizing a true imbalance of electrolytes due to pathological conditions, and as a quality assurance statistic for the technologist. For example, in many types of metabolic acidosis, the anion gap is typically increased due to a deficit of bicarbonate ions and the presence of organic acids, such as acetoacetic acid, lactate, salicylate, formate, or glycolate. Calculation of the anion gap and other parameters can help to narrow the cause of metabolic acidosis to production of organic acids or metabolites versus situations of electrolyte loss and imbalance, such as gastrointestinal or renal loss.[13] Circumstances that cause an increase in sodium relative to a deficiency of anions such as bicarbonate will also increase the anion gap. A decreased anion gap may be due to situations that decrease sodium relative to an excess of chloride and bicarbonate. A finding of a decreased anion gap may occur with an occasional patient sample but rarely in consecutive patient samples. More commonly, a decreased anion gap is an indication of technical problems. When potassium or sodium electrodes are in need of calibration or maintenance, the anion gap may be decreased in several consecutive patient samples. Subsequent quality control results would likely indicate a need to reject patient results at that time until the technical problem is resolved.[15]

Case Scenario 6-7 Pseudohyponatremia? A Problem With Analysis

Follow-Up

Considering the electrolyte and anion gap results obtained, the technologist answered the following question: When does lipemia, a relatively common occurrence in nonfasting patients, cause methodological interferences for electrolytes? Indirect ISE analysis of electrolytes first dilutes the sample to eliminate interference from normal amounts of protein and other constituents not desired in the analysis. However, in extreme hyperproteinemia or hyperlipidemia, this dilution will create a technical interference in sodium levels. The anion gap may calculate as a value lower than normal as another clue that the result needs to be reviewed for interferences. Direct ISE systems measure electrolytes in undiluted samples. This methodology will not be subject to falsely lowered sodium or chloride levels due to volume replacement by a large presence of chylomicrons or paraproteins. Since the analysis was performed by direct ISE, technical interference from the lipemia was ruled out. Also, the anion gap was increased rather than decreased in these results, which correlates with a decreased amount of anions when compared with the measured cations. ●

CASE SCENARIO 6-8

Nephrogenic Diabetes Insipidus: Critical Values

While analyzing samples from the psychiatric unit, the technologist noticed some startling electrolyte results. The technologist verified that the patient identification data were in agreement on the sample, requisition, and barcode. She also compared the laboratory results with previous results of this patient over the past 7 days and noted that the electrolyte results had been abnormal in the past, but not as profoundly abnormal as they now were. The protocol for results such as those produced from this specimen directed the technologist to notify the charge nurse or resident for that unit when critical patient values are obtained. The technologist released the results through the computerized laboratory information system (LIS) immediately and called the unit to bring the results to the attention of the attending physician. The laboratory results are list below.

Test	Current	3 Days Ago	5 Days Ago
BUN (mg/dL)	22	20	22
Creatinine (mg/dL)	1.8	1.8	1.9
Na (mmol/L)	155	148	150
K (mmol/L)	4.9	4.6	4.8
Cl (mmol/L)	121	118	119
Bicarbonate (mmol/L)	22	20	22
Osmolality (mOsm/kg)	245	236	242
Urine Na (mg/day)	24	19	NA
Urine specific gravity	1.006	1.007	NA

Case Scenario 6-8 **Nephrogenic Diabetes Insipidus: Critical Values** *(continued)*

Reference ranges for urine sodium are

Male	40–220 mg/day
Female	27–287 mg/day

Reference range for urine specific gravity: 1.005–1.030

NA = not available

Electrolyte Critical Values

In order to classify electrolyte abnormalities, one must compare results to the reference ranges and be mindful of critically high or low levels. Critical values indicate a life-threatening situation is ensuing due to the electrolyte abnormality. They are typically established at each institution, but an example of critical values is listed below.

Na: 120–160 mmol/L
K: 2.8–6.2 mmol/L
Cl: 80–120 mmol/L
tCO$_2$: 10–40 mmol/L

> **THE TEAM APPROACH**
> Critical values indicate life-threatening situations. Laboratory staff must bring such information to the attention of a responsible health-care provider, such as a nurse, physician assistant, or physician, so that the situation may be immediately evaluated.

Abnormal Sodium Levels

Hypernatremia is caused by renal and nonrenal disorders. A common nonrenal cause is hypotonic dehydration from severe diarrhea, extensive burns, or excessive sweating without proper fluid replacement. Infants, the elderly, and other patients not able to ingest sufficient amounts of water, and who are not properly hydrated, will also experience hypernatremia. Renal loss of water, such as in nephrogenic diabetes insipidus, can also cause hypernatremia. Serum osmolality and urinary sodium levels can help to differentiate renal loss of water versus nonrenal causes.[14]

Hyponatremia is caused by renal and nonrenal causes also. Salt-losing renal nephritis, renal tubular acidosis, or syndrome of inappropriate antidiuretic hormone secretion (SIADH) are common causes of renal loss of sodium and may be evaluated by testing for the presence of excess urinary sodium and hyperosmolar urine. Certain diuretics, such as thiazine, can cause renal loss of sodium.[22] Increased urine sodium levels usually indicate sodium loss. Chronic renal failure can cause water overload due to inability to regulate water and results in hyponatremia, while nephritic syndrome can cause fluid imbalances and edema with resulting hyponatremia. Urine sodium levels are usually normal or decreased in hyponatremia due to edema. Nonrenal causes of hyponatremia include psychogenic water overload, cellular shift changes from acidosis, and edema secondary to cirrhosis or congestive heart failure.[14]

> **CLINICAL CORRELATION**
> Syndrome of inappropriate antidiuretic hormone secretion (SIADH) is associated with decreased urine volume even with unrestricted fluid intake; increased urine sodium concentration, specific gravity, and osmolality; hyponatremia; and low serum osmolality. In water loading tests, urine/serum osmolality >1.0 may be found. ADH is measured in conjunction with urine and serum osmolality in water loading tests to determine appropriate concentration. SIADH is associated with malignancies, acute central nervous system disease, pulmonary disorders, and certain medications.

Abnormal Potassium Levels

Hyperkalemia may be caused by decreased renal excretion in acute or chronic renal failure, certain diuretics, or hypoaldosteronism or hypocortisolism. Hyperkalemia may also be caused by ion shift, such as the ion shift that is seen in cases of diabetic ketoacidosis or other metabolic acidoses, leukemia, excessive muscle activity, or hemolysis. Finally, hyperkalemia is associated with iatrogenic causes of excessive intravenous or oral therapy.

Hypokalemia is caused by renal loss such as renal tubular acidosis, hyperaldosteronism, hypercortisolism, and certain diuretics. Potassium can also be decreased due to gastrointestinal dietary deficit or loss from severe vomiting, diarrhea, nasogastric suctioning, laxatives, and malabsorption. A cellular shift in cases of insulin overdose and alkalosis can also cause hypokalemia.[23]

RENAL IMPACT ON WATER AND ELECTROLYTES

Refer to Figure 6–1, which shows the anatomy of the nephron and its role in filtration of electrolytes, nutrients, and wastes. Notice that filtration removes the majority of electrolytes, nutrients, and waste products and some water in the glomerulus. Reabsorption of much of the sodium, chloride, potassium, minerals, amino acids, glucose, and the like occurs in the proximal convoluted tubule by passive transport, facilitated diffusion, and active transport. More electrolytes and water are reabsorbed in the loop of Henle. Under hormonal influence of antidiuretic hormone, parathyroid hormone, and aldosterone, reabsorption occurs in the distal convoluted and collecting tubules.

PHYSIOLOGY: HORMONAL AND RENAL CONTROL OF ELECTROLYTES AND MINERALS

Parathyroid hormone regulates mineral levels by causing renal reabsorption of calcium and magnesium in exchange for phosphorus. More phosphorus is excreted in the urine, and is used in the phosphate buffer system, while calcium is reclaimed to the plasma.

Antidiuretic hormone (ADH), also known as vasopressin, is secreted by the hypophysis in response to osmoreceptors in the brain. ADH stimulates the renal collecting ducts to reabsorb water, thus conserving more water in times of water deprivation.

Epinephrine is a catecholamine that raises blood pressure by constricting blood vessels but does not impact upon electrolyte or mineral levels in extracellular fluids.

Aldosterone, a mineralocorticoid secreted by the adrenal cortex, induces the distal convoluted tubules to reabsorb sodium and chloride in exchange for potassium. Since these hormones function in an integrated fashion, they help to maintain homeostasis of minerals and electrolytes by finishing the reabsorption and secretion phase within the kidney.

Electrolyte disturbances according to various disease states are listed below:

1. Dehydration is associated with elevated plasma sodium, plasma osmolality, BUN, total serum protein, and hematocrit. Although many dissolved particles in serum are relatively elevated, these are the most sensitive indicators of dehydration.

2. Acute renal failure causes elevated plasma potassium, magnesium, phosphorus, and creatinine and often decreased plasma calcium, sodium, and bicarbonate levels.

3. Cellular breakdown from hemolysis or trauma or in stored blood samples causes increased plasma potassium, magnesium, and phosphorus.

4. Treatment with insulin following hyperglycemia will cause a drop in plasma potassium and phosphorus.

5. Overtreatment with electrolytes will cause imbalances. For example, overtreatment with potassium in IV fluids or orally will cause hyperkalemia, and overtreatment with sodium will cause hypernatremia and hyperosmolality.

6. Overhydration with IV fluids will cause hyponatremia, hypochloremia, and lowered plasma osmolality.

Water and Electrolytes

Total body water and hydration status of the patient impacts electrolyte concentration due to the compartmentalization of body fluids. Extracellular ion concentrations are sensitive to dilutional effects of excessive hydration or concentration effects of dehydration. Sodium concentration is especially sensitive to hydration status and will vary directly with serum osmolality levels, and inversely with total body water levels. For example, in dehydration, the patient usually has hypernatremia (increased sodium) and hyperosmolality, while in overhydration the plasma sodium and osmolality are decreased. Intracellular ion concentrations, such as potassium concentration, are not as sensitive to hydration status, such as in dehydration.

Osmolality is defined as the concentration of solutes dissolved in a solvent and is usually expressed in units of milliosmoles per kilogram of pure water. In plasma all dissolved particles, including electrolytes, carbohydrates, waste products, vitamins, drugs, and hormones, contribute to osmolality. However, the major contributors to osmolality are sodium, chloride, glucose, urea, proteins, and ethyl alcohol (when present). Sodium makes up roughly half of the plasma osmolality. Plasma or serum osmolality can be estimated with the following formula:

$$1.86 \ (\text{Na [mmol/L]}) + (\text{glucose [mg/dL]}/18) + (\text{urea N [mg/dL]}/2.8) + 9$$

where glucose and urea are converted to mmol/L by the factors listed and 9 represents the typical contribution of ionized proteins, potassium, chloride, and calcium. Urine osmolality is useful in comparison to plasma osmolality in assessment of water regulation in regard to hormonal control and renal function.

Osmometry is the general term for analysis of osmolality. Dissolved particles affect a solution by altering the solution's colligative properties, such as lowering the vapor pressure or lowering the freezing point. These are the properties that can be measured in an osmometer to determine the osmolality of body fluids such as serum or urine, as described in Test Methodology 6–7. Sodium contributes nearly half of the osmolality in normal circumstances, but other solutes, such as urea, glucose, and alcohols, can contribute significantly to osmolality when they are present in excess. Alcohols can't be detected by vapor depression osmometers but can be detected in freezing point depression (FDP) osmometers.

TEST METHODOLOGY 6-7.   OSMOLALITY MEASUREMENT

Osmometry measures differences in the colligative properties of solutions. In a freezing point depression osmometer, a thermistor probe and stirring mechanism come in contact with the sample, which is supercooled to approximately –10°C, which is below the freezing point of the sample. A stirring wire vibrates to initiate freezing to a slush stage, and the heat of fusion warms the solution, causing equilibrium in temperature between freezing and thawing state. Variable resistance is measured, representing freezing point depression. Resistance is measured as a reflection of particles in solution that affect freezing point depression.

The Reaction Principle

Osmolality (in mOsm/kg of H_2O) is determined as the observed freezing point compared to the molal freezing point depression of pure water, –1.86°C.

The Specimen

Serum that is free from cells or gross hemolysis is the specimen of choice. Plasma is generally not measured because of interference of anticoagulants in solution. Other body fluids, such as urine and gastric fluids, may be measured by freezing point depression. Samples are stable if maintained in closed containers and analyzed promptly or refrigerated at 2° to 80°C for up to 24 hours.

Reference Ranges (Adults)

Serum	275–300 mOsm/kg
Urine (24-hour collection)	300–900 mOsm/kg

Case Scenario 6-8 Nephrogenic Diabetes Insipidus: Critical Values

Follow-Up

This patient had sustained polyuria with hypo-osmolar urine, characterized by low specific gravity and low output of sodium. The patient also experienced severe hypernatremia, hyperosmolar serum, and other indications of dehydration. Nephrogenic diabetes insipidus is the likely cause of these findings. A review of the patient's therapeutic drug monitoring revealed lithium concentrations that exceeded the therapeutic index. Lithium toxicity can impair the renal response to antidiuretic hormone (ADH), causing water wasting disease and volume depletion. Serious consequences include severe osmotic pressure changes that can induce further complications. The most immediate effect is swelling on the brain and potential coma. ●

CASE SCENARIO 6-9

Renal Calculi: Kidney Stones

As the technologist walked by the door to the emergency room, she noticed a man who was being helped into the room. The man was almost completely doubled over and obviously in great pain. "Passing another one," was all the man said. Later, the technologist received specimens of blood and urine from

Case Scenario 6-9 Renal Calculi: Kidney Stones *(continued)*

this patient. His complete blood count (CBC) was normal; the blood uric acid concentration was abnormally high. His urine specimen was very dark yellow with a high specific gravity of 1.034, pH of 5.0, and the presence of blood. The microscopic examination of the urine showed a moderate amount of red blood cells and a few white blood cells. Moderate levels of crystals were seen in the urine.

The technologist checked the LIS. The patient had been diagnosed with urate **nephrolithiasis** in the past. The technologist knew that most renal **calculi** are calcium oxalate, calcium phosphate, uric acid, cystine, or a mixture of these substances.[24]

nephrolithiasis - presence of calculi in the urinary tract; urate nephrolithiasis indicates the presence of uric acid in the stone

calculi - any abnormal concretion of precipitated organic materials, commonly called a stone, within the body (singular: calculus)

KIDNEY STONES

Kidney stone formation is predisposed by a number of factors, including dehydration, a high- protein diet, and a sedentary lifestyle. Increased levels of calcium, urate, and oxalate and decreased levels of magnesium may promote stone formation. The solubility of the urine chemicals may be influenced by changes in urine pH. Calcium oxalate is the most common stone found. Stones are associated with conditions in which the urine is highly concentrated.

Uric acid is produced from the cellular breakdown products of the purine nucleosides, adenosine and guanosine. Uric acid is one of several compounds that are sometimes called nonprotein nitrogen (NPN) compounds. Most uric acid is produced from the natural cellular breakdown in the body; some uric acid is produced from the breakdown of dietary purines. Individuals who are producing abnormal levels of cells, such as in a leukemia process, may have high levels of uric acid. Uric acid is filtered through the renal glomerulus and is almost completely reabsorbed in the proximal and distal tubules. At pH levels above 5.57, most uric acid is in the urate form, a chemical form that is soluble in urine. At pH levels below 5.57, levels of uric acid formation increase.

Hyperuricemia is a term used to describe individuals who have increased uric acid in the blood. Such individuals may be asymptomatic, but are at increased risk for associated renal problems. Gout is a disease in which urates are deposited in body fluids. The classic symptoms of gout include gouty arthritis, in which uric acid is deposited in joints. Gout may be due to overproduction of purines or to defects in the metabolic pathways of purine metabolism. Methods of measuring uric acid are presented in Test Methodology 6–8.

✔ **Common Sense Check**
On refrigeration of urine specimens, crystals often form around small preformed crystals or cellular elements in the urine. Stone formation is unusual because large crystal calculi form at body temperature.

TEST METHODOLOGY 6-8.   URIC ACID

Two methods for uric acid measurement are commonly used in the clinical laboratory: uricase and phosphotungstic acid methods.

The Reaction

Uricase Method

$$\text{Uric acid} + H_2O + O_2 \xrightarrow{\text{uricase}} \text{allantoin} + CO_2 + H_2O_2$$

continued

TEST METHODOLOGY 6-8.   URIC ACID (continued)

1. Decrease in absorbance at 293 nm is due to loss of uric acid.
2. Alternate methods have hydrogen peroxide converted to a chromagen using 4-aminophenazone and peroxidase in a second enzyme-catalyzed reaction.
3. Excessive amounts of protein and lipids can interfere with results, and negative interferences often occur with the presence of xanthine and hemoglobin.

Phosphotungstate Method

This method requires a protein-free filtrate for serum or plasma.

$$\text{Uric acid} + \text{phosphotungstic acid} + Na_2CO_2 \xrightarrow{\text{alkaline pH}} \text{allantoin} + CO_2 + \text{tungsten blue}$$

Proteins in normal amounts in serum must be removed to prevent interferences. Glucose, ascorbic acid, glutathione, hemoglobin, and drugs such as acetaminophen and caffeine commonly interfere.

The Specimen

Serum, heparinized plasma, and urine may be tested. Anticoagulants containing fluoride or citrate should not be used. Hemolysis and lipemia should be avoided.

Reference Ranges

Uricase Method

Male	3.5–7.2 mg/dL
Female	2.6–6.0 mg/dL

Phosphotungstate Method

Male	4.2–8.0 mg/dL
Female	3.5–7.3 mg/dL

Values are lower in children.

Case Scenario 6-9 Renal Calculi: Kidney Stones

Follow-Up:

The patient was treated with ultrasound lithotripsy, in which sound waves crush the stones inside the body. The patient walked out of the emergency upright, but may expect to experience reoccurrences of the event. ●

SUMMARY

Renal function can be assessed by analysis of creatinine clearance, serum creatinine, BUN, electrolytes, and other laboratory tests. This information is of great value to physicians and other health-care providers as they monitor for renal disease and responsiveness to therapy in their patients. The problems presented in this chapter offered the opportunity for the reader to learn about renal anatomy and function, as well as diseases of the renal system and their impact upon laboratory indicators. The reader was also introduced to clinical laboratory methodologies for measuring these analytes, including principles of analysis and sources of errors. As members of the health-care team, clinical laboratory scientists contribute objective information for medical decision-making.

EXERCISES

As you consider the scenarios presented in this chapter, answer the following questions:

1. What are the physiological sources of creatinine, uric acid, and urea?

2. What considerations should be made for specimen collection and handling of specimens for serum sodium, potassium, and creatinine and urine creatinine testing?

3. How can creatinine clearance results be used in the differential diagnostic causes of renal insufficiency in a patient?

4. Differentiate typical laboratory results of renal failure versus nephrotic syndrome.

5. What are two preanalytical sources of error that need to be avoided in order to provide accurate creatinine values?

6. What are the key reagents that react with urea, forming a measurable product?

7. What are two preanalytical sources of error that need to be avoided in order to provide accurate urea values?

8. What are the methodological principles of ion-selective electrodes for the analysis of sodium, potassium, chloride, and total carbon dioxide?

9. What are three preanalytical sources of error that should be avoided in order to provide accurate electrolyte results?

10. What is the anion gap given the following laboratory results (shown as mmol/L)? Na = 125; K= 4.5; Cl = 100; tCO_2 = 10?

11. An adult female patient has the following results electrolyte results. Which one is within the reference range?

Na	148 mmol/L
K	3.3 mmol/L
Cl	100 mmol/L
CO_2	35 mmol/L
Calcium, total	11.1 mg/dL
Magnesium	3.8 mmol/L

12. What is the most commonly used formula for calculating osmolality?

13. Describe the conditions that promote the production of nephrolithiasis (kidney stones).

14. Why is the uricase method for uric acid often considered preferable to the phosphotungstic acid method?

References

1. Beers MH, Berkow R: *The Merck Manual of Diagnosis and Therapy*, ed 17. Rahway, NJ: Merck & Co., 1999.
2. Rahn KH, Heidenreich S, Bruckner D: How to assess glomerular function and damage. *J Hypertens* 1999; 17:309–317.
3. Gaspari F, Perico N, Remuzzi G: Measurement of glomerular filtration rate. *Kidney Int Suppl* 1997; 63:S151–S154.
4. Manjunath G, Sarnak MJ, Levey AS: Estimating the glomerular filtration rate: Do's and don'ts for assessing kidney function. *Postgrad Med* 2001; 110:55–62.

5. Schwartz GL: A simple estimate of glomerular filtration rate in children. *Pediatrics* 1976; 58:259–263.

6. American Diabetes Association: Standards of medical care in diabetes—2006. *Diabetes Care* 2006; 29:S4–S42.

7. Sacks DB, et al: Guidelines and recommendations for laboratory analysis in the diagnosis and management of diabetes mellitus. *Clin Chem* 2002; 48(3):436–472.

8. Saha H, et al: Limited value of the fractional excretion of sodium test in the diagnosis of acute renal failure. *Nephrol Dial Transplant* 1987; 2:79–82.

9. Needham E: Management of acute renal failure. *Am Fam Physician* 2005; 72:1739–1746.

10. Stein JH (ed): *Internal Medicine*, ed 4. St. Louis: Mosby–Year Book, 1994.

11. Zarich S, Fang LS, Diamond JR: Fractional excretion of sodium: exceptions to its diagnostic value. *Arch Intern Med* 1985; 145:108–112.

12. Wagner CA, Geibel JP: Acid-base transport in the collecting duct. *J Nephrol* 2002; 15(Suppl 5):S112–S127.

13. Swenson ER: Metabolic acidosis. *Respir Care* 2001; 46:342–353.

14. Kumar S, Tomas B: Sodium. *Lancet* 1998; 352:352.

15. Professional Practice in Clinical Chemistry: A Review. Workshop materials, sponsored by the American Association for Clinical Chemistry and the National Academy of Clinical Biochemists in cooperation with The George Washington University Medical Center. Washington, DC: AACC Press, 1991.

16. Lemann J Jr, et al: Acid and mineral balances and bone in familial proximal renal tubular acidosis. *Kidney Int* 2000; 58:1267–1277.

17. Adedoyin O, et al: Evaluation of failure to thrive: diagnostic yield of testing for renal tubular acidosis. *Pediatrics* 2003; 112:463.

18. Juncos LI, et al: Renal tubular acidosis and vasculitis associated with IgE deposits in the kidney and small vessels. *Am J Kidney Dis* 2000; 35:941–949.

19. Oster JR, et al: Metabolic acidosis with extreme elevation of anion gap: case report and literature review. *Am J Med Sci* 1999; 317:38.

20. Oesch U, Ammann D, Simon W: Ion-selective membrane electrodes for clinical use. *Clin Chem* 1986; 32:1448–1459.

21. Kimura S, et al: Enzymatic assay for determination of bicarbonate ion in plasma using urea amidolyase. *Clin Chim Acta* 2003; 328:179–184.

22. McBride LJ: *Textbook of Urinalysis and Body Fluids*. Philadelphia: JB Lippincott, 1998, p 38.

23. Gennari FJ: Hyperkalemia. *N Engl J Med* 1998; 339:7.

24. Samuell CT, Kasidas GP: Biochemical investigations in renal stone formers. *Ann Clin Biochem* 1995; 32(Pt 2):112–122.

7

The clinical laboratory is an important partner in the assessment of hepatic disorder.

Assessment of Liver Function

Wendy Arneson and Jean Brickell

Six laboratory situations are presented in this chapter to illustrate the role of the clinical laboratory in assessment of liver function. By working through the problems as they are presented, the student will learn about tests for liver function, pathophysiology of liver enzymes, and principles of analysis for protein, liver function tests, and liver enzymes. Preanalytical variations such as specimen collection and handling and other factors that influence the results before analysis will be discussed. Analytical errors or interferences at the time of analysis and postanalytical factors, such as communication of the results, will also be described. The chapter also includes a discussion of the role of the laboratory technician in providing laboratory results that aid in diagnosis and monitoring of liver disorders, common sense tips, definitions of terms, and brief descriptions of pathophysiology and clinical correlations, as well as explanations of the team approach in health care.

OBJECTIVES

Upon completion of this chapter, the student will have the ability to

- Discuss common preanalytical errors resulting from improper specimen collection and handling and commonly encountered sources of interference in ammonia, bilirubin, total serum protein, albumin, alkaline phosphatase, alanine transaminase, and other liver enzyme analyses.

- Explain the role of quality control results in liver enzyme analysis.

- Describe the principles of alanine and aspartate transaminase, alkaline phosphatase ammonia, total and direct bilirubin, urobilinogen, total serum protein, and albumin analyses in terms of key reagents and their role.

- Verify calculation of results when a dilution is required.

- Correlate liver enzyme, bilirubin, ammonia, and serum albumin results with expected previous findings and correlate results with pathology.

- Discuss common sources of discrepancies in patient liver function and enzyme test results, including what appropriate action is needed.

- Discuss situations when it is important to communicate bilirubin or ammonia results to health care providers.

---

icterus - yellowish pigmentation in the blood due to increased bilirubin

jaundice - bilirubin deposits in the skin, mucous membranes, and eyes giving tissues a yellow appearance

✓ **Common Sense Check**
Visual examination of the specimen may act as an indicator or verification of a suspected disorder. In this case, increased yellow pigment may be an indicator of increased levels of the pigment bilirubin in the serum.

CASE SCENARIO 7-1

Hyperbilirubinemia: A Yellow Serum Sample in a Rack of Tubes

The laboratory technologist noticed as he was placing the serum sample cup into the automated chemistry instrument that the serum appeared to have **icterus**. Although the increased yellow color of the serum could be caused by dye that has been ingested by the patient, the most common cause of increased yellowness of the serum is increased bilirubin. When the results of the chemistry test for this patient appeared on the screen, the technologist saw that the total bilirubin for this patient was increased and that other liver function tests were also abnormal. The technologist reviewed the laboratory results on this patient from the past several days (Table 7–1). The patient was diagnosed with obstructive **jaundice**. The laboratory results for the patient are typical of the progress of a patient with this disorder.

Case Scenario 7-1 Hyperbilirubinemia: A Yellow Serum Sample in a Rack of Tubes *(continued)*

TABLE 7-1

Test Results of the Patient With the Icteric Specimen

Test	Reference Range	Results	
		Day 1	Day 2
Total protein (g/dL)	6.4–8.3	7.4	7.2
Albumin (g/dL)	3.5–5.2	4.4	4.1
Total bilirubin (mg/dL)	0.0–2.0	3.5	3.6
Direct bilirubin (mg/dL)	0.0–0.2	2.3	2.1
ALT (U/L)	<45	220	208
Alkaline phosphatase (U/L)	53–128	374	380
GGT (U/L)	<55	178	170
AST (U/L)	<38	190	176
Amylase (U/L)	28–100	94	—

In a patient with obstructive jaundice, the increase in bilirubin is primarily an increase in conjugated bilirubin. The enzymes gamma-glutamyltransferase (GGT), aspartate transaminase (AST), and alanine transaminase (ALT) may be increased by as much as five times the normal value. Alkaline phosphatase may be increased up to three times the upper value of the normal range. For this patient, both total and conjugated bilirubin levels are elevated. Serum enzymes, including GGT, AST, ALT, and alkaline phosphatase, are also increased.

TESTS FOR LIVER FUNCTION

The clinical laboratory offers several tests for the assessment of liver function. The enzymes alkaline phosphatase, ALT, AST, GGT, and 5′-nucleotidase are helpful in the assessment of the proper functioning and inflammatory status of the liver. Because the liver is the site for metabolism of carbohydrate, protein, and lipids, as well as for the synthesis of many proteins, the conjugation of bilirubin, and **detoxification** of drugs and other substances, the liver may be assessed by measurement of total and direct bilirubin, total protein and albumin, cholesterol and triglycerides, and urea and ammonia.[1] Correlation of laboratory results across time is an indication of accuracy and appropriateness of results. In this case, increased levels of enzymes and bilirubin and lowered protein correlate with liver disease. The extent of the increased alkaline phosphatase and the presence of increases in both total and direct bilirubin help to specify this liver disorder as obstructive jaundice.[2–5]

detoxification - removal of waste or toxins from a fluid, rendering it harmless

CLINICAL CORRELATION
Increased enzyme levels, lowered protein, and increased bilirubin correlate with liver disease.

LIVER ANATOMY AND PHYSIOLOGY

The liver, represented in Figure 7–1, is a large, bilobed, complex organ receiving a large amount of blood and nutrients from the gastrointestinal system in order to convert nutrients from the diet into usable or storage forms. It also is a key organ in conversion of toxins for their removal, and in production of bile, an important

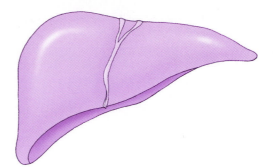

Figure 7–1. The liver is found in the upper right quadrant of the abdomen.

lobules - the microscopic functional units of the liver

parenchymal cells - epithelial liver cells that make bile, bilirubin, and proteins and perform other duties; hepatocytes

fluid to aid in the emulsification of dietary fats prior to their absorption. The liver also contains Kupffer cells as well as tissue lymphocytes and fibroblasts, key contributors in immune defenses.

The liver is composed of a variety of microscopic functional units, called **lobules** (Fig. 7–2). Lobules, comprised chiefly of sheets of hepatic **parenchymal cells** or hepatocytes, are arranged around portal triads and a central vein. The portal vein provides the majority of the incoming blood supply to the hepatocytes via the gastrointestinal system into terminal portal venules. The hepatic artery branches into terminal hepatic arterioles. Together these terminal venules and arterioles, along with small bile ducts, comprise the portal triad. Nutrients from the gastroin-

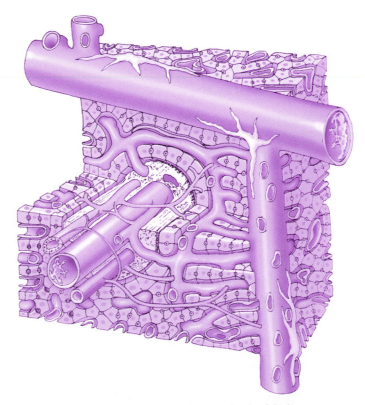

Figure 7–2. The lobule is the functional unit of the liver.

testinal system diffuse into the hepatocytes via **sinusoidal** membranes, where metabolic processes involving proteins, fats, carbohydrates, vitamins, and detoxification occur. The central veins receive the sinuosoidal flow of fluids, which eventually move to the hepatic vein for outflow to the venous circulation. Lymphatic vessels also play a role in removing fluids from the liver. Small bile ducts, or **biliary canaliculi**, are also a part of the lobule and are responsible for carrying the bile out of the liver and eventually to the common bile duct and duodenum.[2]

Hepatocytes are highly organized cells with active organelles, including endoplasmic reticulum, Golgi complex, lysosomes, mitochondria, and microtubules. The smooth endoplasmic reticulum is the site of hepatic drug metabolism, drug detoxification, bilirubin conjugation, and cholesterol synthesis. The rough endoplasmic reticulum with ribosomal complexes is the site for albumin, enzyme, coagulation factor, and other protein synthesis. The Golgi complex receives proteins and modifies them to attach carbohydrates and lipids, forming glycoproteins and lipoproteins. Very low-density lipoprotein is produced in the Golgi complex. The mitochondria are active in oxidative phosphorylation and fatty acid oxidation, while the lysosomes are active in protein breakdown (proteolysis) and other degradation functions. The microtubules and microfilaments help to maintain the hepatocytes' structure and contractile force.

BILIRUBIN METABOLISM

Bilirubin is a degradation product of the heme portion of hemoglobin. Heme is degraded in cells of the reticuloendothelial system, mainly the spleen. The protoporphyrin ring of the heme is opened to the biliverdin form and iron is released. Biliverdin is reduced to produce the yellow-pigmented molecule bilirubin. The bilirubin molecule, a tetrapyrole, has low solubility in water or plasma. When it is released into blood, it is bound to albumin for transport. Covalently bound bilirubin is called delta bilirubin. When the bilirubin-albumin form reaches the liver, it loses albumin and enters the hepatocyte. Within the hepatocyte, the liver enzyme uridyl diphosphate glucuronyltransferase (UDPG-transferase) transfers molecules of glucuronate, a sugar, to the bilirubin molecule. About 85% of bilirubin is conjugated with two molecules of glucuronate to form diglucuronate-bilirubin. Most of the rest of bilirubin is conjugated with one sugar molecule to form monoglucuronate-bilirubin. The addition of the sugar group increases the solubility of the molecule. Figure 7–3 depicts the heme degradation pathway and the formation of bilirubin.

Conjugated bilirubin passes into the intestine through the bile duct, where intestinal bacteria reduce bilirubin to urobilinogen. Some urobilinogen may be reabsorbed through the intestinal mucosa and returned to the portal circulation and the liver. The remaining urobilinogen is excreted into urine or oxidized to form urobilin and excreted in the feces. Urobilin is one component in feces giving its characteristic brown color. Methods of analysis of bilirubin and urobilinogen are shown in Test Methodology 7–1 and Test Methodology 7–2, respectively.

HYPERBILIRUBINEMIA

Bilirubin levels in the blood are increased as the result of several disorders or conditions. These disorders or conditions are categorized into three phases

sinusoidal - forming a small channel for blood in the tissues of the liver or other organs

biliary canaliculi - small ducts or tubes that carry bile out from the liver leading to the small intestine

THE TEAM APPROACH
Laboratory results are just a part of the tools that are available for the assessment of liver function. The patient's signs and symptoms are also important factors. This patient had abdominal pain and noticed a yellowing of the sclera of the eye. An ultrasound scan and radiological imaging indicated the presence of stones in the common bile duct.

TEST METHODOLOGY 7-1.   BILIRUBIN[1]

The three forms of bilirubin (unconjugated, conjugated, and albumin bound) differ in their solubility in water. Testing for the different forms of bilirubin is based upon their differences in solubility. Because conjugated bilirubin and albumin-bound bilirubin (or delta bilirubin[6]) are soluble in water, conjugated bilirubin reacts in a fast or direct reaction with substrates. When an accelerator is used in the reaction, unconjugated bilirubin is solubilized and is measured in the reactant mixture. Therefore, direct bilirubin measures conjugated and albumin-bound bilirubin and total bilirubin, with the addition of the accelerator, measures all forms of bilirubin. Both the Jendrassik-Grof reaction[7] and the Malloy-Evelyn method for measuring bilirubin use diazonium salt to produce a color reaction with bilirubin.

The Reaction

Bilirubin + diazotized sulfanilic acid → azobilirubin

The Jendrassik-Grof method, performed at a pH of 13, measures the blue-colored product at 600 nm. The alkaline reaction produces a more intense color than the equivalent reaction run at a neutral pH. The Malloy-Evelyn method, performed at a pH of 1.3, measures the red-colored product at 560 nm. A sodium benzoate–caffeine mixture or methanol may be used as the accelerator in these methods.

The Specimen

Serum, plasma, spinal fluid, and urine may all be measured by diazonium salt methods. Urine may be measured qualitatively on an absorbent pad. A color change is noted for the assessment of increased bilirubin. The Ictotest© is based upon this method. Hemolysis may falsely decrease bilirubin measurement. Lipemia may falsely elevate bilirubin measurement. Bilirubin may be broken down by light or heat and should be protected from these environmental conditions.

Reference Ranges

Adult bilirubin	0.0–2.0 mg/dL
Adult direct bilirubin	0.0–0.2 mg/dL

TEST METHODOLOGY 7-2.   UROBILINOGEN

The Reaction

Laboratory determination of fecal or urine urobilinogen is based on Ehrlich's reaction, which uses *para*-dimethylaminobenzaldehyde to form a red color. Ascorbic acid may be added to the sample to maintain urobilinogen in its reduced state.[1]

The Specimen

The test requires fresh sample; urobilinogen may be oxidized to urobilin on standing.

Interferences

Urobilin in the sample is reduced by alkaline ferrous hydroxide to urobilinogen. Sodium acetate further reduces other chromogens, which may interfere with Ehrlich's reagent. Bilirubin may interfere with the reaction; significant amounts of bilirubin must be precipitated with barium chloride and removed by filtration.

Reference Ranges

Urine	0.5–4.0 Ehrlich units/day
Feces	75–400 Ehrlich units/day

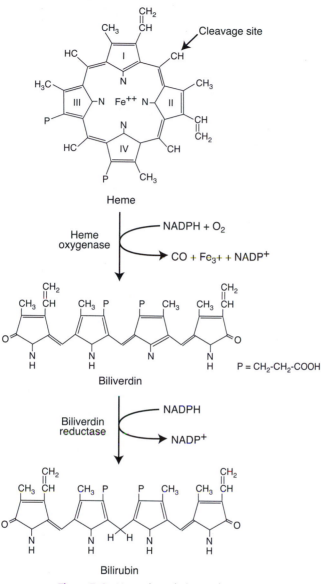

Figure 7–3. Heme degradation pathway.

of bilirubin metabolism, prehepatic, hepatic, and posthepatic. Prehepatic hyper-bilirubinemia is caused by increased hemolysis and increased degradation of heme. Prehepatic hyperbilirubinemia occurs in patients with sickle cell anemia and other hemolytic diseases that cause increased destruction of red blood cells and release of hemoglobin. The typical serum bilirubin pattern of prehepatic hyperbilirubinemia is increased unconjugated bilirubin and normal conjugated bilirubin.

Hepatic hyperbilirubinemia is generally due to defective transport to the liver or conjugation of bilirubin in the hepatocytes. Disorders of transport into the hepatocytes or conjugation disorders result in increased unconjugated bilirubin. Examples of these conditions include Gilbert's and Crigler-Najjar syndromes. Gilbert's syndrome is a hereditary disorder in which there is decreased bilirubin transport into the hepatocytes. Several hepatic hyperbilirubinemic disorders are caused by failure of the liver to conjugate bilirubin. Crigler-Najjar syndrome results from a hereditary deficiency of the UDPG-transferase enzyme. Neonatal jaundice is caused by the inability of the immature liver of the newborn to produce UDPG-transferase. A slight increase in bilirubin in the second and third days of life is a normal response. Damage to hepatocytes by hepatitis, cirrhosis, toxic substances, and other disorders can inhibit conjugation as well. The typical serum bilirubin pattern of hepatic hyperbilirubinemia is increased unconjugated and conjugated bilirubin. Serum enzymes that indicate hepatocellular inflammation and cellular damage within the liver, including ALT and AST, are also often elevated.

Posthepatic hyperbilirubinemia is generally due to a defect in transporting conjugated bilirubin and bile out of the liver. It can involve obstruction of the small canaliculi within the liver, the hepatic bile duct, and the common bile duct leading to the duodenum of the small intestine. Posthepatic hyperbilirubinemia is often called obstructive jaundice. Obstruction of the bile flow can be due to gallstones or to scarring and nodules, such as from cirrhosis or tumors. The typical serum bilirubin pattern of posthepatic hyperbilirubinemia is increased conjugated bilirubin but normal unconjugated bilirubin. Serum enzymes that indicate biliary cell damage, including alkaline phosphatase and GGT, are also often elevated.

Obstructive Jaundice

Obstruction of bile from the liver may be caused by gallstones in the bile duct or a tumor that impedes the flow of bile into the intestine. Increased total bilirubin in the blood of a patient with obstructive jaundice is usually a reflection of increased conjugated bilirubin. Other effects of obstructive jaundice may be defective excretion of lipid substances through bile.

Obstructive jaundice is associated with increased levels of alkaline phosphatase and GGT and increased serum total and direct bilirubin. When the direct bilirubin level is nearing the total bilirubin level, this generally indicates a posthepatic hyperbilirubinemia such as in obstructive jaundice. Sometimes other liver enzymes are elevated as well, indicating hepatic inflammation. Ultrasound and other imaging techniques are needed to locate the source of the obstruction.

Case Scenario 7-1 Hyperbilirubinemia: A Yellow Serum Sample in a Rack of Tubes

Follow-Up

Correlation of laboratory results across time is an indication of the accuracy and appropriateness of the results. In this case, increased enzyme levels and increased bilirubin correlate with liver disease. This liver disorder was specified as obstructive jaundice due to the extent of the increased alkaline phosphatase and the presence of increases in total and direct bilirubin. Other liver enzymes were also elevated, indicating some hepatocellular inflammation was also present.[8] On the third day, the patient passed a gallstone. Laboratory values improved markedly after this event. The patient was advised to undergo gallbladder removal surgery and elected to undergo the surgery. The patient has had no further episodes. ●

Neonatal Hyperbilirubinemia: Why Is the Baby Yellow?

When a clinical laboratory scientist's first nephew was born, her family members told her that the delivery of the full-term infant was normal. All clinical signs and laboratory data were normal in the first few days. By day three, the infant's total bilirubin was 5.8 mg/dL and he appeared jaundiced. Home **phototherapy** was started, along with recording fluid intake, and the baby was monitored daily with serum total bilirubin results. Family members wanted an explanation of the cause for this condition and if this condition likely indicated some inborn liver disorder.

phototherapy - exposure to sunlight or artificial ultraviolet light for therapeutic purposes, such as treating neonatal hyperbilirubinemia

NEONATAL HYPERBILIRUBINEMIA

Neonatal hyperbilirubinemia may result from a variety of conditions, some of which are transient, such as neonatal physiological jaundice of the newborn, and some of which are more serious conditions that cause sustained hyperbilirubinemia in the newborn. Prolonged hyperbilirubinemia often indicates a serious condition in the neonate, such as hemolytic disease of the newborn, biliary atresia, or, in rare situations, idiopathic neonatal hepatitis. Biliary atresia is a rare congenital anatomic obstruction of the biliary ducts and presents as posthepatic jaundice. Idiopathic neonatal hepatitis is a hepatic inflammatory condition of unknown cause and presents as hepatic jaundice, with elevated hepatic enzymes. It is also quite rare.

In the patient, hemolytic disease of the newborn presents as a prehepatic jaundice with a positive direct antiglobulin (Coombs') test. It is most commonly attributed to blood group incompatibility between the expressed blood groups of the mother and the fetus. Rh blood groups are often involved. The disease process develops when the blood cells of the mother come in contact with incompatible cells of the fetus through transfusion or through contact with the infant's blood during pregnancy. The mother's immune system recognizes the incompatible cells as foreign and develops antibodies against them. If the immune process is begun when an infant is delivered, the antibodies will not affect that infant. However, antibody may be directed against blood cells of a subsequent pregnancy if that fetus also expresses an incompatible blood group. Hemolytic disease of the newborn may require exchange transfusion in the neonate if hemolysis is severe.[9]

Phototherapy is often the treatment of choice when bilirubin levels exceed 10 mg/dL since **kernicterus** may occur at levels approaching 20 mg/dL. Phototherapy is a method of treating neonatal hyperbilirubinemia in which the baby is placed periodically under a light source emitting 450-nm wavelength light. Light diffuses through layers of skin and converts unconjugated bilirubin to stable water-soluble forms that can be excreted. The baby's eyes are protected during this process from harmful ultraviolet (UV) and near-UV rays. Kernicterus is a condition in which brain cell nuclei stain yellow and become damaged due to bilirubin or other molecules. High levels of bilirubin are less likely to cause brain damage in adults due to the natural barrier in the brain, called the blood-brain barrier. Kernicterus typically occurs at bilirubin levels greater than 20 mg/dL in infants due to their immature blood-brain barrier. It may result in cerebral palsy, deafness, or mental retardation.

CLINICAL CORRELATION
Biliary atresia is usually a rare congenital disease with anatomic obstruction of biliary ducts.

kernicterus - yellow staining of the lipid-rich meninges of the brain and spinal cord due to bilirubin infiltrates

Physiological Jaundice of the Newborn

When discussing hepatic hyperbilirubinemia earlier in this chapter, it was noted that neonatal jaundice is typically due to the short-term or transient immaturity of the liver. This causes a short-term delay in ability to produce UDPG-transferase for conjugation. In addition, there is higher turnover of neonatal erythrocytes shortly after birth in order to replace fetal hemoglobin (Hb F) with hemoglobin A. This causes an increase in supply of heme for degradation to bilirubin. The reference ranges listed in Test Methodology 7–3 show the slight increase in bilirubin in the first few days of life when compared to the normal adult bilirubin level. This peaks at around 2 to 4 days but may remain elevated for up to 2 weeks.[9]

TEST METHODOLOGY 7-3.   NEONATAL BILIRUBIN[1]

Total bilirubin in the neonate can be measured based on its absorption at 454 nm in phosphate buffer solution of pH 7.4. Oxyhemoglobin, a common molecule found in neonatal serum, absorbs light at 454 and 540 nm. If absorbance is measured with a dual-wavelength narrow bandpass spectrophotometer, neonatal total bilirubin can be determined from the difference in absorbance at these two wavelengths.

The Reaction

Serum is diluted with phosphate buffer at pH 7.4, and absorbance at 454 and 540 nm is determined. Concentration is determined from a standardized curve using adjusted (subtracted) absorbance from the sample.

Interferences

Older pediatric and adult patient samples can't be analyzed by this method due to dietary pigments. Exposure to light will degrade bilirubin in the patient sample as well as in quality control and standard or calibration materials.

The Specimen

Serum and plasma may be used. Hemolysis and lipemia have no effect on the results. Dietary pigments such as carotene will falsely elevate bilirubin measurement but are generally not present in neonates due to their limited diet. Bilirubin may be broken down by light or heat and should be protected from these environmental conditions.

Reference Ranges

Full-term 0–24 hr	2.0–6.0 mg/dL
Full-term 24–48 hr	6.0–10.0 mg/dL
Full-term 3–5 days	4.0–8.0 mg/dL
Premature 0–24 hr	1.0–8.0 mg/dL
Premature 24–48 hr	6.0–12.0 mg/dL
Premature 3–5 days	10.0–14.0 mg/dL

Hyperbilirubinemia may be more pronounced due to blood group differences of mother and child, particularly with group O mothers, who make naturally occurring immunoglobulin M (IgM) anti-A and anti-B antibodies but may also make small amounts of immunoglobulin G (IgG) anti-A and anti-B antibodies, which can enter the maternal-fetal circulation. This generally produces only mild increase in fetal cell turnover but moderate hyperbilirubinemia. Other factors that may influence neonatal hyperbilirubinemia include decreased binding of unconjugated bilirubin to albumin, reabsorption of intestinal meconium, and constituents in mother's milk. Progesterone and other hormones in breast milk as well as beta-glucuronidase may suppress neonatal conjugation of bilirubin. This factor slows excretion of water-soluble forms, thus promoting jaundice. Physiological jaundice of the newborn (PJN) is typically a transient phenomenon, in which jaundice subsides within a few weeks. PJN is associated with increased total and unconjugated bilirubin but near-normal conjugated bilirubin. The serum hepatic enzyme levels are typically normal since there is no associated cell inflammation in PJN.

Methods for analysis of neonatal bilirubin are unique when compared with methods for older pediatric or adult patients. The difference accommodates the smaller neonatal sample size and the less complex nature of neonatal serum. A direct spectrophotometric method is available for smaller neonatal specimens. Analytical interferences due to carotene and other dietary pigments make the method unsuitable for older pediatric or adult bilirubin determinations.

Whether performing neonatal bilirubin testing by a direct spectrophotometric method or a pediatric or adult bilirubin test via a colorimetric method, the specimen must be protected from light and heat. Serum and plasma may be used. Hemolysis and lipemia have no effect on the results with the neonatal method but will affect the diazonium salt methods for bilirubin testing. Dietary pigments such as carotene will falsely elevate neonatal bilirubin measurement, so this method cannot be used for pediatric or adult testing.

> **THE TEAM APPROACH**
> Laboratory results should be called to the attention of the appropriate health care provider if neonatal bilirubin results exceed 10 mg/dL. Release of results needs to comply with institutional and federal guidelines, particularly in regard to confidentiality.

Case Scenario 7-2 Neonatal Hyperbilirubinemia: Why Is the Baby Yellow?

Follow-Up

By day five the baby's total bilirubin was 8.5 mg/dL. Bilirubin levels began declining by day six, returning to reference ranges by the ninth day. Phototherapy was discontinued at that time. Further investigation revealed that the baby's blood type was type A and his mother's blood type was O. The baby was being breastfed. These results correlated with PJN.

CASE SCENARIO 7-3

Elevated Hepatic Enzymes: The Standout Patient

While viewing enzyme results from an automated chemistry instrument, the laboratory technologist noticed that several results from a particular patient appeared to be significantly elevated. The serum was pigmented light amber, a yellowish brown color. She reviewed the laboratory request for this patient and learned the following information: The female patient was 59 years old. Her admitting diagnosis was fever of unknown origin and pruritus (itchy skin). After verifying that the sample was acceptable and quality control was acceptable, the technologist found the results indicated in Table 7–2. Liver biopsy, radiographic imaging, further liver enzyme tests, and liver function tests were pending.

continued

Case Scenario 7-3 Elevated Hepatic Enzymes: The Standout Patient *(continued)*

TABLE 7-2

Test Results of the Patient With Elevated Liver Enzymes

Test	Reference Range	Results	
		Day 1	*Day 2*
IgM (mg/dL)	40–230	425	—
Total biliurubin (mg/dL)	0.0–2.0	2.5	—
Direct bilirubin (mg/dL)	0.0–0.2	0.4	—
ALT (U/L)	<34	145	150
Alkaline phosphatase (U/L)	42–98	803	751
GGT (U/L)	<38	353	—
Rheumatoid factor	Neg	Pos (1:80)	—
Anti-mitochrondrial antibodies	Neg	Pos (1:160)	—

PATHOPHYSIOLOGY OF LIVER ENZYMES

Enzyme analysis is used to aid in diagnosis and treatment of disease. In particular, enzymes that are synthesized within cellular organelles carry out their functions within cells and are released into body fluids when those cells become diseased. Thus, an increase in enzyme activity when compared to the reference range can indicate pathological changes in certain types of cells and tissues. Enzyme activity levels in body fluids can reflect leakage from cells due to cellular injury, or changes in enzyme production rate or actual enzyme induction due to metabolic or genetic states or proliferation of neoplasms. In the latter case, increased enzyme activity can be used as a tumor marker. One aspect of enzyme activity that must be considered is the relative time frame that enzyme activity appears in the blood plasma and how long it remains in relationship to the disorder. For example, some enzymes found in plasma due to tissue necrosis or inflammation rise at such a slow rate that they are not useful for early detection or treatment of the disease. Other enzymes rapidly decline in circulation because of inactivation or metabolism. The clinical utility of enzyme activity in relationship to specific tissue pathology and clinical signs is enhanced when the enzyme activity quickly rises following the onset of the disorder and remains elevated for an adequate time frame, particularly when other clinical signs and symptoms are not sufficient to provide a diagnosis.

Damage to tissue can release different types of enzymes based on their location. For example, mild inflammation of the liver reversibly increases the permeability of the cell membrane and releases cytoplasmic enzymes such as lactate dehydrogenase (LD), alkaline phosphatase (ALP), ALT, and AST, while cellular death (necrosis) will release mitochrondrial sources of ALT and AST.[9] Distribution of these enzymes within specific types of hepatic tissues varies. ALP and GGT are more concentrated in the biliary ducts or tissues of the small ducts (canaliculi), while AST, ALT, and LD are found mainly in structural (parenchymal) hepatic cells. Multiple forms of enyzmes, called isoenzymes, are distributed in several different tissue types. For example, ALP is found in hepatobiliary tissues but also found in

---

CLINICAL CORRELATION

Correlation of patterns of hyperbilirubinemia with enzymes of hepatic origin is useful. Serum bilirubin may often rise later in the course of hepatic disorder. Bilirubin results can still be useful when one considers type of bilirubin elevations and correlations with liver enzymes.

TABLE 7-3

Sources of Liver Enzymes

Hepatocellular	Hepatobiliary	Osteoblasts (Bone)	Intestinal Mucosa	Placenta	Cardiac Muscle	Erythrocytes	Skeletal Muscle
	ALP GGT	ALP	ALP	ALP			
ALT AST LDH					AST LDH	AST LDH	AST LDH

all cytoplasmic membranes of all cells of the body, especially in osteoblasts (bone-forming cells), intestinal mucosa, placenta, and renal tubules. Table 7–3 summarizes tissue origins of key liver enzymes. Methods of analysis for transaminases are presented in Test Methodology 7–4, and for GGT in Test Methodology 7–5.

TEST METHODOLOGY 7-4.   TRANSAMINASES[1]

Aspartate Transaminase

The Reaction

Analysis of aspartate transaminase (AST) can be achieved by a coupled reaction involving pyridoxal-5′-phosphate (P-5′-P) and malate dehydrogenase (MDH) at 37°C:

$$\text{Aspartate} + \text{alpha-oxoglutarate} \xrightarrow{\text{AST, P-5′-P}} \text{oxaloacetate} + \text{glutamate}$$
$$\text{Oxaloacetate} + \text{NADH} + \text{H}^+ \xrightarrow{\text{MDH}} \text{malate} + \text{NAD}^+$$

Decrease in absorbance at 340 nm is determined by continuous monitoring.

The Calculation

The AST level (U/L) is calculated using the following formula:

$$\frac{\Delta A/\text{min} \times 1 \times \text{total volume (mL)}}{0.0063\ \mu\text{mol} \times \text{sample volume (mL)}}$$

If 3.0 mL total volume and 0.2 mL sample volume are used, the activity factor is 2381.

For example: $\Delta A/\text{min} \times 2381 = 0.020 \times 2381 = 48D$ U/L

The Specimen

Serum or heparinized plasma free from hemolysis may be used. Interferences are minimal since the sample is measured at 340 nm, but preanalytical variation can occur due to hemolysis (erythrocyte source of AST), and there may be slight variation due to gender and fasting state. Alcohol and drugs such as opiates, salicylates, or ampicillin may increase AST activity. If temperature is not maintained at a constant 37°C, the rate of the product formation will be inaccurate.

Reference Ranges

Adult male   <35 U/L
Adult female <31 U/L

continued

TEST METHODOLOGY 7-4. TRANSAMINASES[1] (*continued*)

Alanine Transaminase

The Reaction

Analysis of alanine transaminase (ALT) can be achieved by this coupled reaction involving pyridoxal-5′-phosphate (P-5′-P) and lactate dehydrogenase (LDH) at 37°C:

$$\text{Alanine + alpha-oxoglutarate} \xrightarrow{\text{ALT, P-5'-P}} \text{pyruvate + glutamate}$$
$$\text{Pyruvate + NADH + H}^+ \xrightarrow{\text{LD}} \text{lactate + NAD}^+$$

Decrease in absorbance at 340 nm is determined by continuous monitoring.

The Calculations

The ALT level (U/L) is calculated using the following formula:

$$\frac{\Delta A/\text{min} \times 1 \times \text{total volume (mL)}}{0.0063\ \mu\text{mol} \times \text{sample volume (mL)}}$$

If 3.0 mL total volume and 0.2 mL sample volume are used, the activity factor is 2381.

For example: $\Delta A/\text{min} \times 2381 = 0.020 \times 2381 = 48D$ U/L

The Specimen

Serum or heparinized plasma free from hemolysis may be used. Interferences are minimal since the sample is measured at 340 nm, but preanalytical variation may occur due to moderate hemolysis (erythrocyte source of ALT), loss of stability over time, and slight variation due to gender. Certain drugs and alcohol may also increase ALT activity. Maintaining substrate concentration in excess, as well as stable temperature, are also critical for accurate enzyme analysis. Stability of the enzyme activity can be maintained by refrigeration of the sample for up to 3 days and freezing the sample for up to 30 days.

Reference Ranges

Adult male	<45 U/L
Adult female	<34 U/L

TEST METHODOLOGY 7-5. GAMMA-GLUTAMYLTRANSFERASE

The Reaction

Analysis of gamma-glutamyltransferase[1] (GGT) can be achieved by this coupled reaction at 37°C:

$$\text{gamma-glutamyl-}p\text{-nitroanalide + glycylglycine} \xrightarrow{\text{GGT, pH 8.2}}$$
$$\text{gamma-glutamylgylcylglycine + }p\text{-nitroaniline}$$

Increase in absorbance at 405 nm is determined by continuous or endpoint monitoring.

The Calculations

The GGT level (U/L) is calculated using the following formula:

$$\frac{\Delta A/\text{min} \times 1 \times \text{total volume (mL)}}{0.00987\ \mu\text{mol} \times \text{sample volume (mL)}}$$

If 2.4 mL total volume and 0.2 mL sample volume are used, the activity factor is 1216.

For example: $\Delta A/\text{min} \times 1216 = 0.020 \times 1216 = 24D$ U/L

TEST METHODOLOGY 7-5. GAMMA-GLUTAMYLTRANSFERASE *(continued)*

The Specimen

Serum or heparinized plasma that is free from hemolysis may be used. Maintaining substrate concentration in excess, as well as stable temperature, are critical for accurate enzyme analysis. Stability of the enzyme activity can be maintained by refrigeration of the sample for up to 3 days and freezing the sample for up to 30 days.

Reference Ranges

Adult Male	<55 U/L
Adult female	<38 U/L

Correlation of patterns of hyperbilirubinemia with serum enzymes may also be helpful. For example, prehepatic jaundice, as indicated by relatively normal serum conjugated bilirubin, increased unconjugated bilirubin, and increased urinary urobilinogen, correlates with normal serum levels of hepatocellular and hepatobiliary enzymes, with the exception of LDH and possibly AST. These two enzymes are found in erythrocytes so, in situations of increased red cell breakdown, these enzyme concentrations are elevated in the serum. Hepatic jaundice, indicated by increased serum conjugated and unconjugated bilirubin and increased urinary urobilinogen, correlates with increased serum levels of hepatocellular enzymes. Posthepatic jaundice, as indicated by relatively normal serum unconjugated bilirubin, increased conjugated bilirubin, and decreased urinary urobilinogen, correlates with pronounced elevations of hepatobiliary enzymes but normal to slightly elevated serum levels of hepatocellular enzymes.

ANALYTICAL ASPECTS OF LIVER ENZYMES

Multiple forms of enzymes exist, particularly when an enzyme is composed of two or more polypeptide chains or subunits. This unique composition of protein isomers, or protomers, can be associated with different distribution within tissues, and unique chemical and physical properties. Multiple forms of enzymes can also be produced as a result of postgenetic modification, such as from metabolism. The term *isoenzyme* refers to forms of the same enzyme that arise from unique gene sequences. Characterization of isoenzymes based on separation techniques can be used to indicate the tissue source of the enzyme activity and correlate with specific diseases. Separation and quantification techniques for isoenzymes and multiple forms of enzymes include zone electrophoresis, ion-exchange chromatography, selective inactivation, and immunoassay methods.

ALP can consist of multiple forms that may arise from a variety of tissues, but rarely are more than two forms found in a particular patient's sample. The enzyme appears to be associated with lipid transport in the intestine and calcium transport in bone. ALP is present at or near the cell membrane. Generally this enzyme is derived from two sources: bone osteoblasts and either liver, intestine, or placenta. Rarely, serum ALP is derived from renal tubules. Table 7–4 lists the common ALP isoenzymes and methods of their separation. Monospecific antisera can be used to specifically measure ALP isoenzymes, including placental and intestinal forms. Overall enzyme activity should be measured prior to isoenzyme analysis (Test Methodology 7–6).

TABLE 7-4

Alkaline Phosphatase Isoenzyme Characteristics

Characteristic	Name of Isoenzyme				
	Hepatic	Bone	Intestinal	Placental	Other
Heat Stability	Stable at 56°C for 30 minutes	Labile: disappears at 56°C within 10 minutes	Intermediate labile: disappears at 56°C within 15 minutes	Stable at 65°C for 30 minutes	Regan isoenzyme: most stable
Electrophoretic Order	Most anodic	Intermediate	Cathodic to bone fraction	Migrates with hepatic or bone forms	Renal isoenzyme: rare but most cathodic
Chemical Inhibition	Moderate inhibition by urea but low inhibition by L-phenylalanine.	Strong inhibition by urea but low inhibition by L-phenylalanine.	Strong inhibition by L-phenylalanine.	Resistance to urea but strong inhibition by L-phenylalanine.	Regan isoenzyme: Strong inhibition by L-phenylalanine.

TEST METHODOLOGY 7-6.   ALKALINE PHOSPHATASE

The Reaction

Analysis of alkaline phosphatase (ALP) can be achieved by the modified method of Bowers and McComb[10]:

$$\text{4-nitrophenyl phosphate} + H_2O \xrightarrow{\text{ALP, Mg2+, pH 10.3}} \text{4-nitrophenoxide}$$

Measure an increase in absorbance at 405 nm at 37°C either as endpoint or continuous monitoring.

The Calculation

The ALP level (U/L) is calculated using the following formula:

$$\frac{\Delta A/min \times 1000 \times \text{total volume (mL)}}{18.7 \text{ mmol} \times \text{sample volume (mL)}}$$

If 3.0 mL total volume and 0.1 mL sample volume are used, the activity factor is 1604.

For example: $\Delta A/min \times 1604 = 0.035 \times 1604 = 56D$ U/L

The Specimen

Serum or heparinized plasma less than 3 hours old may be used. Anticoagulants that remove calcium and magnesium will prevent product formation. Serum samples show increase in activity over time due to increasing alkalinity of the sample, so analysis of fresh samples is preferred. Potentially other serum constituents such as lipids, hemoglobin, or bilirubin that could also absorb light at 405 nm could provide interference. Maintaining substrate concentration in excess, as well as stable temperature, are critical for accurate enzyme analysis.

Reference Ranges

Adult male	53–128 U/L
Adult female	42–98 U/L

Interpretation of Alkaline Phosphatase Results

ALP is found in high concentration in hepatobiliary cells. Inflammation or obstruction of the biliary ducts may cause disruption of these cells, which causes the release of ALP into the circulation. Serum ALP levels of patients who have **cholestasis** may be increased 3 to 10 times the normal levels.

cholestasis - obstruction of the flow of bile; standing bile

OTHER LABORATORY TEST RESULTS THAT CORRESPOND WITH LIVER DISORDERS

Since the majority of proteins found in plasma are synthesized by the liver from amino acids, including serine protease coagulation factors, prothrombin time, serum albumin, and serum protein electrophoresis results can be used to indicate declining liver function. For example, serum albumin decreases and prothrombin time becomes prolonged with liver failure. Protein levels also reflect other disorders, such as those in which essential amino acids are not provided by the diet or in which proteins are lost by the kidneys or gastrointestinal tract.

Proteins and Amino Acids

Proteins and amino acids have unique structures that allow them to participate in some specific types of chemical reactions. The significant amino acids are found in a table in the Appendix. Proteins are polymers consisting of amino acid units. Amino acid units within the protein are joined by peptide bonds, giving the primary structure of proteins. The amino acid unit on the carboxyl end of the protein contains a free carboxyl group that does not participate in peptide bond formation. The amino acid unit on the amino end of the protein contains a free amino group that does not participate in peptide bond formation. These characteristics of proteins, the amino and carboxyl ends, and peptide bonding play a role in the methods of analysis for total serum proteins.

Proteins are ampholytes, and in aqueous solutions they may have positive and negative charges on the same molecule. This property is used to separate protein molecules during electrophoresis. The pH of the solution determines the net charge of the molecule. At different pH environments, hydrogen ions will be gained or lost from the carboxyl and amine ends and from functional groups of residues of the amino acids. Since proteins are composed of different amino acids, different proteins will gain or lose hydrogen ions at different pH environments.

In addition to their properties as ampholytes, proteins also have other representative structural properties based on their polymer makeup and bonding. Fibrous proteins are stringlike in configuration and usually function as structural components of the body, such as fibrinogen and collagen. Most plasma proteins and enzymes are globular proteins, which are spherical in configuration.

Serum contains a large variety of proteins and a large amount of total protein, averaging 7.0 g/dL in the adult. In contrast, protein levels in serum and urine are normally in the microgram or milligram per deciliter range. Methods for measuring proteins in body fluids are based upon the unique structural properties as well as their relative concentration in the body fluids. Total serum protein test methodology is described in Test Methodology 7–7. There are two main types of proteins, albumin and globulins. They are grouped into five classes as determined by their electrophoretic separation: albumin, alpha$_1$ globulins, alpha$_2$ globulins, beta globulins, and gamma globulins. Serum albumin, at around 4 g/dL, makes up roughly half of the total serum proteins. A simple way to assess the balance between the patient's albumin and globulins in serum is to calculate the albumin:globulin, or A/G, ratio. Globulins (G) are calculated as albumin (A) subtracted from total serum proteins. Albumin is then divided by globulin.

TEST METHODOLOGY 7-7.   TOTAL SERUM PROTEIN[1]

Although there are many classic and reference methods for quantification of serum protein, the biuret reaction has become the most commonly used method in the clinical laboratory. The peptide bonds of proteins react with biuret reagent containing Cu^{2+} ions in an alkaline solution to form a violet color measured at 540 nm. Sodium potassium tartrate is a component of the reagent and functions to maintain copper in the correct valence state and in an alkaline solution, while potassium iodide is present as an antioxidant.

The Reaction

Proteins + biuret reagent → violet-colored product (540-nm absorbance)

Interferences

Marked hyperbilirubinemia and lipemia cause interference unless corrected with a serum blank. Marked lipemia should be removed with acetone-pretreated samples. Ambulatory patients exhibit a slight hemoconcentration causing a physiological increase in serum protein by 0.3 g/dL.

The Specimen

Serum, free from lipemia and collected without prolonged tourniquet use, may be used. Plasma can be used, but the reference range must be adjusted upward to account for fibrinogen. Plasma should not be used for protein electrophoresis.

Reference Range

Adult (ambulatory)   6.4–8.3 g/dL

Interpretation of Total Serum Protein Levels

Total serum protein levels are affected by not only changes in one or more of the individual protein levels, but also by changes in plasma water. A variety of conditions cause hyperproteinemia, or increased serum protein. **Hemoconcentration**, or decreased plasma water volume, will cause total serum protein levels to be increased. Dehydration is the usual cause of hemoconcentration, which is secondary to a variety of conditions including diarrhea, severe vomiting, and water deprivation. Increased total serum protein levels can also occur when there is an increase in a variety of immunoglobulins following inflammation or infection or a monoclonal increase in immunoglobulins, such as in multiple myeloma. More information about multiple myeloma, a malignancy of the bone marrow, is found in Chapter 13. Increased total protein can also result from measuring an unexpected protein such as fibrinogen. Serum is derived from clotted whole blood in which fibrinogen is removed in the clotting process. However, if incomplete clotting occurs before centrifugation, some fibrinogen can remain behind in the serum specimen.

Hypoproteinemia, or decreased protein levels in the blood, is often due to hypoalbuminemia, since albumin is the most abundant single protein. Typical causes of

hemoconcentration - relative increase in blood cells due to decrease in plasma water volume

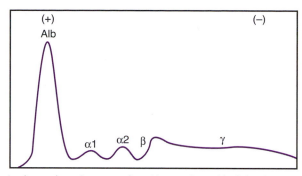

Figure 7–4. Protein electrophoresis pattern found in a patient with cirrhosis. Notice the beta-gamma bridge.

hypoproteinemia are starvation or nutritional deficiency of essential amino acids, renal loss such as in nephritic syndrome, gastrointestinal loss such as in enteropathy, or hepatic failure in which the liver is unable to synthesize proteins.[2]

Serum protein electrophoresis results can also indicate inflammatory states of the liver in which there are elevated gamma globulin protein fractions, especially immunoglobulin A (IgA) and IgM levels. In cirrhosis, protein electrophoresis results show that fast-moving gamma globulins often migrate in the beta to gamma region, causing a beta-gamma bridge. Serum protein electrophoresis principles are discussed in more details in Chapter 13.

Figure 7–4 shows the typical beta-gamma bridge in the **electrophoretic** pattern, and Table 7–5 shows the protein electrophoresis results. The beta-gamma bridge can be seen as a lack of separation of the beta globulins from the gamma globulins. Notice that the beta and gamma globulin results are not reported in separate categories since they migrate in one region.

electrophoresis - a separation technique of different charged molecules in solution in an electrical field of varying potential

Cerebrospinal Fluid Proteins

Cerebrospinal fluid (CSF) is an ultrafiltrate of plasma formed in the choroid plexuses and ventricles of the brain. CSF contains much less protein than serum and cannot be analyzed by biuret reactions or other methods used in measurement of total serum proteins. The proportion of proteins found in CSF is also different than that of serum, with a predominance of low molecular weight proteins such as

---

TABLE 7-5

Protein Electrophoresis Results in a Patient With Cirrhosis

Proteins (mg/dL)	Result	Reference Range
Total protein	6.6	6.4–8.3
Albumin	3.0	3.5–5.2
Alpha$_1$ globulin	0.5	0.2–0.4
Alpha$_2$ globulin	0.6	0.4–0.8
Beta-gamma globulin	2.5	0.5–1.1
		0.6–1.3

These data correspond to the pattern depicted in Figure 7–4.

prealbumin, albumin, and transferrin. Therefore, CSF must be concentrated in order to visualize protein bands on electrophoresis.

Traditional methods for quantitation of CSF protein relied on dye binding methods using Coomassie Brilliant Blue dye or turbidimetric methods using routine spectrophotometry.[11] In turbidimetry, a precipitating reagent, such as sulfosalicylic acid or trichloroacetic acid, is used to lower the solubility of proteins and allow them to precipitate. These reagents precipitate albumin and globulins equally well. Changes in absorbance due to precipitation of the proteins under closely timed reactions are measured spectrophotometrically.[1] Interferences from hemoglobin and drugs that also precipitate in turbidimetry should be considered. The reference range for CSF total protein is 15 to 45 mg/dL. CSF is a difficult sample to obtain and must be handled carefully in preparation, storage, and transport. Refer to Chapter 2 for more details about CSF collection and handling, and to Chapter 13 for details about CSF protein electrophoresis.

Albumin has an important role in maintaining colloidal oncotic pressure and preventing edema. Since water moves freely through cell membranes and into the intravascular space by osmosis, the high concentration of proteins in intravascular fluid allows movement of water into vessels, and normal blood pressure and cardiac output allow circulation to evenly distribute the fluids. If concentration of albumin is significantly decreased, fluids accumulate in interstitial spaces and cause edema. Albumin also serves as a transport molecule for substances such as unconjugated bilirubin and drugs. Serum albumin analysis employs anionic dye binding, while the CSF albumin method is often immunonephelometry.[1] The immunonephelometry method is described in this chapter in more detail later. The common methodology for testing albumin is found in Test Methodology 7–8.

TEST METHODOLOGY 7-8.   ALBUMIN[1]

Serum or plasma albumin methods are based upon structural characteristics. Albumin makes an excellent antigen and can be analyzed by immunoassays such as nephelometry. This is the method of choice for albumin in cerebrospinal fluid. However, other methods such as turbidimetry are also available with chemistry analyzers.[1] A simpler method is used when considering typical serum albumin levels. The routine method is based upon albumin's ionic charge at an acid pH and binding to anionic dyes such bromcresol green (BCG) or bromcresol purple (BCP). In these methods, a colored product forms that absorbs at wavelengths significantly different from the reagent and from typical interfering molecules such as hemoglobin or bilirubin.

The Reaction

$$\text{Albumin} + \text{BCG} \xrightarrow{\text{pH 4.2}} \text{colored product (628-nm absorbance)}$$

Interferences

Marked lipemia causes positive interference unless corrected with a serum blank. Prolonged incubation causes positive interference from $alpha_2$ and beta globulins. Ambulatory patients have hemoconcentration, causing a physiological increase in serum albumin by 0.3 g/dL.

The Specimen

Serum, free from lipemia and collected without prolonged tourniquet use, may be used.

Reference Range

Adult   3.5–5.2 g/dL

Interpretation of Serum Albumin Levels

Albumin levels are affected not only by changes in albumin level, but also by changes in plasma water volume, in a manner similar to effects on total serum protein. In addition to dehydration, fluid redistribution such as in **ascites** may cause hypoalbuminemia as well.[2] Hypoalbuminemia from deficient protein level is due to loss, such as from the gastrointestinal system in malabsorption or protein-losing enteropathy, from the renal system as in glomerulonephritis or nephritic syndrome, or from skin due to severe burns. Hypoalbuminemia can also result from increased catabolism as a result of tissue damage and inflammation, as found in neoplasms or autoimmunity. Decreased serum albumin is also associated with malnutrition and inadequate amino acid intake. Finally, hypoalbuminemia is correlated with declining synthesis in the liver, as associated with cirrhosis or other situations of liver failure.

ascites - accumulation of serous fluid in the abdomen

Other Serum Proteins

There are many other serum proteins to consider. For example, transferrin is involved in the transport of iron in plasma and C-reactive protein is an acute-phase reactant or inflammatory protein. These are listed in Table 7–6 along with their electrophoretic migration category and main physiological function.

TABLE 7-6

Characteristics of Major Serum Proteins

Protein Name	Electrophoretic Category	Main Function
Prealbumin, transthyretin	Most anodic, visible only with certain electrophoretic methods	Transport of the thyroid hormones thyroxine and triiodothyronine; useful as a measurement of nutritional status
Albumin	Most anodic with routine electrophoresis	Transport of bilirubin, drugs; maintenance of colloid oncotic pressure
Alpha$_1$-antitrypsin	Alpha$_1$ globulin	Serine protease (elastase) inhibitor; an acute-phase protein
Alpha$_1$ acid glycoprotein	Alpha$_1$ globulin	Inactivates lipophilic hormones; an acute-phase protein
Alpha-fetoprotein	Alpha$_1$ globulin	Predominant plasma protein of the fetus; a fetal albumin analog
Haptoglobin	Alpha$_2$ globulin	Transports free hemoglobin through the blood to the liver for degradation; an acute-phase protein
Alpha$_2$-macroglobulin	Alpha$_2$ globulin	Protease inhibitor and acute-phase reactant
Ceruloplasmin	Alpha$_2$ globulin	Acute-phase protein; has enzymatic activity and transports copper
Transferrin	Beta globulin	Transport protein for iron
C4	Beta globulin	Complement protein involved in antibody-antigen response and in the destruction of bacteria and viruses; an acute-phase protein

continued

TABLE 7-6 *(continued)*

Characteristics of Major Serum Proteins

Protein Name	Electrophoretic Category	Main Function
C3	Beta globulin	Complement protein that plays a role in immune defense; an acute-phase protein
Beta$_2$-microglobulin	Beta globulin	Light chain of the human leukocyte antigen (HLA) molecule
Beta lipoprotein	Beta globulin	Transports lipids, primarily cholesterol (e.g., low density lipoprotein)
IgG	Gamma globulin	Produced in response to specific infections to destroy toxins and foreign invaders of the body
IgA	Gamma globulin	Secretory immunoglobulin protecting the mucosal surfaces
IgM	Gamma globulin	First antibody produced in response to an infection
C-reactive protein	Gamma globulin	Acute-phase protein that appears in the blood following infection or tissue damage

Individual proteins in serum, other than albumin, are found in low enough concentrations that highly sensitive and specific methods of analysis are required. Immunoassays such as nephelometry are generally utilized since the reaction endpoint can be detected rapidly and with acceptable precision. However, low-affinity antibodies may not react quickly enough to be detected, which somewhat lowers the sensitivity of rate immunoassays.[1]

Nephelometry

Nephelometry relies on the detection and quantitation of forward light scatter due to antigen-antibody complex formation. Patient samples containing protein and specific antibody are allowed to react in a cuvet, with the result being antigen-antibody complex formation. An incident light beam passes through the reaction cuvet and suspended antigen-antibody complexes scatter the light. Rate of particle formation increases until the rate reaches a maximum velocity. At maximum particle formation velocity, the rate of change in intensity of forward-scattered light is measured. Once the maximum rate of change of light scatter is reached, a final measurement is taken, which is proportional to the number of suspended antigen-antibody particles.[1]

Cirrhosis

Cirrhosis is a common and serious disease of the liver resulting from chronic inflammation of the liver. The result is replacement of normal liver tissue with nonfunctional, nodular scar (fibrotic) tissue. Cirrhosis generally involves the entire liver. There are specific types of cirrhosis based on origin and classification and

TABLE 7-7

Diagnostic Indicators of Specific Types of Cirrhosis

Type of Cirrhosis	Causes	Key Tests
Alcoholic cirrhosis	Alcohol	Alcohol, GGT
Primary biliary cirrhosis	Autoimmune	ALP, ALT, anti-mitochondrial antibody
Chronic active viral hepatitis	Viral	ALT, viral antigens
Hemochromatosis	Iron overload	Iron, ferritin, total iron-binding capacity (TIBC)
Wilson's disease	Copper accumulation	Ceruloplasmin, urinary copper
Alpha$_1$-antitrypsin deficiency	Deficiency of alpha$_1$-antitrypsin	Alpha$_1$-antitrypsin
Drug toxicity	Drug overdose, such as with acetaminophen	Specific drug testing

based upon types of nodular tissue, such as micronodular, macronodular, and mixed nodular tissue. Common types of cirrhosis are listed in Table 7–7, along with the main causes and key laboratory tests that are used in the differential diagnosis of cirrhosis. Cirrhosis most commonly arises from chronic alcohol abuse, although chronic viral hepatitis can be a major cause and is more common in some parts of the world.[2] Primary biliary cirrhosis is an unusual cause of chronic liver disease, and its origin lies in chronic inflammation due to autoimmunity. Immunoglobulin levels and autoantibodies may be helpful in diagnosis of primary biliary cirrhosis.[12]

CLINICAL CORRELATION

Cirrhosis is a serious disease of the liver resulting from chronic inflammation and replacement of normal liver tissue with nonfunctional, nodular fibrotic tissue.

Case Scenario 7-3 Elevated Hepatic Enzymes: The Standout Patient

Follow-Up

Several results appeared to be significantly elevated from the patient in Case Scenario 7–3, including alkaline phosphatase, GGT, ALT, total bilirubin, and anti-mitochondrial antibodies (positive to a titer of 1:160). The serum from this patient was pigmented light amber. Her admitting diagnosis was fever of unknown origin and pruritus. Liver biopsy was performed. Based on the laboratory results and clinical findings, including the liver biopsy results, a diagnosis of primary biliary cirrhosis was made and treatment to reduce the inflammation was begun. Liver enzymes were monitored periodically to monitor the success of the therapy. ●

CASE SCENARIO 7-4

Acute Inflammation of the Liver: The Out-of-Range Bilirubin Result

While viewing bilirubin results from an automated chemistry analyzer, the laboratory technologist noticed that the result obtained from one patient sample printed without a specific answer. There was an error message that specified: High. She retrieved the sample, observing that it appeared golden brown.

continued

> **Case Scenario 7-4** Acute Inflammation of the Liver:
> The Out-of-Range Bilirubin Result *(continued)*
>
> The manufacturer's instructions indicated that the upper limit of the total bilirubin procedure is 25.8 mg/dL and that results exceeding that value must be diluted by the operator with purified water and analyzed. The technologist added 40 μL of type I water to 20 μL of patient sample, mixed it well, and placed the diluted sample into the instrument to analyze for total bilirubin. AST, ALT, ALP, and other clinical chemistry tests were pending, as were serology tests for hepatitis virus antibodies and antigens, including hepatitis B surface antigen (HBsAg).
>
> To calculate the corrected bilirubin, the technologist needed to determine the dilution, represented in fraction format, of the sample made by adding 40 μL of water to 20 μL of patient serum. The uncorrected bilirubin result from the diluted sample was 10.5 mg/dL. What is the corrected bilirubin result that should be reported?

A dilution is composed of a volume of diluent and a volume of sample making up a total volume. Since the dilution is an effect on the sample, it is represented as a fraction of sample volume to total volume. The dilution factor is the inverse of this fraction and is used to multiply the result obtained from the diluted sample to indicate the true result of the actual (undiluted) sample.

Let's try the calculations.

$$\text{Diluted bilirubin result} = 10.5 \text{ mg/dL}$$
$$\text{Sample volume} = 20 \text{ μL}$$
$$\text{Diluent volume} = 40 \text{ μL}$$
$$\text{Total volume} = 60 \text{ μL}$$
$$\text{Dilution} = 20 \text{ μL}/60 \text{ μL, which reduces to } 1/3$$
$$\text{Dilution factor is the inverse of } 1/3 = 3/1 \text{ or } 3$$
$$\text{Actual bilirubin} = 3 \times 10.5 = 31.5 \text{ mg/dL}$$

> **✓ Common Sense Check**
>
> Correlation of laboratory results with a suspected disorder may help to clarify unusual results. In this case, increased bilirubin may be an indicator of hepatitis. It is important to always use universal precautions when handling body fluids. Viral hepatitis is highly contagious in body fluids and may enter through mucous membranes such as the eyes, nose, or mouth or through cuts in the skin.

> **■ CLINICAL CORRELATION**
>
> Hepatitis is one of the most common causes of jaundice. It is defined as inflammation of the liver, especially involving the parenchymal liver cells, and correlates with hepatic hyperbilirubinemia, elevated urinary urobilinogen, and elevated hepatocellular enzymes.

Hepatitis

Hepatitis is one of the most common disorders associated with jaundice. It is defined as inflammation of the liver, especially involving the parenchymal liver cells. It is indicated by impairment of bilirubin conjugation and excretion causing elevations of all forms of bilirubin in serum and in urinary bile. Significant elevations of AST and ALT (2 to 75 times normal) and other hepatocellular enzymes are typical in hepatitis.[13,14] Other laboratory and diagnostic tests are needed to determine the specific cause of the hepatitis, including viral and nonviral causes. Common types of acute viral hepatitis are listed in Table 7–8 along with the main causes and key laboratory tests used in the differential diagnosis of acute viral hepatitis.

The origin of viral hepatitis is varied. Acute viral hepatitis is relatively common in occurrence and caused by one of six viral agents: hepatitis A virus (HAV), hepatitis B virus (HBV), hepatitis C virus (HCV), hepatitis delta virus (HDV), hepatitis E virus (HEV), or hepatitis G virus (HGV). These agents produce similar hepatic illnesses but with varied severity. The outcome of viral hepatitis may range from no symptoms (asymptomatic) to acute fatal liver pathology. The hepatitis may remain undetected, also known as subclinical, for years and then present with periods of

TABLE 7-8

Overview of the Common Forms of Viral Hepatitis[6,14–16]

Type of Virus	Epidemiology	Key Tests
HAV: RNA, picor-navirus family	Fecal-oral route	Anti-HAV (IgM) and ALT during acute phase
	3–4-week incubation	Anti-HAV (IgG) for immunity
HBV: DNA, hepadna virus type I	Infected body fluid exposure	HBsAg, anti-hepatitis B core antigen (anti-HBc) (IgM) for acute phase
	4–6-week incubation	Persistent HBsAg, anti-HBc (IgG) for chronic phase
		Anti-HBs (IgG) for immunity
HCV: RNA	Infected body fluid exposure	Anti-HCV
	4–6-week incubation	
HDV: delta RNA virus, coexists with HBV	Infected body fluid exposure	Anti-HDV or HDV RNA and anti-HBc (IgG)

active inflammation. Long-term viral hepatitis may cause cirrhosis or hepatic cancer. People generally become infected with hepatitis virus by exposure to blood and body fluids from an infected person. However, HAV and HEV are food-borne (enterically transmitted).[15] The time frame of clinical indicators can vary dramatically in hepatitis from different viruses as well. Clinical and laboratory features of hepatitis A and B viral agents are illustrated in Figures 7–5 and 7–6, respectively.

Hepatitis can result from nonviral causes as well. Hepatotoxicity is a type of liver inflammation with injury caused by chemicals such as alcohol or drugs. This cause of hepatitis is relatively rare in young adults but common in older patients or those taking certain medications, such as isoniazid for tuberculosis. Other medications associated with hepatotoxicity include phenytoin, cotrimoxazole, and valproic acid. Acetaminophen overdose is a common cause of hepatotoxic hepatitis due to the widespread availability of this nonprescription medication and its toxic effect on the liver when taken in excess. Alcohol can lower the dosage threshold for acetaminophen, causing toxicity to be reached more readily. Other medications can exacerbate preexisting liver conditions, such as methotrexate-induced hepatitis and

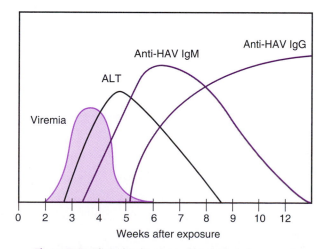

Figure 7–5. Clinical indications of hepatitis A virus over time.

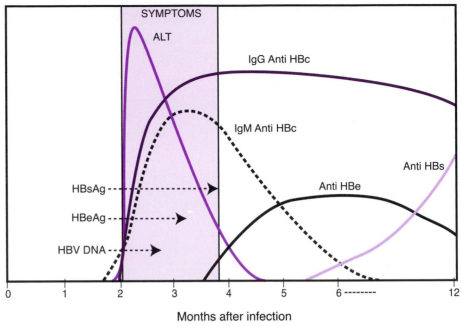

Figure 7-6. Clinical indications of hepatitis B virus over time.

fibrosis secondary to diabetic or alcoholic fatty liver.[6] Certain herbal medications have been associated with liver inflammation as well, including Chinese herbs containing *Lycopodium serratum*, *Teucrium chamaedrys*, and *Larrea tridenta*.[17]

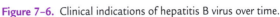

Case Scenario 7-4 Acute Inflammation of the Liver: The Out-of-Range Bilirubin Result

Follow-Up

The total bilirubin is significantly elevated at 31.5 mg/dL (reference range 0.0 to 2.0 mg/dL). ALT and AST were also significantly elevated. The hepatitis serology profile indicated presence of antibody to HAV (IgM). Based on other laboratory results and clinical findings, including the serology results, a diagnosis of acute viral hepatitis type A was made for this patient. Liver enzymes and serology were monitored periodically to monitor the success of the therapy, and the appearance of IgG anti-HAV indicated resolution of the illness and immunity. ●

CASE SCENARIO 7-5

Acute Liver Failure: The STAT Ammonia

A STAT ammonia level was ordered on an 8-year-old male patient in the Pediatric Intensive Care Unit and the EDTA plasma sample was delivered to the clinical chemistry section within 15 minutes in ice water. The result was found

Case Scenario 7-5 **Acute Liver Failure: The STAT Ammonia** *(continued)*

to be 120 µg/dL (reference range 29 to 70 µg/dL venous). The result from 18 hours earlier was found to be 100 µg/dL. The technologist verified that instrument maintenance and acceptable quality control analysis were up to date. The technologist next needs to assess the validity of the sample collection and handling. Following that, the technologist should consider whether this qualifies as a normal comparison and the clinical significance of these two values.

THE TEAM APPROACH

Plasma ammonia levels provide vital information about the potential neurological status of patients in liver failure. Therefore, it is important that results are verified quickly and communicated to the primary health care provider or other health care professionals in order that patient management can begin promptly.

Liver function includes many vital metabolic functions that involve secretory and excretory processes such as detoxification, synthesis of proteins, and catabolism of carbohydrates. As mentioned earlier, several laboratory diagnostic tests can be used to assess liver function, including total and direct bilirubin, total protein and albumin, urea, and ammonia. The role of bilirubin and protein analysis to assess hepatic function has already been discussed.

AMMONIA METABOLISM

Ammonia is produced in parenchymal liver cells during the deamination of amino acids and culminates in the formation of urea. Urea is the major nonprotein nitrogen waste product, further excreted by the kidneys. Thus, in normal conditions, plasma ammonia levels are expected to be low, in the 20-µg/dL range, while urinary urea levels are expected to be higher, such as 20 mg/dL. Some ammonia is also produced in the intestinal tract and skeletal muscles, but the majority of ammonia production is associated with hepatic function.

There are some differences in ammonia levels normally found in venous blood when compared with arterial blood. Venous levels vary significantly from arterial levels due to the rapid removal of ammonia from the circulation by the liver. It is important to indicate if ammonia levels are analyzed from arterial samples and report the results accordingly. Thus, the reference ranges should be determined for venous and arterial samples, if both are frequently provided to the laboratory. Likewise, reference ranges vary for pediatric and adult patients. The typical reference ranges for ammonia nitrogen levels are 90 to 150 µg/dL for newborns, 29 to 70 µg/dL for children, and 15 to 45 µg/dL for adults.

Plasma levels of ammonia will rise when the liver is not functioning properly, such as in Reye's syndrome, inherited deficiencies of metabolic enzymes, cirrhosis, serious drug toxicity, or liver tumors, also known as hepatoma.[6] Excessive nitrogen turnover from gastrointestinal bleeds will contribute a significant amount of plasma ammonia as well.[6] Plasma ammonia levels rise above normal due to inherited deficiencies in enzymes within the urea cycle, particularly those involving lysine and ornithine deamination. Encephalopathy, or damage to the nerves in the brain, is the consequence of rising plasma ammonia levels due to the neurotoxic nature of ammonia. This often results in coma of hepatic origin. Studies have shown that, during periods of declining hepatic function, plasma ammonia levels may increase by as much as five times the upper limit of the reference range.[18] Serial ammonia measurements are most useful to assess the hepatic status and potential risk for hepatic coma.

CLINICAL CORRELATION

Reye's syndrome is a metabolic disorder associated with fatty deposits of the liver and impaired production of urea through the ornithine cycle, causing encephalopathy.

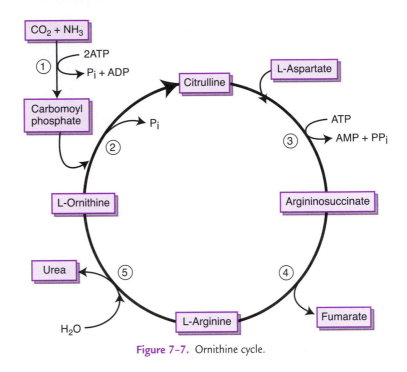

Figure 7–7. Ornithine cycle.

Hepatic Encephalopathy

Reye's syndrome is a metabolic disorder associated with fatty deposits in the liver and impaired production of urea through the ornithine cycle, causing encephalopathy. Figure 7–7 depicts the ornithine cycle. Reye's syndrome is more frequently associated with viral disease of children, especially when treated with medications such as salicylates. When plasma ammonia levels exceed five times the normal level, Reyes's syndrome is often fatal. Elevation of hepatic enzymes such as AST and ALT is also associated with Reye's syndrome.[19–21] The common methodology for testing ammonia is found in Test Methodology 7–9.

TEST METHODOLOGY 7-9.   AMMONIA

Analysis of ammonia can be achieved by enzymatic reaction using glutamate dehydrogenase (GLDH) and coenzyme conversion of NADPH to NADP.[22] Another possible common method for analysis is an ion-selective method in which NH_4^+ from a whole blood sample diffuses through a selective membrane on the selective electrode, causing a pH change in the solution that is detected potentiometrically.[1]

The Reaction

$$NH_4^+ + \text{2-oxoglutarate} + NADPH \xrightarrow{\text{GLDH}} glutamate + NADP + H_2O$$

A decrease in absorbance is measured at 340 nm due to the formation of NADP at 37°C.

---

continued

TEST METHODOLOGY 7-9. **AMMONIA** *(continued)*

Interferences

Interferences are due to preanalytical errors including ammonium heparin anticoagulant, trauma or hemolysis, and an extended time period before the sample is analyzed, which all falsely increase the ammonia level. Analytical errors can arise from ammonia contamination of glassware or water and from sources of ammonia to include ammonium salts, some diuretics, valproic acid, or other drugs. Due to the instability of ammonia and deamination of stored proteins, special quality control samples need to be used for validation of the results.[1] The intake of food generally does not affect plasma ammonia levels, but some IV fluid supplementation, which often provides large intake of amino acids, will increase the plasma ammonia, especially in pediatric patients. Cigarette smoking, or even residual smoke in the air and on clothing, will also cause false increases.

The Specimen

EDTA or (lithium) heparinized plasma that is free from hemolysis may be used. The sample must be separated in a refrigerated centrifuge within 20 minutes of collection and maintained in 0° to 4°C ice water.

Reference Range

Adult Male   15–45 µg/dL venous

Liver Function of the Elderly or Pediatric Patient

Liver function varies with age. For example, hepatic function declines in the elderly as indicated by a slight decline in serum albumin and a slight increase in urea synthesis and detoxification processes. Liver function in pediatric patients is also less than adult hepatic function. In neonates, the liver is not functioning at full capacity, particularly due to the immature hepatic circulation, and plasma ammonia levels are usually higher than 60 µg/dL. Ammonia levels typically remain slightly higher than adult levels until the patient nears the teen years, when the reference range for ammonia is the same as the adult level.

Case Scenario 7-5 Acute Liver Failure: The STAT Ammonia

Follow-Up

The technologist verified that the samples were collected and handled properly. The arterial heparinized whole blood specimens arrived in ice water, were properly labeled, and were centrifuged promptly. The plasma of each specimen was promptly analyzed before changes could occur in the ammonia levels. The ammonia levels from both samples were elevated above the normal reference range for pediatric patients. The two results are significantly different by more than 10% and indicate a rising ammonia level, which indicates hepatic failure and concern for encephalopathy and hepatic coma. Further tests were pending to determine the cause of the hepatic failure, but treatment had begun for encephalopathy. ●

CASE SCENARIO 7-6

**Quality Assurance in the Clinical Chemistry Laboratory:
Why Are All of the Alkaline Phosphatase Results the Same?**

It was a busy day at the Family Practice Clinic laboratory. The technician pulled the computer sheets from the printer to examine the results that were sent from the reference laboratory. The reference laboratory sent laboratory results from specimens drawn the previous day each morning at 6:00 a.m. Each morning, the technician checked in the results and then placed the print sheets into the physicians' boxes.

As the technician logged in the results, she noticed that all the ALP results were approximately the same. She also noticed that all the ALP results were unusually low (Table 7–9). Most of the other clinical chemistry results from these patients were within the reference ranges for the analyte tested. In particular, the liver function tests for these patients were within the reference range for each analyte.

CLINICAL SIGNIFICANCE OF ALKALINE PHOSPHATASE

The ALP results in this case were not physiologically feasible because they were well below the reference range on each patient tested. As discussed earlier in this chapter (see Table 7–3), ALP is present in the cells of most tissues in the body, including the liver, bone, intestinal epithelium, kidney tubules, and placenta. Several isoenzymes of the catalysts are associated with specific tissues and can be used to identify pathological processes in these tissues. The isoenzymes of ALP are differentially sensitive to heat and chemical denaturation (see Table 7–4). The ability to denature some isoenzymes while other forms of the enzyme remain active helps identify and determine the origin of the isoenzymes. Most forms of ALP have optimal activity at a pH of about 10. However, the enzyme is known to have activity over a wide range of pH values.

Serum ALP levels may be increased in diseases in which there is inflammation of the biliary ducts and decreased bile flow. Serum ALP levels may also be increased

TABLE 7-9

Original Test Results from the Reference Laboratory

Test	Reference Range	Patient 1	Patient 2	Patient 3 Day 1	Patient 3 Day 2	Patient 4	Patient 5	Patient 6	Patient 7	Patient 8	Patient 9
Total protein (g/dL)	6.4–8.3	7.1	7.0	7.9	7.6	7.4	7.4	7.1	7.9	6.6	7.2
Albumin (g/dL)	3.5–5.2	4.5	4.2	4.4	4.3	4.7	3.8	4.2	4.8	4.0	4.7
Total bilirubin (mg/dL)	0.0–2.0	0.2	0.4	0.8	0.6	0.4	0.7	0.4	0.8	0.4	0.4
ALT (U/L)	<45	18	28	26	20	40	21	17	20	30	25
ALP (U/L)	53–128	3	3	3	4	4	3	4	4	3	3
AST (U/L)	<35	21	28	23	22	37	32	19	21	45	18

when there is a high amount of osteoblastic activity (cells rebuilding bone). ALP levels of 10 to 25 times normal may be seen in such patients. Most of the ALP that is found in the circulation has its origin in liver or bone tissue cells.

> **Case Scenario 7-6** Quality Assurance in the Clinical Chemistry Laboratory: Why Are All of the Alkaline Phosphatase Results the Same?
>
> **Solving the Problem**
>
> The technician considered many situations regarding the ALP results in order to solve the problem. One consideration was the physiological feasibility of ALP levels of 3 to 4 U/L. Normal turnover rates of liver, bone, intestine, and kidney cells would seem to make such low levels of ALP in the blood impossible. The technician next considered the possibility that specimens from the previous day had been mishandled and that loss of specimen integrity had resulted. The technician knew that bone ALP isoenzyme is sensitive to heat at 56°C. Perhaps the samples had been subjected to heat inactivation during transit from the Family Practice Clinic to the reference laboratory. The resulting specimens would then contain liver isoenzyme as the predominant ALP isoenzyme. The technician rejected this solution for several reasons. She thought that levels of 3 to 4 U/L were low even for liver ALP alone since liver sources should contribute more ALP. She also noticed that other analytes did not seem to have been affected by heat inactivation. Only the ALP seemed to be affected.
>
> The technician decided to perform a **delta check** on ALP. She had results from 2 days earlier for one of the patients (see Table 7–8). She performed a delta check by comparing the two sets of results from the patient and applying a cutoff for normal variation. Delta checks test for results that vary by predetermined ranges or percentages for a patient over time and are appropriate for analytes that normally change slightly from one day to the next. Delta checks should not be used to test laboratory results that normally vary greatly over short periods of time. For example, glucose, phosphate, lactate dehydrogenase, creatine kinase, and aminotransferases are not appropriately monitored by delta checks. Electrolytes, protein, urea, creatinine, ALP, and hemoglobin are all appropriate candidates for delta checks. These checks can often be performed automatically when results are obtained on patient samples analyzed on the same clinical chemistry instrument if the patient ID number does not change. The technician found the delta check for ALP for patient 3 indicated a problem.[24]
>
> The technician then considered a systemic problem in testing. All ALP tests from the previous day appeared to be affected. The technician notified her CLS supervisor, who called the supervisor of the reference laboratory to explain the problem. The technologist supervisor sent a written memo to all physicians of the Family Practice Clinic, informing them that laboratory personnel were confirming laboratory results for ALP tests and that all ALP results would be delayed temporarily in the laboratory until they could be confirmed. The supervisor examined the other computer printouts of test results and found no alert of delta check values following the problem-solving flowchart illustrated in Figure 7–8.

delta check - comparison of concentration of an analyte to values from previous specimens in the same patient; a form of quality assurance

continued

Case Scenario 7-6 Quality Assurance in the Clinical Chemistry Laboratory: Why Are All of the Alkaline Phosphatase Results the Same? *(continued)*

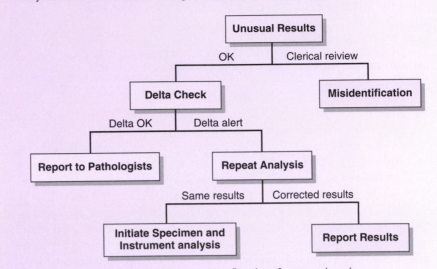

Figure 7–8. Corrective action flowchart for unusual results.

Follow-Up

As part of the specimen and instrument analysis phases of quality assurance, the supervisor of the reference laboratory first examined the quality control results from the night shift on the previous day. The control values for ALP were within the accepted range. The supervisor asked to see the control results for the day shift. These results had not been reviewed by the technician. All ALP control values for the new shift were out of range; all results were reported as 3 or 4 L/U. The technician examined the maintenance log printout for the chemistry analyzer that was used to perform the testing and noted maintenance was performed and no problems were noted. A visual inspection showed that reagent tubing delivering ALP reagent was obstructed by a pinched valve. The computer check for reagent level was malfunctioning. The supervisor asked to have all ALP testing from the previous shift retested. The supervisor notified all clients that current ALP results should not be reported to physicians until the reagent tubing problem was fixed and quality control samples were analyzed and verified to be accurate again. Then the patient samples would be analyzed again for ALP to obtain acceptable results. Corrected results were sent to the Family Practice Clinical laboratory within the day. These results as shown in Table 7–10 were sent to the physicians. ●

SUMMARY

These laboratory situations gave you the opportunity to learn about assessment of liver function and liver diseases. Liver function entails many vital metabolic functions that involve secretory and excretory processes such as detoxification, synthesis of proteins, catabolism of carbohydrates, and others. As mentioned earlier, several laboratory diagnostic tests can be used to assess liver function, including total and direct bilirubin, total protein, albumin, and ammonia levels. Laboratory tests aid in diagnosis and monitoring of hepatic disorders such as hepatitis, cirrho-

TABLE 7-10

Corrected Test Results from the Reference Laboratory

Test	Reference Range	Patient 1	Patient 2	Patient 3		Patient 4	Patient 5	Patient 6	Patient 7	Patient 8	Patient 9
				Day 1	Day 2						
Total protein (g/dL)	6.4–8.3	7.1	7.0	7.9	7.6	7.4	7.4	7.1	7.9	6.6	7.2
Albumin (g/dL)	3.5–5.2	4.5	4.2	4.4	4.3	4.7	3.8	4.2	4.8	4.0	4.7
Total bilirubin (mg/dL)	0.0–2.0	0.2	0.4	0.8	0.6	0.4	0.7	0.4	0.8	0.4	0.4
ALT (U/L)	<45	18	28	26	20	40	21	17	20	30	25
ALP (U/L)	53–128	80	86	98	110	85	62	112	103	78	83
AST (U/L)	<35	21	28	23	22	37	32	19	21	45	18

sis, and neonatal hyperbilirubinemia. Specific evaluation of liver function using assays for bilirubin and ammonia and assessing liver damage using enzymes such as ALT and ALP were discussed. This chapter also conveyed principles of chemical analysis for liver function tests and liver enzymes, including the effect of preanalytical, analytical, and postanalytical factors, while incorporating the scope of practice of the clinical laboratory scientist as a team member in health care.

EXERCISES

As you consider the scenarios presented in this chapter, answer the following questions:

1. What considerations should be made for specimen collection and handling of specimens for bilirubin testing?

2. Describe typical laboratory results of liver function tests for the patient with obstructive jaundice.

3. What are two specific laboratory tests that can be used to determine the source of alkaline phosphatase in patient serum?

4. What are three likely causes of an elevated plasma ammonia level in a pediatric patient?

5. What are three preanalytical sources of error that need to be avoided in order to provide accurate plasma ammonia values?

6. The following liver enzyme results are obtained from an adult male patient: ALT 280 U/L (reference range 0 to 45 U/L), AST 300 U/L (0 to 35 U/L), ALP 150 U/L (53 to 128 U/L). Comparing with the reference ranges for adult males, what might account for these results?

References

1. Kaplan LM, Isselbacher KJ: Jaundice. In Fauci AS, et al (eds): Harrison's Principles of Internal Medicine. New York: McGraw-Hill, 1998.
2. Limdi JK, Hyde GM: Evaluation of abnormal liver function tests. Postgrad Med J 2003; 79:307–312.

3. Black ER: Diagnostic strategies and test algorithms in liver disease. Clin Chem 1997; 43:1555–1560.

4. Dufour DR, et al: Diagnosis and monitoring of hepatic injury I: Performance characteristics of laboratory tests. Clin Chem 2000; 46:2027–2049.

5. Dufour DR, et al: Diagnosis and monitoring of hepatic injury II: Recommendations for use of laboratory tests in screening, diagnosis, and monitoring. Clin Chem 2000; 46:2050–2068.

6. Doumas BT, et al: Delta bilirubin absorption spectra, molar absorptivity, and reactivity in the diazo reaction. Clin Chem 1987; 33:769–774.

7. Jendrassik L, Grof P: Verification of photometric methods for measurement of blood bilirubin. Biochemistry 1938; 297:81.

8. Roche SP, Kobos R: Jaundice in the adult patient. Am Fam Physician 2004; 69:299–304.

9. Beers M, Berkow R: The Merck Manual of Diagnosis and Therapy, ed 17. Rahway, NJ: Merck & Co., 1999.

10. Bowers GN Jr, McComb RB: A continuous spectrophotometric method for measuring the activity of serum alkaline phosphatase. Clin Chem 1966; 12:70–89.

11. Pennock CA, Passant LP, Bolton FG: Estimation of cerebrospinal fluid protein. J Clin Pathol 1968; 21:518–520.

12. Plebani M, et al: Biochemical markers of hepatic fibrosis in primary biliary cirrhosis. Ric Clin Lab 1990; 20:269–274.

13. Balistreri WF: Viral hepatitis. Emerg Med Clin North Am 1991; 9:365–399.

14. Purcell RH: The disease of the hepatitits viruses. Gastroenterology 1993; 104:955–963.

15. Lemon SM: Type A viral hepatitis: Epidemiology, diagnosis, and prevention. Clin Chem 1997; 43:1494–1499.

16. Urdea MS, et al: Hepatitis C: Diagnosis and monitoring. Clin Chem 1997; 43:1507–1511.

17. Stickel F, Egerer G, Seitz HK: Hepatotoxicity of botanicals. Public Health Nutr J 2000; 3(2):113–124.

18. Ansley JD, et al: Quantitative tests of nitrogen metabolism in cirrhosis: Relation to other manifestations of liver disease. Gastroenterology 1978; 75:570–579.

19. Reyes RDK, Morgan G, Garal J: Encephalopathy and fatty degeneration of the viscera: A disease entity in childhood. Lancet 1963; 2:249–252.

20. Johnson GM, Scurletis TD, Carroll ND: A study of sixteen fatal cases of encephalitis-like disease in North Carolina children. N C Med J 1963; 24:464–473.

21. Meites S, Bubis S: Diagnostic quality of laboratory tests as evaluated by graphic comparison of "first test" data, with Reye's syndrome "workup" assays as a model. Clin Chem 1987; 33:100–102.

22. Van Anken HC, Schiphorst ME: A kinetic determination of ammonia in plasma. Clin Chim Acta 1974; 56:151–157.

23. Cembrowski GS: Thoughts on quality control systems: A laboratorian's perspective. Clin Chem 1997; 43:886–892.

24. Lacher DA, Connelly DP: Rate and delta checks compared for selected chemistry tests. Clin Chem 1988; 34:1966–1970.

The clinical laboratory provides objective information for the assessment of risk for cardiac disorders and for management of cardiac disease.

Assessment of Cardiovascular Disorders

Linda S. Gorman

In the past, evaluation of cardiac problems in the laboratory has been used primarily to assess cardiac disease, such as heart attacks or **acute myocardial infarctions (AMIs)**, and offer body chemistry information to aid supportive cardiac therapy. Laboratory information was used to document the occurrence of an AMI and endorse a treatment regimen, such as 24-hour nursing care in the coronary care

acute myocardial infarction (AMI) - sudden heart attack, resulting from dead heart muscle tissue unable to contract in rhythm

unit. More recently, research has shown that risk factors can also be predictive of risk for AMI and other heart disorders such as coronary artery disease. Use of laboratory results still supports diagnosis of AMI but also assesses risk for future cardiac disease through analysis of body chemistry metabolites, such as total cholesterol, high-density lipoprotein cholesterol, and high-sensitivity C-reactive protein. Risk factor assessment enables health-care professionals to educate the patient and to institute activities that will reduce risk for an AMI.

This chapter presents seven patient situations that are pertinent to the role of the clinical laboratory in assessment of cardiac function. By working through the scenarios as they are presented, the student will gain knowledge about the physiology of cardiac health and pathology. Each scenario allows you to examine the laboratory assessment process, including the impact of preanalytical factors, such as specimen collection and handling; the effects of variation on the analytical procedure; and the importance of postanalytical factors, such as communication of results. In this chapter, you will explore your role in providing the laboratory results that aid in diagnosis and monitoring of cardiac disorders and the laboratory assessment of risk factors that help to prevent cardiac disease. The side boxes in this chapter provide common sense tips, definitions of terms, brief descriptions of pathophysiology, and clinical correlations as well as reminders of the team approach in health care. Text boxes within the chapter outline methodology for laboratory assessment of cardiac function.

OBJECTIVES

Upon completion of this chapter, the student will have the ability to

- Identify preanalytical factors that can alter accuracy of laboratory testing for cardiac function.
- Describe testing for cardiac function, such as troponin T and I, CK-MB, LD isoenzymes, hs-CRP, and homocysteine.
- Describe the testing used to assess risk of cardiovascular disease and toxicity to cardioactive medications.
- Describe the current trends and guidelines for reducing cardiovascular disease.
- Assess the predictive values of a cardiac-related clinical laboratory test result for predicting heart disease.

THE FIRST THREE PATIENTS IN THE EMERGENCY DEPARTMENT

The emergency department (ED) at Valley View Memorial Hospital was busy for a Wednesday evening. Three patients of particular concern have arrived and are waiting to see a physician:

1. Joe Smoker, 57 years old, has come to the emergency department complaining of chest pain.
2. Mildred Dodge, a 62-year-old grandmother, was visiting the zoo with her grandchildren when she became dizzy and fainted.
3. Kyle Minute, an athletic 27-year-old, was jogging when he collapsed on the street. He was brought in by ambulance.

These patients will be examined by the medical personnel in the ED, and blood specimens will be sent to the laboratory. From these patients, the student will learn about common cardiac disorders.

CASE SCENARIO 8-1

Acute Myocardial Infarction: The Obese Smoker

Joe Smoker is an overweight 57-year-old white male who was mowing his lawn when he experienced a sharp chest pain along with pain in his left arm. His wife rushed him to the hospital, fearing that he was having a heart attack. In the clinic, the physician examined Joe and sent him for **electrocardiogram (ECG)** and blood work. The blood is processed in the clinical laboratory and the serum is tested for troponins, creatine kinase (CK), and creatine kinase isoenzyme MB (CK-MB).

electrocardiogram (ECG) - tracing of electrical activity of the heart

---

ACUTE MYOCARDIAL INFARCTION

The heart muscle, or **myocardium**, receives its blood flow from three **coronary arteries** rather than from the blood it constantly pumps through its chambers and out to the circulation for the rest of the body. If blood flow from the coronary arteries to the heart muscle is restricted, not enough oxygen reaches the heart. This is termed *ischemia*. It can cause chest pain or **angina**. If blood flow to a portion of the heart muscle is stopped entirely, it can cause cell death, **necrosis**, and heart attack, or acute myocardial infarction (AMI). The precipitating event that leads to blocking of blood flow is a clot or dislodged **plaque** particle that prevents blood flow to tissue. Table 8–1 lists risk factors for the development of cardiovascular disease. In the cellular damage process, troponin leaks from the heart tissue and is released into the bloodstream.[1] Damage to heart muscle fibers releases CK-MB into the bloodstream as well. Other constituents released by damaged heart cells include lactate dehydrogenase isoenzyme 1 (LD1), aspartate transaminase (AST), and electrolytes.[2] Each of these biochemical markers will be discussed in detail.

Several terms are used to describe heart disease, including myocardial infarction and angina **pectoris**. The term *myocardial infarction* focuses on the heart muscle, the myocardium, and the changes that occur in it due to sudden deprivation of circulating blood and oxygen. The main change is necrosis of myocardial tissue due

myocardium - heart muscle

coronary arteries - three major blood vessels supplying blood and oxygen to the heart muscles

angina - chest pain due to inadequate supply of oxygen to heart muscle

necrosis - death of tissue

plaque - accumulated deposits of fat and other substances in the blood vessels causing roughened and narrowed interior surface

pectoris - chest

TABLE 8-1

Risk Factors for Cardiovascular Disease

Smoking
Cholesterol
Elevated blood pressure
Diet and nutrition/weight
Physical activity level
Family history
Gender
Lifestyle

to the interruption of blood flow caused by **atherosclerosis**. Atherosclerosis is hardening, roughing, and narrowing of the blood vessels due to fatty plaque accumulation. This culminates in plugging of the vessel, or a **thrombosis** or blood clot, due to activation of platelets and clotting of blood as it flows past the roughened lining of the vessel. The word **infarction** comes from the Latin word *infarcire*, meaning "to plug up or cram." It refers to the clogging of the artery.

Angina was first described in 1772 by the English physician William Heberden in 20 patients who suffered from "a painful and most disagreeable sensation in the breast, which seems as if it would extinguish life, if it were to increase or to continue." Such patients, he wrote, "are seized while they are walking (more especially if it be uphill, and soon after eating). But the moment they stand still, all this uneasiness vanishes." The word *angina* comes from the Latin verb *angere*, meaning "to choke or throttle." *Angina* is now used interchangeably with *angina pectoris* (the Latin *pectus* = "chest").

Laboratory assays contribute objective information to the assessment of cardiac function. The ECG (or EKG) produces another form of objective information. The ECG tracings represent electrical current as it passes through heart muscle, causing contractions in the upper and lower chambers. Each lead of the ECG represents a tracing of the electrical current as it passes through a different plane of the heart. Cardiac damage, such as that caused by an AMI, produces areas of dead cells within the muscle. Electrical current will not pass through these areas, and the tracing of the area will show abnormalities.

Troponins are contractile proteins found within muscle fibers that help regulate contractions. There are three troponins that work as a complex. They are troponin C (calcium-binding component), troponin I (inhibitory component), and troponin T (tropomyosin-binding component). During the process of muscle necrosis, troponins I and T are released from the dying muscle fibers into the bloodstream. Increases in the concentration of troponins I and T above the reference levels in serum indicate heart muscle fiber damage and necrosis. Serum troponins generally are not elevated with angina or early stages of decreased blood flow before actual muscle fiber death.

Measurement of troponin assays has been a tremendous boon to clinical diagnosis.[3–5] Troponins released from heart muscle remain in the bloodstream from 1 to 14 days after onset of AMI, making them the preferred marker for detection of an AMI.[2,6–9] Troponins, as cardiac markers, appear to have many advantages primarily due to their quick release following heart muscle damage and their longevity in the bloodstream following the heart attack. However, the methods for analysis have been more of a stumbling block than the utility of troponin for cardiovascular events. Test Methodologies 8–1 and 8–2 describe analysis of cardiac troponin I and troponin T.[11,12]

TEST METHODOLOGY 8-1.   TROPININ T

Troponin T is a contractile protein along with other troponin proteins found within muscle fibers, including cardiac myofibrils. Cardiac troponin T (*cTnT*) has unique specificity to cardiac muscle and is released during cardiac muscle damage. It can be measured in serum within 6 hours after AMI with a high degree of sensitivity and specificity. Given the time frame for detecting troponins following AMI, levels elevated above the reference range or medical decision limit reflect irreversible heart muscle damage. Cardiac troponin T is usually measured with an immunoassay method.

TEST METHODOLOGY 8-1. **TROPININ T** *(continued)*

The Reaction Principle

cTnT reacts with the troponin antibody to form a complex. This complex is linked to a dye, enzyme, or chemiluminescent reagent that is linked to a second antibody to allow for quantitation of the cTnT present in the patient's sample. Chemiluminesence is the most sensitive test at this time for cTnT.

The Specimen

Serum; if not analyzed within a few hours, the specimen should be kept frozen for up to 6 months prior to analysis, with steady thawing and mixing prior to analysis.

Reference Range

<0.01 µg/L (highly variable because method-specific)

TEST METHODOLOGY 8-2. **TROPONIN I**

Troponin I is a contractile protein along with other troponin proteins found within muscle fibers, including cardiac myofibrils. Cardiac troponin I (cTnI) has unique specificity to cardiac muscle and is released shortly after cardiac muscle damage. It can be measured in the serum for 1 to 14 days after an AMI with a high degree of sensitivity and specificity. Levels of cTnI above the reference range or medical decision limit reflect irreversible heart muscle damage. The common principle of analysis is by immunoassay.

The Reaction Principle

cTnI also is measured by an immunoassay using anti-troponin monoclonal antibody. Originally the assay patent was owned by a single company, but newer chemiluminescent procedures have enabled automation of this assay as well as the cTnT assay.

The chemiluminescence reaction binds the cTnI to a monoclonal antibody that is attached to the test tube. A second monoclonal antibody with an acridinium-derivative conjugate acts to sandwich the troponin I from the patient sample in this assay. The chemiluminescent signal is then detected and relates to the concentration of cTnI present.

The Specimen

Heparinized plasma with no contamination of buffy coat cells.

Reference Range

0.0–0.05 ng/mL

Historical Biomarkers of AMI

Serum enzymes such as CK, LD, AST, and their isoenzymes have all been used as biomarkers of AMI. Decades ago, they were thought to be sensitive indicators of myocardial necrosis and could be used to correlate with other signs and symptoms such as abnormalities in the ECG pattern. All three of these enzymes, however, are found in other tissues as well, making them less specific to myocardial damage. AST, for example, is also found in skeletal muscle, liver parenchymal cells, and erythrocytes, while CK is found in skeletal muscle, brain tissue, and embryonic or malignant tissue. LD is the least specific of these three enzymes in that it is found in virtually all tissue and is associated with damage to liver, skeletal muscle, cardiac muscle, erythrocytes, renal cells, and many other tissues, as well as ovarian and testicular tumors. In order for these biomarkers to be more specific indicators of AMI, they were analyzed together several times a day over a period of 1 week. Analysis of isoenzymes of CK and LD also provided improved specificity. The goal was to observe the peak and return to normal of these enzymes in order to predict resolution of the heart attack or to monitor for a second cardiac event. The clinical significance of these enzymes as cardiac markers will be discussed in detail next. For more information about the overall significance of serum enzymes and principles of analysis refer to Chapter 1 (Overview of Clinical Chemistry).

Creatinine kinase is composed of two polypeptide chains, B and M, making up three forms: CK-MM, CK-MB, and CK-BB. Distribution of the three isomer forms of CK varies throughout tissue. For example, CK-MM (or CK 3) is found mostly in skeletal muscle tissue, while CK-MB (CK 2) is found mostly in cardiac muscle tissue. CK-BB (CK 1) is associated with brain and nerve tissue but is also an embryonic form found in serum of newborn babies and in malignancies in which tumor cells exhibit characteristics of embryonic cells. Chapter 13 (Malignancy Disorders and Testing) presents more details about tumor markers. The isoenzymes of CK have all been assessed by various methods, including electrophoresis and immunoassay methods.[14] The densitometry scans of electrophoretic patterns of serum CK isoenzymes of healthy individuals and AMI patients are shown in Figure 8–1.

Historically myocardial infarction was detected by looking for the CK isoenzyme CK-MB. This marker is released into circulation from necrotic heart muscle. As the heart muscle becomes damaged, this CK isoenzyme is released into the bloodstream and may be detected for 6 to 18 hours after onset of AMI. The window of detection is quite short, lasting no more than 12 to 18 hours after the heart attack occurred, because of protein degradation mechanisms that eliminate the CK-MB from the blood. Due to this short time frame, often the peak level of CK-MB is missed, leaving in doubt whether a heart attack has occurred or this is an indication of mild heart tissue damage or angina. Many studies have investigated if there is a correlation between the severity of the MI and the level of CK-MB that is measured in the serum. The results have been mixed, but it is easy to understand how more damage might lead to more isoenzymes release. Test Methodologies 8–3 and 8–4 describe analysis of CK and CK isoenzyme MB.[15]

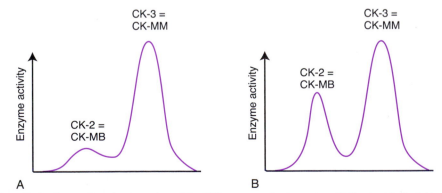

Figure 8–1. Electrophoretic separation of the CK isoenzymes in the serum of (A) a healthy individual and (B) a patient with acute myocardial infarction. Isoenzymes are numbered on the basis of their electrophoretic mobility, with the most anodal form receiving the lowest number.

TEST METHODOLOGY 8-3. CREATINE KINASE

Creatine kinase (CK) is an enzyme that activates creatine in muscle by transferring a high-energy phosphate group in the reaction. The reaction is reversible:

$$\text{Creatine} + \text{ATP} \leftrightarrow \text{creatine phosphate} + \text{ADP}$$

CK is found in highest concentration in heart muscle, skeletal muscle, and brain.

The Reaction

Measurement of CK activity couples the natural reaction with two additional reactions that enable CK activity to be measured. There are two methods for CK measurement.

Method 1

CK

$$\text{Creatine} + \text{ATP} \leftrightarrow \text{creatine phosphate} + \text{ADP}$$

Pyruvate kinase (PK)

$$\text{ADP} + \text{phosphoenolpyruvate} \leftrightarrow \text{pyruvate} + \text{ATP}$$

LD

$$\text{Pyruvate} + \text{NADH} + \text{H}^+ \leftrightarrow \text{lactate} + \text{NAD}^+$$

Decrease in absorbance at 340 nm measures the decrease in NADH and reflects the activity of CK in serum.

Method 2

CK

$$\text{Creatine phosphate} + \text{ADP} \leftrightarrow \text{creatine} + \text{ATP}$$

Hexokinase (HK)

$$\text{ATP} + \text{glucose} \leftrightarrow \text{glucose 6-phosphate} + \text{ADP}$$

Glucose-6-phosphate dehydrogenase (G6PD)

$$\text{Glucose 6-phosphate} + \text{NADP}^+ \leftrightarrow \text{6-phosphogluconate} + \text{NADPH}$$

Interference

Hemolysis may falsely elevate the CK assay. Red blood cells contain adenylate kinase, which catalyzes the production of ADP to ATP; the increased ATP participates in the assay reaction, leading to false increases in CK activity.

The Specimen

Serum, nonhemolyzed, analyzed within a few hours of collection or kept frozen until analysis.

Reference Ranges

Male	46–171 U/L
Female	34–145 U/L

Other historically used AMI biomarkers are LD and its isoenzymes 1 and 2. In particular, these enzymes and isoenzymes carry out their metabolic functions within specific cells, and are released into body fluids when those cells become diseased. Thus, an increase in LD isoenzyme activity can indicate leakage from

TEST METHODOLOGY 8-4.   CREATINE KINASE ISOENZYME MB

Immunoinhibition allows blocking of the M isotope of the CK dimer isoenzymes. Once the M part of the enzyme is blocked, only the CK-B component will react in the typical CK enzyme reaction.

The Reaction

The sample is incubated in the CK-MB reagent, which includes the anti–CK-M antibody. The activity of the noninhibited CK-B is then determined using the following series of reactions:

CK-B

$$ADP + creatine \leftrightarrow creatine\ phosphate + ATP$$

Hexokinase (HK)

$$ATP + glucose \leftrightarrow ADP + glucose\ 6\text{-phosphate}$$

Glucose-6-phosphate dehydrogenase (G6PD)

$$Glucose\ 6\text{-phosphate} + NAD^+ \leftrightarrow 6\text{-phosphogluconate} + NADH + H^+$$

The rate of NADH formation, measured at 340 nm, is directly proportional to serum CK-B activity. This then represents the CK-MB activity in the patient's sample.

The Specimen

Serum

Reference Range

% CK-MB $<3.9\%$ or $<5.0\ \mu g/L$

---

cells due to cellular injury. The level of isoenzyme LD1 compared with LD2 has been used to detect an AMI because of the high concentration of LD1 in cardiac muscle fibers. LD isoenzymes begin to leak out of dying heart muscle cells and are detectable in the serum by 36 hours following a heart attack. Normal LD isoenzyme patterns show that LD2 is greater than LD1. The appearance of more LD1 than LD2, also called the "flipped pattern," is typical of cardiac muscle damage but is nonspecific since it also is associated with red blood cell hemolysis or megaloblastic anemias. The flipped pattern, in which LD1>LD2, lasts up to 3 to 4 days after the heart attack.[13] The densitometry scans of electrophoretic patterns of serum LD isoenzymes of healthy individuals and AMI patients are shown in Figure 8–2. LD levels rise at such a slow rate that they are not useful for early detection or treatment of the disease. This enzyme, however, will remain in the bloodstream for 4 to 7 days after an AMI, enabling clinicians to detect post-AMI conditions in patients who have had mild heart attacks and did not seek diagnosis until several days after the suspected illness.[16] Figure 8–3 presents a graphic depiction of the rise and fall of cardiac markers over the duration of the AMI. The procedure for LD measurement is described in Test Methodology 8–12, found later in this chapter.

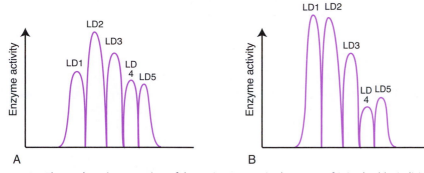

Figure 8–2. Electrophoretic separation of the LD isoenzymes in the serum of (*A*) a healthy individual and (*B*) a patient with acute myocardial infarction.

Case Scenario 8-1 Acute Myocardial Infarction: The Obese Smoker

Follow-Up

Joe Smoker's laboratory results were as follows:

Test	Joe	Reference Ranges
Troponin I (ng/mL)	1.7	0.0–0.05
CK-MB (%)	7	<3.9
CK (IU/L)	275	46–171

All of these cardiac biomarkers are elevated. Given these laboratory results, there is a high likelihood that Joe Smoker had a myocardial infarction. These results, combined with ECG, history, and physical examination, were used to make the diagnosis of AMI. He was moved to the coronary care unit of his hospital, where he stayed for 3 days. His physician ordered a medication regimen of pravastatin (Pravachol), clofibrate, and niacin. Pravachol is a 3-OH-3-methylglutaryl-coenzyme A (HMG-CoA) reductase inhibitor. Pravachol and drugs like it reduce cholesterol synthesis in cells, including the liver, by inhibiting the enzyme responsible for a key step in cholesterol synthesis. Clofibrate-type drugs act to inhibit fatty acid release from the liver and inhibit tissue lipolysis. Niacin and drugs that act to sequester bile acids reduce the formation of very low-density lipoprotein (VLDL) and lead to increases in high-density lipoprotein (HDL) levels.[17,18] These and other **lipoproteins** will be discussed in more detail.

Joe was sent home with instructions for follow-up visits to his cardiologist and his generalist physician. ●

lipoprotein - protein combined with lipid components

```
CK-MB       XXXX*****////////////
LD                          XXXXXXXXXXXXXXXXXXXXXXXX********////// (7 days)
Troponin    XXXXXX******************//////////////////////////////////////////////////////// (14 days)

            0      6      12     18     24     30     36-------96
```

Figure 8–3. Rise and duration of select cardiac markers from time of onset of AMI.

THE TEAM APPROACH

Laboratory analysis contributes objective information for the assessment of cardiac function. The electrocardiogram (ECG or EKG) produces another form of objective information. The tracings of the ECG represent electrical current as it passes through the heart muscle, causing contraction. Each lead of the ECG provides a tracing of the electrical current as it passes through a different plane of the heart. Cardiac damage, such as that caused by an AMI, produces areas of dead muscle cells that do not conduct electricity. ECG tracings will show abnormalities that reflect these areas of dead heart muscle.

ester - compound formed by combination of an organic acid and alcohol with elimination of water

micelle - ultramicroscopic particle

chylomicron - parcel of lipids and proteins made from dietary fats (especially triglycerides) during intestinal absorption

CASE SCENARIO 8-2

Type 2 Diabetes With Cardiac Risk: Mildred Dodge, the Bonbon Eater

Mildred Dodge, at age 62, has had type 2 diabetes mellitus for 12 years. She was at the zoo with her grandchildren when she became faint and dizzy, causing her family to wonder if she was having a diabetic episode. Mildred was brought to the ED for evaluation. She has been taking medication for her diabetes and blood pressure, but this day she had not wanted to take her "water pill" so she could enjoy her grandchildren at the zoo. Table 8–2 provides a review of the symptoms of type 2 diabetes. The ED physician orders blood drawn for glucose, lipids, and electrolytes on Mrs. Dodge. The physician notices she has some odd heart sounds found with the physical examination and orders an ECG as well. The laboratory findings for Mildred Dodge are as follows:

Test	Mildred	Reference Ranges for Age (or Risk Ranges)
Glucose (nonfasting; mg/dL)	235	<200
Total cholesterol (mg/dL)	289	<200
Triglycerides (mg/dL)	434	<150
HDL-cholesterol (mg/dL)	34	>59
hs-CRP (mg/L)	9.56	0.2–9.1

LIPIDS AND LIPOPROTEINS

Lipids are either compounds that yield fatty acids when hydrolyzed or complex alcohols that can combine with fatty acids to form **esters**. For example, cholesterol ester forms from cholesterol and fatty acid. Lipids are carried in the bloodstream by complexes known as lipoproteins. This is because these lipids are not soluble in the plasma water. Thus they travel in **micelle**-like complexes composed of phospholipids and protein on the outside with cholesterol, cholesterol esters, and triglycerides on the inside. The four main types of lipoproteins are **chylomicrons**, VLDL, low-density lipoprotein (LDL), and HDL and are represented in Figure

TABLE 8-2

American Diabetic Association Description of Symptoms of Type 2 Diabetes[21]

Frequent urination
Excessive thirst
Extreme hunger
Unusual weight loss
Increased fatigue
Irritability
Blurry vision

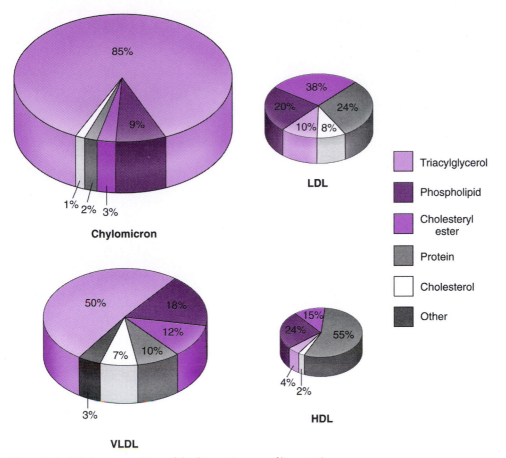

Triacylglycerol

Phospholipid

Cholesteryl ester

Protein

Cholesterol

Other

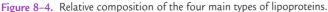

Figure 8–4. Relative composition of the four main types of lipoproteins.

8–4. Each of these has some percentage of cholesterol or triglyceride associated with its **apoproteins** and phospholipids, to make each lipoprotein unique. Triglycerides are the major constituent of chylomicrons and VLDL, while cholesterol is the major lipid associated with LDL and HDL. The cholesterol form most associated with cardiovascular problems when in excess is LDL cholesterol (LDL-C). Thus, the laboratory monitors the total cholesterol, the LDL-C and the HDL cholesterol (HDL-C) in patients at risk for cardiovascular disorders, including pre-AMI patients. Test Methodologies 8–5 through 8–7 describe methods of analysis for total cholesterol, LDL-C, and triglycerides. These four tests are commonly performed together in a lipid panel.

The Role of HDL

Just as there is a ying to a yang, so too is the relationship between the two main forms of lipoproteins. While LDL-C is considered harmful when in excess, the elevation of HDL-C is viewed as a positive cardiovascular biomarker for a patient. Elevated HDL-C has a beneficial effect for the vascular system, due to the role that HDL plays in the body. HDL removes excess cholesterol from tissues and routes it to the liver for reprocessing and/or removal.

apoprotein - the protein portion of a lipoprotein

✓ **Common Sense Check**
Excessive levels of serum chylomicrons are found in patients who have eaten in the past few hours and cause lipemia, or creamy appearance of serum. Lipemia usually indicates the patient has not properly fasted in preparation for the lipid panel or triglyceride test. A lipemic sample is a signal that the fasting status of the patient should be investigated.

TEST METHODOLOGY 8-5.   TOTAL CHOLESTEROL

Testing methods for total cholesterol use cholesterol oxidase reactions along with cholesterol esterase and usually a peroxidase reaction for the "color" or final determination reaction.

The Reaction

Cholesterol Esterase

$$\text{T. cholesterol esters} \rightarrow \text{cholesterol} + \text{free fatty acid}$$

Cholesterol Oxidase

$$\text{Cholesterol} + O_2 \rightarrow \text{cholest-3-ene-4-one} + H_2O_2$$

Peroxidase

$$2\,H_2O_2 + \text{4-aminoantipyrine} \rightarrow 4\,H_2O + \text{chromogen}$$

Interference

Remove sample from red cells after blood clots or plasma has been spun down. The peroxidase assay can be susceptible to increases in uric acid, ascorbic acid, bilirubin, hemoglobin, or other reducing substances. Samples should have only the normal amount of these substances present.

The Specimen

Nonhemolyzed serum or plasma, free from clots. The patient need not be fasting if this is the only lipid test requested. However, if total cholesterol is requested as part of a lipid panel, the patient must be fasting for 10 to 12 hours.

Reference Ranges (Age-Specific)

Male (25–29 year old)	130–234 mg/dL
Female (25–29 years old)	130–231 mg/dL
Based on coronary heart disease risk:	
Child	desirable <170 mg/dL
Adult	desirable <200 mg/dL

TEST METHODOLOGY 8-6.   LDL CHOLESTEROL

LDL cholesterol (LDL-C) may be calculated or measured directly.

Friedewald Calculation or Derived Beta-Quantification

Testing for LDL-C involves a calculation that includes total cholesterol, HDL cholesterol (HDL-C), and triglyceride (TG) values using the formula:

$$\text{LDL-C} = \text{total cholesterol} - [\text{HDL-C} + (\text{TG}/5)]$$

where TG/5 approximates the VLDL cholesterol concentration in the sample.

Interference

Cannot be used for TG over 400 mg/dL

Sample Calculation

Total cholesterol = 350 mg/dL; triglycerides = 150 mg/dL; HDL-C = 30 mg/dL

$$\text{LDL-C} = 350 - [30 + (150/5)] = 350 - (30 + 30) = 350 - 60 = 290 \text{ mg/dL}$$

TEST METHODOLOGY 8-6. **LDL CHOLESTEROL** *(continued)*

Specimen

None required for this portion, but 10- to 12-hour fasting serum specimen for lipid panel.

Reference Ranges (Age-Specific)

Male (25–29 years old)	70–165 mg/dL
Females (25–29 years old)	71–164 mg/dL

National Cholesterol Education Program risk factors (adult male):

Optimal	<100 mg/dL
Near optimal	100–129 mg/dL
Borderline high	130–159 mg/dL
High	>160 mg/dL
Very high	>190 mg/dL

Direct Measurement of LDL-C

With the advent of homogeneous reagents, LDL-C is now measured using the cholesterol reaction along with reagents that block the contribution of HDL and VLDL to the resulting answer. In the homogeneous LDL assay, detergents block the other two lipoprotein cholesterol products from forming colored chromogens. Only the LDL-C forms a colored chromogen that can be measured spectrophotometrically by automated systems or designated analyzers.

The Specimen

Serum, plasma. The patient need not be fasting if this is the only lipid test requested. However, if total cholesterol is requested as part of a lipid panel, the patient must be fasting for 10 to 12 hours.

Reference Ranges (Age-Specific)

Male (25–29 years old)	70–165 mg/dL
Females (25–29 years old)	71–164 mg/dL

National Cholesterol Education Program risk factors (adult male):

Optimal	<100 mg/dL
Near optimal	100–129 mg/dL
Borderline high	130–159 mg/dL
High	>160 mg/dL
Very high	>190 mg/dL

TEST METHODOLOGY 8-7. **TRIGLYCERIDE**

Triglycerides are composed of three fatty acids and a glycerol moiety. Analyzing a serum or plasma sample for triglycerides typically involves four reactions.

The Reaction

Lipase (Bacterial)

$$\text{Triglycerides} \rightarrow 3 \text{ fatty acids} + \text{glycerol}$$

Glycerol Kinase

$$\text{Glycerol} + \text{ATP} \rightarrow \text{glycerol-3-phosphate} + \text{ADP}$$

continued

> **TEST METHODOLOGY 8-7.   TRIGLYCERIDE** (*continued*)
>
> *Pyruvate Kinase*
>
> $$ADP + phosphoenol\ pyruvate \rightarrow ATP + pyruvate$$
>
> *Lactate Dehydrogenase*
>
> $$NADH + H^+ + pyruvate \rightarrow NAD + lactate$$
>
> **The Specimen**
>
> Serum, fasting 10 to 12 hours.
>
> **Reference Ranges (Age-Specific)**
>
> | | |
> |---|---|
> | Male (25–29 years old) | 45–204 mg/dL |
> | Females (25–29 years old) | 42–159 mg/dL |
>
> National Cholesterol Education Program risk factors (adult male):
>
> | | |
> |---|---|
> | Optimal | <150 mg/dL |
> | High | 150–199 mg/dL |
> | Hypertriglyceridemic | 200–499 mg/dL |
> | Very high | >499 mg/dL |

> ✓ **Common Sense Check**
>
> If a lipid panel (total cholesterol, triglycerides, HDL-C, and LDL-C) is requested, a fasting (10–12 hours) specimen is needed to prevent interferences from dietary fats, including chylomicrons. The total cholesterol portion of this lipid panel can be performed on a nonfasting specimen but provides limited information without the other three lipid and lipoprotein results.

Physiological Changes in Lipid and Lipoprotein Levels

High HDL-C levels are seen in premenopausal women, persons who exercise regularly, and those who maintain a low but healthy weight. Insulin, estrogen, and thyroxine (T_4) have an inverse relationship with total cholesterol levels. When estrogen levels are higher, as in women who menstruate, the total cholesterol level is lower, preferably 200 mg/dL. The HDL-C level is also elevated in menstruating women, while the LDL-C tends to be lower.[19] Test Methodology 8–8 describes the method of analysis for HDL-C.

> **TEST METHODOLOGY 8-8.   HDL CHOLESTEROL**
>
> Testing for HDL cholesterol (HDL-C) using either precipitation methods or homogenous assays.
>
> ### The Precipitation Reaction
>
> The precipitation methods use either dextran sulfate, polyethylene glycol (PEG), or phosphotungstic acid with magnesium chloride ($MgCl_2$) to precipitate LDL and VLDL lipoproteins from a fasting serum sample, leaving HDL in the supernatant. This HDL supernatant is then assayed for cholesterol. The resulting answer (in mg/dL) represents the amount of HDL in the serum sample.
>
> The supernatant is tested for cholesterol concentration.
>
> #### Interference
>
> Chylomicrons from nonfasting specimens will interfere in these precipitation methods.
>
> #### The Specimen
>
> Serum, plasma (depending on the precipitating reagent used); 10 to 12 hours fasting.

TEST METHODOLOGY 8-8. **HDL CHOLESTEROL** *(continued)*

Reference Ranges (Age-Specific)

Men (25–29 years old)	31–63 mg/dL
Women (25–29 years old)	37–83 mg/dL

National Cholesterol Education Program risk factors (adult male):

Low risk	>59 mg/dL
High risk	<40 mg/dL

The Homogeneous Reaction

Homogeneous HDL-C assays do not use precipitation, nor do they require a centrifugation separation step. This improves the yield of HDL recovered from the specimen.

One method uses an antibody to apolipoprotein B-100 to bind LDL and VLDL in the sample. This leaves the HDL-C to react with the second reagent, which contains enzymes and substrate for cholesterol analysis.

In a second method, a synthetic polyanion reagent binds the sites on VLDL and LDL particles, blocking their products from forming cholesterol colored products. The second reagent added has detergent, enzymes, and substrate that react with the HDL-C in the sample. Only the HDL particle cholesterol is allowed to form a colored product and be measured.

The Specimen

Serum, plasma (depends on the method used).

Reference Ranges (Age-Specific)

Men (25–29 years old)	31–63 mg/dL
Women (25–29 years old)	37–83 mg/dL

National Cholesterol Education Program risk factors (adult male):

Low risk	>59 mg/dL
High risk	<40 mg/dL

Diabetes and Cardiac Disease

The American Diabetic Association states that type 2 diabetics can develop cardiac complications, especially patients who have had this disease over a long period of time and who demonstrate lipid abnormalities. Diabetics often have low HDL-C levels with elevated LDL-C and triglyceride levels. The National Cholesterol Education Program (NCEP) committee states that diabetics with elevated cholesterol develop plaque formation in their blood vessels leading to narrowing of the vessel **lumen**. In type 2 diabetics who exhibit elevated triglyceride levels, the cholesterol level needs to be less than 200 mg/dL and the LDL-C level needs to be maintained at 100 mg/dL or less in order to provide a low risk for plaque formation in the blood vessels. Because type 2 diabetics cannot move glucose from the bloodstream into the tissues for metabolism as efficiently as the nondiabetic person, they convert the excess glucose into fatty acid chains (in the liver) and make more triglycerides. The triglycerides enter the bloodstream, and the diabetic must use them as an energy source in place of glucose. Depending on the efficiency of cellular mobilization of these triglycerides, the diabetic patient will often exhibit excess triglycerides in the bloodstream, leading to most of the blood vessel damage we associate with excess triglycerides.[20]

lumen - space within a tube, such as a blood vessel or the esophagus

A summary of the American Heart Association description of factors that can lead to cardiovascular problems such as AMI in type 2 diabetes is provided below[21]:

- Being insulin resistant (about 9 out of 10 patients have insulin resistance)
- Being obese (about 50% of men and 70% of women who have diabetes are obese)
- Having a lifestyle that does not involve significant physical activity
- Having low HDL ("good") cholesterol levels and high triglyceride levels
- Having an increased prevalence of high blood pressure

National Cholesterol Education Program

The NCEP provides guidelines for evaluation of lipid panel results in regard to risk factors for cardiovascular problems. HDL (good) cholesterol protects against heart disease, so for HDL, higher numbers are better. An HDL-C level less than 40 mg/dL is considered abnormally low and a major risk factor because it increases the risk of developing heart disease. HDL levels of 60 mg/dL or more help to lower risk for heart disease. High amounts of triglycerides can also raise risk of heart disease. Individuals with triglyceride levels that are borderline high (150 to 199 mg/dL) or high (200 mg/dL or more) may need treatment. Type 2 diabetics often exhibit elevated cholesterol, triglycerides, and LDL-C with low HDL-C. Decreasing the LDL-C level is necessary to decrease the risk of cardiovascular disease in the type 2 diabetic. Table 8–3 shows the NCEP lipid range guidelines for cardiovascular risk factors in type 2 diabetics.

C-Reactive Protein

C-reactive protein (CRP) is a sensitive acute-phase protein, an important but non-specific aspect of the immune response. That is, CRP appears in the blood following infection or tissue damage. Its name is derived from the discovery that it binds to the cell wall of the C-polysaccharide of *Streptococcus* organisms, which helps phagocytic cells to destroy these and other pathogens. It also binds to tissue break-

TABLE 8-3

National Cholesterol Education Program Guidelines for Lipid Ranges of Cardiovascular Risk Factors in Type 2 Diabetics[22]

Total Cholesterol Level	Category
Less than 200 mg/dL	Desirable
200–239 mg/dL	Borderline high
240 mg/dL and above	High

LDL Cholesterol Level	LDL Cholesterol Category
Less than 100 mg/dL	Optimal
100–129 mg/dL	Near-optimal/above optimal
130–159 mg/dL	Borderline high
160–189 mg/dL	High
190 mg/dL and above	Very high

down products released following myocardial infarction, stress, surgery, trauma, and infection and aids in resolution of inflammatory responses. Older methods of analysis for CRP were based on immunoassays that were sensitive to measuring concentrations in the 0.5- to 2.0-mg/L (0.05- to 0.2-mg/dL) range. Newer methods are more sensitive and are capable of detecting amounts as low as 0.1 to 0.3 mg/L (0.01 to 0.03 mg/dL). CRP levels greater than 8.6 mg/L (0.86 mg/dL) are generally released 6 to 12 hours following AMI. One of these new high-sensitivity C-reactive protein (hs-CRP) methods of detecting CRP is described in Test Methodology 8–9.

TEST METHODOLOGY 8-9. HIGH-SENSITIVITY C-REACTIVE PROTEIN

The Reaction Principle

Measurement of a high-sensitivity C-reactive protein (hs-CRP) complex by light scatter is facilitated by linking the antibody to latex particles. Light scatter is more controlled and reproducible in automated systems using this approach.

hs-CRP (sample) + anti-CRP antibody → complex

Standardization problems are being corrected by an ongoing study by the Centers for Disease Control and Prevention. At present, it is recommended to take two measurements spaced 2 weeks apart, average them, and use the value to monitor risk for atherosclerosis inflammation. If the hs-CRP value is greater than 10 mg/L, the sample is invalid. High values are due to the presence of active infection or another inflammatory stimulus that has elevated the CRP.

The Specimen

Serum, plasma (nonfasting is acceptable).

Reference Ranges

Male	0.3–8.6 mg/L
Female	0.2–9.1 mg/L

Case Scenario 8-2 Type 2 Diabetes With Cardiac Risk: Mildred Dodge, the Bonbon Eater

Follow-Up

Mildred's laboratory results show that her glucose was elevated, as were her total cholesterol, triglycerides, and hs-CRP. These results indicate medication changes may be needed to better control her glucose levels. Mildred is also exhibiting hypertriglyceridemia, as may be common with type 2 diabetes. In these patients, inadequate or poorly functioning insulin leads to more triglyceride formation in the liver, hypertriglyceridemia, and more utilization of triglycerides by the tissues for energy. Increased demand leads to more triglyceride mobility from the liver to the tissues.[14]

With the mobilization of triglycerides, there is an increase in VLDL cholesterol (VLDL-C), which also elevates the total cholesterol. There is a

> **CLINICAL CORRELATION**
> Type 2 diabetics lack insulin and have increased serum cholesterol, VLDL-C, and LDL-C.

continued

Case Scenario 8-2 **Type 2 Diabetes With Cardiac Risk: Mildred Dodge, the Bonbon Eater** *(continued)*

reduction in the level of HDL-C, which means less removal of LDL-C. The LDL-C deposits as plaque in the blood vessels, narrowing and decreasing blood flow to all tissues and especially to coronary arteries.

The elevated LDL-C levels in Mrs. Dodge may lead to atherosclerosis, or hardening and obstruction of her coronary blood vessels, and possibly lead to heart attacks.

Mrs. Dodge's hs-CRP level was elevated, which indicates an acute inflammation possibly from cardiac origin. With elevated lipid values and this elevated hs-CRP, Mrs. Dodge needs to be monitored with ECG and other cardiac tests for heart muscle damage. This event at the zoo may have been an early warning sign for her and her physician to make changes to better manage the diabetes and hyperlipidemia conditions. The ECG performed on Mrs. Dodge based on the chest pains she experienced showed that she had angina but had not experienced heart muscle death, abnormal heart rhythm, or heart attack yet. With her elevated lipoprotein and inflammatory values, she will need to be placed on medication to prevent her heart ailment from becoming more serious.

Statin drugs are capable of inhibiting HMG-CoA reductase, the enzyme in the committed step of cholesterol synthesis. This enzyme catalyzes the conversion of 3-OH-3-methylglutaryl-CoA to mevalonate, a precursor to the formation of cholesterol.[1] When HMG-CoA reductase is inhibited, such as by statin medications, less cholesterol is formed. Statin drugs are very effective in reducing cholesterol, but in some patients the drugs cause harmful side effects such as muscle weakness and pain. Patients taking statin drugs should be monitored with periodic serum CK and CK-MM levels, with removal of the drug when muscle pain or CK-MM elevations unrelated to other pathology are present.[18] ●

statin - medication used to control hypercholesterolemia by affecting metabolism of cholesterol

Primary and Secondary Hyperlipoproteinemia

Elevations of LDLs and HDLs can rarely result from inborn errors of metabolism such as enzyme or apoprotein deficiencies or, more commonly, from secondary causes or underlying diseases. Generally, secondary diseases are ruled out first before investigation into primary disorders begins. Some of the secondary diseases and medications that cause hyperlipoproteinemia have already been discussed, including diabetes mellitus, blood pressure medication, and certain estrogen hormone replacement therapies. Other disorders that can increase total cholesterol, LDL, and triglyceride levels include nephrotic syndrome, chronic renal failure, hepatic disorders including biliary obstruction, other acute and transient stress-related conditions, and medications such as corticosteroids.

Hypertriglyceridemia can result from enzyme deficiency or from abnormal forms of VLDL. One fairly common condition of triglyceride excess is familial hypertriglyceridemia (FHTG). In FHTG, the particle size but not the amount of VLDL is usually large. There is also increased cholesterol content of the VLDL particles but normal levels of LDL-C and apoproteins associated with LDL. These patients may be prone to acute pancreatitis. One notable cause of primary hypertriglyceridemia is deficiency in **lipoprotein lipase** activity. This enzyme is found

lipoprotein lipase - enzyme that catalyzes hydrolysis of triglycerides found on chylomicrons and VLDL in peripheral cells and the liver and converts dietary fats in the form of chylomicrons to remnants for the uptake of triglycerides in the liver. When lipoprotein lipase is absent, dietary fats are not properly metabolized, and circulating levels of chylomicrons cause lipemic serum even in a fasting state and serum triglyceride levels that are well in excess of 500 mg/dL. These patients are also prone to acute pancreatitis and skin and eye disorders.

CASE SCENARIO 8-3

Apolipoprotein A Deficiency: The Jogger

Kyle has come to the ED due to chest pain while jogging in his neighborhood. Kyle is a 33-year-old white male who normally jogs 3 to 5 miles several times a week. His past medical history is unremarkable, and he has regular annual check-ups, including routine physicals, complete blood count (CBC), and serum glucose, blood urea nitrogen (BUN), creatinine, electrolyte, and protein levels. Kyle has never had a serum cholesterol or lipid panel analysis but, due to the chest pain he recently experienced, the physician requests a cardiac panel, CBC, and ECG.

The ECG shows some abnormalities typical of angina, while the CBC is within normal reference ranges. The lipid panel, however, shows the following results:

Test	Kyle	Reference Ranges (or Risk Ranges)
Total cholesterol (mg/dL)	172	<200
Triglycerides (mg/dL)	122	<150
HDL-C (mg/dL)	0	>59
LDL-C (mg/dL)	148	<100
hs-CRP (μg/L)	4.1	<0.3

Given these results, the physician asks for a repeat of the lipid profile, particularly because the HDL-C is absent. The second set of laboratory results are comparable to the first, confirming absent HDL-C. Additional tests of Kyle's heart and blood vessels were performed, including **cardiac catheterization**, in which a small flexible tube is inserted into a vein or artery and is guided into the heart to detect pressures and patterns of blood flow and for injection of dye to observe images of the heart and coronary arteries. The results of Kyle's cardiac catheterization show a 70% blockage of one coronary artery and 50% blockages in the other two coronary arteries. Kyle's lack of detectable HDL-C was investigated further by assaying his blood for apoproteins A-I, A-II, B-100, C-I, C-II, C-III, and E. The results showed

- ApoA-I: absent
- ApoA-II: low
- ApoE: normal
- ApoC-III: normal
- ApoB-100: normal
- ApoC-I: normal
- ApoC-II: normal

cardiac catheterization - insertion of thin, flexible tube into the heart and coronary arteries for detecting blood pressure and flow and taking images

TABLE 8-4

Apoproteins

Lipoprotein	Associated Apoprotein
Chylomicrons	B-48, A-II, C-I, C-II, C-III, E
LDL	B-100
HDL	A-I, A-II, A-IV, C-I, C-II, C-III, E
VLDL	B-100, C-I, C-II, C-III, E, A-I

Apoproteins

Apoproteins are the proteins associated with the four main lipoproteins functioning as transport proteins for the lipids. Apoproteins, which are proteins made by the liver, are packaged with the VLDL and HDL as they are released from the liver. In the circulation, cells containing lipoprotein lipase metabolize VLDL, leading to LDL formation, which results in the release of apoproteins C and E, while keeping the apoprotein B-100. The loose apoproteins can be taken up by circulating HDL particles or they can be degraded into their amino acid constituents. The main types of apoproteins (A-I, A-II, B-48, B-100, C-I, C-II, C-III, and E) are listed in Table 8–4 along with the main lipoproteins associated with each apoprotein.

Apoproteins, like most proteins, have a genetic basis. Rather than a single chromosome containing the genetic code for all the apoproteins, the biological basis of each apoprotein is spread over different chromosomes. Apoprotein A-I and A-IV as well as apoprotein C-III are genetically housed on chromosome 11.[23–25] Apoprotein A-I is the major apoprotein on the HDL particle, making up 90% of the apoprotein found in HDL. Apoprotein A-I is a cofactor for the enzymatic action of **lecithin:cholesterol acyltransferase (LCAT)**, an enzyme in the circulation that esterifies a fatty acid to a cholesterol molecule. Transport of excess cholesterol by HDL can be facilitated by LCAT esterifying the cholesterol and making it less soluble. The cholesterol ester quickly enters the HDL particle to find a **hydrophobic** environment. Apoprotein A-IV also activates LCAT and so, as part of the HDL apoprotein array, assists in removing cholesterol excesses. Apoprotein C-III is an inhibitor of lipoprotein lipase, the enzyme responsible for hydrolysis of triglycerides in chylomicrons to form remnants, or of VLDL to form LDL.

Chromosome 2 has the code for both apoprotein (apo) B-100 and apoB-48.[26,27] ApoB-100 is attached to VLDL when it leaves the liver. In the degradation of VLDL to LDL, the apoB-100 stays attached. As the major apoprotein on the LDL particle, apoB-100 is the recognition point for the cell to recognize an LDL particle. Once the LDL is engulfed by the cell and broken into its constituent parts, the apoB-100 is degraded into its amino acids. ApoB-48 is attached to chylomicrons coming from the intestinal absorption of fats. As the chylomicron is degraded in the circulation, the apoB-48 stays attached. When the liver recognizes a chylomicron remnant, the liver engulfs the remnant and the apoprotein. Degradation of these products results in liver uptake of dietary fats.[26] Test Methodology 8–10 describes an immunoassay method of analysis for apoproteins.[28,29]

Apoproteins C-I, C-II, and E share chromosome 19 as their code location and share similar functions.[20,30] ApoC-I activates LCAT and is located on chylomicrons and VLDL and HDL lipoproteins. ApoC-II is an important cofactor for

lecithin:cholesterol acyltransferase - an enzyme that esterifies a fatty acid to cholesterol

hydrophobic - water insoluble

TEST METHODOLOGY 8-10. APOPROTEINS

Apoproteins can be measured by antigen-antibody assays in which antibody to a specific apoprotein is used to complex with the "antigen" apoprotein and no other. Enzyme-linked immunosorbent assays (ELISAs) use two antibodies to "sandwich" the apoprotein of interest.

The Reaction

In the antigen-antibody (Ab) assay, where X = any apoprotein, such as apoprotein A-I:

$$ApoX + Ab \leftrightarrow Ab\text{-}apoX$$
$$Ab\text{-}apoX + Ab_2 \text{ complex} \leftrightarrow Ab\text{-}apoX\text{-}Ab_2$$

The Specimen

Serum, plasma.

Reference Ranges

ApoA-I	94–199 mg/dL
ApoB-100	55–125 mg/dL

Other assays use different methods.

lipoprotein lipase. ApoC-II is also found on chylomicrons, VLDL, and HDL in the circulation. Apoprotein E is located on the same three lipoproteins as C-I and C-II, and its function is to aid in the uptake of chylomicron remnants by the liver. ApoE, genetically, has three alleles (e2, e3, and e4) that can combine in twos to make three possible apoE expressions. The combinations can be e2/2, e2/3, e2/4, e3/3, e3/4, and e4/4. The isoforms of apoE that are seen are labeled apoE2, apoE3, and apoE4. The apoE2 within chylomicrons and VLDL remnants shows a lower binding affinity with liver receptors than does the apoE3 form, which is associated with decreased clearing of chylomicrons and VLDL remnants from the bloodstream. ApoE4 has an increased affinity for the receptors to the point that they block the liver receptors with their binding. ApoE3 isoforms are highest in frequency and have a normal clearing rate for chylomicron and VLDL remnants.[20,25] Figure 8–5 shows the relationship of the apoproteins and metabolism.

Hypoalphalipoproteinemia

The absence or a nondetectable level of apoprotein A-I is exhibited by a severely decreased or absent level of HDL-C. This was the true in the case of Kyle Minute. A condition in which the apoprotein A-I is absent is called Tangier's disease or hypoalphalipoproteinemia. This condition leads to elevated LDL in the circulation with no viable HDL action to remove cholesterol from the tissues. Apoprotein A-I is the major apoprotein associated with HDL and is necessary for the enzyme LCAT to function. LCAT joins a fatty acid to cholesterol, an alcohol, to make a cholesterol ester. These cholesterol esters can be packaged into the HDL particles for transport to the liver, causing the HDL particle to go from disk shape to spherical shape in the circulation. When apoprotein A-I is absent, LCAT is unable to function and esterification of cholesterol is diminished. Plaque buildup and blockage of blood vessels from excessive LDL-C levels can occur and lead to coronary

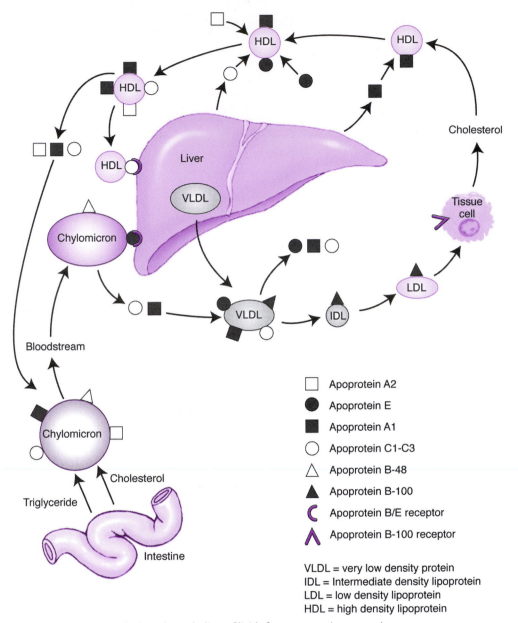

Figure 8–5. Liver synthesis and metabolism of lipids from apoprotein perspective.

heart disease (CHD). Heart aliments related to hypoalphalipoproteinemia include atherosclerosis, myocardial infarctions, and strokes, as well as some circulation problems seen as peripheral neuropathies.[23,30]

Hyperbetalipoproteinemia

Other genetic variants of apoproteins common to people of European descent include hyperbetalipoprotein or familial defective apoB-100, in which there is an absence of normal apoprotein B-100 due to an amino acid substitution in the B-100 structure. With an abnormal structure of apoprotein B, there is a lack of

LDL uptake by the steroid-generating tissues because of poor receptor specificity. This leads to deposition of cholesterol esters in tissues, hepatomegaly, and even loss of eyesight due to clouding of the cornea.[26,27,31] Heterozygote variants have some normal apoB-100 and therefore exhibit less severe problems. A pattern for a patient with hyperbetalipoproteinemia would be as follows:

Test	Result	Low Risk Category
Total cholesterol (mg/dL)	300	<200
Triglycerides (mg/dL)	150	<150
HDL-C (mg/dL)	52	>59
LDL-C (mg/dL)	218	<100

Abnormalities With Apoprotein E

Variants of apoprotein E may have significance for atherosclerosis, **Alzheimer's disease**, and **cerebrovascular accidents** such as strokes. The phenotype E4/E4 may well be associated with Alzheimer's disease, the progressive neurological disease characterized by profound memory loss and confusion.[25,32] Variants of apoE may have importance in characterizing a type of hyperlipoproteinemia in which there are elevated intermediate-density lipoprotein (IDL) levels, demonstrating a broad pre-beta band with an electrophoretic procedure. The phenotype for this elevated IDL is often described as the isoform apoE2 homozygote.[32-34]

Alzheimer's disease - progressive brain disorder with deterioration of mental capacity affecting memory and judgment

cerebrovascular accident - stroke or sudden loss of blood flow to the brain due to obstruction or clot in the blood vessels

CLINICAL CORRELATION
Apoprotein E isoform E4 has been associated with Alzheimer's disease, while apoprotein E isoform E2 heterozygosity can be a marker for increased atherosclerosis and possible stroke and myocardial infarction.

Case Scenario 8-3 Apolipoprotein A Deficiency: The Jogger

Follow-Up

Kyle's absence of apoprotein A-I led to an increase in the atherosclerotic process resulting in coronary artery blockage. Kyle met with a nutritionist to learn about diet changes and was prescribed medications to lower his LDL cholesterol by his physician. Kyle was counseled that he was at risk for bypass surgery if the coronary arteries continued to develop plaque deposits. His exercise program was considered an advantage, so he was sent for an exercise consult with the physical therapy department for modifications to help lower his LDL cholesterol. The statin medication he was prescribed was necessary to lower his LDL even though his total cholesterol was less than 200 mg/dL. The relationship between elevated LDL cholesterol and increases in atherosclerosis has been shown through numerous studies, with the Framingham study being one of the earliest examinations of this problem. ●

Abetalipoproteinemia

Absence of lipoproteins containing apolipoprotein B, including LDL and VLDL, is a rare genetic disorder. People with abetalipoproteinemia have extremely low levels of total cholesterol and the vast majority is HDL-C. They also have low levels of triglycerides. The disorder becomes evident in infants with fat absorption problems and difficulty in weight gain and growth. Characteristic of these individuals is red blood cell membrane defects, including acanthocytes, or thorn-shaped erythrocytes. Without treatment, these children develop severe vision, neurological, and mobility problems.[14]

CASE SCENARIO 8-4

Congestive Heart Failure: Joe Returns

Several months have passed since Joe Smoker had an AMI, but he has not been following the protocols prescribed by his physician. Joe takes blood pressure and anticoagulant medicine, but his diet has slipped back to his old habits of eating saturated fats, fried foods, and red meat. Joe's exercise program stopped once the physical therapy visits were no longer covered by his insurance. On a recent clinic visit to the cardiologist, the physician encourages him to follow the treatment regimen and to get some regular exercise or "pay the consequences, Joe." Joe assures Dr. Jordan he will, leaves the office, and lights up a cigarette.

About 6 months later, Joe is experiencing difficulty in breathing. His wife rushes him to the emergency department, fearing another heart attack. The ED is quite busy at this time, but they bring Joe into an examination room for evaluation. Blood work is sent to the laboratory with orders for cardiac markers and therapeutic drug monitoring (TDM) of his medication. A b-type natriuretic peptide (BNP) assay is also ordered to check for heart versus pulmonary congestion.

Patients who have had severe or repeated myocardial infarctions (MIs) are at risk for developing congestive heart failure (CHF). Congestive heart failure is the condition in which the heart is unable to pump out the required volume of blood and fluid accumulates in the chest. In left-sided CHF, the left ventricle has weakened because of muscle damage often secondary to MI. A weakness in the left ventricle leads to edema of the tissues because more blood enters the heart from the veins than leaves through the arteries. Edema is most evident first in the extremities, such as the ankles and legs. In addition, capillary circulation is slower, with water and waste products accumulating. The collected blood leads to expansion and enlargement of the ventricle. Symptoms of CHF include edema, increased blood pressure, shortness of breath and easy fatigue, dizziness, difficulty in walking short distances, and compromised renal function as blood pressure rises and circulation becomes diminished. CHF can result from not following treatment plans at the first sign of heart disease.[35,36]

NATRIURETIC PEPTIDES

The body's natural reaction to the fluid expansion in CHF is to release brain or b-type natriuretic peptide (BNP) from the heart muscle of the left ventricle.[35] Release of this peptide hormone acts on the kidneys to increase excretion of the fluid. This helps to decrease the cellular edema and the load on the left ventricle of the heart. BNP serum levels are typically greater than 100 pg/mL in patients with CHF. Other causes of cellular edema, including pulmonary edema, do not cause an elevation of BNP. Thus, BNP is a specific marker of edema due to heart failure.[35–37] BNP is one of three peptides that can be released from the heart muscle. Atrial natriuretic peptide (ANP) is released from atrium heart muscle to affect the sodium level of the fluids. While aldosterone encourages conservation of sodium, ANP stimulates sodium release. CNP, or c-type natriuretic peptide, affects the central nervous system and is believed to be a neuropeptide.[35] BNP increases the urine output of the kidney, typically in association with compensation for fluid accumulation associated with CHF.

Case Scenario 8-4 Congestive Heart Failure: Joe Returns

Follow-Up

The blood results for Joe Smoker reveal the following:

Test	Joe	Reference Ranges
CK-MB (%)	<5	<3.9
CK total (IU/L)	183	46–171
Troponin I (ng/mL)	0.45	<0.5
BNP (pg/mL)	185	<100*

*Instrument-specific range.

Since the troponin I and CK-MB levels are below the medical decision limits, the ED physician reassures Mrs. Smoker that Joe is not having a heart attack. However, the elevated BNP indicates Joe has CHF. The physician counsels Joe to stop smoking, increase his exercise level, eat a diet low in fat, and take his medications. He provides information on a smoking cessation program and refers Joe back to his cardiologist for continued therapy. ●

CASE SCENARIO 8-5

Silent Myocardial Infarction: Woman at Risk

At the same time as Joe is being evaluated in the ED, Lindsey Walters, a 62-year-old woman from Dr. Jordan's office, enters the ED by ambulance. Her husband says she fell down some stairs at their home and injured her right leg. He also reveals that Lindsey had some chest pain and discomfort in her left arm a couple of days ago, but did not let him call her physician. She thought she might have some indigestion and so brushed away her husband's concerns. The ED team taking care of Lindsey finds her semiconscious but responsive to their questions. They order a chemistry metabolic profile, a CBC, and right leg x-rays to determine what may be wrong with Lindsey. The treating physician also requests cardiac markers on Lindsey.

WHY WOMEN AND MEN EXPERIENCE DIFFERENT RISK FOR HEART ATTACKS

The Food and Drug Administration (FDA) and American Heart Association suggest that women are protected from heart attacks due to lipid plaque before they reach menopause. Estrogen levels in younger women are typically a factor causing them to maintain high levels of HDL in most situations. Once menopause occurs, women experience a reduction in HDL as their estrogen levels decline. Postmenopausal women are at the same risk for coronary artery disease and heart attack as men, particularly if they have risk factors of smoking, elevated cholesterol, elevated triglycerides, family history, and/or elevated blood pressure.[9,10,17,18]

It has only been through recent research that the effect of lowered estrogen levels in postmenopausal women with coronary artery disease has become evident. Previously risk of heart attacks was not studied in women because it was not considered a common event. Also, there currently is evidence that women do not express the same physical symptoms of a heart attack as do men. Women may have a "silent heart attack" in which they feel milder and less specific chest pain than men. Women having heart attacks complain of indigestion, abdominal pain, even lower back pain. These are not the characteristic midchest pain and pain radiating up the left arm and neck that are common in men. Because of the difference in or milder symptoms, women tend to ignore the possibility that they are having a heart attack.

DELAYED DIAGNOSIS OF AMI

Delay in seeking a diagnosis renders CK and CK-MB useless as markers of AMI because of their quick resolution to normal values within 48 hours after the onset of MI. In the past, LD isoenzymes were used to indicate that a heart attack had occurred when the patient did not seek treatment immediately. Test Methodologies 8–11 and 8–12 describe LD and LD isoenzyme methods of analysis. Problems with specificity of LD and LD isoenzyme results were discussed earlier. Newer, more specific tests such as troponin assays are currently recommended.[14]

Troponin assays offer increased opportunities to detection "silent heart attacks" in patients, especially women. Elevated serum troponin levels can be sustained for 14 days after onset of AMI, making this marker invaluable in detecting heart attacks in those patients who do not have the typical symptoms. Troponin I or T is replacing LD isoenzymes studies, CK total, and CK-MB detection as the marker of choice for cardiac dysfunctions as seen in AMIs.[2,3,7]

✓ **Common Sense Check**

Hemolysis causes visible red pigmentation to the serum or plasma when the ruptured red blood cells release hemoglobin, LD, and other substances from the cells. A hemolyzed specimen should be rejected and re-collected in a manner than minimizes chances for hemolysis, which would falsely increase LD and LD1.

TEST METHODOLOGY 8-11.   LACTATE DEHYDROGENASE

This serum enzyme test was used historically to detect myocardial damage following delay in seeking diagnosis and treatment of a heart attack. It also is used to detect elevations in serum levels associated with cellular liver damage, megaloblastic anemias, and certain tumors.

In the LD reaction, lactate is the substrate that the LD converts to pyruvate in the presence of NAD, which converts to NADH. This reaction is read at 340 nm spectrophotometrically.

The Reaction

$$\text{Lactate} + \text{NAD} \leftrightarrow \text{pyruvate} + \text{NADH}$$

The Specimen

Serum, nonhemolyzed and analyzed within a few hours or kept refrigerated, not frozen.

Reference Range

180–360 IU/L

TEST METHODOLOGY 8-12. LACTATE DEHYDROGENASE ISOENZYME

There are five isoenzymes of LD, which is a tetramer using a combination of H and/or M subunits. The LD1 isoenzyme has four H units, while the LD5 has four M units. A flipped pattern in which more LD1 is present than LD2 is associated with cardiac muscle damage following myocardial infarction as well as hemolytic or megaloblastic anemia. The LD isoenzymes can be separated by electrophoresis, or the LD1 and LD2 isoenzymes can be isolated out using antigen-antibody reactions. Automation of the isoenzyme separation can be accomplished using antigen-antibody reactions.

The Reaction

Serum + anti-LD-M → serum (H) + complexed LD-M–anti-LD-M
Assay serum (H) for LD content = concentration of LD1

The Specimen

Serum.

Reference Ranges

LD1	14–26 (% of total LD)
LD2	29–39%
LD3	20–26%
LD4	8–16%
LD5	6–16%

Case Scenario 8-5 Silent Myocardial Infarction: Woman at Risk

Follow-Up

Radiographic (x-ray) images showed that Lindsey broke her ankle, so a cast was applied to her foot and calf for 6 weeks. Her clinical laboratory results obtained during the ED visit showed the following:

Test	Lindsey	Reference Ranges
CK total (IU/L)	157	34–145
CK-MB (%)	3.0	<3.9% of total CK
LD total (IU/L)	503	180–360
LD1/LD2	1.0	0.5–0.8
Troponin (ng/mL)	1.2	0.0–0.5

Her troponin level was elevated, indicating that she had experienced an AMI but delayed in seeking diagnosis. Because of the time frame, troponin was the only cardiac marker that still showed a clear indication that an MI had occurred. The CK-MB was within normal limits because it returns to normal level after peaking 18 to 24 hours post-MI. The LD flip was not clear cut, although the LD1 was at the same level as the LD 2, indicating that the LD1 was elevated. Pinpointing the MI using the LD isoenzymes alone would not be sufficient evidence of an MI given its lack of specificity to cardiac muscle damage. The troponin level is clearly above the upper limit of the reference range and so demonstrates that an MI has occurred.

continued

Case Scenario 8-5 **Silent Myocardial Infarction: Woman at Risk** *(continued)*

Current recommendations by national experts, including the American Association of Clinical Chemists, advise the use of serum troponin levels in place of LD isoenzymes for diagnosis of delayed MI.[1]

Lindsey was admitted to the hospital and supportive treatment was given. Her "silent MI" was treated with supportive care and observation. Dr. Jordan, her physician, prescribed medications, diet, and exercise. ●

CASE SCENARIO 8-6

Medication Toxicity: Age-Related Drug Distribution

Ambrose Peterson is an 81-year-old, retired school teacher. He has been seeing Dr. Jordan for heart and blood pressure problems for 10 years. Mr. Peterson lives at the Middle Brook assisted living facility. Previous laboratory results obtained at the physician's office included a BUN of 45 mg/dL (reference range 8 to 23) and creatinine of 1.8 mg/dL (0.8 to 1.3). Mr. Peterson takes digoxin, a diuretic, and blood pressure medication.

It has been 6 months since Mr. Peterson has had a cardiologist office visit. He is currently being sent to the ED by ambulance because he shows symptoms of extreme disorientation. He is thrashing his arms and his body movements are aggressive. Ambrose is vomiting, confused, and complaining about the light hurting his eyes. At the ED, the physician reviews his history. Mr. Peterson is taking digoxin for his heart, diuretic medicine for his kidney, and blood pressure medications. The physician orders some clinical chemistry tests, a CBC, and a serum digoxin level. Digoxin is a cardioactive medication that helps to maintain strong pumping action and regular rhythm of the heart muscle contractions. The laboratory results are

Test	Ambrose	Reference Ranges (Age-Specific)
Digoxin (ng/mL)	2.2	0.5–1.5
BUN (mg/dL)	62	8–23
Creatinine (mg/dL)	2.8	0.8–1.3
Potassium (mmol/L)	4.9	3.5–4.5
CBC	Normal	

DIFFERENCES IN ELDERLY PATIENTS

Elderly patients may have electrolyte distribution that differs from younger adults. This difference in distribution of water and electrolytes can adversely affect the elderly when taking certain medications, such as diuretics and blood pressure medications. Many diuretics can affect electrolyte levels, especially sodium (Na^+) and potassium (K^+) distribution and excretion. Diuretic medications affect the kidneys and cause excretion of potassium. Replacement of potassium is needed in many elderly patients in order to maintain electrolyte balance and heart pacemaker rhythm. Blood pressure medications also may lead to sodium changes if there is a water imbalance due to the diuretics and potassium losses. In particular, plasma sodium levels may rise due to excessive water and potassium loss associated with diuretic medications.[38]

Kidney function declines in the elderly due to a natural decrease in glomerular filtration rate. However, BUN and creatinine levels in the elderly usually remain within normal reference ranges due to the loss of body mass that also occurs with aging. Renal insufficiency can be common in the elder and can complicate drug excretion. This must be taken into consideration when health-care professionals consider the drug dosage in elderly patients and utilize therapeutic drug monitoring (TDM). Renal clearance of digoxin is normally 50% to 80% with a half-life, or decline to half its amount after absorption and distribution to the tissues, of 36 hours. When renal function declines, as seen in the elderly, the level of digoxin in the circulation remains elevated longer. The half-life has been known to increase to 5 days in patients with renal insufficiency over the typical 36 hours when renal function is normal. Digoxin levels correlate with tissue levels but are higher in tissue than blood.[39,40] Digoxin is secreted by glomerular filtration but also by the renal tubular cells via a special pump that facilitates digoxin excretion.[38] Chapter 6 (Assessment of Renal Function) contains more information about kidney function tests.

Distribution of digoxin is also affected by the change in body fat typical in the elderly. As body fat declines in an older patient, the drug distribution (including digoxin) shifts from fat stores to interstitial spaces and higher drug serum concentrations are seen. The usual adequate dose of digoxin is now potentially high enough to be toxic in the elderly patient due to the lack of body fat where the drug is usually sequestered. If the elderly patient also has renal insufficiency, drug toxicity becomes more likely because of less renal elimination. More details about the effect of digoxin and the requirements of TDM can be found in Chapter 14 (Therapeutic Drug Monitoring and Toxicology).

Case Scenario 8-6 Medication Toxicity: Age-Related Drug Distribution

Follow-Up

Ambrose Peterson is now exhibiting digoxin toxicity in the ED, including vomiting and confusion because of decreased body fat with less tissue distribution of the drug. He also has declining renal function as indicated by elevated urea nitrogen, creatinine, and potassium. His blood digoxin levels are increased to toxic levels most likely due to a combination of both situations. Drug dosage changes and monitoring of this patient need to take into account his increasing renal insufficiency.

In the ED, it is evident that Mr. Peterson is dehydrated. His elevated potassium and urea nitrogen may also be related to that dehydration. The digoxin toxicity is treated with digoxin-specific Fab fragments to bind the interstitial digoxin and neutralize its effects.[39] This treatment is known to cause hypokalemia, so the ED closely monitors Mr. Peterson's electrolytes. His potassium at first elevates to 5.8 mmol/L and then decreases to 2.7 mol/L (reference range 3.5 to 4.5). The ED staff closely monitors Mr. Peterson and gives him supportive IV fluids. Laboratory monitoring of his electrolytes and other chemistries continues for several days as the digoxin toxicity is corrected and electrolyte levels return to normal. ●

CASE SCENARIO 8-7

The Clot Thickens: Joe Returns Again

One month later, Joe is examined by Dr. Jordan and has his BNP level checked. The BNP is still high at 125 pg/mL (reference range <100 pg/mL). Dr. Jordan orders serum Lp(a) and homocysteine tests. Lp(a) and homocysteine are independent risk factors for cardiac disease.

Lipoprotein (a)

Lipoprotein (a) (Lp(a)) is unique among the lipoproteins. It is thought to be an unusual type of LDL particle with an apoprotein a attached to the apoprotein B. Because there is variability in the structure of apoprotein a, it is very difficult to assay and detect all the possible variants. The uniqueness of Lp(a) is also related to its similarity to plasminogen. Plasminogen, when converted to plasmin in the blood, is instrumental in degrading the incidental clots that are formed periodically in blood vessels. When plasmin is not available, little clots become big ones and can lead to blood vessel occlusions. High Lp(a) levels inhibit plasmin formation by attracting the plasminogen activators and blocking their action. Thus, high levels of Lp(a) are an independent risk factor for patients. If patients have elevated levels of Lp(a), their blood tends to clot.[41] Test Methodology 8–13 describes a method of analysis for Lp(a).

TEST METHODOLOGY 8-13.   LIPOPROTEIN (a)

This enzyme-linked immunosorbent assay (ELISA) assay uses a polyclonal antibody specific to lipoprotein (a) (Lp(a)) and a monoclonal antibody with specificity for apoprotein B. After an incubation step, an enzyme-conjugate is attached to a second antibody to apo-B. When substrate is added the enzyme catalyzes the formation of product that is read spectrophotometrically.

The Reaction

$$\text{Ab–apo-a} + \text{Ab-apoB} + \text{sample} \leftrightarrow \text{apo-a–apoB complex}$$
$$+ \text{Ab}_2\text{-enzyme} \rightarrow \text{new complex} + \text{substrate} \rightarrow \text{product}$$

The Specimen

Serum.

Reference Range

<30 mg/dL

Homocysteine

Homocysteine is also an independent risk factor for cardiac disease. Often this marker is prominent in a family at risk for cardiac disease, but some evidence has linked it to men at risk who already exhibit some cardiac problems. Homocysteine and Lp(a) together are a strong predictors of coronary artery disease in women.[41] Homocysteine is an intermediate in the pathway between methionine and cysteine. Homocysteine along with folic acid will form cysteine, a necessary sulfur-containing amino acid. Then, at times of low methionine concentrations, homocysteine will convert to methionine. Homocysteine is a clinically significant marker of homocytinuria and for folic acid deficiency, but its recognition as a cardiac risk factor marker is more recent.[14] Test Methodology 8–14 describes a method of analysis for homocysteine.

TEST METHODOLOGY 8-14.   HOMOCYSTEINE

All forms of homocysteine (Hcy) are reduced to free homocysteine. Reduced homocysteine binds with fluorescent-labeled antibody (F-Ab) to form a complex. Fluorescence is detected that relates directly to the amount of homocysteine present in the patient's serum.

The Reaction

$$Serum + reducing\ agent \rightarrow serum\text{-}Hcy$$

$$Serum\text{-}Hcy + F\text{-}Ab\text{-}Hcy \rightarrow F\text{-}Ab\text{-}Hcy\text{-}serum$$

Read fluorescence either in a polarization device or a fluorometer.

The Specimen

Serum.

Reference Range

<5 µmol/L

Case Scenario 8-7 The Clot Thickens: Joe Returns Again

Follow-Up

Joe's blood results showed that his homocysteine level was 27 µmol/L (reference range <15 µmol/L) and his Lp(a) was 25 mg/dL (<30 mg/dL). This indicates an elevated homocysteine level but normal Lp(a) level in his serum. Dr. Jordan told Joe that men who smoke and have high homocyteine levels are at risk for coronary artery disease and blood clots. Given Joe's history of cardiac problems, he will need to change his diet and lifestyle. Dr. Jordan also decided to continue anticoagulant therapy to decrease Joe's risk of clots and a possible embolism.[42] ●

SUMMARY

These patients illustrate the laboratory's role in assessing cardiovascular risk, congestive heart failure, cardiogenic drug toxicity, and acute myocardial infarction. As we followed Joe, you could see how one patient's cardiac problems can become complicated over time due to the progression of the illness. Joe showed diagnoses of AMI with progression to CHF and risk for clotting and embolism. Mildred showed cardiac complications that can occur with type 2 diabetes. The role of apoproteins in lipid metabolism and cardiac risk was demonstrated in the case of Kyle Minute. Gender differences in cardiac presentation were shown through

Lindsey Walters, who had angina, while age differences and drug toxicity were shown in the case of Ambrose Peterson. These patients help us to see the importance of laboratory assessment in aiding other health-care providers with the information they need to treat and advise the patient.

EXERCISES

As you consider the scenarios presented in this chapter, answer the following questions:

1. List the recommended tests for myocardial infarction and explain the role of each in the detection of that condition.

2. Describe the specimen requirements for testing for troponins, a lipid profile, and cardiac enzymes.

3. Describe the influence of diabetes on cardiac disease.

4. Describe the methods used to assay for CK, CK-MB, cardiac troponins, and LD.

5. Describe the methods of the cholesterol, triglyceride, and HDL cholesterol analyses, including sources of interferences.

6. Describe the role of apoproteins in cardiac assessment.

7. Describe the importance of renal function testing and therapeutic drug monitoring when drug toxicity is suspected in elderly cardiac patients.

8. Describe laboratory markers for CHF and the inflammatory stage of MI.

9. Explain the importance of hs-CRP, homocysteine, and Lp(a) for the assessment of cardiac disease.

References

1. Rosalki SB, et al: Cardiac biomarkers for detection of myocardial infarction: perspectives from past to present. *Clin Chem* 2004; 50:2205–2213.

2. Costa MA, et al: Incidence, predictors, and significance of abnormal cardiac enzyme rise in patients treated with bypass surgery in the Arterial Revascularization Therapies Study (ARTS). *Circulation* 2001; 104:2689.

3. Reddy GC, et al: Cardiac troponin-T and CK-MB (mass) levels in cardiac and non-cardiac disease. *Ind J Clin Biochem* 2004; 19(2):91–94.

4. Katus HA, et al: Development of in vitro characterization of a new immunoassay of cardiac troponin T. *Clin Chem* 1992; 36:386–393.

5. Christenson RH, et al: Cardiac troponin I measurement with the ACCESS® immunoassay system: analytical and clinical performance characteristics. *Clin Chem* 1998; 44:52–60.

6. Di Serio F, et al: Analytical evaluation of an automated immunoassay for cardiac troponin I: the Vidas Troponin I assay. *Clin Chem* 2003; 10:1363–1368.

7. Bachmaier K, et al: Serum cardiac troponin T and creatine kinase-MB elevations in murine autoimmune myocarditis. *Circulation* 1995; 92:1927–1932.

8. Aviles RJ, et al: Troponin T levels in patients with acute coronary syndromes with or without renal dysfunction. *N Engl J Med* 2002; 346:2047–2052.

9. Katus HA, et al: Diagnostic efficiency of troponin T measurements in acute myocardial infarction. *Circulation* 119, 83:902–912.

10. Vikenes K, et al: Cardiac biochemical markers after cardioversion of atrial fibrillation or atrial flutter. *Am Heart J* 2000; 140:690–695.

11. Ripoll E, et al: Evaluation of a new chemiluminescent, microparticle-based assay for troponin I on ARCHITECT instrument system. Poster presented at the Euromedlab meeting, Glasgow, May 8–12, 2005.

12. Wu AH, et al: Cardiac troponin-T immunoassay for diagnosis of acute myocardial infarction. *Clin Chem* 1994; 40:90–907.

13. Heeschen C, et al: Evaluation of a rapid whole blood ELISA for quantification of troponin I in patients with acute chest pain. *Clin Chem* 1999; 45:1789–96.

14. Burtis CA, Ashwood ER (eds): *Tietz Fundamentals of Clinical Chemistry*, ed 5. Philadelphia: WB Saunders, 2001.

15. TECO Diagnostics: Technical bulletin on CK-MB reagent set. Anaheim, CA: TECO Diagnostics, 2001.

16. Cleveland Clinic: List of blood tests for determining risk of coronary artery diseases. Available at *www.clevelandclinic.org/heartcenter/pub/guide/tests/labtests/testscad.htm*

17. Singh V: New ATP III lipid guidelines update for patients at high risk for cardiovascular events. July 2005. Available at *www.emedicine.com*

18. Nachimuthu S, Varghese C: Statins: Cardiovascular disease regression and plaque stabilization. June 2005. Available at *www.emedicine.com*

19. Lusis AJ, et al: Regional mapping of human chromosome 19: organization of genes for plasma lipid transport (APO C1, -C2, and -E and LDLR) and the genes *C3*, *PEPD*, and *GP1*. *Proc Natl Acad Sci U S A* 1986; 83:3929–3933.

20. American Diabetes Association: Diagnosis and classification of diabetes mellitus. *Diabetes Care* 2004; 27(Suppl 1):S5–S10.

21. American Heart Association: Available at *www.americanheart.org* (accessed March 30, 2006).

22. Expert Panel on Detection, Evaluation and Treatment of High Blood Cholesterol in Adults: Executive summary of the third report of the National Cholesterol Education Program Expert Panel on Detection, Evaluation and Treatment of High Blood Cholesterol in Adults (Adult Treatment Panel III). *JAMA* 2001; 285:2486–2497.

23. Cohen JC, et al: Multiple rare alleles contribute to low plasma levels of HDL-cholesterol. *Science* 2004; 305:869–872.

24. Chroni A, et al: Deletions of helices 2 and 3 of human apoA-I are associated with severe dyslipidemia following adenovirus-mediated gene transfer in apoA-I-deficient mice. *Biochemistry* 2005; 44:4108–4117.

25. Masson LF, McNeill G, Avenull A: Genetic variation and the lipid response to dietary intervention: a systematic review. *Am J Clin Nutr* 2003; 77:1098–1111.

26. Aguilar-Salinas CA, et al: Apoprotein B-100 production is decreased in subjects heterozygous for truncations of apoprotein B. *Arterioscler Thromb Vasc Biol* 1995; 15:71–80.

27. Chan DC, et al: ATP-binding cassette transporter G8 gene as a determinant of apolipoprotein B-100 kinetics in overweight men. *Arterioscler Thromb Vasc Biol* 2004; 24:2188.

28. Fu M, et al: Competitive enzyme immunoassay for human serum apolipoproteins C1, C11 and C111. *Clin Chim Acta* 1987; 167:339–340.

29. Stein AV, Myers GL: Lipids, lipoproteins, and apolipoproteins. In Burtis CA, Ashwood ER (eds): *Tietz textbook of clinical chemistry*, ed 2. Philadelphia: WB Saunders, 1994, pp 1085–1087.

30. Liu L, et al: Effects of apolipoprotein A-1 on ATP-binding cassette transporter A-1 mediated efflux of macrophage phospholipid and cholesterol. *J Biochem* 2003; 278:42976–42984.

31. Online Mendelian Inheritance in Man: Abetalipoproteinemia (alternative titles: acanthocytosis, Bassen-Kornzweig syndrome, apolipoprotein B deficiency, microsomal triglyceride transfer protein deficiency, MTP deficiency). Available at *www.ncbi.nlm.nih.gov/entrez/dispomim.cgi?id=200100* (accessed September 2005).

32. Jong MC, Hofker MH, Havekes LM: Role of ApoCs in lipoprotein metabolism: functional differences between ApoC1, ApoC2, and ApoC3. *Arterioscler Thromb Vasc Biol* 1999; 19:472–484.

33. Moreno JA, et al: The effect of dietary fat on LDL size is influenced by apolipoprotein E genotype in healthy subjects. *J Nutr* 2004; 134:2517–2522.

34. Gylling H, Kontula K, Miettinen TA: Cholesterol absorption and metabolism and LDL kinetics in healthy men with different apoprotein E phenotypes and apoprotein B Xba I and LDL receptor Pvu II genotypes. *Arterioscler Thromb Vasc Biol* 1995; 15:208–213.

35. Mitchell JE, Palta S: New diagnostic modalities in the diagnosis of heart failure. *J Natl Med Assoc* 2004; 96:1424–1430.

36. Lubarsky L, Mandell K, Coplan NL: B-type natriuretic peptide: practical diagnostic use for evaluating ventricular dysfunction. *Congestive Heart Fail* 2004; 10:140–143.

37. Squire LI, Davies JE, Ng LL: Reference ranges for natriuretic peptides for diagnostic use are dependent on age, gender, and heart rate. *Eur J Heart Fail* 2003; 10:599–606.

38. Dec GW: Digoxin remains useful in the management of chronic heart failure. *Med Clin North Am* 2003; 87:317–337.

39. Marik PE, Fromm L: A case series of hospitalized patients with elevated digoxin levels. *Am J Med* 1998; 105:110–115.

40. Wofford JL, Ettinger WH: Risk factors and manifestations of digoxin toxicity in elderly. *Am J Emerg Med* 1991; 9(2 Suppl 1):11–15.

41. Foody JM, et al: Homocysteine and lipoprotein (a) interact to increase CAD risk in young men and women. *Arterioscler Thromb Vasc Biol* 2000; 20:493–499.

42. Tanne D, et al: Prospective study of serum homocysteine and risk of ischemic stroke among patients with pre-existing coronary heart disease. *Stroke* 2003; 34:632–636.

9

The clinical laboratory is an important partner in the assessment of respiratory disorders.

Assessment of Respiratory Disorders

Joshua R. Schuetz and Wendy Arneson

Arterial blood gases and oxygen saturation provide vital information to clinicians and members of the health-care team. In some settings the respiratory care technologist collects and analyzes the arterial blood gases, while in other settings laboratory personnel perform collection and/or analysis. Since these results are so important in assessing the vital status of the patient and for treatment, it is necessary to have a teamwork approach when dealing with arterial blood gas testing.

OBJECTIVES

Upon completion of this chapter, the student will have the ability to

■ Discuss sample preparation for arterial blood gas analysis and co-oximetry.

■ Calculate H_2CO_3, HCO_3^-, oxygen capacity, and oxygen content.

■ Correlate arterial blood gas, oxygenation, and carboxyhemoglobin results with previous findings and with pathology of acid-base and oxygenation disturbances.

■ Discuss sources of discrepancy in terms of preanalytical and analytical errors in arterial blood gases, oxygen, and carboxyhemoglobin testing.

■ Discuss main steps needed for sample collection of arterial and venous samples by laboratory and other appropriate personnel.

■ Explain the typical causes, signs, symptoms, and laboratory indicators of respiratory illnesses, including chronic bronchitis, adult respiratory failure, and neonatal respiratory distress.

CASE SCENARIO 9-1

Arterial Blood Gas Collection and Specimen Handling: The Case of the Pink Patient With a Dark Blood Sample

The medical technologist was asked to collect and analyze arterial blood gases from a 54-year-old male recovering from coronary artery bypass graft (CABG) surgery, 1 hour after he was weaned from the ventilator. His **ventilation** rate and coloration appeared relatively normal. Results obtained from the blood gas analysis are as follows:

Test	Patient	Reference Ranges
pH	7.33	7.35–7.45
P_{CO_2} (mm Hg)	49	35–48
P_{O_2} (mm Hg)	58	83–108
HCO_3^- (mmol/L)	25	19–24

Looking at these results, the technologist considered preanalytical and analytical variations, including typical specimen collection and handling requirements and sources of interferences.

---

ventilation - air exchange between lungs and gases inhaled and exhaled; designated as V

COLLECTION AND HANDLING OF ARTERIAL BLOOD GASES

The specimen for blood gases and pH should be arterial or arterialized capillary blood collected in heparinized plastic containers including syringes and capillary tubes. All air bubbles should be removed, and the needle replaced or the ends of the capillary tube fitted with a tight-fitting cover. Air bubbles frequently form during syringe collection but must be expelled before mixing the specimen. The container should hold the correct amount of heparin (0.05 mg heparin/mL blood) and, after blood is added, it should be mixed well and be properly labeled with identification verified against the patient's identification. The specimen must be placed in ice water until analysis, unless it is analyzed immediately at the patient's bedside. Temperatures warmer than 4°C allow cell glycolysis to continue in the whole blood specimen, resulting in falsely decreased pH and partial pressure of oxygen (PO_2) and falsely increased partial pressure of carbon dioxide (PCO_2). Syringes with lyophilized heparin are available for use but must have an adequate amount of blood added to maintain the correct blood-to-anticoagulant ratio. Normal venous blood is darker red than normal arterial blood in appearance. Arterial blood generally fills automatically into the syringe due to the higher blood pressure found within arteries, without the need to pull back on the barrel of the syringe.

Air bubbles should be expelled immediately after the sample is drawn and should not be mixed into the sample. Failure to remove the air bubbles causes contamination, which will falsely increase pH and PO_2 and decrease PCO_2. This is due to the concentration gradient of gases in air compared to blood. Atmospheric air contains much more O_2 and much less CO_2 than the typical arterial or venous blood sample. Since gases pass to the area of lower pressure by simple diffusion, air exposure will decrease PCO_2 in the blood sample due to its *escape to* the air. Air contamination in the blood specimen will produce a false increase in PO_2 due to oxygen leaving the air and *dissolving into* the blood. The loss of CO_2 also causes the pH to become more alkaline. Thus, air bubbles contaminate whole blood samples and, if not removed promptly, will cause erroneous results.[1]

In blood gas and pH specimen collection, preanalytical errors to avoid include identification and handling problems. For example, variations in the anticoagulant, air exposure, and exposure to warm temperatures during transport of the specimen all cause preanalytical errors. Specifically, too much heparin causes decreased PCO_2 and variable PO_2 levels. Inadequate amounts of heparin or improper mixing of the heparin into the specimen causes clots to form that make analysis of the sample difficult or impossible in most flow-through systems. The correct amount of heparin is 0.05 mg heparin/mL blood and is available in prepared syringes. The wrong type of anticoagulant, such as EDTA or citric acid, will alter the pH and affect the gas distribution as well.[1] The effects of air contamination, a common preanalytical error, have been previously discussed. Specimens not analyzed immediately within the first 30 minutes must be maintained in ice water and analyzed within 1 hour of collection. In warmer temperatures and over time, cell glycolysis in heparinized whole blood can continue, allowing erythrocytes to use up oxygen and produce carbon dioxide and organic acids.[2]

QUALITY ASSESSMENT AND IMPROVEMENT FOR ARTERIAL BLOOD GASES

Analytical and postanalytical errors can occur with blood gas analysis as well. Analytical errors involve the actual technique of blood gas and pH analysis in an instrument that has had improper maintenance, inadequate reagent, and poor or loss of calibration. Verification of acceptable analytical processes should be made with

PCO_2 - partial pressure of dissolved carbon dioxide gas as related to carbonic acid (H_2CO_3); sometimes expressed as PCO_2

✓ **Common Sense Check**
A specific protocol should be followed for the proper identification of patients prior to collection of blood and for specimen labeling. For example, an identification band is an ideal way to indicate the patient's name, identification number, room number, and physician. Other factors relevant to blood gas analysis, including time, date, and ambient air or assisted ventilation parameters, should be recorded on the test requisition at the time of blood collection.

THE TEAM APPROACH

Often the blood gas results may be reported directly to the patient's nurse, physician assistant, or respiratory care therapist, who, as part of the health-care team, will assist the clinician. A system of reporting must be developed within the institution so that critical values are verbally reported and documented along with an electronic or written report while maintaining patient privacy.

THE TEAM APPROACH

When critical results are obtained for arterial blood gases, it is important to quickly verify that there are no errors and then communicate the results to the patient's nurse and/or physician. Many laboratories have a logbook to record the time, date, patient name and identification number, result, who called, and to whom the result was given in addition to the usual reporting through a laboratory information system.

daily analysis of quality control samples and periodic internal and external quality control samples for validation. Test Methodology 9–1 describes analysis of arterial blood gases and sources of interferences. Postanalytical errors involve all required aspects following analysis during the reporting of patient's test results.[2] Postanalytical errors include poor turnaround time or poor timeliness of analysis and reporting without age-adjusted reference ranges or correct units or rounding of data. Using an inadequate method of reporting routine results is also a postanalytical error that can cause erroneous results.

TEST METHODOLOGY 9-1. ARTERIAL BLOOD GAS ANALYSIS, pH, AND CALCULATIONS[2]

A blood gas analyzer measures multiple parameters using a series of electrodes and spectrophotometric measurements. Earlier models used carbon dioxide and air tanks to calibrate the partial pressure of oxygen, or Po_2, and carbon dioxide, or Pco_2, but newer instruments use tonometered aqueous gas solutions. Oxyhemoglobin and other hemoglobin forms are determined from a standardized spectrophotometer, calibrated with a total hemoglobin standard. Quality control samples are generally commercially prepared aqueous tonometered solutions rather than whole blood, in order to maintain stability.

The Reaction Principle

pH

Potentiometric reaction of an indicator electrode that selects for H^+ with a specific glass membrane and measures potential versus reference electrode of calomel or Ag/AgCl with a saturated AgCl salt bridge; voltage change due to H^+ is measured.

Pco_2

Modified pH electrode using potentiometry with Teflon or silicon semipermeable membrane that selects for CO_2 gas and containing H_2O/bicarbonate buffer that produces H^+ as a result of carbon dioxide reacting with water to form carbonic acid, bicarbonate ions, and H^+; voltage change due to H^+ is measured.

Po_2

Polarographic Clarke electrode with polypropylene selective semipermeable membrane that allows O_2 to diffuse through and be reduced at the platinum cathode in a KCl/phosphate buffer solution, with oxidation occurring at the Ag anode; change in current is measured.

So_2

Saturated O_2 measured as oxyhemoglobin versus total hemoglobin by spectrophotometer taking multiple absorbance readings at various wavelengths; O_2 hemoglobin/total hemoglobin is measured.

Interferences

The sample should be properly anticoagulated and well mixed to avoid clots for continuous flow method of sample delivery. Carryover is avoided by a wash step. The analyzer need frequent calibration with automated and semiautomated calibration as indicated by manufacturer's recommendations. The pH electrode and to some degree other gases need to be maintained at 37°C. Excess protein buildup on the pH electrode or membranes will decrease sensitivity, which necessitates cleaning with periodic bleach solution, proteolytic enzyme application, or replacement membranes. Disposable electrodes and/or membranes maintain electrode function.

continued

TEST METHODOLOGY 9-1.   ARTERIAL BLOOD GAS ANALYSIS, pH, AND CALCULATIONS[2] *(continued)*

The Specimen

Heparin-coated syringe containing well-mixed arterial whole blood and placed in ice water if not analyzed within a few minutes. An air bubble often forms during collection and must be expelled immediately before recapping the syringe. Radial or brachial arterial (wrist) sites are used. Preanalytical errors to avoid: too much heparin, which dilutes blood and increases PCO_2; air in sample, which falsely increases O_2 and decreases CO_2; sample not kept on ice, which allows cell glycolysis to occur, which falsely decreases O_2 and increases CO_2; poorly mixed or clotted sample, which causes variable results; and venous blood rather than intended arterial blood; which causes near-normal pH but CO_2 and O_2 both close to 45 mm Hg.

The Calculations

$$H_2CO_3 = PCO_2 \times 0.0301$$
$$\text{HCO}_3^- \text{ given pH and } PCO_2 \text{ values: pH} = 6.1 + \log \text{HCO}_3^-/(PCO_2 \times 0.0301)$$

The Henderson-Hasselbalch equation is used for calculating the pH in blood by using the dissociation constant and the ratio of HCO_3^- to H_2CO_3. When two of the three parameters are known, the third parameter can be calculated. This is the preferred method for calculating HCO_3^- rather than the formula for estimating it from total CO_2.

Reference Ranges

Analyte	Reference Range	Critical Values
pH	7.35–7.45	7.20–7.60
PCO_2 (mm/Hg)	35–48	25–60
PO_2 (mm/Hg)	83–108	<40
HCO_3^- (mmol/L)	19–24	10–40

Calculations in Arterial Blood Gas Analysis

Given arterial pH and PCO_2, the formula to solve for bicarbonate is derived as follows:

$$\text{pH} = \text{pK}_a + \log (\text{HCO}_3^-/PCO_2 \times 0.0301)$$
$$\text{pH} - \text{pK}_a = \log (\text{HCO}_3^-/H_2CO_3)$$
$$\text{inv. log (pH} - \text{pK}_a) = \text{HCO}_3^-/H_2CO_3$$
$$\text{inv. log (pH} - \text{pK}_a) \times H_2CO_3 = \text{HCO}_3^-$$

For example, calculate HCO_3^- given pH 7.50 and PCO_2 of 30 mm Hg.

$$7.50 = 6.1 + \log [\text{HCO}_3^-/(30 \times 0.0301)]$$
$$7.50 = 6.1 + \log (\text{HCO}_3^-/0.9)$$
$$1.4 = \log (\text{HCO}_3^-/0.9)$$
$$\text{inv. log } 1.4 = (\text{HCO}_3^-/0.9)$$
$$25 = (\text{HCO}_3^-/0.9)$$
$$25 \times 0.9 = \text{HCO}_3^- = 23 \text{ mmol/L}$$

Base excess (BE) is best determined from a nomogram or the van Slyke equation.

Case Scenario 9-1 Arterial Blood Gas Collection and Specimen Handling:
The Case of the Pink Patient With a Dark Blood Sample

Follow-Up

The medical technologist was asked to collect and analyze arterial blood gases from a 54-year-old male recovering from CABG surgery, 1 hour after his ventilator was discontinued. His ventilation rate and coloration appeared relatively normal. Considering the results that were obtained, including the slightly elevated carbon dioxide and significantly decreased oxygen level, the technologist evaluated the process for preanalytical and analytical variations, including typical specimen collection and handling requirements and sources of interference.

The specimen appeared very dark red and had only filled the syringe slowly, so the technologist had provided suction with the syringe by drawing back on the barrel during collection. This specimen therefore is most likely venous, as indicated by the relatively normal pH and PCO_2 but low PO_2. This sample should be redrawn, taking care to collect from an artery and retest before reporting. ●

Arterial Collection

Some suggestions for assuring collection from an artery including feeling for a pulse, inserting the needle at that pulse point, and observing that the syringe fills without the need to provide negative pressure by pulling back on the barrel of the syringe. Arterial pressure is high enough to fill the syringe without negative pressure being applied.[1,4] When analyzing a specimen collected by someone else, the technologist should discuss with that person how the specimen was collected to determine if a venous sample is likely, particularly if this patient has a normal appearance and respiration. Indicate that results can't be reported until a proper arterial sample is collected since the reference ranges are determined with arterial samples.

Venous Versus Arterial Samples

We will now discuss in greater detail why the oxygen values are significantly different in venous versus arterial blood, including the role of the cardiovascular and respiratory system in oxygenation and acid-base status.

Understanding the basic interpretation of arterial blood gases is valuable in helping to evaluate validity of obtained results and in recognizing the importance of critical values. This chapter will take you through a step-by-step approach to interpreting arterial blood gases (ABGs). The cases presented will illustrate and help you learn the concepts. There are five main evaluations we need to consider in interpreting ABGs in the clinical setting:

1. Acid-base status
2. Alveolar ventilation
3. Oxygenation status
4. O_2 transport
5. Carboxyhemoglobin

CASE SCENARIO 9-2

Chronic Bronchitis: Blue Bloater or Pink Puffer Patient?

A 62-year-old Caucasian female with a history of 80 pack-years of cigarette smoking and shortness of breath has the following paired arterial blood gas results upon admission:

Test	Patient: Room Air	Patient: 2 L O_2	Reference Ranges
pH	7.32	7.33	7.35–7.45
P_{CO_2} (mm Hg)	56	58	35–48
P_{O_2} (mm Hg)	52	68	83–108
Bicarb (mmol/L)	32	32	19–24
O_2 sat. (%)	88	92	94–98
CO (%)	0	0	0–2.5

ACID-BASE STATUS

Disorders of acid-base status are classified by pH (alkalosis or acidosis) and based on the primary origin of the disorder (metabolic or respiratory). For example, a metabolic disorder such as diabetes can cause acidosis, or below-normal blood pH due to accumulation of organic acids such as acetoacetic acid secondary to excessive fat metabolism. Chapter 4 (Diabetes and Other Carbohydrate Disorders) describes this phenomenon in more detail. Another example is when the kidneys lose the ability to remove metabolic waste products, resulting in metabolic acidosis from uremia. Chapter 6 (Assessment of Renal Function) describes this and other renal causes of metabolic acid-base disorders.

Metabolic Acid-Base Disturbances

Common causes of metabolic acidosis include metabolic diseases such as diabetic ketoacidosis; uremia; renal tubular acidosis; lactic acidosis; gastrointestinal loss of bicarbonate, fluid, and potassium; or exposure to certain toxins that cause blood pH to fall below normal. Another example of metabolic acidosis arises from hypotension secondary to dehydration, which leads to poor tissue **perfusion**, lactic acid formation, and fluid and electrolyte imbalance. Metabolic alkalosis can stem from vomiting or gastric suction, low potassium or chloride levels (electrolyte imbalance), and liver cirrhosis with ascites, corticoid excess, and massive blood transfusion.[5] These conditions are not categorized as acute or chronic.

perfusion - passage of blood through the vessels of a particular organ; designated as Q

Respiratory Acid-Base Disturbances

Respiratory acidosis can result from diseases of the respiratory system that cause carbon dioxide gas retention. Respiratory alkalosis can result from respiratory or systemic diseases that cause hyperventilation and carbon dioxide deficit. Respiratory acid-base disturbances are often classified as acute or chronic. These will be discussed in more details in the following paragraphs. Table 9–1 provides a review of primary acid-base disorders.

TABLE 9-1

Metabolic Indicators of Primary Acid-Base Disorders

Metabolic acidosis	Loss of $[HCO_3^-]$ or addition of $[H^+]$
Metabolic alkalosis	Loss of $[H^+]$ or addition of HCO_3^-
Respiratory acidosis	Increase in P_{CO_2}
Respiratory alkalosis	Decrease in P_{CO_2}

anion gap - the unmeasured anions in plasma present with bicarbonate and chloride to balance sodium and potassium cations

Henderson-Hasselbalch equation - equation that relates pH of blood plasma to equilibrium of salt (HCO_3^-) and weak acid (H_2CO_3)

diuretic - agent that promotes urine formation

ureterosigmoidostomy - implantation of the ureter into the sigmoid colon to eliminate wastes when the urinary system is unable

carbonic anhydrase inhibitors - compounds that reduce the secretion of H^+ ions through alkalinization of the urine; drugs that are commonly used to treat glaucoma

hypoperfusion - decreased passage of blood through vessels of an organ

alveolar ventilation - effective air exchange between alveoli and blood

Approach to Interpreting Acid-Base Disturbance

In order to interpret acid-base disturbances, the following five factors are considered: pH, HCO_3^-, P_{CO_2}, **anion gap**, and assessment for compensation. The first step is to determine if the patient is acidemic or alkalemic, based on pH. Second, the primary disorder is determined by evaluating HCO_3^- and P_{CO_2}. There is a direct relationship of pH to bicarbonate based on the **Henderson-Hasselbalch equation**, compared with the inverse relationship of pH to P_{CO_2} and carbonic acid. If HCO_3^- is elevated and pH is elevated, there is metabolic alkalosis. If both are decreased, there is metabolic acidosis. Next, one must look at the P_{CO_2} in the context of the HCO_3^-. If HCO_3^- is within the normal reference range and P_{CO_2} is elevated but the patient is acidotic, the condition is respiratory acidosis. If bicarbonate is within the normal reference range and P_{CO_2} is decreased but the patient is alkalotic, the condition is respiratory alkalosis. Next determine the anion gap, using standard formulas described in earlier chapters, to determine the etiology of metabolic acidosis. In metabolic acidosis and mixed acid-base disorders, the anion gap is significantly elevated. Finally the pH, HCO_3^-, and P_{CO_2} are considered to determine if compensation is as expected based on the typical ratio of 20:1 for bicarbonate to carbonic acid. For example, both decreased HCO_3^- and P_{CO_2} should produce a slightly decreased or nearly normal pH if they are in metabolic acidosis compensation. To determine the actual ratio of bicarbonate to carbonic acid, P_{CO_2} is converted to H_2CO_3 using the relationship $P_{CO_2} \times 0.03 = H_2CO_3$.[5]

Classification of metabolic acidosis can be based on a normal anion gap versus an elevated anion gap. For example, metabolic acidosis with a normal anion gap is associated with renal diseases such as proximal or distal renal tubular acidosis, renal insufficiency with HCO_3^- loss, and hypoaldosteronism with potassium-sparing **diuretics**. Other causes include loss of alkali due to diarrhea or **ureterosigmoidostomy** or ingestion of **carbonic anhydrase inhibitors**, such as the medications used to treat glaucoma.[5] Metabolic acidosis with a high anion gap is generally due to addition of acid from ketoacidosis; lactic acidosis from **hypoperfusion** or decreased circulation; toxic ingestions of aspirin, ethylene glycol, or methanol; or renal insufficiency.

Compensation for metabolic acidosis or alkalosis is achieved initially by the respiratory system. Respiratory compensation for acidosis means that the lungs increase the level of **alveolar ventilation**, which raises the pH toward normal. The increased ventilation eliminates or blos off CO_2, which eliminates carbonic acid. Also, the presence of acidosis normally increases respiratory drive. The respiratory system compensates for a metabolic defect. In metabolic alkalosis, some decrease in ventilation occurs but the P_{CO_2} generally remains normal since respiratory compensation doesn't occur until alkalosis has been severe and prolonged. Compensation for metabolic alkalosis is less complete since hypoventilation is not a naturally

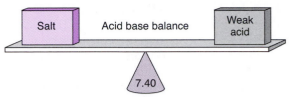

Figure 9–1. To maintain acid-base balance and provide a neutral blood pH, there is approximately 20 times more salt (bicarbonate) than weak acid (carbonic acid). Both components contribute to acid-base balance.

sustainable condition. Figure 9–1 depicts the relative ratio of carbonic acid and bicarbonate salt required in order to maintain balance and provide a neutral blood pH of 7.40.

VENTILATION AND P_{CO_2} RELATIONSHIP

Ventilation is inversely proportional to the resulting P_{CO_2}. Ventilation increases in response to a drop in plasma and cerebrospinal fluid (CSF) pH detected by the respiratory center in the medulla. The respiratory center responds rapidly to CSF pH in relationship to plasma pH. Elevated pH associated with metabolic alkalosis causes a less predictable decrease in ventilation and elevated P_{CO_2}, only when alkalosis is severe and prolonged.

Likewise, the kidneys compensate for a primary respiratory defect. The respiratory system can never completely compensate for a metabolic defect, but renal compensation can almost be complete. Respiratory compensation attempts to maintain pH in a reasonable range. You can use the following crude formula to gauge pH and P_{CO_2} changes: The pH changes 0.1 unit for every 10 mm Hg change of P_{CO_2}, moving in opposite directions.[5]

In acid-base disturbances of respiratory origin, the kidneys provide compensation through control of bicarbonate and other electrolyte levels. Commonly respiratory acid-base disturbances are classified as acute or chronic, which is determined in two ways. First the bicarbonate level is compared to its reference range, and secondly pH is compared to CO_2 changes. For example, the kidneys compensate for respiratory alkalosis by excreting bicarbonate ions, but it takes at least 24 hours before changes are observed. Hence, if the bicarbonate levels are normal, the acid-based disturbance is an acute event. In addition, one should see an approximate change of 0.1 pH unit for every 10 mm of CO_2 change. For example, a pH of 7.40 is within the reference range and corresponds to a P_{CO_2} of 40, also within the reference range. However, a pH of 7.50, which is 0.10 pH unit higher than 7.40, corresponds to a P_{CO_2} of 30 mm Hg, which is 10 units lower.[5]

Various terms and calculations, such as **alveolar P_{O_2}**, **F_{IO_2}**, respiratory quotient, and alveolar-to-arterial gradient (**A-a gradient**), are used to help determine the lungs' ability to transfer oxygen. Since the gases exist in a certain volume and create pressure, water vapor pressure and barometric pressure are considered in assessment and treatment of the patient. The gaseous exchange between the lungs and the circulatory system takes into account ventilation, perfusion, and respiratory quotient.

In order to determine the A-a gradient, one must consider partial pressure of gases dissolved in the body fluids. *Alveolar P_{O_2}* is the partial pressure of oxygen gas found in **alveoli**. The *fraction of inspired oxygen*, or F_{IO_2}, is the amount of oxygen

---

✓ **Common Sense Check**
If the respiratory compensatory effort of the patient is effective, the P_{CO_2} should be the same as the decimal value of the pH. In other words, for a pH of 7.28, the P_{CO_2} level would be 28 mm Hg.

alveolar P_{O_2} - P_{AO_2}; the partial pressure of carbon dioxide gas in the alveolar sacs

F_{IO_2} - amount of oxygen available to breath

A-a gradient - alveolar-to-arterial gradient, which assesses alveolar ventilation

alveoli - air sacs at the end of air ducts in the lungs and in contact with capillaries that allow gases to diffuse in or out (singular: alveolus)

⬡ **THE TEAM APPROACH**
Respiratory care therapists, physician assistants, and clinicians utilize arterial blood gas values such as P_{CO_2} and P_{O_2} to determine alveolar-to-arterial gradient and assess for ventilation/perfusion ratio problems, diffusion defects, or shunts.

available for a patient to breath. This is often quantified as a percentage. For example, since room air is 21% oxygen, the F_{IO_2} would be 21%. *Alveolar ventilation* is the effective air exchange between the alveoli (the air sacs) and the blood. The *respiratory quotient* is the molar ratio of carbon dioxide production to oxygen consumption and is determined to be a constant number, 0.8. The *water vapor pressure* at human body temperature is 47 mm Hg. *Barometric pressure* is determined with a barometer and is reported in millimeters of mercury (mm Hg). These factors all help to define the interaction of the lungs with the circulatory system.

In addition to determining the acid-base disturbance, one should consider if acute-on-chronic CO_2 retention is occurring and if hypoxia is present. A patient has partially compensated respiratory acidosis if the bicarbonate is high. This is considered a chronic defect since the kidneys take 48 hours to 5 days to retain bicarbonate and compensate for the pH. When pH remains decreased after 5 days, there is evidence of CO_2 retention.

OXYGENATION STATUS

Oxygen status relates to P_{O_2}, the partial pressure of dissolved oxygen in plasma, as well as oxygen saturation (S_{O_2}). **Hypoxia**, decreased oxygen supply to the tissues, is typically determined based on arterial P_{O_2}. Physiological mechanisms of hypoxia include hypoventilation, low fraction of inspired oxygen provided (F_{IO_2}), ventilation/perfusion mismatch, anatomic **shunt** in heart or lungs, or problems with diffusion.[5]

In regard to perfusion, erythrocytes have a transit time in the pulmonary capillary bed of 0.8 seconds. In the tissues where capillaries and veins exchange gases, **mixed venous oxygen saturation** is generally 75% while normal oxygen saturation of arteries or arterialized capillaries is close to 100%. The time frame is only 0.2 second for oxygen saturation to reach 100% in erythrocytes during transit across the pulmonary capillary bed.[5] There is always sufficient time to fully saturate the erythrocytes with oxygen even with the worse diffusion defects. Hence, hypoxia cannot be explained on the basis of capillary or alveolar diffusion defects. Diffusion, however, contributes to hypoxia when exercise occurs because of the decreased transit time of erythrocytes across the pulmonary capillary bed compared to the increased demand for oxygen. In diffusion defects, there is a near-normal resting O_2 level but decreased oxygen level with exercise. This exercise desaturation is not unique to but commonly associated with diffusion defects.

Oxygen transport is based on oxygen status and hemoglobin molecules' ability to deliver oxygen to the tissues. Several values are used to represent oxygen transport, including oxygen-carrying capacity, oxygen saturation, and oxygen content. In order to fully understand these terms, it is best to characterize them with formulas and practice the calculations of oxygen-carrying capacity and oxygen content.

Oxygen-Carrying Capacity and Content

One gram/dL of hemoglobin can hold about 1.34 mL of oxygen when 100% saturated. Thus, 1.34 multiplied by g/dL of hemoglobin is the formula for *oxygen-carrying capacity*.[4] For example, with a hemoglobin of 16 g/dL, the oxygen-carrying capacity = 1.34×16, or 21.44. The formula used to calculate *oxygen content* is $(1.34 \times hemoglobin) \times$ oxygen saturation (S_{O_2}). For example, in a patient with a hemoglobin of 16 g/dL,

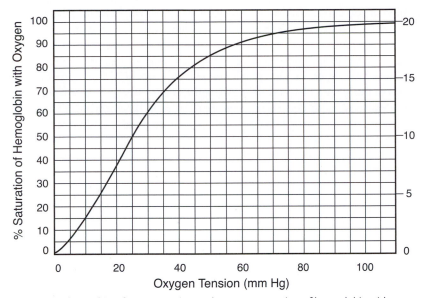

Figure 9–2. Relationship of oxygen tension and percent saturation of hemoglobin with oxygen.

While breathing room air (SO_2 of 0.88), oxygen content = (1.34 × 16) × 0.88 = 18.87

On 2 L of oxygen and 0.92 SO_2, oxygen content = (1.34 × 16) × 0.92 = 19.72

On 50% FIO_2 and an SO_2 of 1.0, oxygen content = (1.34 × 16) × 1.0 = 21.44

Notice that increasing the FIO_2 to 50% doesn't significantly increase the oxygen content. This is because the relationship between oxygen saturation and measured PO_2 is nonlinear. This phenomenon requires that you are familiar with the *oxygen dissociation curve*, as illustrated in Figure 9–2.

The relationship between *oxygen tension* (PO_2, in mm Hg) and saturation of hemoglobin with oxygen is positive and sigmoidal. The hemoglobin molecule can retain or release oxygen to the tissues at different rates depending upon certain conditions such as pH, PCO_2, temperature, or 2,3-diphosphoglycerate (2,3-DPG) levels. In general, as pH decreases or as PCO_2, temperature, and/or 2,3-DPG levels increase, the oxygen dissociation curve shifts to the right, indicating that the hemoglobin molecule has a lower affinity for oxygen. This *shift to the right* of the hemoglobin-oxygen dissociation curve means that, as the percentage saturation of hemoglobin increases, so does oxygen tension. But the increase in oxygen tension is minimal until the hemoglobin nears 85% saturation with oxygen. A left shift, with increased affinity of hemoglobin for oxygen, is associated with a decreased oxygen tension as the saturation of hemoglobin with oxygen decreases. This is found with conditions of high pH, low PCO_2 or 2,3-DPG levels, or the presence of carboxyhemoglobin.

Shift to the Right

A shift to the right of the hemoglobin-oxygen dissociation curve means that the affinity of hemoglobin for oxygen is lowered, and the midway point of the curve, the **p50**, will be increased. The p50 is the oxygen tension when the hemoglobin is 50% saturated with oxygen. It is a measure of the hemoglobin-oxygen affinity, or

p50 - the midway point of the hemoglobin-oxygen dissociation curve, representing the oxygen tension (in mm Hg) when the hemoglobin molecules are 50% saturated with oxygen

the ability of the arterial blood to release oxygen to the tissues. The hemoglobin molecule readily gives up the oxygen it is carrying so that oxygen is able to diffuse into the tissues. The deoxyhemoglobin is then free to act as a buffer by picking up H^+. High levels of P_{CO_2} derived from cellular metabolism result in the formation of more H_2CO_3, which in turn produces HCO_3^- and H^+. The deoxyhemoglobin continues to buffer the H^+. A shift to the right occurs when tissues become acidotic following exercise, with decreased perfusion, or at high altitudes. This also occurs in anemia and, as long as 2,3-DPG levels remain high, the patient does not suffer serious effects of hypoxia.

Oxygen-carrying capacity is decreased when the patient is anemic, a condition in which the patient has a low hemoglobin level. Oxygen delivery also depends on cardiac output, the amount of arterial blood delivered from the left side (or right side of the heart). Oxygen extraction by the tissues depends upon oxygen content and mixed venous oxygen saturation. Hemodynamic monitoring is the process of assessing O_2 delivery and extraction using measurements taken by a pulmonary artery catheter (Swan-Ganz catheter) and is commonly assessed in critical care patients.

RESPIRATORY DISORDERS

As a result of chronic obstructive pulmonary disease (COPD), patients have irreversible structural changes in the lung causing problems in ventilation and specifically an inability to exhale air rapidly. This results from a variety of causes, including long-term cigarette smoking, inhalation of toxic particles or gases, severe asthma, and autoimmune diseases. Two specific diseases that fall within the COPD category are **emphysema** and **chronic bronchitis**.[5]

Patients with COPD are at risk to develop CO_2 retention because their alveolar ventilation is inadequate to maintain normal P_{CO_2} levels. These patients retain CO_2, which initiates renal compensation. That is, the kidneys retain HCO_3^- in an effort to return the pH to normal. Renal compensation causes long-standing increase in bicarbonate and plasma carbon dioxide. Pulmonary function test (PFT) results of patients with COPD indicate reduced expiratory flow rates.[5]

At one end of the COPD spectrum is the patient we may call the "pure" emphysematic patient. Structural changes in the lung cause a loss of elasticity in the terminal airways and alveoli. Additionally, the surface area of the alveoli is reduced due to loss of alveolar wall integrity and air trapping. These theoretical pure emphysema patients have been described as "pink puffers." That is, their appearance is usually thin, their **work of breathing** (WOB) is high, but because of their increase work effort, they maintain adequate oxygenation and appear pink, rather than **cyanotic**, or bluish.[5]

At the other end of the COPD spectrum is the patient with chronic bronchitis. These patients have been labeled "blue bloaters" because of their clinical appearance. They are usually overweight or **edematous**, and have a bluish discoloration of the skin and mucus membranes due to hypoxia with cyanosis. The pathophysiology of chronic bronchitis is one of chronic airway irritation with excess secretion from mucus glands leading to chronic infections and airway obstruction. These patients have ventilation-perfusion (V/Q) mismatching that leads to chronic hypoxia and CO_2 retention, not corrected by the increase in the work of breathing. The chronic hypoxia may lead to pulmonary artery hypertension and eventual right

emphysema - chronic pulmonary disease marked by abnormal increase in the airspaces and destructive changes in their walls

chronic bronchitis - long-standing irritation and inflammation of the respiratory ducts

work of breathing - effort needed to inhale and exhale

cyanotic - characterized by bluish appearance due to lack of tissue oxygenation

edematous - puffed up due to visible accumulation of fluids

heart failure, termed **cor pulmonale**. They also exhibit markedly reduced expiratory flow rates on pulmonary function tests, hence the designation **obstructive** pulmonary disease.[5]

Chronic Bronchitis

Patients with chronic bronchitis are typically overweight or edematous, and have a bluish discoloration of the skin and mucus membranes due to hypoxia with cyanosis. The causes of chronic bronchitis are chronic airway irritation from cigarette smoke, for example, with excess secretion from mucus glands leading to chronic infections and airway obstruction. These patients have chronic hypoxia, as indicated by low SO_2 and PO_2, and CO_2 retention, as indicated by increased bicarbonate and PCO_2.

The respiratory drive in the central nervous system responds to abnormal pH and carbon dioxide levels based on chemoreceptors. Ventilation changes to attempt compensation when these levels deviate only slightly from normal. Likewise, hypoxic drive receptors are located within the carotid and aortic bodies, the anatomic chemoreceptors. Hypoxic drive does not activate until arterial PO_2 falls below 55 mm Hg. What this means is that the hypoxic drive isn't involved if baseline arterial PO_2 is above 55 mm Hg. If a COPD patient presents with a chronically elevated PCO_2, then the respiratory drive has been activated and CO_2 is not the primary stimulation to ventilation changes. In addition, when low O_2 levels are present the hypoxic drive is activated.[5]

Case Scenario 9-2 Chronic Bronchitis: Blue Bloater or Pink Puffer Patient?

Follow-Up

A 62-year-old Caucasian female with history of 80 pack-years of cigarette smoking and shortness of breath has blood gas analysis performed. Paired blood gas results revealed a compensating respiratory acidosis, due to a decrease in pH and an increase in both bicarbonate and PCO_2. Chronic CO_2 retention with low PO_2 was also found, indicating a V/Q mismatch. COPD is the likely disorder based on history of cigarette smoking. Other diagnostic tests, including chest x-ray, were performed to confirm the diagnosis.

The initial therapy for this patient was a low-flow FIO_2 oxygen such as 2 L O_2 by nasal cannula. The shunt component of V/Q mismatch is easily correctable by supplemental oxygen. The oxygen-carrying capacity and the hypoxic drive are two issues to be considered when determining how much oxygen to be given. Oxygen-carrying capacity is not significantly improved when PO_2 is over 60 mm Hg. This can be visualized by reviewing the O_2 dissociation curve. The hypoxic drive may be induced by patients with chronic carbon dioxide retention, when oxygen tension is low. Indiscriminate administration of oxygen can worsen CO_2 retention. Complications of COPD are conditions that worsen the hypoxia, including congestive heart failure, acute bronchitis, pneumonia, pneumothorax, and pulmonary embolism. They induce V/Q mismatch. ●

---

cor pulmonale - right-sided heart failure

obstructive - causing blockage

THE TEAM APPROACH

Although emphysema and chronic bronchitis have different pathological definitions, most COPD patients have an admixture of both diseases. History and physical examination are of paramount importance in understanding the disease presentation in any particular patient. Clinicians often have to expect blood gas results that reflect complicated chronic acid-base disturbances and provide treatment accordingly.

THE TEAM APPROACH

In chronically hypoxic patients, significant changes occur in 2,3-DPG levels that contribute to a right shift in the oxyhemoglobin dissociation curve so that one cannot predict exactly at what level the hypoxic drive activates. Therefore, respiratory care therapists and clinicians adjust oxygen levels slowly, with incremental changes in oxygen therapy while observing changes in oxygen status, to determine at what level the hypoxic drive remains.

CLINICAL CORRELATION

Generally, known chronic COPD patients with CO_2 retention do not require more than 1–2 L/min of O_2 given by a nasal tube or 24%–28% air entrainment mask (AEM), also known as a Venturi mask, for O_2.

CASE SCENARIO 9-3

Acute Respiratory Failure: Pain Medication Made Things Worse

The respiratory care therapist collected arterial blood from the 75-year-old Caucasian male with a history of 120 pack-years of cigarette smoking and worsening shortness of breath. The patient arrived to the hospital by ambulance. Arterial blood gas results are shown below.

Test	Patient: Room Air	Patient: 2 L O_2	Reference Ranges
pH	7.37	7.25	7.35–7.45
Pco_2 (mm Hg)	56	82	35–48
Po_2 (mm Hg)	55	62	83–108
Bicarb (mmol/L)	30	32	19–24
SO_2 (%)	90	94	94–98
CO (%)	0	0	2.5

These indicate chronic CO_2 retention compared to last year's blood gas results. Other cardiac or respiratory complications were ruled out, but overdose of pain medication was suspected.

Acute-on-Chronic CO_2 Retention

THE TEAM APPROACH
Respiratory care therapists determine the alveolar-to-arterial (A-a) gradient using arterial blood gas values to assess if ventilation/perfusion (V/Q) mismatch is present.

ARDS - respiratory distress syndrome of the adult; acquired respiratory failure

CLINICAL CORRELATION
A large A-a gradient indicates the patient may have V/Q mismatch, diffusion defect, or a shunt. The fraction of inspired oxygen, Po_2 and Pco_2, and A-a gradient can be correlated, taking into consideration conditions of barometric and water vapor pressure. A negative value indicates an error in Fio_2.

As described earlier, chronic CO_2 retention occurs when the kidneys are unable retain sufficient bicarbonate to balance with the primary elevation of carbon dioxide, and restore the pH. In other words, the pH remains acidotic. Causes for acute-on-chronic CO_2 retention can be worsening V/Q mismatch with demand for increased effort, shutting off the hypoxic drive, or respiratory depressants such as sleeping pills or antianxiety medications. Congestive heart failure, acute bronchitis, pneumonia, and pneumothorax, as discussed earlier, all worsen the V/Q mismatch with demand for increased respiratory effort.[5] Acute-on-chronic carbon dioxide retention is associated with the general condition of acute respiratory distress syndrome (**ARDS**).

Sleeping pills or antianxiety medications, taken chronically as abused drugs, depress the respiratory center when taken in large amounts and cause acute-on-chronic CO_2 retention. These drugs include barbiturates, such as phenobarbital or secobarbital; opium derivatives, including morphine and oxycodone; ethyl alcohol; and many others. Noncompensatory respiratory acidosis and serious hypoxia can result.

The A-a oxygenation gradient, in simplified form, is

$$\text{A-a} = \text{alveolar } Po_2 \text{ (PAo}_2\text{)} - \text{arterial } Po_2 \text{ (Pao}_2\text{)}$$

The alveolar partial pressure of dissolved carbon dioxide gas ($PAco_2$) is determined by the following formula:

$$PAo_2 = (BP - WVP) \times Fio_2 - (Pco_2/RQ)$$

in which barometric pressure (BP) = 760 mm Hg, water vapor pressure (WVP) = 47 mm Hg, FIO_2 = 21% ambient air, and respiratory quotient (RQ) = 0.8 under normal conditions. Alveolar PCO_2 is generally the same as arterial PCO_2 (PaO_2), and a low value suggests increased alveolar ventilation. The units may be expressed in mm Hg or torr (1 mm Hg = 1 torr).

The A-a gradient is normally 4 to 20 mm Hg. A widened A-a gradient indicates that the patient may have a V/Q mismatch, a diffusion defect, or a shunt.[5] In simple terms, this means that there is something wrong with the patient's lungs that need an explanation, such as pneumonia or another complicating respiratory illness.

The A-a gradient can be calculated using the following formula:

$$A\text{-}a = [(BP - WVP) \times FIO_2] - (PCO_2/RQ) - PO_2$$

For example, given ABG values of pH = 7.28, PCO_2 = 29 torr, PO_2 = 81 torr, the following steps are used to determine the A-a gradient:

$$BP - WVP = 760 - 47 = 713 \text{ torr}$$
$$713 \times FIO_2 \, (0.21\%) = 149.7 \text{ torr}$$
$$PCO_2/RQ = 29/0.8 = 36 \text{ torr}$$
$$149.7 - 36 = 133.7, \text{ rounded to } 134 \text{ torr}$$
$$A\text{-}a = 134 \text{ torr} - 81 \text{ torr} = 53 \text{ torr}$$

For another example, with ABGs of pH = 7.25, PCO_2 = 82, and PO_2 = 62:

$$A\text{-}a = [(760 - 47) \times 0.21] - (82/0.8) - 62 = -14.5 \text{ torr}$$

The negative number obtained is not possible and indicates an error in one of the measured blood gas parameters. Individual steps are as follows:

$$760 - 47 = 713 \text{ torr}$$
$$713 \times 0.21 = 150 \text{ torr}$$
$$82/0.8 = 102.5 \text{ torr}$$
$$150 - 102.5 = 47.5 \text{ torr}$$
$$47.5 - 62 = -14.5 \text{ torr}$$

Shunts, fistulas, and atelectasis are all complications of acute respiratory distress syndrome. An anatomic shunt was described earlier as a passage between two natural channels such as blood vessels. There can be shunted and nonshunted areas of the lung or the heart. It is easy to understand an anatomic shunt in cardiac causes because of the anatomy of the four chambers of the heart and the large blood vessels leading into and out of the heart. Likewise, in an alveolar-venous fistula, there is an abnormal passage between the alveoli and the venous circulation, when the exchange should be between capillaries and alveoli. Diffuse alveolar atelectasis with continued perfusion is common in ARDS. This means that there is collapse of the airways but blood continues to circulate in capillaries adjacent to the airways.

Focal atelectasis may be due to lack of alveolar surfactant, while **diffuse** atelectasis may be due to anesthesia.

CLINICAL CORRELATION
An anatomic shunt is a passage between two natural channels such as blood vessels. There can be shunted and nonshunted areas of the lung or the heart. An alveolar-venous fistula is also a shunt in which there is an abnormal passage between the alveoli and the venous circulation, when the exchange should be between capillaries and alveoli.

focal - present in one small area

atelectasis - partial or complete lung collapse due to obstruction of the airway

diffuse - present over a large area

Case Scenario 9-3 Acute Respiratory Failure: Pain Medication Made Things Worse

Follow-Up

The patient with a history of cigarette smoking and COPD now exhibits long-term carbon dioxide retention, hypoxia, and worsening of respiratory acidosis with incomplete compensation. This is termed *acute-on-chronic* carbon dioxide retention. The drug testing and patient history revealed excessive intake of OxyContin, a synthetic narcotic, for chronic upper back pain. This medication was causing acute respiratory distress.

Treatment options need to take into consideration that nonshunted areas in the lung do not compensate for shunted portions on 100% O_2. From your understanding of the O_2 dissociation curve, you realize that, once equilibration has been reached with hemoglobin saturation, more O_2 can only be added as dissolved O_2, and this is usually insignificant. The shunted areas then will actually add a venous admixture to the saturated blood in the nonshunted areas, prolonging hypoxia. Further and frequent blood gas monitoring will be necessary while respiratory treatments are given. ●

CASE SCENARIO 9-4

Neonatal Respiratory Distress: The Grunting Baby

The neonatal nurse in charge of analyzing capillary blood gases in the neonatal intensive care unit indicated that it was difficult to obtain a nonclotted specimen from a new patient. The patient, a premature infant, had difficulty in breathing. The technologist in charge of the point-of-care (POC) blood gas analyzer verified that the instrument was functioning properly and advised the nurse to warm the infant's heel, obtain a free-flowing drop of blood, and twist the capillary thoroughly immediately to adequately mix the heparin in with the whole blood. This sample did not clot, and results were obtained that indicated the baby had decreased pH, increased P_{CO_2}, and decreased P_{O_2}. The baby had already received intratracheal treatments for lung immaturity.

Fetal Lung Maturity

phosphatidyl choline - phosholipid lung surfactant; also known as lecithin

Pneumocytes, specialized alveolar cells in the lungs, produce pulmonary surfactants containing phospholipids such as **phosphatidyl choline**, cholesterol, and protein. The surfactants coat the alveolar epithelium and reduce surface tension in the alveolar wall during exhalation. This is one of the final developmental stages of the fetus prior to birth. Infants born prematurely at less than 37 weeks or weighing less than 2500 g frequently experience respiratory distress from lack of lung maturity, particularly due to the immature pneumocytes. The alveoli collapse during exhalation when there is insufficient surfactant, which results in overinflation of the remaining airways. This process is termed *focal atelectasis*. This condition progresses, causing decreased oxygenation of the collapsed alveoli and cyanosis and respiratory distress in the neonate. This condition was formerly known as hyaline membrane disease. Respiratory distress can be treated with surfactants given into the trachea at birth as well as prenatal therapies aimed at enhancing lung surfactant production prior to birth.[5] Chapter 12 (Reproductive

Endocrinology and Neonatal Testing) presents a detailed description of fetal lung maturity testing.

Respiratory Distress Syndrome

Respiratory distress syndrome is a condition of atelectasis due to alveolar collapse. In neonates, as described already, it is due to premature lungs, and in particular lack of lung surfactant. The infant develops rapid, difficult respirations, sometimes with grunting sounds, within a few hours of delivery. Amniotic fluid testing can reveal decreased phosphatidyl glycerol or other phospholipids. The extent of atelectasis and respiratory failure worsens with time. Carbon dioxide retention, decreased pH, increased P_{CO_2}, and worsening respiratory acidosis occur. Hypoxia, decreased SO_2, and P_{O_2} may start out mild but progress if treatment doesn't commence. Hypoxia occurs due to lack of oxygenation in the collapsed alveoli. Providing oxygen and treating the acidosis is necessary to sustain life in the neonate with respiratory distress syndrome.[5]

In respiratory distress syndrome of the adult (ARDS), the respiratory failure is associated with acute pulmonary injury from aspiration or infectious pneumonia, for example.[6] Shock, burns, and near-drowning are other causes of ARDS. This can actually occur in children or adults but is termed ARDS to distinguish it from neonatal respiratory distress. At the cellular level, the most likely cause of progression of the disease is inflammatory products, including leukocytes, prostaglandins, and fibrosis, which reduce the amount of lung surfactant activity. Cells and collagen accumulate, causing severe scarring, poor respiratory function, and hypertension and V/Q problems.[7] The arterial blood gases initially indicate very low P_{O_2}, normal or low P_{CO_2}, and elevated pH causing respiratory alkalosis.[8] Chest x-ray can reveal pulmonary changes, including edema, but these may lag behind the severity of the blood gas results. Eventually acidosis can result from prolonged hypoxia, particularly if treatment is not adequate. Further effective treatment would need to take place after ruling out heart failure by taking pulmonary arterial blood pressure readings. Pulmonary embolism is ruled out by angiography, while a bronchoalveolar lavage may be needed to provide a culture to rule out certain types of infections. Complications of ventilation can also prevail, such as gram-negative bacterial infections.[5]

ANALYSIS OF OXYGENATION

Oxyhemoglobin (O_2Hb) can be measured using a co-oximeter, a dedicated spectrophotometer. Oxyhemoglobin exhibits peak absorbance at 585 and 540 nm, while deoxyhemoglobin (HHb) peaks at 594 nm. **Total hemoglobin** is generally a sum of oxyhemoglobin and deoxyhemoglobin. The formula used to calculate SO_2 is the proportion of oxyhemoglobin within the total hemoglobin concentration. In this formula, c represents concentration and Hb represents hemoglobin.

$$\text{Total hemoglobin} = cO_2Hb + cHHb$$
$$SO_2 = [cO_2Hb/(cO_2Hb + cHHb)] \times 100\%$$

Errors in this calculation of SO_2 arise if significant levels of dysfunctional forms of hemoglobin, such as carboxyhemoglobin, are present. If only normal hemoglobin forms of hemoglobin are present, then the SO_2 is close to O_2Hb, and the terms are sometimes used interchangeably. The O_2Hb is similar to the term *fraction of oxyhemoglobin* (FO_2Hb). FO_2Hb is defined as the fraction of oxyhemoglobin com-

oxyhemoglobin (O_2Hb) - the combined form of hemoglobin with oxygen; a measure of the utilization of the potential oxygen transport capacity

total hemoglobin - a measure of potential oxygen transport capacity

pared to total hemoglobin. Total hemoglobin in this regard refers to all forms of hemoglobin, including dysfunction forms (dysHb) such as carboxyhemoglobin or methemoglobin, and is equal to $cO_2hb + cHHb + cdysHb$. Dysfunction forms of hemoglobin can be measured with the co-oximeter based on absorbance peaks at unique wavelengths compared with O_2Hb and HHb. The equation below depicts fraction of oxyhemoglobin compared to total hemoglobin.

$$FO_2Hb = [cO_2Hb/(cO_2hb + cHHb + cdysHb)] \times 100\%$$

Transcutaneous monitoring of oxygen saturation, also known as pulse oximetry, has been used for many years in pediatric and critical care patients since monitoring can be continuous and noninvasive. It operates on the principle that oxyhemoglobin found in capillary blood of warmed skin can be measured spectrophotometrically. Only certain regions of skin have capillary beds close enough to the surface that light can diffuse through, absorb into the blood, and transmit or reflect light back through diodes. Fingers and toes in adults and infants can be used for assessing capillary oxyhemoglobin levels. Infrared light is used to warm the skin and increase capillary circulation, stimulating arterial blood. Light of two different wavelengths is passed through capillaries close to the skin in the digits in order to estimate cO_2Hb and cHHb. Light is absorbed by the blood. Photosensors detect light reflected back from oxyhemoglobin and relate it to percent SO_2. Because this method does not estimate dysHb forms, it overestimates SO_2 when dysfunctional forms of hemoglobin are present. Errors also occur with decreased circulation, anemia, or even excessive movement of the digit during the measurement process. Similar reference ranges are used for pulse oximetry as for arterial oxygen saturation. The advantage of this method of estimating oxygen saturation is that it is noninvasive.

Other invasive methods of determining arterial blood gas and oxygen status have been developed over the years, including transcutaneous (percutaneous) electrodes for measuring P_{O_2}, pH, and P_{CO_2} as well as **ex vivo** blood gas analysis. In ex vivo blood gas analysis, blood circulates to an external machine that measures blood gases and oxygenation by the usual methods of electrodes and spectrophotometry but then is returned to the patient. This method requires an indwelling catheter and anticoagulation of the arterial lines in order to assure that blood clots are not returned to the patient.[9] It is therefore invasive but since the blood is recirculated to the patient, the problem of depleting blood volume in the infant or anemic adult is overcome.[10]

transcutaneous - through the skin, not invading the body through a puncture; percutaneous

ex vivo - outside of a living being

Case Scenario 9-4 Neonatal Respiratory Distress: The Grunting Baby

Follow-Up

The neonatal nurse in charge of analyzing capillary blood gases in the neonatal intensive care unit had difficulty getting a nonclotted specimen from a premature infant. After some guidance from the charge technologist, blood gas results were obtained that indicated the baby had decreased pH, increased P_{CO_2}, and decreased P_{O_2}. The baby had received treatments for lung immaturity. This patient exhibited respiratory acidosis and decreased oxygen levels as typical of a patient with neonatal respiratory distress or hyaline membrane disease. Since the lungs need additional surfactant in order to prevent airway

Case Scenario 9-4 Neonatal Respiratory Distress: The Grunting Baby *(continued)*

collapse, the increased respiration was not effective in compensating for carbon dioxide retention. Lactic acidosis from poor oxygenation is likely to ensue, along with combined metabolic and respiratory acidosis. Providing oxygen and treating the acidosis is necessary for this infant. ●

CASE SCENARIO 9-5

Possible Carbon Monoxide Poisoning: The Nauseated Patient With Cherry Red Lips

A venous heparinized whole blood sample was transported on dry ice and analyzed within 15 minutes of draw time by co-oximetry in the ED laboratory. The results are shown below:

Test	Patient	Reference Ranges
Carboxyhemoglobin (%)	9	0–2.5
Oxyhemoglobin (%)	92	94–98 (arterial)
Methemoglobin (%)	1	0.4–1.2
Sulfhemoglobin (%)	0	0–0.5

The clinical laboratory scientist found out the following information when reporting the results to the patient's physician assistant. The patient is a 35-year-old nonsmoking firefighter who suffered a minor injury on the job. Other laboratory data were also obtained: red blood cell count of $4.8 \times 10^6/\mu L$ (reference range 4.3 to 5.7), hemoglobin 13.9 g/dL (13.5 to 17.3), and hematocrit 41% (39 to 49). The blood cell morphology was normal. Random urinalysis and routine serum chemistry testing results were all within normal reference ranges. Exposure to a toxic gas was suspected due to occupational hazard.

TOXIC GASES

Table 9–2 provides a summary of the most commonly encountered toxic gases.

Cyanide Poisoning

A relatively rare but serious toxic gas forms from cyanide exposure. Firefighters and other people coming in contact with burning plastic or synthetic materials in an

TABLE 9-2	
Toxic Gases and Their Sources	
Toxic Gas	**Source**
Cyanide	Fires of synthetic materials (carpets and insulation in walls)
Carbon monoxide	Incomplete combustion of organic matter

industrial accident or any type of large interior fire can inhale cyanide gas along with other toxins. Some of the toxicity is accounted for by the volatile nature of cyanide poisoning. This property of cyanide gas is also used in some methods of analyses. Toxic effects of cyanide gas can be screened with a microdiffusion method or quantified in plasma with an ion-selective electrode. Cyanide gas forms when cyanide ions combine with acid. Inhalation of cyanide gas causes the majority of the gas to bind with hemoglobin and only a small amount to remain in plasma. Cyanide ions bind to Fe^{3+} in hemoglobin and mitochondrial cytochromes, causing competitive blockage resulting from inhibition of oxidative phosphorylation. Cellular hypoxia, respiratory failure, and possible coma and death from heart failure result from cyanide toxicity. A common misconception is that the individual and even the health-care providers examining the patient may detect an odor similar to almonds that indicate presence of cyanide gas. This is not a reliable indicator as many people are unable to detect this odor.[11]

Carbon Monoxide Poisoning

Carbon monoxide (CO) is the most commonly encountered toxic gas. It is an odorless gas that is a by-product of incomplete combustion of carbon, such as from burning of natural gas, gasoline, or other petroleum products. It is present in exhaust from automobile engines or natural gas furnaces or water heaters. It also is a product of structure fires, and so a commonly encountered toxin in firefighters. It is a by-product of cigarette smoking both for the smoking individual and for those inhaling secondhand smoke. People become exposed through these routes, especially from auto exhaust, gas leaks, or secondhand smoke.

Minimal amounts of carbon monoxide dissolve in the aqueous or lipid layer of tissues or fluids. Most of the carbon monoxide, like oxygen, binds to hemoglobin and myoglobin. However, carbon monoxide has a much stronger affinity for hemoglobin than does oxygen. The resulting compound that forms is termed *carboxyhemoglobin.*

Rarely, carboxyhemoglobin is formed from the metabolism of other chemicals. An unusual source of CO exposure is from inhalation of paint remover containing dichloromethane, which is metabolized to carbon monoxide in the body. Also, trace amounts of carboxyhemoglobin form in moderate to severe cases of hemolytic anemia and in gastrointestinal (GI) bleeding, further complicating those conditions.

Distribution of Gases via Circulation of Erythrocytes

There are normal forms of hemoglobin, which are capable of reversibly binding to oxygen, and abnormal forms, which are not. Oxyhemoglobin and deoxyhemoglobin are normal forms, while carboxyhemoglobin, methemoglobin, and sulfhemoglobin are abnormal forms. Oxyhemoglobin (O_2Hb) makes up 95% or more of hemoglobin in normal circumstances. Deoxyhemoglobin (HHb) is the reduced form found normally in small amounts that is capable of binding O_2 to become oxyhemoglobin. Carboxyhemoglobin (COHb) is an abnormal form with a strong affinity for hemoglobin, which limits oxygen content of blood. Methemoglobin (MetHb) and sulfhemoglobin are abnormal forms of hemoglobin containing oxidized iron (Fe^{3+}) that cannot bind oxygen. They are formed by certain drugs or chemicals.

Pathological Effects of Carbon Monoxide

Hemoglobin combines with CO at a rate of 210 times the affinity of oxygen, thus preventing the formation of further oxyhemoglobin. Carboxyhemoglobin also increases the affinity of hemoglobin for oxygen that has already formed as oxyhemoglobin. Thus, a shift to the left in the oxygen-hemoglobin dissociation curve occurs. In Figure 9–1, the resulting oxygen saturation can be visualized as Po_2 levels that fall to the left of this curve.[12] This relationship between oxyhemoglobin and Po_2 is characterized by the p50. As affinity of hemoglobin for oxygen increases, p50 decreases. Generally CO doesn't affect Po_2 levels as readily as it affects SO_2 and O_2 content levels.

The normal carboxyhemoglobin level is 0% but, due to environmental exposure to air pollutants, people may have a reference interval of 0% to 2.5%. The reference range should be determined by the laboratory to reflect the typical patient population it encounters since geographic location impacts upon the reference range. People who live in rural areas may only have COHb levels of up to 1.5%, but those in urban areas or moderate smokers often have COHb levels of up to 6%. Heavy smokers may have carboxyhemoglobin levels of 8% to 9%. Generally if COHb levels are less than 5%, there are few or no pathological effects. However, the elderly, young children, and those with chronic illnesses may suffer ill effects even at this level.

Once carboxyhemoglobin levels reach 10%, most people suffer symptoms of tissue hypoxia but often do not exhibit the classic bluish tinged skin and mucous membranes often associated with hypoxia. Patients may exhibit cherry red lips and nailbeds. Hypoxia has the greatest impact on organs that consume more oxygen, the brain and the heart. However, delayed central nervous system and cardiac symptoms make it difficult to correlate with actual carboxyhemoglobin levels. Table 9–3 lists the physiological effects of carboxyhemoglobin levels.

Interpretation of levels must be related to the time of exposure, total hemoglobin level of the patient, age and general health of the patient, and his or her smoking status. Delayed development of neuropsychiatric *sequelae* such as personality changes, memory impairment, or motor disturbances may result from elevated COHb. These neurological conditions do not always correlate well with carboxyhemoglobin levels, or even with length of exposure, but usually do correlate with lapse of consciousness.

The treatment of a patient with carboxyhemoglobinemia involves providing more oxygen to the patient. The half-life ($t_{1/2}$) of carboxyhemoglobin in patients

TABLE 9-3	
Pathological Effects of Carbon Monoxide	
COHb Levels	**Signs, Symptoms, and Effects**
<10%	Headache possible
10%–20%	Shortness of breath upon exertion
30%	Headache, irritation, and impaired judgment
40%–50%	Severe headache, confusion, collapse
60%–70%	Respiratory failure, unconsciousness
80%	Rapidly fatal
>80%	Instantly fatal

breathing ambient (20% oxygen) air is generally 6 hours, but the half-life of COHb decreases if higher concentrations of oxygen are provided. For example, the $t_{1/2}$ of carboxyhemoglobin is 1.5 hours if the patient breathes 100% oxygen and is 25 minutes if the patient is placed in a hyperbaric chamber. Use of a hyperbaric chamber is recommended to treat patients once the carboxyhemoglobin level exceeds 25%.[13]

Analysis of Carboxyhemoglobin

Detection of CO can be (1) indirectly through the release of CO gas and measurement in a Conway microdiffusion system, (2) directly through the release of CO gas from the hemoglobin complex using gas chromatography, or (3) by estimation of carboxyhemoglobin by absorbance peaks. The Conway microdiffusion system is a qualitative method for screening for CO gas poisoning. This method is rarely used since it has poor specificity and sensitivity. A more definitive carboxyhemoglobin method is needed for adequate assessment of the patient's status.

The reference method for carboxyhemoglobin is gas chromatography. Whole blood is mixed with potassium ferricyanide, which releases free CO. The molecular sieve column separates carbon monoxide from other gases in the reaction and detects it by thermal conductivity. A reducing catalyst, such as nickel, can increase the sensitivity of this method and allow for flame ionization detection. This direct method of measuring carboxyhemoglobin is sensitive but time consuming and requires highly trained technologists to perform the analysis. A fume hood is necessary in order to safely handle the gas standards and to determine the carboxyhemoglobin capacity. This method is more accurate and precise at low concentrations of carboxyhemoglobin, particularly at concentrations below 3% of the total hemoglobin.

Indirect Analysis of CO in a Venous Whole Blood Sample

The principle of the most commonly used carboxyhemoglobin method of analysis is the measurement of the absorbance peaks with the use of a co-oximeter. This method is sometimes termed an *estimation method* of carbon monoxide since CO gas is not released from the hemoglobin prior to analysis. Instead, carbon dioxide attached to hemoglobin is measured. A co-oximeter is a narrow bandpass (<2 nm) spectrophotometer that can measure absorbance at various wavelengths. This method is rapid, convenient, accurate, and precise at COHb levels greater than 3%. The instrument is relatively inexpensive and routinely calibrated with a hemoglobin standard, in contrast with the chromatographic method. Since other abnormal hemoglobins also exhibit absorbance peaks at 541 nm, carboxyhemoglobin must be differentiated from methemoglobin and sulfhemoglobin by further steps in the analysis. Methemoglobin and sulfhemoglobin exhibit a peak absorbance at 630 nm, while carboxyhemoglobin does not. Addition of potassium ferricyande is used to convert MetHb to cyanmethemoglobin, which no longer exhibits an absorbance peak at 630 nm. Sulfhemoglobin continues to absorb light strongly at 630 nm after addition of potassium ferricyanide. MetHb is verified by a second peak absorbance at 600 to 626 nm since oxyhemoglobin has little or no absorbance at these wavelengths. Test Methodology 9–2 describes this method of analysis using an automated instrument.

TEST METHODOLOGY 9-2. CARBON MONOXIDE AND OXYGEN SATURATION BY CO-OXIMETRY

The Reaction Principle

The principle of the most commonly used method for carboxyhemoglobin is measurement of the absorbance peaks using a co-oximeter with a tungsten lamp capable of emitting light from 690 to 300 nm and in particular for wavelengths in the 500- to 650-nm range. The monochromator is capable of selecting for 541, 555, 600, 626, and 630 nm. The specimen must contain hemoglobin in order to quantify the percentage of carboxyhemoglobin compared to total hemoglobin. Whole blood that has been diluted with sodium hydrosulfite is added to the sample, which releases the hemoglobin and converts oxyhemoglobin to deoxyhemoglobin but having no effect on carboxyhemoglobin (COHb). The diluted sample is introduced into a cuvette, and specific wavelengths of light are transmitted through the sample in the cuvette to the photodetector. Absorbances are measured at 555 and 541 nm for deoxyhemoglobin and COHb, respectively. The absorbance ratio at 541/555 nm after sodium hydrosulfite treatment is equal to the percentage of carboxyhemoglobin (% COHb). Calculations are performed by the microprocessor so that % SO_2 and % COHb will be displayed on the LED readout and printed.

Interferences

There are false increases in COHb from Hb F, lipemia, and methylene blue. Increases of 4% to 7% are from Hb F due to hemoglobinopathies, such as beta thalassemia major. Methylene blue is a treatment for methemoglobinemia, which causes variable interference in co-oximetry. Gas chromatography should be used for analysis of carboxyhemoglobin levels after methylene blue is given. Co-oximetry spectroscopy is highly sensitive for quantification at levels greater than 2% to 3%. Below that level, imprecision is too great. This method is not sensitive enough to detect trace levels of carboxyhemoglobin that are typically present in hemolytic anemias, GI bleeding, or other causes of endogenous carboxyhemoglobin production. Gas chromatography is required to accurately analyze carboxyhemoglobin at levels less than 3%.

The Specimen

Heparinized whole blood is preferred, but EDTA whole blood may also be used. Blood samples must be kept covered, contain no air bubbles, and be well mixed, properly labeled, and maintained in 2° to 4°C (ice water) and analyzed within 4 hours. Clotted blood can be used for forensic purposes but must be homogenized and not exposed to air during processing. Postmortem blood or blood containing denatured hemoglobin can't be used. Syringes with lyophilized heparin are available but must have adequate amount of blood added to maintain the correct blood-to-anticoagulant ratio, and proper mixing is required to prevent clots.

Reference Ranges

COHb, adult nonsmoker	0–2.5%
COHb, adult smoker	0–9%
SO_2	94–98%

Reference ranges for COHb can vary with environmental exposure and smoking habits. For example, the overall reference range is 0% to 2.5% but 0% to 1.5% is often used for a nonsmoking, rural dwelling patient. Up to 4% to 5% is typical for a moderate smoker, while 8% to 9% is common in heavily smoking patients. Carboxyhemoglobin levels greater than 10% to 20% are considered toxic, and levels greater than 50% are generally lethal.

Determining p50

The p50 can be determined from a nomogram that includes measured and estimated SO_2. The SO_2 can be estimated by software algorithms programmed into many blood gas analyzers using measured pH and PO_2 values. This method is inaccurate if dysfunctional forms of hemoglobin, such as hemoglobin S, are present. If estimated SO_2 is larger than the measured SO_2, the p50 will be increased compared with normal. Similarly, if the estimated SO_2 is less than measured SO_2, the p50 will be decreased. Normal p50 is 25 to 28 mm Hg. The reference method for measuring p50 is a complicated process called **tonometry**. This is rarely performed and only in a few reference laboratories.

tonometry - measurement of dissolved gases in a solution in order to standardize the partial pressure or tension of carbon dioxide and oxygen

Case Scenario 9-5 Possible Carbon Monoxide Poisoning: The Nauseated Patient With Cherry Red Lips

Follow-Up

The 35-year-old nonsmoking firefighter who suffered a minor injury on the job had a carboxyhemoglobin of 9% (reference range 0% to 2.5%), oxyhemoglobin of 92% (94% to 98% arterial), and negligible methemoglobin and sulfhemoglobin levels. This level of carboxyhemoglobin is above the reference range for a nonsmoker and indicates some environmental exposure to carbon monoxide but not enough to begin intensive treatment. The patient most likely will require ventilation with ambient air (free from smoke). There are expectations of a return to normal reference ranges for all parameters within the next 12 hours. ●

CASE SCENARIO 9-6

Correlation of POC Blood Gas Analyzer With Bench-Top Instrument: Are We Comparing Apples to Oranges?

The new clinical chemistry technical supervisor is asked to evaluate the use of the Instrumentation Laboratory (IL) GEM Premier 3000™ point-of-care blood gas analyzer for use by the respiratory care department and by personnel in surgery, and also to compare its patient results to those from the Radiometer ABL™ bench-top blood gas analyzer. The new analyzer also may be used as a backup instrument when the laboratory analyzer is inoperable. Prior to performing a method evaluation of the new instrument and method comparison study of both instruments in order to determine validity, the technical supervisor is asked to first report on advantages and shortcomings of use of the GEM Premier 3000.

Clinical Laboratory Improvement Amendments of 1988 (CLIA) - quality standards for all clinical laboratories to ensure the accuracy, reliability, and timeliness of patient test results regardless of where the test was performed; the Centers for Medicare and Medicaid Services regulates all laboratory testing (except research) performed on humans in the United States

PROFICIENCY TESTING AND OTHER QUALITY ASSURANCE ISSUES

The specific **Clinical Laboratory Improvement Amendments (CLIA)**[14] recommendations for accuracy and precision of arterial blood gases and pH are found in Table 9–4.

TABLE 9-4

CLIA Reliability Requirements for Arterial Blood Gases

Test	Precision	Accuracy	Total Allowed Error
P_{CO_2}	1.3 mm Hg	4.0 mm Hg	5.0 mm Hg
P_{O_2}	$0.75 \times SD$	$2.25 \times SD$	$3.0 \times SD$
pH	0.01	0.03	0.04

SD = standard deviation.

Medical decision limits are critical threshold levels for therapeutic decisions and patient management (Table 9–5). These are also the levels for which precision and accuracy should be checked in samples. This is useful information when monitoring a currently used instrument, choosing quality control levels, or evaluating a new method.[14]

There are published expectations for **delta checks** of many chemical analytes. These can be used in monitoring quality assurance for preanalytical and analytic errors in that patient samples are used as internal controls by checking with previous results from that same patient. However, arterial blood gases and pH vary too quickly to be of use for a true delta check. If ventilation conditions have changed significantly, comparing with the previous arterial blood gas results will not be valid.

delta check - comparison of concentration of an analyte to values from previous specimens in the same patient; a form of quality assurance

Role of the Clinical Laboratory Scientist When the Blood Gas Analyzer Is Not Located in a Centralized Laboratory

Point-of-care testing (POCT) is the analysis of patient samples at or near the location of the patient. POCT is also known as near-patient testing, ancillary testing, bedside testing, and decentralized testing. One of the many applications of POCT is blood gas and pH analysis, a particularly useful application when critical results need to be in the physician's hands within minutes of the patient's acid-base status change. While most POCT is waived testing, arterial blood gases are not waived and must be performed by trained individuals with completion of specific educational requirements. Federal regulation through CLIA and accreditation bodies such as the **Joint Commission for Accreditation of Healthcare Organizations (JCAHO)** require a technical consultant with a minimum of 2 years of laboratory experience to monitor quality assurance and external proficiency of the instrument results. The most likely person to fit this educational standard is an

point-of-care testing (POCT) - testing that does not require specimen preparation and provides rapid results at or near the patient's location

Joint Commission on Accreditation of Healthcare Organizations (JCAHO) - accreditation organization for health-care facilities in order to continuously improve safety and quality of health care

TABLE 9-5

Medical Decision Limits for Arterial Blood Gases

Test	Lower Limit	Upper Limit
P_{CO_2}	35 mm Hg	50 mm Hg
P_{O_2}	30 mm Hg	80 mm Hg
pH	7.35	7.45

experienced medical technologist or clinical laboratory scientist. This person is responsible for the technical and scientific oversight of testing. Educational requirements for the technical consultant are a bachelor's degree and 2 years of laboratory training and experience in nonwaived testing.[15] The role of technical consultant for nonwaived testing is to oversee quality management. The director and technical consultant are not required to be on-site at all times of testing. Quality management includes the following:

1. Have procedures that assure proper patient preparation and specimen identification and integrity; and that monitor and evaluate the testing process and quality management system.
2. Have a procedure manual (manufacturer's package insert may be acceptable).
3. Follow manufacturer's instructions for performing the test.
4. Test a positive and negative control each day that patient samples are tested (package insert may provide flexibility).
5. Enroll and participate in proficiency testing (if available).
6. Identify and correct problems, and record remedial actions taken.
7. Maintain test requests and laboratory records for 2 years.
8. Undergo biennial inspection. Laboratory may choose to have inspections conducted by either the Center for Medicare and Medicaid Services (CMS) or private accrediting organizations.

POINT-OF-CARE TESTING FOR BLOOD GASES

Advantages of POC blood gas analyzers include rapid turnaround time, simplified maintenance using consumable pieces, and frequent automated calibration with each patient sample. Total turnaround time is rapid, often less than 5 minutes, since the instrument is close to the patient's side and no sample transport time is involved. Often the analysis dwell time is short as well. This means that medical decisions can be made more quickly, especially when dealing with critical results. Maintenance has been simplified in these POC analyzers to include sensors that monitor reagent and waste levels and expiration dates of reagents and electrodes. Some hand-held devices have virtually eliminated maintenance other than cleaning and replacement of batteries and consumable cartridges. Miniaturized electrodes in cartridge format make maintenance easier. Often electrode maintenance involves disposing of electrodes rather than membrane changes. Automated calibration and internal checks on quality control (QC) results are possible with many analyzers. Some blood gas analyzers have QC software programmed with Westgard rules and the capability of storing QC results so that using paper logs of daily QC charts is not necessary. Less sample handling is required with POCT prior to analysis, which can lessen some preanalytical errors.

POC blood gas analyzers have disadvantages to include cost of consumables, variances with the bench-top analyzers, and the training limitations of health-care personnel who may be performing actual patient POC testing. Disposable elements of an instrument often make application easier but are costlier than components that are reused and often can be purchased only from one vendor. Cost per test is usually more than non-POC testing depending on the amount of consumable supplies. Cost/benefit ratios can help to determine if POC blood gas analyzers are worthwhile for an institution. Due to the ease of operation, training is often minimal, but that does not eliminate all sources of error in POC blood gas analysis. Separation of the instrument from the laboratory may make maintenance of

THE TEAM APPROACH

Nonwaived (formerly labeled moderately complex) testing requires that only personnel with specific education and training be allowed to perform those laboratory tests. That does not preclude nonlaboratory personnel such as nurses, physician assistants, and respiratory care personnel from performing arterial blood gas analysis.

quality assurance issues difficult. The most common problems arise with lack of documentation by nonlaboratory personnel when QC or sample testing failure occurs.[16]

Preanalytical Variations in POC Blood Gas Analysis

It is assumed that POCT eliminates preanalytical errors since the time from patient specimen collection to testing is shortened. But not all preanalytical errors are avoided, including use of the correct anticoagulant, avoiding dilution of sample with excessive heparin or IV solutions, clots, improper mixing, or inadequate patient sample identification. Many of the new POC blood gas devices include bar-code readers that provide reliable, error-free confirmation of patient identification at the bedside. This should help to limit medical errors due to misidentification, the most serious of which is performing procedures on the wrong patient. Positive identification of the patient at the bedside is the most crucial step.[17]

Analytical Variations in POC Blood Gas Analyzers

Some analyzers may not have temperature control devices, so samples must be analyzed immediately while at 37°C. This generally isn't a problem unless the patient has a high fever or recently received cooling intervention in surgery. Some POC analyzers are more sensitive to clots, which easily disable the analysis. Since the specimen is collected and analyzed immediately, some nonlaboratory personnel do not recognize the importance of properly mixing the syringes or capillary tubes in order to distribute the heparin throughout the sample and prevent clotting. Certain patients, particularly those recently treated with vitamin K or those who have naturally quick clotting times, will have clotted specimens in a period of 1 minute or less, which poses a problem of clotted samples yielding no results. Although less commonly a problem, some analyzers are not able to interface with laboratory information systems (LIS), and a permanent record of results is difficult to obtain. Thermal printer papers can degrade quickly when exposed to light and handling. Most POC analyzers will interface with the LIS, but this is an important consideration when choosing an instrument.[18]

Analytical errors have been reduced but not eliminated. Most POC instruments are designed to be simple to operate and to automate calibration. But it is often difficult for nonlaboratorians to recognize the importance of analyzing QC samples, which ensures adequate calibration status or instrument function prior to patient analysis. Stability of calibration verified through electronic parameters and internal sensors has made these instruments more reliable and simpler to operate, but the technical consultant must periodically monitor calibration information and QC results in order to verify reliability of daily testing. Also, patient samples tested between QC samples must be validated on individual merit. These issues point to the need for clear-cut policies, protocols, and training for collection of samples, operation of the instrument, and reporting of results. Otherwise, preanalytical, analytical, and postanalytical errors are quite likely to occur.

Newer, simpler POC blood gas analyzers have been developed, including the EasyStat by Medica® blood gas monitor. Most maintenance with this instrument is simplified, with minimal help needed from a service representative or biomedical engineer. One reason for this is a smaller number of analytes in its menus than other analyzers to capitalize on simplicity and minimize cost per test. On another note of simplification, this analyzer has customizable interfaces to prevent extraneous information for data input or retrieval, which should simplify use. This feature is found with Nova's Stat Profile Critical Care Xpress family of analyzers. Users can customize up to 30 different panels and name them whatever they want. These analyzers have configuration and flexibility similar to that found with a desktop computer.[18]

The Radiometer America ABL 700™ series of bench-top blood gas analyzers also allows users to create customized data input fields with drop-down boxes for all patient populations, such as neonates or adult intensive care patients. All data input can be done directly at the analyzer instead of at an LIS or other data-management workstation, eliminating an extra step for the user. This instrument is also known for a wide number of tests offered with a very small whole blood sample requirement. There is conserving of patient blood, which is critical for neonatal samples.[2]

A variety of POC blood gas and pH analyzers is available in the clinical laboratory. Table 9–6 lists some of the more readily available instruments.

Case Scenario 9-6 Correlation of POC Blood Gas Analyzer With Bench-Top Instrument: Are We Comparing Apples to Oranges?

Follow-up

The new technical supervisor is asked to evaluate the use of the IL GEM Premier 3000 POC blood gas analyzer for respiratory care and in surgery compared to the Radiometer ABL bench-top blood gas analyzer. It also may be used as a backup instrument when the laboratory analyzer is inoperable. She learned about both instruments by consulting with manufacturer's information and discussing with a sales and technical representative from each company. ●

Comparison of POC and Bench-Top Analyzers

The GEM Premier 3000 POC blood gas analyzer measures pH, PCO_2, and PO_2 by the same methodologies as the bench-top analyzers described earlier in this chapter. Additional analytes deemed vital for critical care can also be measured with this analyzer. Users of this instrument must have a password in order to use the instru-

---

TABLE 9-6

Common POC Analyzers of Blood Gases

Company	Instrument Model(s)
Abbott	i-STAT 1
Bayer	Rapidpoint 400
ITC	IRMA TRUpoint
Instrumentation Laboratory	Synthesis; GEM Premier 3000
Nova Biomedical	Stat Profile pHOx; Stat Profile Critical Care Xpress
Radiometer	ABL5 and ABL77, ABL700
Roche	cobas b 121, cobas b 221 with OMNILINK

ment, with the ability to lock out unidentified or untrained users. This helps to ensure that only proficient trained users are operating the instrument. It is a closed system in that it requires that specific supplies and reagents, including the cartridges of electrodes, be purchased only from the manufacturer, adding to the cost per test due to lack of competition between vendors. Multiuse electrode cartridges are available in units of 75, 150, 300, 450, and 600 test cartridges. These cartridges have a shelf-life of 6 months at room temperature but approximately 2 weeks after installation on the instrument. The manufacturer describes the instrument as free from maintenance, but it requires discarding the cartridge and replacing it with a new one, rather than reusing and inserting membranes and refilling as was customary with blood gas analyzers of the past. Calibration with two different levels of standards occurs every 4 hours automatically with internal standard solutions, rather than gas tanks. One standard solution is checked for calibration stability before each patient test sample is analyzed. Aqueous solutions for QC samples are stored internally in the instrument and analyzed automatically and periodically after calibration. QC rules are programmed into the instrument, and results are evaluated automatically with decisions about the instrument's validity made automatically. This is termed *intelligent quality management* (IQM) by the manufacturer. Samples are manually identified or introduced into the device with barcode entry. Arterial, venous, or capillary whole blood heparinized samples can be used, requiring 135 µL total sample volume. Clots are detected with sensors and, when present, results are not printed. Patient sample carryover is minimized due to self-wiping probes. Dwell time in the instrument is less than 2 minutes, with 15 patient samples per hour as the maximum test volume. Patient temperature correction is available. Results print from an internal printer or from an external computer printer. Results can be interfaced to the hospital or LIS as well. Previous results from patients can be retrieved. Trouble-shooting of instrument problems can be provided by the company via the Internet.

The Radiometer ABL is a bench-top blood gas analyzer that measures pH, P_{CO_2}, and P_{O_2} and calculates many parameters, including **base excess**. Users of this instrument may have a password in order to use the instrument, with the optional ability to lock out unidentified users. It is a closed system in that it requires that specific supplies and reagents, including the electrodes, be purchased from the manufacturer. The test volume for electrodes is limited mainly by the life of the electrode, 2 years. The manufacturer describes the instrument as needing minimal monthly maintenance and around 5 hours annual maintenance with electrodes reused and inserting membranes, which helps to keep the cost per test less than with POC devices. Calibration with two different levels of standards occurs every 4 hours automatically, with gas tanks providing the mix of oxygen and carbon dioxide gases. One standard solution is checked for calibration stability every 30 minutes. Use of compressed gas tanks adds a safety considerations in that they must have a pressure regulator, be secured to the wall to prevent tipping and possible explosions, and be kept away from sources of combustion, with annual safety inspections conducted by the institution. Aqueous solutions for QC samples can be used and analyzed periodically after calibration manually by the user with programmed identification information. QC rules are programmed into the instrument, and results are evaluated automatically with decisions about the instrument's validity made automatically. Samples are manually identified or introduced into the device with barcode entry. Arterial, venous, or capillary whole blood heparinized

base excess - concentration of titratable base in a solution with pH 7.40 and P_{CO_2} of 40 mm Hg

samples can be used, requiring 85 μL total sample volume. The sample probe must be manually wiped, and clots are detected with sensors. Dwell time in the instrument is less than 1 minute, with 30 patient samples per hour as the maximum test volume. Temperature correction is available when patient body temperature is not 37°C, as is the testing temperature. Results print from an internal printer or from an external computer printer. Results can be interfaced to the hospital or laboratory information system as well. Previous results from patients can be retrieved. Trouble-shooting of instrument problems can be provided by the company and with detailed onboard diagnostics.

Advantages and Disadvantages of the POC Blood Gas Analyzer

Some advantages of the POC blood gas analyzer are the simplicity of operation with essentially no maintenance. Since there are no gas tanks for calibration and QC and calibration tonometered fluids are inside of the instrument, calibration and validation is ongoing and easy. There is also the ability to restrict usage by untrained personnel who do not have a password. There is automatic clot detection, which prevents results from printing out and requires resampling or re-collection. Some disadvantages of using the GEM Premier 3000 in this role include the cost per test, which is much higher than bench-top instruments due primarily to the disposable electrode and reagent cartridges. The turnaround time is a little slower than the bench-top instrument, which is mainly a problem in high-volume situations. The ease of operation encourages nonlaboratory personnel to operate the instrument, requiring oversight in documentation and sample collection training, the most common problems identified in POC blood gas analysis.

The next step before introducing this analyzer, when it is purchased, is to perform validation studies, including systematic error studies for accuracy, random error or precision studies, and method comparisons between the two different analyzers to assess for differences in results obtained. If the new instrument is deemed valid and the method comparison does not indicate vast differences in results, the standard operating procedure can be written, training can begin, and the new analyzer can be implemented into surgery and onto respiratory care therapists' carts. Chapter 2 (Quality Assessment) contains details about how to perform the method validation and comparison studies.

SUMMARY

Arterial blood gases and oxygen saturation provide vital information to clinicians and members of the health-care team. In some health-care settings, nonlaboratory personnel collect and/or analyze arterial blood gases. Federal regulations require that a technical consultant, such as a medical technologist with 2 years of laboratory experience, oversee quality management of this testing. Understanding the basic interpretation of arterial blood gases is valuable in helping to evaluate validity of obtained results and in recognizing the importance of critical values. This chapter included a step-by-step approach to performing relevant calculations of acid-base and oxygenation status, interpreting arterial blood gases, and avoiding preanalytical, analytical and postanalytical variations.

EXERCISES

As you consider the scenarios presented in this chapter, answer the following questions:

1. Given arterial pH and P_{CO_2}, derive the formula so that you can solve for carbonic acid and then bicarbonate.

2. What are three possible causes for preanalytical errors in arterial blood gas results?

3. Explain the typical causes, signs, symptoms, and laboratory indicators of chronic bronchitis.

4. Explain the principle for indirect analysis of carbon monoxide gas toxicity in a venous whole blood sample.

5. What might be the effect on a P_{CO_2} result of a sample that contains too much heparin?

6. Describe the potential arterial blood gas results from a clotted specimen.

7. Explain why arterial blood cannot be kept at room temperature for prolonged period of time (such as longer than 30 minutes) for blood gas analysis.

8. Given a pH of 7.33, P_{CO_2} of 54, and P_{O_2} of 88, calculate carbonic acid and bicarbonate results using the Henderson-Hasselbalch equation.

9. Given the results obtained from question number 8, classify the acid-base status.

References

1. Elser RC: Quality control of blood gas analysis: a review. *Respir Care* 1986; 31:807–816.
2. Ward K, et al: *Clinical Laboratory Instrumentation and Automation: Principles, Applications and Selections.* Philadelphia: WB Saunders, 1994.
3. Radiometer America, Inc: Operating manual of Radiometer ABL 700™. Westlake, OH: Radiometer America, Inc., 2001.
4. American Thoracic Society: *ATS pulmonary function laboratory management and procedure manual.* New York: American Thoracic Society, 1998.
5. Shapiro BA, Peruzzi WT, Kozelowski-Templin R: *Clinical application of blood gases,* ed 5. St. Louis: Mosby–Year Book, 1994.
6. Raffin TA: Indications for arterial blood gas analysis. *Ann Intern Med* 1986; 105:390–398.
7. Demling RH: Current concepts on the adult respiratory distress syndrome. *Circ Shock* 1990; 30:297–309.
8. Schumacker PT, Cain SM: The concept of a critical oxygen delivery. *Intensive Care Med* 1987; 13:223–229.
9. McKinley BA, Parmley CL: Clinical trial of an ex vivo arterial blood gas monitor. *J Crit Care* 1998; 13:190–197.
10. Dubois J, et al: Ex vivo evaluation of a new neonatal/infant oxygenator: comparison of the Terumo CAPIOX Baby RX with Dideco Lilliput 1 and Polystan Safe Micro in the piglet model. *Perfusion* 2004; 19:315–321.
11. Campbell A: Hospital management of poisoning in victims suffering from smoke inhalation. *Emerg Nurse* 2000; 8(4):12–16.
12. Beers M, Berkow R: *The Merck Manual of Diagnosis and Therapy,* ed 17. Rahway, NJ: Merck & Co., Inc., 1999.
13. Brent J: What does the present state of knowledge tell us about the potential role of hyperbaric oxygen therapy for the treatment of carbon monoxide poisoning? *Toxicol Rev* 2005; 24:145–147.

14. U.S.Department of Health and Human Services: Medicare, Medicaid and CLIA programs: regulations implementing the Clinical Laboratory Improvement Amendments of 1988 (CLIA). Final rule. *Fed Regist* 1992; 57:7002–7186.

15. U.S. Food and Drug Administration: Clinical Laboratory Improvement Amendment of 1988. Available at *www.fda.gov/cdrh/CLIA/index.html*

16. Ford A: Blood gas traps. *CAP Today*, September 2003. Available at *www.cap.org/apps/docs/cap_today//ctarchive_2003.html*

17. Aller RD: Blood gas analyzer basics—and beyond. *CAP Today*, September 2002. Available at *www.cap.org/apps/docs/cap_today/surveys/0203_SRSlinking.pdf*

18. Kadidio K: Evolution of blood gas testing. *Adv Med Lab Professionals* November 3, 2003.

The clinical laboratory assesses biochemical markers of nutritional and digestive health and disease.

10

Assessment of Nutrition and Digestive Function

Maria G. Boosalis and Jean Brickell

This chapter explores the role of laboratory personnel as collaborators in the assessment of nutritional status and gastrointestinal function. The chapter offers a discussion of laboratory tests that aid in the diagnosis and treatment of malabsorption and other digestive problems. Scenarios illustrate the use of laboratory results in these types of assessments. Two scenarios are presented from the perspective of the registered dietitian in the form of a complete nutritional assessment—anthropometric, biochemical, clinical, dietary, and environmental, or A through E assessment.[1] The chapter is divided into two sections: 1) the role of the laboratory in nutritional assessment from the perspective of the registered dietitian and a clinical laboratory sciences student, and 2) the role of the laboratory in assessing digestive disorders from the perspective of laboratory personnel. The side boxes in this chapter provide common sense tips, definitions of terms, brief descriptions of pathophysiology, and clinical correlations as well as reminders of the team approach in health care. Text boxes within the chapter outline methodology for laboratory assessment of nutrition and digestive function.

OBJECTIVES

Upon completion of this chapter, the student will have the ability to

■ Discuss ways in which the laboratory assists the dietitian in the assessment of nutritional disorders and evaluation of nutritional therapy.

■ Discuss the biochemical markers of nutrition in health and disease.

■ Describe laboratory testing that may be used to assess nutritional and digestive status.

■ Describe common preanalytical errors resulting from improper specimen collection and handling for tests of biomarkers that are used for the assessment of nutrition and digestive function.

■ Discuss commonly encountered sources of interference in biochemical analysis of nutrition and digestive function.

■ Correlate laboratory results of biomarkers with nutritional and digestive disorders.

Nutrition

Nutritional status of the patient is assessed by a health care team. The team consists of primary health-care providers, nurses, registered dietitians, laboratory personnel, pharmacists, social workers, physical therapists, occupational therapists, nuclear medicine technicians, and other specialists in health care. The laboratory contributes to this team effort by providing biochemical markers of nutritional or digestive function or dysfunction.

A Registered Dietitian (RD) is a food and nutrition expert who has met the minimum academic and professional requirements to qualify for the credential "RD."[2] Some RDs may hold additional certifications in specialized areas of practice, such as pediatric or renal nutrition, nutrition support, and diabetes education, that are awarded through the Commission on Dietetics Registration (CDR), which is the credentialing agency for the American Dietetic Association (ADA), and through other medical and nutrition organizations that are recognized within the profession. Given the education and training required, the RD is the member of the health-care team who is qualified to determine, address, and meet all nutrient needs of an individual.

The RD is trained to perform a complete nutritional assessment that includes gathering data from five separate areas: **anthropometric** measures, biochemical analyses, clinical history and physical examination, dietary profile, and information

anthropometric - literally means the "measure of man"; type of measurement also referred to as body composition analysis

TABLE 10-1

The Nutritional Assessment

	Example of Data That May Be Gathered	Primary Responsibility
Anthropomorphic measures	Height and weight Weight history Waist circumference Body mass index (BMI)	Nurse
Biochemical analyses	Identification and concentration of body fluid macronutrients and micronutrients	Laboratory personnel
Clinical information	Current and past medical history Physical examination Medications	Primary health-care provider

Dietary Profile	Food intake:
	  24-hour recall
	  Food frequency questionnaire
	Food preparation and storage
	Calculation of the total nutrient content of food intake (total kilocalories; grams of protein, fat, carbohydrate; and milligrams/micrograms of vitamins, minerals)
		Dietitian

Environmental Information	Context in which nutritional decisions are made:
	  Income/financial status
	  Employment/lifestyle pattern
	  Physical resources relative to food
	  Purchasing, preparation, and/or storage
	  Physical/lifestyle activity
	  Psychosocial-familial support
	  Belief systems
		Dietitian/social worker

macronutrient - a chemical element or substance, such as carbohydrates, proteins, and fats, required in relatively large quantities in the diet

micronutrient - organic compound, such as a vitamin, or chemical element essential in minute amounts in the diet

malnutrition - disease-promoting condition resulting from either an inadequate or excessive exposure to nutrients

✓ **Common Sense Check**
Waist circumference is an estimate of abdominal obesity. Abdominal obesity (android distribution) is more closely associated with the development and progression of disease than is hip obesity (gynoid distribution). Individuals with abdominal obesity resemble apples, while individuals with hip obesity more closely resemble pears.

on the environment in which the individual lives as well as his or her lifestyle. Different types of information are gathered from each of these categories. Each piece of information contributes to the assessment and determination of nutrient needs and requirements of the patient. Table 10–1 lists data that are collected in a nutritional assessment.

Interpretation of anthropomorphic values, such as height, weight, and waist circumference, reflect body composition. The body mass index (BMI), a calculation based on height and weight, is an indicator of total body fat. Extremes of total body fat are related to the development of cardiovascular disease, diabetes, cancer, and other chronic disorders.

The laboratory provides measures of biochemical assessment of **macronutrient** and **micronutrient** status. Macronutrient assessment includes identification and analysis of the concentration of proteins, lipids, and carbohydrates and the derivatives of these compounds. Both total protein and individual protein status may be useful in determining **malnutrition**; measurement of specific proteins, such as albumin and thyroxine-binding prealbumin (TBPA) (also known as transthyretin), provides information about the duration of malnutrition. Measurement of the essential fatty acids, total cholesterol, lipoproteins, and triglycerides establish the nutritional status of these important nutrients. Carbohydrate nutritional status may be evaluated through laboratory testing of fasting glucose, glycated hemoglobin, and tolerance to glucose loading. Micronutrient status may be assessed through laboratory testing of plasma levels of vitamins and minerals and through functional testing of the processes to which micronutrients contribute. Functional laboratory testing includes the assessment of the organs, such as the kidney, liver, heart, and bone, which may be affected by inadequate nutrition.

The dietitian employs all categories of information for the determination of current nutritional status and for the determination of the nutritional care plan. The nutritional care plan is based on an individual's age, gender, current state of health, and nutrition-related diagnosis. Concurrent pathology, such as obesity, diabetes, cardiovascular disease, or hypertension, as well as organ function will influence the plan. The dietitian instructs the individual on the implementation of the nutritional care plan and continues to follow up on these nutritional recommendations and work closely with the health-care team to assure compliance.

Malnutrition may occur in one category or several categories of **essential nutrients**. **Energy malnutrition** may occur with deficient intake of carbohydrates, lipids, and proteins. Carbohydrates and lipids are important sources of calorie requirements in the body. Protein malnutrition may be caused by poor diet or by insufficient nutritional support of hospitalized patients. Twenty amino acids are important to human body function. Eight of these amino acids cannot be made by the adult human and are essential nutrients. These eight are isoleucine, leucine, lysine, methionine, phenylalanine, threonine, tryptophan, and valine. Nutritional deficiency of these essential amino acids will cause severe malnutrition. Humans are also unable to produce two important fatty acids, linoleic acid and linolenic acid. These fatty acids must be included in the diet. Fatty acid deficiency may cause skin, immune system, and circulatory system disorders.

Support of the patient with nutritional deficiencies includes oral therapy that is rich in energy and protein foods, tube feeding directly into the gastrointestinal tract, and parenteral feeding directly into the circulatory system.

NITROGENOUS BIOMARKERS OF NUTRITIONAL STATUS

Biochemical measurements of such compounds as creatinine, albumin, retinol-binding protein, transferrin, and transthyretin provide a quantitative measure of nutritional status. Creatinine is a waste product of muscle metabolism. Measurement of the concentration of creatinine in serum or the excretion of creatinine in urine provides an assessment of total body muscle mass for individuals with normal renal function. Muscle mass is a reflection of proper protein nutrition. Several proteins are used as markers of nutritional status. Because proteins have short half-lives in the body, they are indicators of nutrition over relatively short time spans. Albumin is the protein in highest concentration in plasma, and has a half-life of 18 to 20 days. Hypoalbuminemia is an indicator of protein deficiency; however, albumin concentration is also affected by other physiological changes and disease states of the patient, so albumin concentration must be carefully assessed for nutritional status. Retinol-binding protein correlates well with protein-energy status of the patient. However, retinol-binding protein concentration is affected by glomerular

THE TEAM APPROACH
The clinical laboratory provides the B for Biochemical information for the A through E assessment of nutritional status by the Registered Dietitian.

essential nutrients - molecules that are required for metabolism but cannot be produced by the body; required in the diet

energy malnutrition - nutritional deficiency caused by inadequate intake of calories, proteins, or both, seen in children under age 5 years or persons undergoing stress of major illness; also called protein-calorie malnutrion

filtration rate, so assessment of this protein must also be carefully evaluated. Transferrin is the protein that acts as a carrier protein for iron. It has a half-life of 8 days, which makes it a sensitive marker of recent protein-energy nutritional status. Iron concentration must be taken into consideration when evaluating nutritional status based upon transferrin concentration. Transthyretin, or TBPA, is the protein that acts as a carrier for thyroid hormones. Its short half-life of 1-2 days makes it a sensitive marker for protein-energy nutritional status. Thyroid hormone level must be taken into consideration when evaluating nutritional status based upon transthyretin concentration. The use of multiple biochemical markers for nutritional status gives a more accurate picture of nutritional status than relying upon the measurement of only one marker. Several indices use multiple markers for calculating nutritional status.

Nitrogen balance is the measurement of the difference between nitrogen intake and excretion. A positive nitrogen balance is recommended for therapy of certain disorders, such as wound healing, as well as during periods of anabolism or growth. Since most nitrogen is excreted in urine, nitrogen balance may be estimated by measurement of urinary urea nitrogen. Renal status will affect this measurement and must be taken into consideration when using urinary urea nitrogen as an assessment tool.

Immunocompetence is also affected by nutritional status. Malnutrition is associated with progressive decline of immune function. Total lymphocyte levels, T lymphocyte levels, immunoglobulin levels, and complement levels are all affected by protein malnutrition. The loss of immunocompetence will lead to infections. *Candida* and other opportunistic infections may be acquired following the loss of immunocompetence due to malnutrition.

The best assessment of nutritional status is the use of a combination of measurements from several categories, such as weight measurement, BMI, and biochemical markers. Albumin, transferrin, TBPA (transthyretin), urine urea nitrogen, and immune markers all give quantitative measurements for the assessment of nutritional status. Table 10–2 lists proteins that are relevant to nutritional assessment, their half-life and chief function.[3] Table 10–3 lists reference ranges for these nutritional biomarkers.

nitrogen balance - difference between the amount of nitrogen ingested and that excreted

CLINICAL CORRELATION
Protein-losing enteropathy is the abnormal loss of protein into the gastrointestinal tract, which may be due to any disease that causes extensive ulceration of the intestinal mucosa.

Nephropathy is a disease of the kidney that may include inflammation and degenerative and sclerotic lesions of the kidney. The disease is characterized by decreased proteins, including albumin, transferrin, and TBPA (transthyretin), because of abnormal loss of proteins through the kidney.

TABLE 10-2

Plasma Protein Indicators of Nutritional Status

Plasma Protein	Half-Life	Function
Albumin	18–20 days	Maintains osmotic pressure and is carrier of hydrophobic molecules in plasma
Transferrin	8–9 days	Carrier protein for iron in plasma
Transthyretin (thyroxine-binding prealbumin, prealbumin)	2–3 days	Carrier protein for thyroid hormones in plasma, carrier for retinol-binding protein
Retinol-binding protein	12 hr	Transports vitamin A in plasma; binds non-covalently to prealbumin
Insulin-like growth factor, somatomedin	2–6 hr	Have metabolic effects similar to insulin; sensitive to nutritional variation while free from the effects of inflammation

TABLE 10-3

Reference Ranges for Biomarkers of Nutritional Status

Biomarker	Reference Range
PROTEINS	
Albumin	3.5–5.2 g/dL
Transferrin	200–360 mg/dL
Transthyretin	20–40 mg/dL
Retinol-binding protein	3.0–6.0 mg/dL
Insulin-like growth factor I	135–449 ng/mL
VITAMINS	
Vitamin A	30–60 µg/dL
Vitamin D	25(OH)D: 10–65 pg/mL
	1,25(OH)D: 15–60 pg/mL
Vitamin E	0.5–1.8 mg/dL
Vitamin K	0.13–1.19 ng/mL
Vitamin B_1	Whole blood: 90–140 nmol/L
	RBCs: 280–590 ng/g hemoglobin
Vitamin B_2	Serum: 4–24 µg/dL
	RBCs: 10–50 µg/dL
Vitamin B_6	EDTA plasma: 5–30 ng/mL
Niacin	24-hour urine: 2.4–6.4 mg/day
Folate	Serum: 2.6–12.2 µg/L
	RBCs: 103–411 µg/L
Vitamin B_{12}	206–678 ng/L
Biotin	0.5–2.20 nmol/L
Pantothenic acid	Whole blood: 344–583 µg/L
	24-hour urine: 1–15 mg/day
Vitamin C	0.4–1.5 mg/dL
TRACE ELEMENTS	
Chromium	0.7–28.9 µg/L (whole blood)
Copper	Male: 70–140 µg/dL
	Female: 80–155 µg/dL
Selenium	63–160 µg/L
Zinc	80–120 µg/dL

VITAMINS

The word vitamin was coined by Funk to describe vital amines—substances necessary for life.[4] However, not all vitamins are amines. Vitamins are organic compounds required in trace amounts in the diet for health, growth, and reproduction. Vitamins play an important role in nutrition as micronutrients. When vitamin levels are deficient, severe complications to bones, teeth, blood clotting, and nerve function can occur. Some vitamins can become toxic in increased amounts. Vitamins are classified on the basis of their solubility. Fat-soluble vitamins differ from water-soluble vitamins in that they must have carrier molecules that transport them through blood and they are stored in body adipose tissues for longer periods of time. Water-soluble vitamins have a shorter life span in the body and are usually not stored but excreted through urine. Many water-soluble vitamins function as coenzymes in metabolic reactions. Table 10–4 lists the important fat-soluble and water-soluble vitamins, their functions, diseases that result from deficiencies and

TABLE 10-4

Vitamins

	Function	Disease	Laboratory Assessment
FAT-SOLUBLE VITAMINS			
Vitamin A Retinol Retinal Retinoic acid	Required for normal vision and immune function	*Deficiency:* degeneration of eyes and skin *Toxicity:* abdominal pain, headaches, skin roughness	Fluorospectrophotometry, immunoassay, HPLC
Vitamin D Ergocalciferol Cholecalciferol	Calcium and phosphorus metabolism Maintains bone structure	*Deficiency:* rickets, osteomalacia *Toxicity:* hypercalcemia	Immunoassay, HPLC
Vitamin E Tocopherol	Antioxidant of unsaturated fatty acyl groups of membrane phospholipids Protects membranes	*Deficiency:* hemolytic anemia due to fragility of RBC membranes *Toxicity:* antagonistic to vitamin K, may enhance the effect of coumarin therapy, resulting in hemorrhage	Erythrocyte hemolysis functional test, GC, HPLC
Vitamin K Phylloquinones	Required for synthesis of clotting factors II, VII, IX, and X Coumarins act by interfering with the activation of vitamin K	*Deficiency:* hemorrhagic disease, increased clotting time	Immunoassay, HPLC, prothrombin time functional test
WATER-SOLUBLE VITAMINS			
Vitamin B_1 (thiamine)	Coenzyme of metabolic reactions	*Deficiency:* beriberi	Fluorospectrophotometry, HPLC, transketolase functional test
Vitamin B_2 (riboflavin)	Component of coenzymes FMN and FAD for redox reactions	*Deficiency:* general metabolic defect	Fluorospectrophotometry, HPLC, glutathione reductase functional test
Vitamin B_6 (pyridoxine)	Coenzyme of metabolic reactions	*Deficiency:* general metabolic defect	HPLC, tyrosine decarboxylase functional test
Niacin (nicotinic acid)	Component of coenzymes, NAD and NADP for redox reactions	*Deficiency:* pellagra	Fluorospectrophotometry
Folate	Carrier of one-carbon groups for metabolic reactions	*Deficiency:* megaloblastic anemia	Competitive binding protein, HPLC

continued

TABLE 10-4 *(continued)*

Vitamins

	Function	Disease	Laboratory Assessment
Vitamin B$_{12}$ (cyanocobalamin)	Complexes with intrinsic factor to pass through the intestinal mucosa Involved in the synthesis of methionine and conversion of methylmalonate to succinate	*Deficiency:* megaloblastic anemia, pernicious anemia	Competitive binding protein, immunoassay
Biotin	Prosthetic group for carboxylation reactions	*Deficiency:* vomiting, anorexia, dermatitis	Microbiological functional assay
Pantothenic acid	Component of carrier molecules such as coenzyme A and acyl protein carrier	*Deficiency:* general metabolic defect	Microbiological functional assay, immunoassay, GC, HPLC
Vitamin C (ascorbic acid)	Cofactor of protocollagen Aids the synthesis of cartilage, dentin, and bone Reducing agent for hydroxylation reactions	*Deficiency:* scurvy, inability to form connective tissue	Fluorospectrophotometry, photometry

excesses, and typical laboratory methods for measuring them.[5] Table 10–3 lists reference ranges for these nutritional biomarkers.

The diet is the main source for most vitamins. Vitamin A is found in the yellow pigment of most vegetable and fruits. Fish, eggs, liver, and some dairy products are sources for vitamin D; many foods, such as milk, are fortified with vitamin D. Vitamin E may be found in vegetable oils. Vitamin K is supplied by plants, and may also be produced by some bacteria. The dietary sources for most water-soluble vitamins are leafy green vegetables, cereal grains, and animal tissue, especially organ meats. The predominant source for vitamin B$_{12}$ is animal products, such as meat, milk, and eggs. Citrus fruits, berries, and tomatoes are sources for vitamin C.

TRACE ELEMENTS

Trace elements are vital to normal function and are necessary for restoring health during the recovery phase from a disease. If trace elements become depleted secondarily to an illness, further complications arise that also may be life threatening. As the term implies, trace minerals are necessary in the diet in small amounts. They often function as enzyme cofactors. Zinc, copper, selenium, and chromium are considered trace minerals.

TABLE 10-5

Trace Elements

Element	Function	Disease	Laboratory Assessment
Chromium	Promotes insulin action	Glucose intolerance	AAS
Copper	Component of redox reactions and cytochrome reactions	Menkes disease	AAS
		Wilson's disease	Functional assay of superoxide dismutase and cytochrome c oxidase
		Indicated in inflammatory reactions	
Selenium	Protects against oxidative stress	Associated with increased instance of cancer and cardiopathy	AAS
	Constituent of enzymes		
Zinc	Constituent and cofactor of enzymes	General metabolic defect, including growth retardation and poor wound healing	AAS

CLINICAL CORRELATION

Wilson's disease is a defect of copper transport from the liver resulting in overload of copper in liver and brain. Menkes disease is an X-linked recessive disorder in which defective transport of copper from mucosal cells results in copper deficiency.

Zinc is absorbed through the intestine from the dietary nutrients. It is transported in blood with albumin or alpha$_2$ macroglobulin carriers and finally excreted in feces or pancreatic secretions. The concentration of zinc is higher in erythrocytes than in plasma or serum. Copper is also absorbed through the intestine from dietary substances. It travels through blood bound to albumin or histidine for transport to the liver. Most copper is incorporated as ceruloplasmin, an acute-phase reactant. A deficiency of copper results in decreased hemoglobin and collagen production.

Care must be taken in specimen collection and processing of the trace minerals to prevent contamination by environmental elements. Laboratory methodology for the measurement of the concentration of trace minerals must be highly sensitive to low concentrations of analyte. Trace metals are measured by a variety of methods, including atomic absorption spectrophotometry (AAS) and mass spectrometry (MS). Levels of trace minerals in body specimens are affected by physiological factors, such as inflammatory response and liver function, and other factors, such as nutrition, age, gender, and smoking. The results of laboratory analysis of trace elements must be interpreted with consideration of patient demographics and history. Table 10–5 lists common trace elements, diseases that result from their deficiencies, and methods for measuring these elements. Table 10–3 lists reference ranges for these nutritional biomarkers.

Nutritional Disorders

The following scenarios explore team efforts in diagnosing and monitoring nutritional disorders.

spider angioma - a form of tumor, usually benign, consisting of blood vessels or lymph vessels

esophageal varices - tortuous dilatation of veins of the esophagus

gastritis - inflammation of the gastric mucosa

CASE SCENARIO 10-1

Alcoholic Liver Disease: Nutritional Effects of Alcohol Substance Abuse

Mr. Green was having trouble seeing at night. At the Veterans Administration (VA) Clinic, he told the physician that he had recently lost weight and lacked energy to follow his usual pursuits. The physician noted that Mr. Green was a 58-year-old white male who has drunk a six-pack of beer most days of the week on and off for the last 10 years. A visit to the eye clinic at the VA Clinic ruled out anatomic disease of the eye.

The physician suspected that the night blindness was due to his poor diet. In particular, the physician was concerned about vitamin A deficiency. Mr. Green was referred to the dietitian at the clinic to assess this aspect of his diet and because of his history of alcohol abuse, weight loss, and suspected poor dietary intake. The dietitian performed a complete nutritional assessment. His nutritional assessment showed him to be a 5-foot 10-inch, 145-pound man with a BMI of 20.8 kg/m^2 (normal for his height and weight). His history and physical examination included difficulty seeing at night, normal blood pressure, **spider angioma**, **esophageal varices**, and mild **gastritis**.[6]

The 24-hour recall dietary recall evaluation showed poor overall intake, high sugar and caffeine consumption, few to no fruit or vegetables in his diet, poor and inconsistent intake of high-quality protein, and no dairy consumption. An environmental assessment revealed a man who lives alone, is unemployed, and is divorced with no children. The assessment did not reveal religious beliefs that would influence dietary intake. Mr. Green was a 2-pack/day smoker. He was taking nonsteroidal antiinflammatory medication for a sore back. Biochemical markers were as follows:

Marker	Result	Reference Range
Hemoglobin (g/dL)	14.2	14–18
Hematocrit (%)	42.4	42–52
Red blood cell count ($\times 10^6/\mu$L)	4.80	4.7–6.1
White blood cell count BC ($\times 10^3/\mu$L)	4.5	4.8–10.8
Platelet count (/μL)	152,000	130,000–400,000
Mean corpuscular volume (fL)	88.3	80–94
Mean corpuscular hemoglobin (pg)	29.7	27–31
Mean corpuscular hemoglobin concentration (%)	33.6	33–37
Creatinine (mg/dL)	0.9	0.9–1.3
BUN (mg/dL)	10	6–20
Na (mEq/L)	140	136–145
K (mEq/L)	4.0	3.5–5.1
Cl (mEq/L)	102	98–107
Carbon dioxide (mEq/L)	25	23–29
AST (U/L)	42	<35

Case Scenario 10-1 Alcoholic Liver Disease: Nutritional Effects of Alcohol Substance Abuse *(continued)*

Marker	Result	Reference Range
ALT (U/L)	49	<45
GGT (U/L)	64	<55
Bilirubin, total (mg/dL)	1.8	0.0–2.0
Albumin (g/dL)	3.0	3.5–5.2
Serum iron (μg/dL)	52	50–170
Transferrin saturation (%)	21	20–50
Ferritin (ng/mL)	42	20–250
Transthyretin (mg/dL)	17	20–40
Zinc (μg/dL)	64	80–120
Vitamin A (μg/dL)	42	30–60
Fecal occult blood	Positive	Negative

The results of Mr. Green's dietary evaluation and biochemical analysis suggested a dietary problem. Mr. Green's history of alcohol abuse put him at risk for anemia, zinc deficiency, electrolyte imbalance, protein-calorie malnutrition, and liver and renal dysfunction. The biochemical analysis revealed decreased circulating levels of albumin, transthyretin, and zinc. Circulating liver enzyme levels were slightly increased, suggesting a developing liver problem, whereas circulating levels of electrolytes, creatinine, and blood urea nitrogen (BUN) were all within reference limits. The complete blood count and iron studies were within normal limits, but on the low side of normal. Circulating levels of vitamin A were also within reference ranges. His 24-hour dietary recall showed a deficiency of protein, kilocalories, and zinc. As evidenced by the positive fecal occult blood result, he is experiencing a mild loss of blood, which accounts for his iron-deficiency anemia. It is not uncommon for chronic alcoholics to experience gastrointestinal blood loss due to gastritis, peptic ulcer, or esophageal varices.

VITAMIN A METABOLISM

There are three active forms of vitamin A: retinol, retinal, and retinoic acid. All three forms are derived from dietary sources, mainly beta carotenoids. In the small intestine, enzymes convert beta carotenoids to retinol. As it passes through the intestinal mucosal cell, retinol is esterified and transported in this form to the liver. When the body needs vitamin A, free retinol is released from the liver bound to retinol-binding protein. Bound to TBPA (transthyretin), this complex travels through blood to the target cell. Retinol-binding protein binds with specific receptors on the target cell and another protein, cytosol-retinol–binding protein. This action transfers retinol into the cell. In **rods** of the eye, retinol is oxidized to retinal. This aldehyde form of vitamin A combines with **opsin** to form **rhodopsin**, a photopigment of vision. Figure 10–1 diagrams vitamin A metabolism with regard to opsin.

rods - the slender sensory bodies in the retina of the eye, which respond to faint light

opsin - the protein portion of the rhodopsin molecule in the retina of the eye

rhodopsin - the glycoprotein opsin of the rods in the retina, which combines with retinal to form a functional photopigment responsive to light

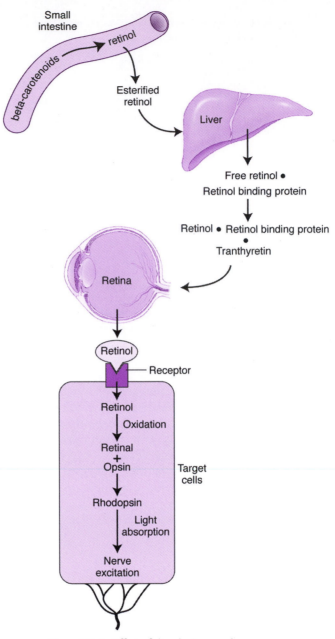

Figure 10–1. Effect of vitamin A on opsin.

Case Scenario 10-1 Alcoholic Liver Disease: Nutritional Effects of Alcohol Substance Abuse

Discussion

Mr. Green's night blindness problem was examined from the perspective of vitamin A metabolism. Mr. Green's normal status of vitamin A, coupled with his protein and zinc deficiency, suggest that his symptoms of night blindness may be due to a deficiency of the transthyretin-retinol–binding protein complex

> **Case Scenario 10-1** Alcoholic Liver Disease: Nutritional Effects
> of Alcohol Substance Abuse *(continued)*
>
> for vitamin A (retinol) or to an inability to convert retinol to retinal. Liver dis-
> ease, such as that caused by alcohol abuse, decreases the synthesis of protein.
> Zinc supplementation has been shown to be helpful in preventing macular
> degeneration and may be involved in the oxidation of retinol to retinal.[7] An
> early hypothesis for this finding is based upon the competition of alcohol with
> retinol for the enzyme alcohol dehydrogenase, which is necessary for oxidation
> of retinol to retinal and to retinoic acid. Zinc is a cofactor of many alcohol
> dehydrogenases. However, the dehydrogenase that oxidizes retinol is zinc
> independent.[8,9] It is possible that one of the other enzymes that is involved
> in the visual cycle is also zinc independent,[10] or that zinc is a cofactor of one
> of the enzymes that catalyzes the production of the carrier proteins of vitamin
> A. Zinc plays a key role in protein and DNA synthesis.

Vitamin A Night Blindness

A combined deficiency in carrier protein and zinc can affect vitamin A function,
due to inadequate transport of substrate and inability to convert substrate to active
molecule. In this case, the eye does not receive enough retinal to ensure normal
function, and the result is night blindness.[11] The action of vitamin A on the eye is
dependent upon concentration of dietary substrates of the active forms of vitamin
A, enzyme catalysts and their cofactors, and transport proteins. Assessment of the
function of vitamin A must include examination of all of these factors.

> **Case Scenario 10-1** Alcoholic Liver Disease: Nutritional Effects
> of Alcohol Substance Abuse
>
> **Follow-Up**
>
> Mr. Green was counseled to stop drinking and select a healthier diet. Since
> Mr. Green lives alone with no available social support, a high-protein, high-
> kilocalorie diet along with dietary supplement was recommended to meet his
> nutritional needs. The dietitian explained how to select and prepare foods to
> improve overall dietary quality, using his microwave only. She also recom-
> mended a multivitamin and mineral supplement, including zinc, to improve his
> overall dietary intake. Elemental zinc supplement was also recommended, for
> the short term, to improve his current zinc status. Since zinc supplementation
> may interfere with copper absorption and thereby cause a compromise in cop-
> per status, the recommended multivitamin and mineral supplement also con-
> tained the recommended intake of copper[12] to prevent a possible deficiency.
> He was scheduled for routine follow-up visits with both his primary health-
> care provider and the dietitian, at which time he will have repeat analysis of
> protein concentration, copper, and zinc. In particular, TBPA (transthyretin)
> concentration will be monitored, as a measure of short-term changes in pro-
> tein status and to determine the success of his nutritional therapy. A complete
> blood count will also be performed to monitor anemia. Liver and renal func-
> tion tests will also be monitored periodically to assess possible consequences
> of his chronic alcoholism on his liver and renal function. ●

CASE SCENARIO 10-2

Dietary Assessment of the Elderly: Mrs. Jansen's Anemia

The dietitian met with 83-year-old Mrs. Jansen and her daughter, Margaret. Mrs. Jansen had been referred to the dietitian as part of an assessment of her increasing weakness and pallor.

Margaret took her mother to the primary care physician when she found that her mother appeared thinner and more disoriented then when she last saw her. Mrs. Jansen told the physician that her legs were swelling and that she had lost weight in the last few months. She appeared pale and unsteady on her feet. Her daughter noticed that her mother had become slightly forgetful.

Upon questioning, Mrs. Jansen said that she had not noticed rectal bleeding and had no history of gastric surgery. Mrs. Jansen stated that she was not taking medication and did not drink alcohol.

Mrs. Jansen's blood pressure, pulse, and temperature were normal. She appeared alert and answered the physician's questions appropriately. No abnormalities were noted in her lungs, heart, or abdomen. A neurological examination showed normal responses. The physician ordered blood tests and referred Mrs. Jansen to the dietitian. Her biochemical markers were as follows:

Marker	Result	Reference Range
Hemoglobin (g/dL)	11	12–16
Hematocrit (%)	34	37–47
Red blood cell count ($\times 10^6/\mu L$)	3.12	4.2–5.4
White blood cell count ($\times 10^3/\mu L$)	4.9	4.8–10.8
Platelet count ($/\mu L$)	131,000	130,000–400,000
Mean corpuscular volume (fL)	109	81–99
Mean corpuscular hemoglobin (pg)	35	27–31
Mean corpuscular hemoglobin concentration (%)	34	33–37
Red cell morphology	Normochromic, microcytic; no blast forms	
Reticulocytes (%)	0.3	0.5–1.5
Fecal occult blood	Positive	Negative

The results of the blood test showed that Mrs. Jansen had a macrocytic anemia, as evidenced by the high mean corpuscular volume, without increased red blood cell production, as evidenced by the low reticulocyte count. Her anemia did not appear to be caused by gastrointestinal bleeding.

Using the algorithm shown in Figure 10–2, further tests were ordered to assess the causes of the low hemoglobin and macrocytic appearance of the red blood cells. Laboratory tests were ordered for liver and thyroid function and for the assessment of vitamin B_{12} and folate.

Case Scenario 10-2 **Dietary Assessment of the Elderly: Mrs. Jansen's Anemia** *(continued)*

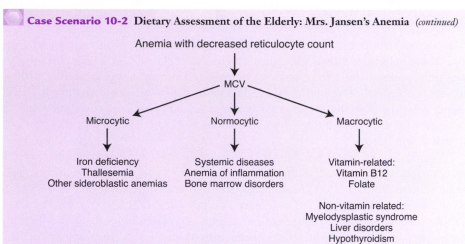

Figure 10–2. Algorithm for assessing anemia with decreased reticulocyte count.

The dietitian's assessment showed that Mrs. Jansen had had an unintentional weight loss of 10 pounds over the last 3 months. Her dietary survey revealed a diet that consisted mainly of processed foods with no vitamin supplementation. She did very little cooking, eating foods out of the box or container. Her diet consisted of a high intake of simple carbohydrates, such as cookies, chips, crackers, and sweetened breakfast cereals; minimal intake of red meat, poultry, or fish; only one serving per day of dairy foods; and a high intake of caffeine from coffee with sugar and nondairy creamer. Mrs. Jansen lived alone and, because of her arthritis, she had difficulty moving around her house and cooking for herself.

She was a widow whose children and grandchildren lived in distant states. She was on a limited income, with a small support system of older women in her local area and children who called once a month and lived over 15 hours away by car. She did not drive and lived in an area that lacked resources for elders.

The results of the follow-up laboratory tests and dietary assessment suggested a nutritional deficiency of folate. The low TBPA (transthyretin) concentration also suggested a poor-quality diet.

Marker	Result	Reference Range
Bilirubin, total (mg/dL)	0.64	0.0–2.0
Alkaline phosphatase (U/L)	78	53–141
AST (U/L)	24	<31
ALT (U/L)	23	<34
TSH (IU/mL)	7.0	0.5–8.9
T_4 (μg/dL)	5.7	5.0–10.7
Serum iron (μg/dL)	52	50–170
Transferrin (mg/dL)	205	160–340
Ferritin (ng/mL)	24	10–120
Vitamin B_{12} (ng/L)	220	206–678
Serum folate (μg/L)	1.5	2.6–12.2
RBC folate (μg/L)	70	103–411
Transthyretin (mg/dL)	15	20–40
Fecal occult blood	Negative	Negative

VITAMIN-RELATED MACROCYTIC ANEMIA

Macrocytic anemia may be caused by vitamin deficiencies of folic acid or vitamin B_{12}. Many cells need vitamin B_{12}, including nerve cells and blood cells. Inadequate vitamin B_{12} gradually affects **sensory nerves** and **motor nerves**, causing neurological problems to develop over time. The neurological effects of vitamin B_{12} deficiency may be seen before anemia is diagnosed. Folate is a coenzyme that is necessary for one-carbon transfers in metabolism. Folate deficiencies also result in hematologic affects.

Vitamin B_{12} is a water-soluble vitamin that functions as a coenzyme for several enzyme reactions in human metabolism, including the conversion of methylmalonyl coenzyme A (CoA) to succinyl-CoA and the conversion of homocysteine to methionine. Vitamin B_{12} is a required cofactor for DNA synthesis. Impaired DNA synthesis results in ineffective red, white, and platelet blood cell production. Deficiency of this coenzyme affects production of blood cells, resulting in anemia, and myelination of the central nervous system, resulting in the neurological symptoms, such as dementia, that are typical of the disease.[13]

Vitamin B_{12} is obtained through the diet from sources such as meats and eggs. In the small intestine, vitamin B_{12} becomes bound to **intrinsic factor**, a glycoprotein that is secreted by **parietal cells** of the gastric mucosa. Receptors for intrinsic factor on the ileal mucosa bind the complex, allowing vitamin B_{12} to be absorbed into portal blood. Through the circulation, the vitamin is transported to the liver, where it is stored, being released back into the circulation as needed. Failure to produce intrinsic factor results in **pernicious anemia**, a deficiency of blood vitamin B_{12} resulting from the inability to absorb the vitamin through the intestinal mucosa.

Since absorption of vitamin B_{12} in humans depends on intrinsic factor, diseases that interfere with the secretion or activation of intrinsic factor also result in vitamin B_{12}-related anemia. Pernicious anemia is caused by an inability to absorb vitamin B_{12} through the ileum and into the blood. Although bacteria in the large intestine produce vitamin B_{12}, it is not absorbed into the bloodstream from this site. Pernicious anemia may be caused by destruction of the gastric mucosa, autoimmunity against gastric parietal cells, or an autoimmunity against intrinsic factor. Vitamin B_{12} deficiency may result from defects other than loss of function of intrinsic factor. Diseases of the small intestine that cause malabsorption, such as ileal resection, may cause vitamin B_{12} deficiency. Vegetarians who consume no foods of animal origin are also at risk of vitamin B_{12} deficiency due to insufficiency of this vitamin in their diet. Test Methodology 10–1 describes a common method of analysis for vitamin B_{12}.

sensory nerves - nerves of the sensory organs

motor nerves - nerves that control movement

intrinsic factor - glycoprotein that is secreted by the parietal cells of the gastric mucosa; necessary for the absorption of dietary vitamin B_{12} through the intestinal mucosa

parietal cells - cells of the stomach that secrete hydrochloric acid and intrinsic factor

pernicious anemia - autoimmune disease in which antibodies affect intrinsic factor and cause vitamin B_{12} deficiency

---

TEST METHODOLOGY 10-1.   VITAMIN TESTING IN THE CLINICAL LABORATORY: VITAMIN B_{12}

Vitamins may be measured by direct or indirect methods. Vitamin concentration level may be measured directly by spectrophotometric, fluorometric, immunoassay, and high-pressure liquid chromatography methods. Vitamin function may be assessed by measuring the reaction or process in which the vitamin participates. For example, vitamin K

continued

TEST METHODOLOGY 10-1.   VITAMIN TESTING IN THE CLINICAL LABORATORY: VITAMIN B$_{12}$ *(continued)*

may be assessed by measuring the prothrombin time, an overall assessment of the components of blood clotting. Vitamin B$_1$ may be assessed functionally by examining the enzyme reaction that is catalyzed by transketolase in which vitamin B$_1$ is important as the precursor of the coenzyme thiamine pyrophosphate. Vitamin B$_{12}$ may be functionally assessed by measuring the concentration of methylmalonic acid and homocysteine. Serum methylmalonic acid will be increased in response to decreased vitamin B$_{12}$, since the conversion of methylmalonic acid to succinyl-CoA is blocked. Homocysteine may also be increased since the vitamin is required for production of methionine from homocysteine. The presence of vitamin may be assessed by placing an unknown specimen in the presence of a microbial agent, which has a growth requirement for the vitamin. Growth of the microbial agent infers presence of the vitamin in the specimen.

Competitive protein-binding techniques are common methods for measuring the concentration of vitamin B$_{12}$ and other vitamins.

The Reaction Principle

In the competitive protein-binding technique for vitamin B$_{12}$, patient vitamin B$_{12}$ is first released from serum binding proteins by denaturing the protein. Free patient vitamin B$_{12}$ competes with labeled vitamin B$_{12}$ for binding sites on nonhuman intrinsic factor. Vitamin that is bound to intrinsic factor is separated from free vitamin through absorption of the free vitamin onto dextran-coated charcoal. Alternately, intrinsic factor may be bound to a solid phase such as a bead or magnetic particle. The amount of unbound, labeled vitamin reflects the amount of unlabeled patient vitamin B$_{12}$.

The Specimen

Serum.

Reference Range

206–678 ng/L

Vitamin B$_{12}$ deficiency may result from infestation of intestinal parasites such as *Diphyllobothrium latum* that compete for the vitamin, stomach removal surgery or ileal resection, **celiac sprue**, **Crohn's disease**, or drugs such as alcohol, neomycin, or *para*-acetylsalicylic acid.

Folic acid is present in foods such as green vegetables, liver, and yeast. Folate is taken into cells in a methylated form. This form must be demethylated, a process that is mediated by vitamin B$_{12}$. The functions of vitamin B$_{12}$ and folic acid are linked. In the conversion of homocysteine to methionine, vitamin B$_{12}$ is a coenzyme in the reaction in which a methyl group is transferred by folic acid. Folic acid is a B vitamin required for the production of normal red blood cells through its effects on the conversion of deoxyuridine monophosphate to thymidine monophosphate. This early step in the metabolic pathway affects the production of pyrimidine molecules.[14,15] Test Methodology 10–2 describes a common method of analysis for folate.

celiac sprue - malabsorption syndrome resulting from intolerance to dietary wheat proteins

Crohn's disease - inflammatory disease of the gastrointestinal tract that can lead to intestinal obstruction

TEST METHODOLOGY 10-2.   FOLATE ANALYSIS

Because folate is required in the metabolism of homocysteine, folate may be functionally assessed by measuring the concentration of homocysteine. In the absence of folate, homocysteine will be increased since the folate is required for production of methionine from homocysteine. A deficiency of either vitamin B_{12} or folate can cause increased homocysteine concentrations. Decreased folate may cause low vitamin B_{12} concentrations because of metabolic blocks. Serum folate levels measure recent folate deficiency, while erythrocyte folate is a reflection of folate concentration over the life span of a red blood cell (RBC), 120 days. Competitive protein-binding techniques are common methods for measuring the concentration of folate. High-pressure liquid chromatography (HPLC) is also used to measure folate concentration.

The Reaction Principle

Patient folate competes with labeled reagent folate for binding sites on a protein, such as beta lactoglobulin. After separation, unbound label is measured as an indicator of the competition of patient folate.

The Specimen

Serum or whole blood.

Reference Ranges

Serum folate (μg/L)	2.6–12.2
RBC folate (μg/L)	103–411

Testing Strategies for Macrocytic Anemia

The testing strategy for diagnosing vitamin-related macrocytic anemia is based upon the assessment of each aspect of vitamin function.[16-18] Tests may include

- Complete blood count (CBC) results that show low hematocrit and hemoglobin with elevated mean corpuscular volume (low red blood cell count with large-sized red blood cells) and peripheral blood smear in which red blood cells may appear large and distorted.
- Reticulocyte count, with a normal or low count indicating normal or low red blood cell production.
- Measurement of the concentration of vitamin B_{12} and folate in the blood.
- Test for methylmalonic acid in the serum as an indicator of vitamin B_{12} deficiency.
- Test for homocysteine as an indicator of folate function.
- Test for gastric hydrochloric acid; lack of gastric HCl is an indirect measure of lack of intrinsic factor as it is due to atrophy of gastric cells.
- Test for intrinsic factor antibodies. Blocking antibody prevents vitamin B_{12} from binding to intrinsic factor; binding antibody prevents the vitamin B_{12}–intrinsic factor complex from binding to the ileum. Seventy percent of pernicious anemia patients have these antibodies.
- If antibody studies are negative (30%), a Schilling test is performed (Test Methodology 10–3) for below-normal serum vitamin B_{12} concentration
- Bone marrow examination for myelodysplasia if the diagnosis is unclear.

TEST METHODOLOGY 10-3. SCHILLING TEST

The Schilling test is a test for vitamin B_{12} absorption. The test requires the cooperation of both the laboratory and the nuclear medicine department. The test is used to differentiate the three main causes of vitamin B_{12} deficiency: dietary deficiency, malabsorption of B_{12}, and pernicious anemia. The Schilling test is a two-step procedure. If results in the first step indicate normal absorption, there is no need to perform the second step of the test.

The Procedure

Step 1

The patient must be fasting. The patient should not have taken any exogenous vitamin B_{12} for 2 days prior to the test. The patient is instructed to begin the test by emptying his or her bladder. A 0.5- to 1.0-μg oral dose of radiolabeled B_{12} is then administered. Within 2 hours, the patient is injected with a "flushing" dose of 1000 μg of unlabeled B_{12}. The purpose of the flushing dose is to saturate all the B_{12} receptor sites in the tissue and plasma so that labeled B_{12} absorbed in the gut will be in excess and will be excreted in the urine, where it can be measured by the laboratory. A 24-hour urine collection is begun after both doses of B_{12} have been administered. All urine for the next 24 hours is added to the collection container, which is kept refrigerated. After the 24-hour urine collection is complete, the amount of radiolabeled B_{12} is measured. If the amount of labeled B_{12} measured in the urine exceeds 7.5% of the oral dose, absorption is considered normal and the test is complete. The deficiency is considered dietary. If the results are <7.5%, then Step 2 is performed.

Step 2

This step distinguishes between pernicious anemia and other causes of malabsorption. Step 2 repeats the doses of B_{12} from Step 1, but adds intrinsic factor along with the oral dose of labeled B_{12}. The 24-hour urine collection is repeated for measurement of the radiolabeled B_{12}. If the labeled B_{12} in the urine from Step 2 is >7.5%, then the malabsorption has been corrected by the addition of the intrinsic factor and the diagnosis is pernicious anemia. If the results are ≤7.5%, the results indicate another cause of malabsorption, such as *Diphyllobothrium latum* infection or celiac sprue.

Interferences

The test is not accurate in the presence of renal disease. The patient may be able to absorb the vitamin B_{12}, but renal output is not sufficient to excrete the excess, causing false-positive test results. Patients who have had gastric bypass surgery, achlorhydria, or hypochlorhydria may be able to absorb vitamin B_{12} given in the Schilling test, but may not be able to absorb B_{12} in foods. This leads to confusion when trying to interpret results with respect to the patient's clinical picture.

Incomplete urine collection will cause false-positive test results. Vitamin B_{12} administered other than in the test will alter the results.

The Specimen

24-Hour urine collection.

Reference Ranges

Results of radiolabeled vitamin B_{12} at Step 1 of procedure:

> >7.5% indicates dietary deficiency

Results of radiolabeled vitamin B_{12} at Step 2 of procedure:

> >7.5% indicates pernicious anemia
> ≤7.5 % suggests another cause of malabsorption

Case Scenario 10-2 Dietary Assessment of the Elderly: Mrs. Jansen's Anemia

Follow-Up

As described in her nutritional assessment, Mrs. Jansen is at risk for poor nutrition. This limitation is further evidenced by results of her biochemical analysis, including reduced hemoglobin and hematocrit, increased mean corpuscular volume, and decreased transthyretin. Normal circulating levels of vitamin B_{12} and decreased levels of folate suggest that the anemia is a result of folate deficiency.

Mrs. Jansen was prescribed a vitamin supplement with folate and was referred for home care. Her complete blood count, reticulocyte count, and folate were repeated in 2 weeks with improved results. She steadily improved over the next 6 months. Since folate treatment could mask a vitamin B_{12} deficiency, Mrs. Jansen will be followed with both folate and vitamin B_{12} laboratory evaluation if macrocytic anemia returns, since folate treatment may mask a vitamin B_{12} deficiency. Mrs. Jansen now lives with her daughter, who is able to monitor her dietary intake and medications. ●

PHYSIOLOGICAL AND NUTRITIONAL CHANGES WITH AGE

Elders in general are at a greater risk for malnutrition than younger adults for several reasons. Physiological changes that often accompany aging, including decreased stomach acid, decrease in mobility, dentition problems, muscle weakness, osteoarthritis, osteoporosis, and gastrointestinal motility, may compromise acquisition, preparation, absorption, and metabolism of food. Multiple medications, both prescription as well as over-the-counter drugs, may also alter intake of foods or interfere with nutritional status. Physical limitations that compromise the acquisition and preparation of food, such as osteoarthritis, osteoporosis, decreased muscle weakness, impaired mobility, and decreased cognitive ability, may also lower confidence in food preparation.

Normal physiological changes of age must be considered when interpreting laboratory results of the elderly. As organs and tissues age, function may be lost. Renal function starts to diminish early into adulthood. Diminishing glomerular filtration coupled with changes in the resorption ability of the nephron tubule result in increased normal ranges for blood creatinine, urea nitrogen, and glucose concentrations for this special population. Aging may also be associated with decreased muscle mass and decrease liver, respiratory, and immune function. The laboratory should consider providing relevant reference ranges for biochemical markers for these systems. Decreases in hormone concentration of this age group are modulated by decreased degradation and excretion of hormone and metabolic products. In women, estrogen levels decrease with menopause with a concurrent rise in pituitary gonadotropins.

There are some physiological differences between elderly adults and other age groups that affect laboratory reference ranges (Table 10–6).

TABLE 10-6

Physiological Differences in the Elderly

Analyte	Reference Range	
	Elderly	Other Adult
Albumin (g/dL)	3.2–4.6	3.5–5.2
Alkaline phosphatase (U/L)		
Male	56–119	53–128
Female	53–143	42–98
Carbon dioxide (mmol/L)	23–31	
Chloride (mEq/L)	98–111	
Cholesterol (mg/dL)		
Male	166–88	
Female	167–291	
Creatinine (mg/dL)		
Male	0.8–1.3	
Female	0.6–1.2	
Creatinine clearance	Decreases approximately 6.5 mL/min/1.73 m^2 per decade	
17-Ketosteroids	Decreases with age (24-hour urine collection)	
Sodium (mEq/L)	132–146	136–145
T$_3$ (ng/dL)	40–181	70–204
T$_4$ (µg/dL)	5.0–1.7	
Male		4.6–10.5
Female		5.5–11.0
Urea nitrogen (mg/dL)	8–23	6–20
Uric acid (mg/dL)		
Male	4.2–8.0	4.4–7.6
Female	3.5–7.3	2.3–6.6

CASE SCENARIO 10-3

Prediabetes and Metabolic Syndrome: Apples and Pears

As the glucose levels appeared on the computer screen, the clinical chemist asked the CLS student to identify those that were normal and those that might indicate diabetes. The student noted that several results were higher than normal but not yet in the range that would indicate possible diabetes. He knew that these results were in the impaired fasting glucose or impaired glucose tolerance range. "Do these patients have prediabetes?" he asked.

The chemist pointed to one result, a fasting glucose level of 111 mg/dL. "Follow up on this patient. Evaluate the laboratory results for assessment of prediabetes and metabolic syndrome. If the glucose is abnormal, what other laboratory results may be abnormal?" he asked.

The student found that the glucose level had been drawn from Mr. Layne, a 47-year-old man who had been treated for hypertension for 6 years. His blood

continued

Case Scenario 10-3 **Prediabetes and Metabolic Syndrome: Apples and Pears** *(continued)*

pressure on this visit was 126/82 mm Hg. His family history included family members who had been diagnosed with hypertension, type 2 diabetes, and heart disease. For his height, Mr. Layne was obese and had been steadily gaining weight over the last year. His physician had noted that Mr. Layne declined help with the development of an exercise plan. Mr. Layne's examination findings included

Waist circumference (in.)	45
BMI (kg/m^2)	34

A lipoprotein profile on Mr. Layne's blood was drawn on the same day as the glucose level. The results were as follows:

		References for age and gender
HDL cholesterol (mg/dL)	30	Optimal > 50 mg/dL
Triacylglycerol (mg/dL)	187	Optimal < 150 mg/dL
LDL cholesterol (mg/dL)	133	Optimal < 100 mg/dL
Total cholesterol (mg/dL)	199	Desirable < 200 mg/dL

A week later, the student noticed that a fresh blood specimen was drawn on Mr. Layne. Mr. Layne's fasting glucose was 114 mg/dL, and a 2-hour glucose challenge test result was 170. These tests confirmed the assessment of prediabetes and ruled out a diagnosis of diabetes. Mr. Layne was also screened for assessment of metabolic syndrome. Mr. Layne's low high-density lipoprotein (HDL) level, high triglyceride level, waist circumference, hypertension, and glucose intolerance confirmed the assessment of metabolic syndrome.

PREDIABETES AND METABOLIC SYNDROME

Prediabetes is defined by results of laboratory analysis for fasting glucose that fall into the impaired fasting glucose range, or by results of laboratory analysis for a 2-hour glucose challenge that fall into the impaired glucose tolerance range, or by laboratory results that exhibit both impaired fasting glucose and impaired glucose tolerance (Table 10–7). Impaired fasting glucose is defined as a glucose level that is above the upper limit of normal and below the lower limit that defines diabetes, 100 to 125 mg/dL. Impaired glucose tolerance is defined as a glucose level that is above the upper limit of normal and below the lower limit that defines diabetes, 140 to 199 mg/dL. The term *prediabetes* is now preferred over "impaired fasting glucose" or "impaired glucose tolerance."[19]

The American Diabetes Association recommends screening for prediabetes for individuals who are 45 years old or older and have a BMI that suggests obesity (BMI ≥ 25 kg/m^2). Screening is also suggested for individuals who are less than 45 years old but obese and have other risk factors, such as family history of diabetes, or ethnicity that is associated with diabetes or hypertension. For individuals who meet the requirements for screening, screening should be repeated every 3 years.[19]

The assessment of metabolic syndrome is based on risk factors for the development of metabolic disorders, such as cardiovascular disease and type 2 diabetes[20] (Table 10–8).

Waist circumference is an estimate of abdominal obesity. Abdominal obesity (android distribution) is more closely associated with the development and progres-

TABLE 10-7

Definition of Prediabetes

	Fasting Plasma Glucose (mg/dL)	2-Hour Plasma Glucose (mg/dL)
Normal (for the assessment of diabetes)	<100	<140
Prediabetes	100–125	140–199
Diabetes	≥126	≥200

The assessment of prediabetes should be confirmed by testing on a second day.

sion of disease than is hip obesity (gynoid distribution). Individuals with abdominal obesity resemble apples, while individuals with hip obesity more closely resemble pears. The risk factors that define metabolic syndrome are associated with insulin resistance.

An assessment of prediabetes or metabolic syndrome indicates risk for disease, but is not diagnosis of the disease in itself. These assessments are intermediate stages in many of the disease processes and have been associated with the progression of insulin resistance. Early assessment of the disease process may assist the medical community in preventing or delaying disease. Several studies have shown the efficacy of early assessment and prevention of disease once identified.

A study performed by Tuomilehto and associates identified middle-aged, obese subjects with impaired glucose tolerance. These individuals were divided into two groups; the control group received minimal diet and exercise counseling, while the test group received individualized weight control therapy through diet and exercise planning. There was greater than 50% reduction in the development of diabetes in the test group compared to the control group.[21]

TABLE 10-8

Definition of Metabolic Syndrome from National Cholesterol Education Program Adult Treatment Panel III

Risk Factor	Defining Level
Abdominal obesity (defined by waist circumference)	
Men	>102 cm (>40 in.)
Women	>88 cm (>35 in.)
Triacylglycerol	≥150 mg/dL
HDL cholesterol	
Men	<40 mg/dL
Women	<50 mg/dL
Blood pressure	≥130 mm Hg systolic or ≥ 85 mm Hg diastolic
Fasting glucose	≥110 mg/dL

Diagnosis is made when three of five risk factors are present.

Source: Expert Panel on Detection, Evaluation and Treatment of High Blood Cholesterol in Adults: Executive summary of the third report of the National Cholesterol Education Program Expert Panel on Detection, Evaluation and Treatment of High Blood Cholesterol in Adults (Adult Treatment Panel III). *JAMA* 2001; 285:2486–2497.

protocol - a formal plan or expectation concerning the actions of those involved in patient care

A study by the Diabetes Prevention Program provided further information about individuals who were obese and showed glucose intolerance. Three intervention treatment groups were studied. One group received diet and exercise counseling; one received medication; and the third received a placebo. As compared to the third group, the first group had over 50% reduction in diabetes and the second group has over 30% reduction in diabetes. Other studies have shown that individuals who are identified with impaired glucose metabolism may prevent or delay the onset of type 2 diabetes through lifestyle modification and appropriate medication.[22–25]

Prediabetes and metabolic syndrome are also associated with high triglycerides, low HDL, hypertension, and the development of cardiovascular disease. The association of these states with cardiovascular risk is discussed in the Chapter 4, Diabetes and Other Carbohydrate Disorders.

The assessment of prediabetes and metabolic syndrome are examples of **protocols** that are designed to be used to prevent disease rather than to diagnose disease. Health providers may identify individuals who are at risk for future disease and implement therapy and medication that will help slow progression to chronic disease such as diabetes and cardiovascular disease.

Case Scenario 10-3 **Prediabetes and Metabolic Syndrome: Apples and Pears**

Follow-Up

The next time that the student was in the laboratory, he searched for additional information about Mr. Layne. Mr. Layne was referred to a registered dietitian for nutritional therapy and received instructions for an exercise program. The primary objective or goal for the clinical treatment of an individual with metabolic syndrome is first, to reduce the risk of clinical atherosclerotic disease, and second, to decrease the risk of developing type 2 diabetes mellitus. Generally, reducing the risk for the former involves reducing the major risk factors: cigarette smoking and low-density lipoprotein (LDL) cholesterol, blood pressure, and/or plasma glucose levels.[26] Due to the likely presence of abdominal obesity, weight loss is a necessary first step. ●

Digestive Disorders

In addition to information about nutrition, the clinical laboratory also provides information about digestion. Specialized chemical analysis provides objective information about gastric output, digestive enzymes, and intestinal absorption to help the physician evaluate and treat digestive disorders.

THE GASTROINTESTINAL TRACT

lumen - space within a tube, such as a blood vessel or the esophagus

Nutrients are digested in the human body extracellularly, outside of cells. Digestive enzymes are secreted from cells lining the **lumen** of the organs of the digestive tract. The digestive enzymes, or exocrine secretions, hydrolyze large molecules in food into small, soluble molecules that can be transported across the lining of the gastrointestinal tract into blood and hence to body cells as nutrients.

Nutrients are ground into finer particles by the teeth, partially digested by amylase from the salivary glands, and carried by **peristalsis** along the esophagus and into the stomach. **Chief cells**, parietal cells, and mucus-secreting cells line the lumen of the stomach. Chief cells synthesize and secrete pepsin and pepsinogen, the precursor to pepsin. Pepsin is a proteolytic enzyme that degrades polypeptide chains by cleaving peptide bonds. Parietal cells produce hydrochloric acid and intrinsic factor. Hydrogen ions are secreted by active transport across the parietal cell membrane via a transmembrane protein called H^+-ATPase. Through this process, the pH of the stomach may reach levels below pH of 1. Hydrogen ion secretion is stimulated by the hormone gastrin, which itself is produced by the cells of the **pyloric** region of the stomach and the **duodenum**. As previously mentioned, intrinsic factor is a protein that binds and helps transport vitamin B_{12} through the lining of the intestine to blood. Very little absorption of nutrients into the circulatory system occurs in the stomach. The contents of the stomach are mixed and liquefied and passed into the duodenum, the first section of the small intestine.

Both the gallbladder and the pancreas drain into the duodenum. The gallbladder drains bile, which contains bile acids and bile pigments produced by the liver, into the duodenum. The release of bile from the gallbladder is stimulated by the hormone **cholecystokinin**. Bile acids contain lipids that have been conjugated to hydrophilic groups to make them more soluble in the water-based fluids of the intestinal system. Bile pigments consist of the breakdown products of hemoglobin, which has metabolized by the liver. The color of the bile pigments contributes to the brown color of feces.

The pancreas contains both exocrine and endocrine cells. Pancreatic fluid contains sodium bicarbonate, which neutralizes the acidic gastric fluid, increasing the pH to approximately 8. Pancreatic proteolytic enzymes attack proteins that are carried in the gastric fluid. Arginine- and lysine-containing peptides are cleaved by trypsin; tyrosine-, phenylalanine-, and tryptophan-containing peptides are cleaved by **chymotrypsin**; **elastase** cleaves peptide bonds associated with alanine and serine; and **carboxypeptidase** removes amino acids at the C-terminal of peptides. Pancreatic **nucleases** hydrolyze nucleic acids, which are also contained in the gastric fluid, into smaller, more absorbable units. The secretion of pancreatic fluid into the duodenum is regulated by gastrointestinal hormones. **Secretin** controls the release of sodium bicarbonate, and cholecystokinin controls the release of the catabolic enzymes. The pancreatic hormones, produced in the islets of Langerhans, also contribute to nutrient degradation. Amylase breaks down starch polymers into monosaccharides, and lipase hydrolyzes triglycerides into fatty acids and monoglycerides.

Final digestion of nutrients occurs within the villi, which line the lumen of the small intestine. Peptidases and **disaccharidases** break their substrates into amino acids and monosaccharide subunits that are small enough to be absorbed through the lining of the intestine and into the lymphatic and circulatory systems. Nutrients travel to the liver, adipose tissue, and other organs, where they are further processed.

Nutrients that are not absorbed through the small intestine mucosa pass into the large intestine. This undigested material consists of mainly of water and cellulose. Resident bacteria of the large intestine complete the degradation process. The chief function of the large intestine is the reabsorption of water from the undigested material. Failure to reabsorb water causes watery diarrhea, while absorption of too much water may produce constipation.

peristalsis - wavelike movement that occurs involuntarily in hollow tubes of the body

chief cells - secretory cells that line the gastric glands and secrete pepsin or its precursor, pepsinogen

pyloric - pertaining to the distal portion of the stomach or to the opening between the stomach and duodenum

duodenum - the first part of the small intestine that is adjacent to the pyloric region of the stomach

cholecystokinin - hormone secreted by the upper small intestine that stimulates contraction of the gallbladder and pancreatic secretion

chymotrypsin - digestive enzyme produced by the pancreas that, with trypsin, hydrolyzes proteins to peptones or amino acids

elastase - an enzyme that dissolves elastin

nuclease - an enzyme that participates in the hydrolysis of nucleic acids

THE TEAM APPROACH
The assessment of gastrointestinal disorders requires a multidisciplinary approach. Evaluation is based upon patient history, physical examination, imaging studies, and laboratory markers of disease. In general, laboratory tests do not make the diagnosis in digestive disease but support the clinical impression and contribute objective information for monitoring prognosis and treatment. Laboratory results contribute to assessment of malabsorption, inflammation, and tumorous processes of the gastrointestinal tract.

carboxypeptidase - a pancreatic enzyme that hydrolyzes peptides from the C-terminal end

secretin - hormone secreted by duodenal mucosa; stimulates sodium bicarbonate secretion by the pancreas and bile secretion by the liver

disaccharidases - enzymes that hydrolyze the glycolic bond of disaccharides

flatulence - excessive gas in the stomach and intestines

steatorrhea - failure to digest or absorb fats in the gastrointestinal tract

✔ **Common Sense Check**
The first check for intestinal malabsorption of fat is stool appearance. Stool that contains excess amounts of fat appears greasy and pale.

MALABSORPTION

Malabsorption is the consequence of a variety of disorders. Such consequences may disrupt the digestion of a specific nutrient, such as carbohydrate or lipid, or may be of a more general nature. Symptoms of malabsorption are caused both by the effects of water absorption from nondigested substances and by nutritional deficiencies in tissue cells. Symptoms include weight loss, bruising, **flatulence**, bloating, and diarrhea. The effects of malabsorption may be manifested as abnormal amounts of undigested materials in stool. A common consequence of malabsorption is **steatorrhea**, which may present as greasy, pale stools or stools that have a normal appearance. The laboratory tests for fat in stool both qualitatively and quantitatively.

Inflammatory diseases of the gastrointestinal tract may be of nonspecific or unknown origin. Bacterial, viral, and parasitic etiology must be considered. Onset is often sudden with nausea, vomiting, abdominal cramps, and diarrhea. Vomiting that causes excessive fluid loss may produce metabolic alkalosis with hypochloremia. Severe diarrhea may cause acidosis. Either vomiting or diarrhea may result in severe dehydration and renal failure. Rehydration is an important supportive treatment.[27,28]

Nutritional deficiencies vary depending upon the severity of disease and the area of the gastrointestinal tract that is involved. Specific deficiencies result in specific diseases. Iron deficiency results in microcytic anemia, folic acid deficiency results in megaloblastic anemia, and calcium deficiency may be caused by vitamin D deficiency or impaired absorption of calcium. Malabsorption of fats may cause impaired absorption of fat-soluble vitamins such as vitamin K.

Laboratory tests such as disaccharidase levels, D-xylose absorption test, fecal fat analysis, breath tests, iron studies, and folic acid and vitamin B_{12} tests contribute to the clinical picture of malabsorption of nutrients. Test Methodologies 10–4 through 10–6 describe laboratory testing of fecal fats, D-xylose, and lactose/hydrogen (lactose breath test).

TEST METHODOLOGY 10-4.   FECAL FAT ANALYSIS

Normal fecal lipids consists of 60% fatty acids, 30% sterols, and 10% triacylglycerols. Increased fecal fats are clinically significant to the assessment of pancreatic insufficiency and small intestine disorders. Fecal fat is also increased in biliary obstruction. Direct measurement of fecal fat is used to establish a diagnosis of malabsorption. Steatorrhea is evidence of fat malabsorption but is not always present.

The Reaction Principle

Qualitative analysis for fecal fat employs fat-soluble stains, such as Sudan III and Sudan IV, to stain fat globules on a microscopic slide preparation of stool. The stained stool is examined for stained oil droplets. Triacylglycerols stain more readily than fatty acids with these stains. Undigested meat particles will also stain, but may be distinguished by their rectangular, striated appearance. Fecal fat may be analyzed qualitatively by gravimetric measurement. The fecal specimen is acidified to obtain deionized fatty acids. Lipids are extracted into an organic solvent. The solvent is evaporated and the residue is weighed.

continued

TEST METHODOLOGY 10-4.   FECAL FAT ANALYSIS (continued)

The Specimen

Qualitative Analysis

Random stool specimen.

Quantitative Analysis

A 72-hour collection is recommended. Specimen is collected into a preweighed container. Specimen and container are weighed to determine the total weight of collection.

Reference Ranges

Qualitative reference range: 40–50 droplets per HPF

Quantitative reference range: ≤6 g/day (fecal fat may also be reported as percentage of total fecal weight)

TEST METHODOLOGY 10-5.   D-XYLOSE

A D-xylose absorption test is an indirect but specific method for assessing mucosal absorption of the small intestine. D-Xylose is not normally present in blood or urine and digestive enzymes are not necessary for its metabolism. Normally, approximately 60% of D-xylose taken in an oral dose will pass through the intestinal mucosa and, over time, into the circulatory system, eventually to be excreted into urine. Low absorption of xylose will occur in disorders of the small intestine, such as intestinal malabsorption, Crohn's disease, celiac disease, AIDS, pellagra, and ascariasis.

The Reaction Principle

Several spectrophotometric procedures are available for laboratory measurement of xylose. Xylose is measured by heating the protein-free specimen to convert xylose to a furfural, then combining the product with a chromagen for measurement by spectrophotometry. An *o*-toluidine procedure is also available for xylose, with differential absorbance at 630 nm.[29]

The Specimen

Patient Preparation

The patient fasts overnight. D-Xylose is given by mouth. Either a 5-g or a 25-g dose is given. The 5-g dose is less likely to cause nausea or diarrhea, but is less sensitive for detecting malabsorption.

Procedure

Urine is collected over the next 5 hours.

Reference Ranges

For proper interpretation of the results, the urine output must be adequate and glomerular filtration rate must be normal. Reference ranges below describe the 5-g dose and amount recovered in a 5-hour urine collection.

Reference	≥1.4 g
Borderline	1.2–1.4 g
Abnormal:	<1.2 g

TEST METHODOLOGY 10-6.   LACTOSE BREATH TEST

The production of hydrogen (H_2) by bacterial fermentation of carbohydrate substrate in the colon is the basis for the lactose breath test. The test measures the changes in breath hydrogen concentration prior to and after the ingestion of lactose. Normally, very little hydrogen is detectable in the breath. Individuals who suffer from lactose malabsorption produce increased amounts of hydrogen because undigested lactose passes from the small intestine into the large intestine unmetabolized. In the large intestine, bacteria ferment the lactose to gases, including hydrogen. The hydrogen is absorbed from the large intestine and carried through the blood to the lungs, where it is exhaled.

The Reaction Principle

H_2 is measured by gas chromatography or electrochemical hydrogen analyzer.

The Specimen

A baseline sample is tested for H_2. The patient drinks a lactose-loaded beverage. Breath samples are tested for H_2 at 1, 2, and 3 hours postingestion.

Reference Range

Reference intervals are method dependent. An increase of ≥ 20 ppm (parts per million) is considered to be evidence of lactose malabsorption.[30-33] In a healthy individual, the difference between the H_2 breath baseline and postingestion samples will be small. Some patients with lactose malabsorption will produce methane from lactose. Both methane and H_2 should be measured.

CASE SCENARIO 10-4

Zollinger-Ellison Syndrome: The Gastrinoma

Seven samples were submitted for gastric fluid analysis on patient Richard Wilson. The laboratory technologist measured the pH and titratable acid for each specimen and calculated the basal and peak acid outputs. Both the basal and peak acid outputs were very high.

Basal acid output (mEq/hr)	30
Peak acid output (mEq/hr)	75

The technologist noted that Mr. Wilson's serum gastrin level of 170 pg/mL was also high (reference range for an adult: 25 to 90 pg/mL). A gastrin stimulation test showed marked increase (320 pg/mL) after administration of secretin.

GASTRIC FLUID ANALYSIS

Analysis of gastric fluid is useful in assessment of gastrointestinal disorders to evaluate hyperchlorhydria or hypochlorhydria. Gastric fluid analysis is useful in assessing gastrin-secreting tumors such as those in Zollinger-Ellison syndrome, evaluating gastric hyperacidity, and diagnosing achlorhydria. Test Methodology 10–7 describes the procedure for performing gastric acid testing.

TEST METHODOLOGY 10-7.   GASTRIC ACID

The Reaction Principle

Gastric pH is measured with a calibrated pH meter. Acid output is determined by titrating the gastric fluid with NaOH to determine the milliequivalents per milliliter (mEq/mL) of hydrogen ion.

The Specimen

Patient Preparation

Medications that may affect gastric secretion are discontinued for 24 hours prior to testing. The patient fasts overnight.

Procedure

The stomach is intubated. A basal specimen is aspirated. A gastric acid stimulant, such as pentagastrin, is administered subcutaneously or intramuscularly. Six specimens are collected every 15 minutes for 90 minutes.

Test and Calculations

Volume, pH, titratable acid, and acid output are reported. The specimen consists of 25 mL of gastric fluid. Of this fluid, 5 mL is titrated to pH 7.0 with 10 mL of 0.1N NaOH. The acid output is

$$0.1 \text{ mEq/mL} \times 10 \text{ mL} = 1 \text{ mEq}$$

$$\text{Acid} = 1 \text{ mEq/5 mL, or 0.2 mEq/mL}$$

The specimen consists of 25 mL, so

$$\text{Acid output of the specimen} = 0.2 \text{ mEq/mL} \times 25 \text{ mL, or 5 mEq}$$

The peak output is the average of the two consecutive collections with the highest free acid. The peak output is expressed in milliequivalents per hour (mEq/hr).

Reference Ranges

Basal volume   10–100 mL
Stimulated volume   40–350 mL

	Basal Acid Output	Peak Acid Output
	(mEq/hr)	(mEq/hr)
Reference	<5	5–20
Gastric ulcer	<5	5–20
Duodenal ulcer	5–15	20–60
Zollinger-Ellison syndrome	>20	>60

Gastrin measurement is also useful in determining causes of gastric abnormalities. Some patients with ulcer disease will have mildly elevated serum gastrin levels. The gastrin stimulation test following secretin injection can help distinguish patients with **gastrinoma** and Zollinger-Ellison syndrome from patients with secondary causes of elevated gastrin levels. In clinical chemistry, the only well-indicated routine use of gastrin assays is in the diagnosis of gastrinomas, such as in the Zollinger-Ellison syndrome.[34–37] Test Methodology 10–8 describes the procedure for gastrin analysis.[38,39]

gastrinoma - gastrin-secreting tumor

TEST METHODOLOGY 10-8. GASTRIN STIMULATION

Basal value of gastrin is determined as the average concentration of the two samples drawn before secretin administration. The maximal increase in gastrin is determined as the maximal value of gastrin after secretin administration.

The Reaction Principle

Gastrin secretion is evaluated by immunoassay, usually enzyme-linked immunosorbent assay (ELISA). Test methodology for gastrin secretion should measure all forms of gastrin.[40]

The Specimen

Patient Preparation

The patient fasts overnight.

Procedure

Two fasting specimens are drawn. Secretin is administered intravenously. Specimens are drawn at 2, 5, 10, 15, 20, and 30 minutes after injection of secretin. Serum is separated from cells and frozen if the test will not be performed immediately.

Reference Ranges

Reference	No or mild maximal increase
Zollinger-Ellison syndrome	Maximal increase ≥200 pg/mL

■■ CLINICAL CORRELATION

Laboratory results are helpful in assessing the consequences of tumorous processes of the gastrointestinal tract. The most reliable test for Zollinger-Ellison syndrome is immunoassay measurement of serum gastrin; levels over 150 pg/mL are diagnostic, and in some patients levels may exceed 1000 pg/mL. Clinical characteristics and hypergastrinemia are specific; however, hypergastrinemia can be found in hypochlorhydric states, such as pernicious anemia, and in renal insufficiency, which is associated with decreased clearance of gastrins. Duodenal gastrinomas are visualized about 50% of the time and pancreatic tumors 75%–90% of the time by ultrasound.

multiple endocrine neoplasia - one of several inherited endocrine gland syndromes caused by a defect in tumor suppressor genes

---

Case Scenario 10-4 Zollinger-Ellison Syndrome: The Gastrinoma

Discussion

Previously Mr. Wilson had been diagnosed with multiple duodenal ulcers. Most recently, he complained of severe abdominal pain and diarrhea. On the basis of his symptoms and biochemical studies, his physician made a diagnosis of gastrinoma of Zollinger-Ellison syndrome.

ZOLLINGER-ELLISON SYNDROME

Zollinger-Ellison is a syndrome that is caused by a gastrin-producing tumor, or gastrinoma. High levels of gastrin cause overproduction of stomach acid, and the high acid levels lead to multiple ulcers in the stomach and small bowel. The gastrinoma may occur in the stomach, pancreas, lymph node, or mesentery. Multiple tumors may occur. About one-half to two-thirds of single gastrinomas are malignant tumors that most commonly spread to the liver and lymph nodes near the pancreas and small bowel. Nearly 25% of patients with gastrinomas have multiple tumors as part of a condition called **multiple endocrine neoplasia** type I (MEN I). MEN I patients have tumors in their pituitary gland and parathyroid glands in addition to tumors of the pancreas. Zollinger-Ellison syndrome is suspected in patients with relevant clinical history, x-ray evidence of ulceration, and an excessive gastric acid secretion.[41]

> **Case Scenario 10-4** **Zollinger-Ellison Syndrome: The Gastrinoma**
>
> **Follow-Up**
>
> H$^+$, K$^+$-ATPase inhibitor was given to reduce parietal cell H$^+$ secretion. The inhibitor alleviates symptoms and promotes ulcer healing. Mr. Wilson's progress will be follow by his physician. If the tumor spreads, chemotherapy will be considered to reduce tumor mass. Total **gastrectomy** will be considered for treatment failure. ●

gastrectomy - surgical removal of part or all of the stomach

CASE SCENARIO 10-5

Pancreatic Insufficiency: The Patient With Cystic Fibrosis

Pam was 18 years old and just entering college. She had been diagnosed with cystic fibrosis when she was 6 years old. As a toddler, she had trouble gaining weight and often complained of stomachache. She was diagnosed with cystic fibrosis when she became seriously dehydrated. A **sweat test** for chloride was performed at that time; the positive result confirmed the physician's suspicion that she had cystic fibrosis. Pam's parents helped her start chest physical therapy to clear her lungs of the thick mucus that is produced as a consequence of the disease and gave her pancreatic enzyme supplements to help her digest and absorb food at a normal rate. As Pam grew older, she monitored her own symptoms for progression of the disease. At each meal, she took pancreatic enzymes.

However, during orientation week at college, Pam found it difficult to maintain her usual routine. She forgot to take pancreatic supplements at several meals and started to experience symptoms of stomach pain and vomiting. She also had a slight temperature and was sweating. She immediately saw her physician, who ordered laboratory tests to evaluate pancreatic function. The tests showed diminished pancreatic function, as evidenced by decreased amylase, and defective fat absorption, as evidenced by decreased serum cholesterol and increased stool fats.

sweat test - test for cystic fibrosis that involves measuring the subject's sweat for abnormally high sodium chloride content

Test	Result	Reference Range
Amylase (U/L)	22	28–100
Lipase (U/L)	8	<38
Cholesterol (mg/dL)	90	140–200
Qualitative fecal fat (droplets per HPF)	>100	40–50

CYSTIC FIBROSIS

Cystic fibrosis is an inherited, autosomal recessive disease that affects nearly all **exocrine glands** in the body. The disease is characterized by chronic obstructive pulmonary disease, pancreatic insufficiency, and abnormally high sweat electrolytes. The gene that causes the disease encodes for a membrane-associated protein called

exocrine glands - glands that secrete externally through ducts

the cystic fibrosis transmembrane regulator (CFTR). CFTR appears to be part of a cyclic AMP–regulated chloride channel, which regulates chloride and sodium transport across epithelial membranes. The disease causes the exocrine glands to become obstructed by viscous material. The blockage leads to cellular damage within the tissue. Blockage of the pulmonary bronchi with thick mucus is associated with recurrent or chronic pulmonary infections. Pancreatic insufficiency leads to poor digestion and poor growth pattern with a deficiency of fat-soluble vitamins. Excessive sweating leads to episodes of hypotonic dehydration and circulatory failure. In arid climates, infants may present with chronic metabolic alkalosis. Salt crystal formation on the skin is an indicator of cystic fibrosis.[28]

Pancreatic insufficiency occurs as the result of abnormally viscous fluid, causing decreased amylase and lipase activity, decreased trypsin and chymotrypsin levels, and lowered bicarbonate level. Fat in the stool, measured qualitatively or quantitatively, is an indirect test of decreased fat absorption and decreased pancreatic exocrine function. Pancreatic insufficiency may also affect glucose metabolism through delayed insulin response. The patient may also show the effects of the disease through reduced blood levels of carotenoids, vitamins A and E, essential fatty acids, and cholesterol. Laboratory results aid the assessment and differentiation of pancreatic insufficiency, pancreatic cancer, and pancreatic inflammation. Test Methodologies 10–9 and 10–10 describe the analysis of serum amylase and lipase, respectively.

TEST METHODOLOGY 10-9.   AMYLASE

Amylase is a hydrolase that catalyzes the breakdown of starch, glycogen, and some oligosaccharides. Calcium is a necessary cofactor in the reaction. Animal amylases, called alpha amylases, break down the alpha-1,4 glycosidic linkages in these substrates, producing glucose, maltose, and dextrins, which contain the branched products of degradation. Amylase is produced in the pancreas and salivary glands. Small amounts of amylase are also found in the small intestine and skeletal muscle. The finding of increased concentrations of amylase in blood and urine is clinically significant to the diagnosis of pancreatitis. Hyperamylasemia is also found in nonpancreatic disorders such as salivary gland tumor, mumps, perforated peptic ulcer, renal insufficiency, and diabetic ketoacidosis. Low levels of serum amylase may indicate pancreatic insufficiency such as found in cystic fibrosis.

The Reaction

Laboratory reactions that are used to measure concentrations of amylase in body fluids start with a starch or oligosaccharide, such as maltopentose or maltotetraose, as substrate. The oligosaccharide maltopentose is shown in the reaction below. The amylase-catalyzed reaction is coupled with an enzyme reaction that uses NAD^+ as a coenzyme.

Alpha Amylase Alpha Glucosidase

$$\text{Maltopentose} \rightarrow \text{maltotriose} + \text{maltose} \rightarrow \text{glucose}$$

Hexokinase

$$\text{Glucose} + \text{ATP} \rightarrow \text{glucose 6-phosphate} + 5 \text{ ATP}$$

Glucose-6-Phosphate Dehydrogenase

$$\text{Glucose 6-phosphate} + NAD^+ \rightarrow \text{6-phosphogluconolactone} + NADH + H^+$$

The reaction is measured by the change in absorbance of NAD^+ at 340 nm.

continued

TEST METHODOLOGY 10-9.   AMYLASE *(continued)*

The Specimen

Serum, heparinized plasma, and urine may be tested. Anticoagulants, such as EDTA, citrate, or oxalate, should not be used because of their effect on the cofactor, calcium. Lowered pH may affect the stability of urine amylase; therefore, the pH of stored urine must be maintained at 7.

Reference Ranges

Reference intervals are method dependent. The reference intervals below are common:

Serum (U/L)	28–100
Urine (IU/L)	1–17

TEST METHODOLOGY 10-10.   LIPASE

Lipase enzymes catalyze the hydrolysis of glycerol esters of long- chain fatty acids. Lipase hydrolyzes dietary triacylglycerol at the ester bonds at carbons 1 and 3 of the molecule to produce monoacylglycerols and fatty acids. Lipase acts at the interface between water and lipid, or substrate; therefore, the substrate must be in an emulsion, such at that found in association with bile salts. A cofactor, called colipase, is required for the reaction. Lipase is produced by the pancreas. Small amounts of lipase are also found in small intestine and stomach. The finding of increased concentrations of lipase in body fluids is clinically significant to the diagnosis of pancreatitis. Hyperlipemia is also found in non-pancreatic disorders, such as perforated peptic ulcers and intestinal obstruction.

The Reaction

Laboratory analysis of lipase measures the fatty acid that is produced by the catalysis of lipase.

Lipase at pH 8.6–9.0

$$\text{Triacylglycerol} + H_2O \rightarrow \text{2-monoacylglycerol} + \text{fatty acids}$$

Fatty acid produced by the reaction may be measured in several ways:
1. Increased turbidity of the product occurs as the result of increased fatty acids. The reaction can be measured by turbidometry.
2. Fatty acid production may also be coupled to reactions that can be measured by spectrophotometry or fluorometry.

The Specimen

Serum may be tested. Hemolysis will inhibit lipase activity.

Reference Range

Reference intervals are method dependent. The reference interval below is common with turbidometric methods.

Serum (U/L)	<38 U/L

The diagnosis of cystic fibrosis is made by clinical symptoms and positive sweat chloride test. People with cystic fibrosis have unusually large amounts of chloride in their sweat when compared to reference ranges of healthy individuals, due to the CFTR defect. **Iontophoresis** is used to facilitate sweating with the drug **pilocarpine**. The sweat is collected on sterile gauze over a period of a few minutes and later analyzed for the amount of chloride present.[27] Genetic analysis can be used to

iontophoresis - introduction of a drug through intact skin by the application of a direct electric current

pilocarpine - a muscarinic alkaloid drug that can induce sweating

counsel families for gene carrier status. The serum concentration of immunoreactive trypsin is elevated in newborns with cystic fibrosis. Measurement of this enzyme is the basis of cystic fibrosis newborn screening programs.

Case Scenario 10-5 Pancreatic Insufficiency: The Patient With Cystic Fibrosis

Follow-Up

The goals of therapy for cystic fibrosis patients are the maintenance of nutritional status and prevention of further cellular damage. Pam's therapy was directed by her physician in conjunction with nutritionists and nurses. Pam was counseled to take pancreatic enzyme replacement capsules with all meals, continue her chest physical therapy, and take antibiotics to decrease the risk of lung infection.

Pam registered for classes in the clinical molecular biology program, in hopes of working in a research laboratory to study the gene mutation that causes her own disease. ●

CASE SCENARIO 10-6

Electrolyte Disturbance in Acute Vomiting:
Does Mr. Vijay Have Metabolic Alkalosis?

The technologist working in the emergency department (ED) satellite laboratory had been asked to collect blood specimens from an 80-year-old male patient, Mr. Vijay, since the nurse had difficulty collecting a nonhemolyzed sample. The patient's veins were difficult to palpate, and he was not very responsive or cooperative with the venipuncture technique. The patient was not combative, however, and the venipuncture was successful. The technologist collected the specimens for basic chemistry profile and CBC. Mr. Vijay's preliminary diagnosis was severe vomiting for 6 hours. Laboratory test results were as follows:

Test	Result	Reference Range (Age-Specific)
Sodium (mmol/L)	149	136–145
Potassium (unit)	3.6	3.5–5.1
Chloride (mmol/L)	108	98–107
CO_2 (mmol/L)	30	22–28
BUN (mg/dL)	48	8–23
Hematocrit (%)	52	37–51
Hemoglobin (g/dL)	16.5	12.6–17.2
Anion gap (mmol/L)	14.6	7–15

The technologist verified that no error codes printed out with the analysis results. Although some of the values were abnormal compared to the reference ranges, the electrolytes were balanced, based on the anion gap, and values correlated with the preliminary diagnosis. Results were reported promptly following the laboratory protocol for the ED. It was noted that none of the values was at a critical or alert level.

GASTRIC FLUIDS AND ELECTROLYTE LEVELS

Gastric fluid is rich in hydrochloric acid and electrolytes, including potassium. Acute loss of gastric fluid from vomiting causes loss of ions, including hydrogen and potassium. Metabolic alkalosis results from loss of hydrochloric acid and fluid volume depletion.[27] It is characterized by increased plasma bicarbonate and total carbon dioxide levels. Hypokalemia is also common with metabolic alkalosis, especially when resulting from gastric fluid loss, such as in vomiting, pyloric obstruction, or gastrointestinal suction. Loss of gastric fluid also depletes plasma fluid volume, causing dehydration. Dehydration causes some analytes to be relatively increased, including sodium, chloride, and blood urea nitrogen, illustrating the inverse relationship between water and chemical constituents in the plasma. Sodium is a sensitive indicator of plasma fluid level since it makes up roughly half of the total plasma concentration. Thus, when plasma water level decreases, plasma osmolality and sodium levels increase.[42]

Case Scenario 10-6 **Electrolyte Disturbance in Acute Vomiting: Does Mr. Vijay Have Metabolic Alkalosis?**

Follow-Up

Mr. Vijay, who has been vomiting for 6 hours, has developed electrolyte and acid-base disturbance. The electrolyte disturbances typical with severe vomiting are hypokalemia, hypernatremia, and increased total CO_2. This was found to be true in this case as well, considering that the serum potassium level is on the low side of the normal reference range. The physicians determined that he has a history of heart problems and was feeling dizzy and lethargic. His eyes appeared sunken and he complained of a dry mouth, typical of dehydration. He walked unsteadily and complained also of muscle aches. He was thirsty but unable to retain food or fluid. A neighbor brought Mr. Vijay to the hospital, where examination showed that his blood pressure was low and his pulse and respirations were rapid. By talking with the neighbor and the patient, the physician found that the patient lives alone but has meals brought in to his home on weekdays. Since the patient arrived on a weekend, the physician suspected that he was eating leftover food from earlier in the week that was not adequately refrigerated or reheated, resulting in common *Staphylococcus* food poisoning. This illness is generally short lived and self-limiting except in the elderly or those susceptible to electrolyte disturbances. Treatment involved restoring fluid and electrolyte balance with intravenous fluids, providing medication to counteract nausea and vomiting, and restoring normal intake of food by mouth. ●

OTHER ELECTROLYTE DISTURBANCES RESULTING FROM GASTROINTESTINAL DISTURBANCES

Intestinal Loss

Other gastrointestinal illnesses can cause fluid and electrolyte loss as well. Diarrhea is associated with increased gastrointestinal motility and decreased absorption of water and electrolytes in the colon. The result is loss of bicarbonate, sodium, potassium, and chloride. Metabolic acidosis results from the loss of bicarbonate. Treatment involves replacing fluids and electrolytes in order to reverse the acid-base and electrolyte disturbance.[28]

Bulimia Nervosa

This condition is characterized by recurrent episodes of binge eating followed by self-induced vomiting, use of laxatives and/or diuretics, and vigorous dieting or fasting to overcome the effects of excessive eating. It is associated with adolescent and young adult females more than any other group, even though it can occur at any age. Bulimia can cause several ill effects, including electrolyte imbalance, especially potassium depletion from vomiting and laxatives. Life-threatening consequences can arise from the hypokalemia and metabolic alkalosis, with resulting cardiac arrhythmia and shock. Fluid and electrolyte replacement can reverse the acute hypokalemia if administered early. The psychological aspects of the illness require long-term treatment in order to prevent relapses.[28]

SUMMARY

The role of the laboratory in nutritional and digestive assessment was addressed through several scenarios in this chapter. In particular, the effects of protein and mineral deficiencies were discussed in the context of alcoholic liver disease and malnutrition of the elderly. Acute disorders have an effect on mineral and electrolyte balance as well as other nutritional markers. Dietary plans and other interventions can help treat malabsorption from cystic fibrosis and the hyperlipidemia and glucose intolerance of metabolic syndrome. In these disorders, laboratory data provide vital information for the diagnosis and treatment of disease.

EXERCISES

As you consider the scenarios presented in this chapter, answer the following questions:

1. List protein laboratory tests that are used as sensitive indicators of malnutrition and describe the use of these tests to assess short-term and long-term nutritional status.
2. Describe the roles and functions of vitamins and trace elements in the physiology of the human body.
3. Discuss the principle of the Schilling test.
4. Discuss the etiology of lactose intolerance and list laboratory tests that are useful in the diagnosis of this disorder.
5. Define steatorrhea and describe three laboratory tests that are used to assess this condition.
6. Explain the etiology of cystic fibrosis and describe the association of this disease with pancreatic insufficiency.
7. State the chemical reaction that is catalyzed by the enzyme lipase.
8. State the chemical reaction that is catalyzed by the enzyme amylase.
9. Define metabolic syndrome, using five diagnostic criteria.
10. Define prediabetes, using three diagnostic criteria.

References

1. Boosalis MG, Stiles NJ: Nutritional assessment in the elderly: Biochemical analyses. *Clin Lab Sci* 1995; 8:31–33.
2. American Dietetics Association: Who is a registered dietitian? (2006). Available at *http://www.eatright.org*
3. Lee DL, Nieman C: *Nutritional Assessment*, ed 3. New York: McGraw-Hill, 2003.
4. Briggs GM, Calloway DH (eds): *Bogert's Nutrition and Physical Fitness*. Philadelphia: WB Saunders, 1979.
5. Roberts WL, McMillin GA, Burtis CA, Bruns DE: Reference information for the clinical laboratory. In Burtis CA, Ashwood ER, Bruns DE (eds): *Tietz Textbook of Clinical Chemistry*, ed 4. St. Louis: Elsevier Saunders, 2006.
6. The Cleveland Clinic: Alcoholic liver disease (revised 2004). Available at *http://www.clevelandclinicmeded.com/diseasemanagement/gastro/ald/ald1.htm*
7. Newsome DA, et al: Oral zinc in macular degeneration. *Arch Ophthalmol* 1988; 106:192–197.
8. Duester G: Involvement of alcohol dehydrogenase, short chain dehydrogenase/reductase, aldehyde dehydrogenase, and cytochrome p450 in the control of retinoids signaling by activation of retinoic acid synthesis. *Biochemistry* 1996; 535:1221–1227.
9. Perrson B, Krook M, Jornvall H: Short-chain dehydrogenases/reductases. *Adv Exp Med Biol* 1995; 372:383–395.
10. Saari JC Retinoids in photosensitive systems. In Sporn MB, Roberts AB, Goodman DS (eds): *The Retinoids: Biology, Chemistry and Medicine*. New York: Raven Press, 1994.
11. Bates J, McClain CJ: The effect of severe zinc deficiency on serum levels of albumin, transferrin, and prealbumin in man. *Am J Clin Nutr* 1981; 34:1655–1660.
12. U.S. Department of Agriculture, Food and Nutrition Information Center: Dietary reference intakes (DRI) and recommended dietary allowances (RDA) (modified January 24, 2006). Available at *http://www.nal.usda.gov/fnic/etext/000105.html*
13. Lee GR, et al: Megaloblastic anemias: Disorders of impaired DNA synthesis. In *Wintrobe's Clinical Hematology*, vol 1. Philadelphia: Lippincott Williams & Wilkins, 1999.
14. Harmening DM: *Clinical Hematology and Fundamentals of Hemostasis*, ed 3. Philadelphia: FA Davis, 2001.
15. McKenzie SB: Megaloblastic and nonmegaloblastic microcytic anemias. In *Clinical Laboratory Hematology*. Upper Saddle River, NJ: Pearson Education, Inc, 2004.
16. ARUP Laboratories: Megaloblastic anemia (revised 2006). Available at *http://www.arupconsult.com*
17. Irvine WJ: Immunoassay of gastric intrinsic factor and the titration of antibody to intrinsic factor. *Clin Exp Immunol* 1966; 1:99–118.
18. Rothenberg SP, et al: Autoantibodies to intrinsic factor: Their determination and clinical usefulness. *J Lab Clin Med* 1971; 77:476.
19. American Diabetes Association: Diagnosis and classification of diabetes mellitus. *Diabetes Care* 2004; 27(Suppl 1):S5–S10.
20. Expert Panel on Detection, Evaluation and Treatment of High Blood Cholesterol in Adults: Executive summary of the third report of the National Cholesterol Education Program Expert Panel on Detection, Evaluation and Treatment of High Blood Cholesterol in Adults (Adult Treatment Panel III). *JAMA* 2001; 285:2486–2497.
21. Tuomilehto J, et al: Prevention of type 2 diabetes mellitus by changes in lifestyle among subjects with impaired glucose tolerance. *N Engl J Med* 2001; 344:1343–1350.
22. Knowler WC, et al: Reduction in the incidence of type 2 diabetes with lifestyle intervention or metformin. *N Engl J Med* 2002; 346:393–403.
23. Buchanan TA, et al: Preservation of pancreatic β-cell function and prevention of type 2 diabetes by pharmacological treatment of insulin resistance in high-risk Hispanic women. *Diabetes* 2002; 51:2796–2803.
24. Chiasson JL, et al: Acarbose for prevention of type 2 diabetes mellitus: The STOP-NIDDM randomized trial. *Lancet* 2002; 359:2072–2077.
25. Pan XR, et al: Effects of diet and exercise in preventing NIDDM in people with impaired glucose tolerance: The Da Qing IGT and Diabetes Study. *Diabetes Care* 1997; 20:537–544.
26. Short RJ, Sahebzamani FM, Brownlee HJ: Case study: Screening and treatment of prediabetes in primary care. *Clin Diabetes* 2004; 22:98–100.

27. Hill PG: Gastric, pancreatic, and intestinal function. In Burtis CA, Ashwood ER, Bruns DE (eds): *Tietz Texbook of Clinical Chemistry*, ed 4. St. Louis: Elsevier Saunders, 2006.

28. Beers M, Berkow R: *The Merck Manual of Diagnosis and Therapy*, ed 17. Rahway, NJ: Merck & Co., 1999.

29. Goodwin JF: Method for simultaneous direct estimation of glucose and xylose in serum. *Clin Chem* 1970; 16:85–91.

30. Fleming SC: Evaluation of a hand-held hydrogen monitor in the diagnosis of intestinal lactose deficiency. *Ann Clin Biochem* 1990; 27(Pt 5):499–500.

31. Bruno MJ, et al: Simultaneous assessments of exocrine pancreatic function by cholesteryl-[^{14}C]octanoate breath test and measurement of plasma p-aminobenzoic acid. *Clin Chem* 1995; 41:599–604.

32. Fleming SC: Evaluation of a hand-held hydrogen monitor in the diagnosis of intestinal lactase deficiency. *Ann Clin Biochem* 1990; 27:499–500.

33. Duan LP, et al: Clinical evaluation of a miniaturized desktop breath hydrogen analyzer. *Z Gastroenterol* 1994; 32:575–578.

34. Lambert JR: The stomach and duodenum: Gastritis, duodenitis and peptic ulceration. In Shearman DJC, et al (eds): *Diseases of the Gastrointestinal Tract and Liver*, ed 3. New York: Churchill Livingstone, 1997, pp 217–262.

35. Tietz NW (ed): *Clinical Guide to Laboratory Tests*, ed 3. Philadelphia: WB Saunders, 1995, pp 262–263.

36. Jensen RT: Gastrin-producing tumors. *Cancer Treat Res* 1997; 89:293–334.

37. Wolfe MM, Jensen RT: Zollinger-Ellison syndrome: Current concepts in diagnosis and management. *N Engl J Med* 1987; 317:1200–1209.

38. Hilborne LH, Eckfeldt JH: Pancreatic and gastrointestinal function. In Howanitz JH, Howanitz PJ (eds): *Laboratory Medicine—Test Selection and Interpretation*. New York: Churchill Livingstone, 1991, pp 85–105.

39. Tietz NW (ed): *Clinical Guide to Laboratory Tests*, ed 3. Philadelphia: WB Saunders, 1995, pp 258–259.

40. Goetze JP, Rehfeld JF: Impact of assay epitope specificity in gastrinoma diagnosis. *Clin Chem* 2003; 49:333–334.

41. Medline Plus Online Medical Encyclopedia: Zollinger-Ellison syndrome (revised Oct. 4, 2006). Available at *http://www.nlm.nih.gov/medlineplus/encyclopedia.html*

42. Coslovsky R, Bruck R, Estrov Z: Hypo-osmolal syndrome due to prolonged nausea. *Arch Intern Med* 1984; 144:191–192.

11

The clinical laboratory is a vital member of the health-care team in the assessment of endocrine disorders.

Endocrine Disorders and Function

Wendy Arneson, Karen Chandler, and Jean Brickell

homeostasis - state of dynamic equilibrium of the internal environment of the body that is maintained by processes of feedback and regulation in response to external or internal changes

Classically, hormones were named to describe their synthesis by glandular tissue and ability to arouse activity in another part of the body. Further study of hormones has revealed just how wide-reaching are their sites of synthesis and distribution and their roles within the body. When **homeostasis** is disturbed, a variety of serious consequences result, including problems with growth and development and even life-threatening metabolic problems. These endocrine disorders are a main focus in this chapter, which includes a discussion of the role of the laboratory in Cushing's syndrome, Addison's disease, pheochromotocytoma, thyroid and parathyroid disorders, and diabetes insipidus. Case scenarios will illustrate the role of laboratory testing in diagnosis, treatment, and monitoring of patients with endocrine disorders. The side boxes in this chapter provide common sense tips, definitions of terms, brief descriptions of pathophysiology, and clinical correlations as well as reminders of the team approach in health care. Text boxes within the chapter outline methodology for laboratory assessment of nutrition and digestive function.

OBJECTIVES

Upon completion of this chapter, the student will have the ability to

- Describe the chemical makeup of specific hormones as they relate to methods of analysis.
- Compare advantages and disadvantages of current methodologies for hormone analysis to include principle of analyses, specimen requirements specificity, and sources of interferences.
- Differentiate primary and secondary hormonal disorders in terms of causes and typical laboratory results.
- Correlate patient endocrine test results with clinical pathology.
- Describe communication that may be necessary with appropriate members of the health-care team to include requesting clarification of unexpected test results, verification of patient preparation or sample collection for suspected discrepancies, and reporting test results according to accepted practice for routine, emergency, and critical values.

CASE SCENARIO 11-1

Cushing's Syndrome: The Woman With the Buffalo Hump

While reviewing the workload for the day, the clinical laboratory scientist (CLS) working in the special chemistry section of the laboratory noticed that a cortisol specimen for Mrs. Jones was missing. Her physician had requested that specimens be collected for cortisol analysis at 8:00 a.m. and 8:00 p.m. Her diagnosis is possible Cushing's syndrome. It is now 7:00 a.m. on the next day, and the CLS discovers that the 8:00 p.m. cortisol was never drawn. After a search for the missing specimen, the phlebotomist suggests that the laboratory draw the second specimen at 8:00 a.m. today and submit the two 8:00 a.m. cortisol results in place of the 8:00 a.m. and 8:00 p.m. cortisol. What would be the most appropriate course of action? In order to answer this question correctly, we must first study the characteristics of hormones in general and cortisol in particular.

ENDOCRINOLOGY

Endocrinology is the study of hormones and disorders associated with abnormalities of these hormones. Hormones are substances that serve as vehicles for intracellular and extracellular communication. Historically, hormones have been defined as chemical substances that are produced by a gland in one part of the body, are secreted into the bloodstream, and act on a target organ elsewhere. This has been found to be an oversimplification as hormones are often produced in more than one site and can be transported by mechanisms other than the circulation. In addition, hormones have been found to act on neighboring cells and sometimes even on the very cells in which they were produced.

There are many variations in the actions of hormones and similar chemicals. A few of the most common types of hormonal action include endocrine, paracrine, autocrine, juxtacrine, exocrine, and neuroendocrine actions. Endocrine hormones are synthesized in one location and released into the bloodstream. They typically bind to a specific receptor at a site distant from their production. Paracrine hormones are synthesized in endocrine cells and released into the interstitial space. These hormone acts on neighboring cells. Autocrine hormones are synthesized in endocrine cells and typically act on a receptor in the cell of origin. Juxtacrine hormones are synthesized in endocrine cells and act on adjacent receptor cells by direct cell-to-cell contact. Exocrine chemicals are synthesized in endocrine cells and released into the gut. Neuroendocrine hormones are synthesized in cells of the nervous system and released into the blood circulation. They typically interact with receptors of cells at a site distant from their production.

Classification of Hormones

Hormones can be classified into three basic chemical types: **steroids**, proteins, and amines. These contrasting chemical types result in differences in transport, mechanism of action, and metabolic characteristics. Steroid molecules are lipid in nature. Once these hormones are produced and travel to their site of action, they immediately diffuse through the cell membrane due to the lipid bilayer. They are water insoluble, and therefore the greatest concentration of hormone is bound to a carrier molecule, which is protein in nature. An example of a protein carrier molecule is cortisol-binding globulin. The plasma half-life of steroids is relatively long and usually ranges from 4 to 120 minutes.[1]

Protein and amine hormones are somewhat similar to each other. Protein hormones are either peptides or glycoproteins in nature. Most are synthesized as larger molecules or prohormones, which are then cleaved to produce a smaller, active molecule. Protein hormones are water soluble and not bound to carrier molecules for transportation in blood. The half-life of the peptide hormones is much shorter than the steroid hormones. Typical plasma half-life is 4 to 40 minutes.[1] Amine hormones are derived from amino acids and share properties found in both the steroid- and protein-based hormones. For example, the catecholamines tend to have characteristics similar to the protein hormones. They circulate unbound to carrier molecules and have a short half-life. In contrast, thyroxine tends to have a relatively long half-life and circulates bound to a carrier molecule.[1]

Hormones differ not only in their chemical makeup but in the way in which they produce a response at their target tissue. Some hormones interact with specific receptors, which have a high affinity for the hormone molecules. These receptors

steroids - high-molecular-weight compounds with carbon atoms in a four-ring structure similar to cholesterol

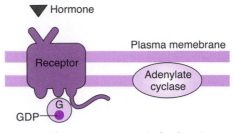

Figure 11–1. G protein family action.

provide for target organ specificity. The hormone-receptor complex activates the target cell to begin the biochemical reactions that ultimately produce the observed biological response. However, the location of these receptors is different depending on the biochemical nature of the hormone.

Protein and catecholamine hormones cannot cross cell membranes and therefore interact with cellular receptors located on the surface of the cell membrane. The action of binding to receptor initiates the reactions that lead to the production of a second-generation messenger, which then mediates the hormone's effect on intracellular enzymes and/or gene expression. Two major classes of membrane-bound receptors include the G protein family and the protein kinases. The G protein receptors use guanine nucleotide-binding proteins (G proteins) as the interface with target proteins.[1] Figure 11–1 illustrates the interaction of protein hormones and G protein receptors.

Hormone Receptors

Hormone receptors are monomeric proteins with an extracellular domain and a cytoplasmic domain. The extracellular portion binds the hormone while the intracellular portion binds the G protein. For some hormones, binding with their receptor activates adenylate cyclase, which then catalyzes the formation of cyclic AMP (cAMP) from ATP. In order for this reaction to occur, several conformational steps must occur. When the stimulatory hormone binds to the receptor, G protein associates with the hormone-receptor complex. Guanine diphosphate (GDP) then dissociates from the G protein and is replaced by cytoplasmic guanine triphosphate (GTP). The G protein–GTP complex then associates with adenylate cyclase. This causes the rapid conversion of ATP to cAMP. Cyclic AMP then diffuses throughout the cell and activates cAMP-dependent protein kinases, which consist of two regulatory subunits and two catalytic subunits. When cAMP binds to the regulatory dimer, the catalytic subunits are released and become activated phosphorylating enzymes. These enzymes regulate the activity of other intracellular proteins. When cAMP is removed, the regulating dimer reassociates with the catalytic subunits, thereby shutting down the enzyme activity.[2]

Protein kinase receptors contain intrinsic hormone–activated tyrosine kinase activity. These receptors serve as direct catalysts of phosphorylation reaction. No intracellular second messengers are needed. The insulin receptor is an example of a protein kinase receptor. It has two alpha subunits and two beta subunits joined by disulfide bridges. The alpha subunit is extracellular, and this is where the hormone attaches to the receptor. The beta subunits have an ATP binding site and

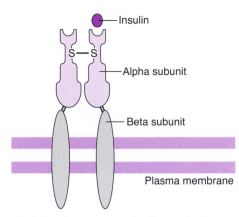

Figure 11–2. Insulin as an example of a protein kinase receptor.

a catalytic kinase domain. Modulation of this activation involves tyrosine auto-phosphorylation, serine/threonine phosphorylation by protein kinase and cAMP, and conformational changes. Tyrosine autophosphorylation is stimulatory, while serine/threonine phosphorylation by protein kinase and cAMP is inhibitory. Conformational changes may produce stimulation or inhibition.[3] Figure 11–2 illustrates the interaction of insulin hormone and protein kinase receptors.

Steroid and thyroid hormones are capable of entering the target organ cell and binding with intracellular receptors. The majority of these hormones are bound to carrier proteins, with a small amount found in the free form. Steroid hormones are large organic molecules that are synthesized for cholesterol. Steroid hormones bind to an inactive receptor located in the cytoplasm or nucleus. When the hormone binds to the specific receptor, a shape change occurs and the receptor becomes activated. The receptor complex binds to nuclear DNA at sites called *hormone response elements*. The bound and free hormones are in dynamic equilibrium, and only the free form can enter the cell. This is the "biologically active" form. Aromatic amine hormones, which are steroid-like molecules, are sometimes transformed further to a more active form by peripheral nonendocrine cells. An example of this is thyroxine, which is converted to the more potent form, triiodothyronine, by peripheral cells. Steroid and thyroid hormones act in a similar fashion in that thyroid hormones bind to specific chromatin receptors in the nucleus. Binding to nuclear sites causes a chemical change, which leads to activation or repression of gene transcription.

The quantity and responsiveness of hormone receptors may increase or decrease in response to various stimuli. Exposure of receptors to high concentrations of hormone may decrease the number and affinity of surface receptors. This effect has been given various names, including **downregulation** and **desensitization**. This phenomenon is seen in obesity, where high levels of insulin occur, as illustrated in Figure 11–3. This results in a decreased sensitivity of cells to insulin in many obese individuals.

The binding of a hormone to its receptor may also influence the affinity of neighboring receptor sites by causing decreased sensitivity of nearby receptors. An increase in receptor occupancy tends to decrease the affinity of the unoccupied receptors. Therefore, there is lower sensitivity of the receptors at higher hormone levels.

downregulation - inhibition or suppression of the normal response of an organ or system

desensitization - lowering of responsiveness

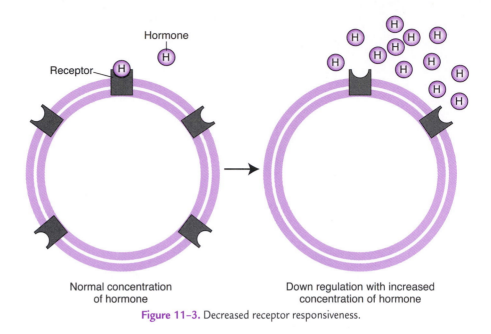

Figure 11–3. Decreased receptor responsiveness.

Other types of receptor modulation also occur in which numbers or responsiveness of receptors change. For example, angiotensin induces the presence of receptors. Normally, hormones only influence their own receptors, but some hormones can influence other receptors. Another example is estrogen, which increases the binding of other hormones, including oxytocin. In addition, some hormones may have varying affinity levels, such as strong affinity for their own receptors and a weaker affinity for receptors of another hormone. This phenomenon is called *specificity spillover.* At normal levels, specificity spillover does not cause problems, but at elevated levels a multiorgan response may occur. Cortisol is an example of such a hormone in that it ordinarily exhibits a glucocorticoid effect.[1] However, at high levels cortisol can produce the same effect as an excess of mineralcorticoids as well.

Hormone production is influenced by many factors besides receptors. It is a dynamic process in which circulating levels of hormones tend to vary within set physiological limits. Hormonal control is an important mechanism of maintaining appropriate hormone levels. The hypothalamus and anterior pituitary glands are important in the regulation of many hormones. The hypothalamus produces several neurosecretory factors that stimulate or inhibit the release of corresponding hormones from the anterior pituitary. The hormones from the anterior pituitary then act on other target endocrine glands, which produce other hormones, which provide feedback. Figure 11–4 shows the overall interaction of the hypothalamus, the anterior pituitary, and a target endocrine gland, the adrenal cortex. It depicts the hypothalamic response to subnormal levels of circulating free cortisol, secreting corticotropin-releasing hormone (CRH; also known as corticotropin-releasing factor [CRF]). CRH stimulates the anterior pituitary to release adrenocorticotropic hormone (ACTH) or adrenocorticotropin, which in turn stimulates the adrenal cortex to release cortisol and to some degree aldosterone. When cortisol levels exceed normal levels, through negative feedback they influence the hypothalamus and pituitary gland to discontinue release of CRH and ACTH. This cycle continues so that the steady-state level of cortisol is maintained.

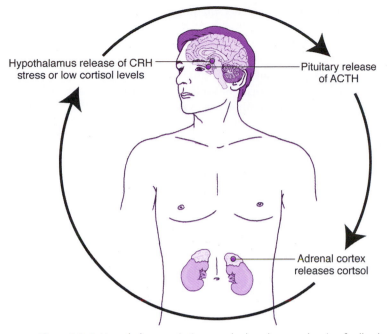

Hypothalamus release of CRH
stress or low cortisol levels

Pituitary release
of ACTH

Adrenal cortex
releases cortsol

Figure 11–4. Hypothalamus, pituitary, and adrenal cortex showing feedback.

Feedback Control

Feedback control mechanisms play a major role in the regulation of hormone levels and are an important feature of the endocrine system. Feedback control mechanisms are systems in which the function of one hormone (A) affects the function of another hormone (B). Feedback control mechanisms can be either positive or negative in nature. **Negative feedback** control mechanisms occur when the concentration of hormone A causes a decrease in hormone B. This is the principal mechanism for hormone level regulation.

Negative feedback can exhibit three main types of actions. Negative feedback can act directly to change the hormone level itself, it can cause a change in a related physiological response, or it can occur indirectly via another hormone. For example, when high concentrations of cortisol circulate in the bloodstream, receptors in the hypothalamus suppress the release of CRF, which in turn suppresses release of ACTH by the pituitary gland. When circulating levels of cortisol fall below the threshold level, the hypothalamus is again stimulated to produce CRF, which in turn stimulates release of ACTH. This cycle of "turning off and turning on" of hormone release helps to maintain normal levels of hormones and hormonal functions and is sometimes compared to the thermostat that regulates the heating/cooling cycles in your home.

Positive feedback control mechanisms occur when the function of hormone A results in an increase in hormone B. Positive feedback control is less common and rarely operates in isolation. It is usually a part of a more complex control mechanism, which involves other regulatory factors. In Chapter 12 (Reproductive Endocrinology and Fetal Testing), you will see an example of positive feedback when increasing levels of estradiol cause an increase in luteinizing hormone just prior to ovulation. The interaction of various endocrine glands will be discussed,

negative feedback - stabilizing a process by reducing its rate or output when its effects are too great

positive feedback - enhancing the output when the effects are not at optimum

tertiary level - a third level in a hierarchy, such as the hypothalamus in the endocrine system

including the role of the hypothalamus, the pituitary, and target glands such as the testes or ovaries.

The hypothalamus is composed of neuroendocrine tissue in the mesencephalon, and it has a variety of hormone receptors within many of its cells. It provides a **tertiary level** of control and stimulation of the target organ glands by secreting releasing hormones, usually peptide hormones that respond to lower than normal levels of target organ hormone. For example, the hypothalamus responds to low levels of cortisol by secreting CRH. Although CRH has many functions, its primary function is to stimulate the adenohypophysis to produce ACTH.

Other factors that may influence circulating hormone levels include the nervous system, biorhythms, and stress levels. The hypothalamus may receive neural signals from other hormones or releasing factors in the brain. This allows the brain to fine-tune control mechanisms. Some hormones are produced within the nervous system, such as oxytocin, and secreted by the posterior pituitary. The tissues of the adrenal medulla are neuroendocrine and respond to stimuli from the nervous system. In addition, many feedback mechanisms involve the hypothalamus. Biorhythms are cyclic occurrences in physiology. Rhythmic secretion of hormones is an important factor of many endocrine systems. The rhythms can vary over minutes, hours, days, or weeks. Changes occurring over an approximate interval of 24 hours are termed *circadian* or **diurnal variations**. These cycles may be influenced by light or sleep.

diurnal variations - changes in chemical levels during the day, especially when comparing two different times

A characteristic example of the rhythmic secretory cycle is seen with ACTH. ACTH levels peak about 8:00 a.m. and then gradually fall during the day. The lowest point is usually reached late in the evening, with 8:00 p.m. used as a standard of comparison. These changes in ACTH levels cause resulting changes in cortisol levels since ACTH stimulates the secretion of cortisol from the adrenal cortex. This variation makes it necessary for physicians who wish to assess ACTH and cortisol levels to request two blood samples, typically at 8:00 a.m. and 8:00 p.m. In contrast, surges of growth hormone occur during periods of sleep. For many hormones, multiple samples may be necessary to determine the true hormone status of the patient. Stress is another factor that can influence hormone levels. Stress increases the concentration of hormones such as ACTH, cortisol, and growth hormone.

THE PITUITARY GLAND

hypophysis - pituitary or master endocrine gland

neurohypophysis - the posterior or back portion of the pituitary gland

adenohypophysis - anterior lobe, or front portion, of the pituitary; sometimes called the master endocrine gland

tropins - stimulating protein hormones

The pituitary gland, or **hypophysis**, is composed of two segments, the **neurohypophysis** and **adenohypophysis**. The adenohypophysis, also known as the anterior pituitary, provides the secondary level of control and stimulation. It produces and secretes stimulating hormones, or "**tropins**," usually glycoprotein hormones. The neurohypophysis, or posterior pituitary, is closely associated with the hypothalamus and is connected to it via a stalk. It primarily stores and releases certain hormones produced by the hypothalamus, including antidiuretic hormone and oxytocin. The anterior pituitary is sometimes referred to as the master gland, due to the many hormones it secretes, including thyroid-stimulating hormone (TSH) or thyrotropin, ACTH, reproductive hormones such as follicle-stimulating hormone and luteinizing hormone, and many others. For example, the adenohypophysis produces ACTH to stimulate the cortex region of the adrenal gland to produce and secrete cortisol. Tables 11–1 and 11–2 summarize the main roles of hormones produced by the pituitary gland.

TABLE 11-1

Effects of the Anterior Pituitary Hormones

Growth Hormone (GH)	Adrenocorticotropic Hormone (ACTH)	Thyroid-Stimulating Hormone (TSH)	Luteinizing Hormone (LH)	Follicle-Stimulating Hormone (FSH)	Prolactin (PRL)
Promotes growth	Stimulates the adrenal cortex	Stimulates the thyroid to release thyroid hormones	Controls reproductive functions	Controls reproductive functions	Milk production

THE ADRENAL GLANDS

The two adrenal glands are located immediately anterior to the kidneys. Each adrenal gland consists of two distinct regions, an inner adrenal medulla surrounded by the adrenal cortex. Figure 11–4 depicts the location of the adrenal glands in comparison to the kidneys. Although the adrenal glands are organized into a single gland, the medulla and cortex are functionally different endocrine organs, and have different embryological origins. The adrenal medulla derives from the outermost germ layer of an embryo, forming **ectoderm** (neural crest), while the cortex develops from the **mesoderm**, or middle layer. The cortex produces steroids such as cortisol and corticosterone (both glucocorticoids), dehydroepiandrosterone, and mineralcorticoid steroids such as aldosterone; both of the latter are somewhat under response to ACTH release from the anterior pituitary.

Cortisol Synthesis

Cortisol, also known as hydrocortisone, is produced in the adrenal cortex under ACTH stimulation of the **zona fasciculata** and **zona reticularis** in the adrenal glands. Cortisol is synthesized from a series of enzyme-catalyzed biochemical reactions beginning with cholesterol, a **cyclopentanoperhydrophenanthrene** structure, forming first delta-5-pregnenolone, a 21-carbon atom structure (Figs. 11–5 and 11–6). The precursor steroid immediately prior to cortisol in the synthetic pathway is 11-deoxycortisol. These organic molecules with 21 carbon atoms and a hydroxyl group at the 17th carbon are termed **17-hydroxycorticosteroids (17-OHCS)**

TABLE 11-2

Effects of Hormones Stored in the Posterior Pituitary

Antidiuretic Hormone (ADH) or Vasopressin	Oxytocin
Causes the body to conserve water	Stimulates uterine contraction and ejection of milk

ectoderm - the outermost of the three primary germ layers of an embryo, forming neural tissue

mesoderm - middle of the three primary germ layers of an embryo, the source especially of bone, muscle, connective tissue, and dermis

zona fasciculata - middle of the three layers of the adrenal cortex that consists of radially arranged columnar epithelial cells

zona reticularis - innermost of the three layers of the adrenal cortex that consists of irregularly arranged cylindrical masses of epithelial cells

cyclopentanoperhydrophenanthrene - an organic molecule with 17 carbon atoms composed of three six-sided rings (the phenanthrene portion) and one five-sided ring

17-hydroxycorticosteroids (17-OHCS) - 21-carbon atoms with a hydroxyl group at the 17th carbon atom

Cholesterol

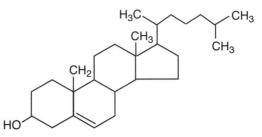

Figure 11–5. Cyclopentanoperhydrophenanthrene ring structure.

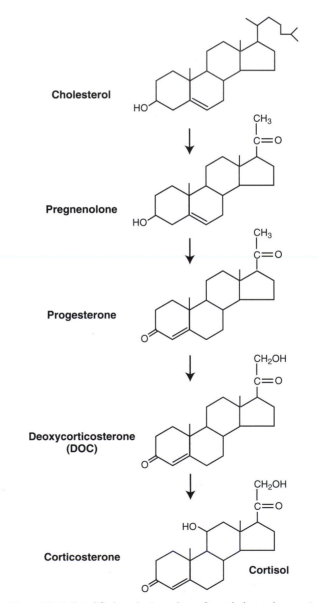

Figure 11–6. Simplified synthetic pathway from cholesterol to cortisol.

and include 17-alpha-hydroxypregnenolone, 17-alpha-hydroxyprogesterone, 11-deoxycortisol, and cortisol.[4]

Cortisol Activity

Cortisol is the main **glucocorticoid**, meaning it affects carbohydrate and fat metabolism, while mineralcorticoids affect mineral or electrolyte balance. In actuality, cortisol has some minor role in mineral and electrolyte balance and some of the **mineralocorticoids** do exhibit an effect on carbohydrate metabolism. The general term *glucocorticoid* refers to the chief property of the steroid. Cortisol raises blood glucose levels by suppressing secretion of insulin, inhibiting peripheral cell uptake of glucose, and promoting hepatic glucose synthesis. Glycogen synthesis and protein catabolism are also induced in the liver. Fatty acids are produced in larger amounts due to cellular lipase activation, with an uneven impact upon adipose cells. For example, adipose accumulates in the trunk of the body but depletes along with muscle mass in the arms and legs. Anti-inflammatory properties of cortisol include suppression of cytokines, release of leukocytes from the bone marrow but inhibition of their egress through capillary walls, and depletion of eosinophils and T lymphocytes. When cortisol is secreted in large amounts, it induces poor wound healing, bruising, and immunosuppression during infections. Cortisol also affects body water by regulation of water migration into extracellular fluids and through renal excretion. The effect is that excessive levels of cortisol cause accumulation of water in the face and other visible areas of the body.[5]

DISEASES OF THE ADRENAL CORTEX

When the cortex region of the adrenal gland is overfunctioning, it is often due to a secreting **adenoma**, a benign hormone-secreting tumor. Primary hypercortisolism is the name of this disorder because the disease resides in the primary organ of this endocrine structure, the adrenal cortex. It is associated with increased levels of cortisol throughout the day, loss of diurnal variation, and decreased levels of ACTH. ACTH is low due to the negative feedback response of the pituitary gland, which is functioning normally in primary hypercortisolism. Hypercortisolism in the adult is characterized by hyperglycemia and changes in fat and water distribution. Other characteristics include bruising and poor wound healing, weight gain, weakening of bones, and depression. The weight gain tends to be located in the middle of the body with accompanying muscle wasting, known as **truncal obesity**. Fat accumulation on the upper shoulders and collar bone causes a hump on the upper back and jutting forward of the neck and head. This unusual fat distribution is sometimes called a **buffalo hump**. Finally, fluid and tissue accumulation around the face tends to make it round in appearance and is termed "moon face." This disorder is named Cushing's syndrome after Dr. Harvey Cushing, a surgeon who first characterized hypercortisolism. Cushing's syndrome may occur as a result of treatment with corticosteroids, which is the most common nonadrenal cause. It may also occur secondary to a benign hormone-secreting pituitary adenoma. In pituitary origins there is increased ACTH along with cortisol. Other possible causes of mild but transient hypercortisolism in the adult include chronic alcoholism, stress, and obesity. These mild forms may not exhibit all of the signs and symptoms, and hypercortisolism can revert to normal if the patient is given certain suppressing agents, such as **dexamethasone**.[6]

glucocorticoids - adrenal cortical hormones primarily active in protecting against stress and affecting protein and carbohydrate metabolism

mineralocorticoids - steroid molecules that influence blood electrolyte levels

adenoma - a benign tumor of glandular origin

truncal obesity - weight gain in the middle of the body rather than including the arms or legs

buffalo hump - fat accumulation on upper shoulders and collar bone causing the neck and head to jut forward

dexamethasone - a synthetic glucocorticoid used to determine the cause of hypercortisolism

CLINICAL CORRELATION
Cushing's disease is secondary hypercortisolism associated with adenomas of the pituitary causing adrenal hyperplasia, with increased ACTH and cortisol levels. The disease, named after Dr. Cushing, is different from Cushing's syndrome. High doses of dexamethasone, a synthetic glucocorticoid, when given overnight, will cause suppression of pituitary output of ACTH and a lowered 8:00 a.m. cortisol level.

CLINICAL CORRELATION
Certain medications, stress, or obesity will cause elevated plasma cortisol levels, but 24-hr urinary free cortisol levels are generally normal. Dexamethasone in low dosage given overnight will suppress ACTH, followed by suppression of cortisol output (<3 µg/dL at 8:00 a.m.).

CLINICAL CORRELATION

Hypercortisolism due to ectopic ACTH syndrome is generally a result of malignancy (e.g., small cell lung carcinoma). It is characterized by high levels of plasma and 24-hour urinary free cortisol, and no suppression of plasma cortisol when given low-dose or high-dose dexamethasone in overnight treatments.

THE TEAM APPROACH

Computed tomography or other diagnostic imaging performed by a radiological technician is necessary to determine the location of ectopic ACTH-producing tumors.

✓ Common Sense Check

When multiple specimens are obtained from the same patient over time, it is important to properly transcribe the correct time to the specimen containers and to all results so that a mix-up doesn't occur.

Case Scenario 11-1 Cushing's Syndrome: The Woman With the Buffalo Hump

Follow-Up

While reviewing the workload for the day at 7:00 a.m., the CLS working in the special chemistry section of the laboratory noticed that a cortisol specimen on Mrs. Jones was missing. Her physician had requested that the laboratory draw specimens for cortisol analysis at 8:00 a.m. and 8:00 p.m. to confirm a possible diagnosis of Cushing's syndrome. After a search for the missing specimen, it is discovered that the 8:00 p.m. cortisol was never drawn. The phlebotomist suggests that the laboratory draw the second specimen at 8:00 a.m. today and submit the two 8:00 a.m. cortisols in place of the 8:00 a.m. and 8:00 p.m. cortisol. The CLS thinks of four possible courses of action:

1. Agree with the phlebotomist to collect the 8:00 a.m. specimen today and then run both 8:00 a.m. specimens.
2. Analyze the cortisol that was collected at 8:00 a.m. and cancel the second collection since the physician only needs to see what the patient's cortisol level is in the morning.
3. Collect a second sample at 11:00 a.m. today along with other tests that were ordered and run it with the 8:00 a.m. sample, as that will give the physician the cortisol level at two different times and that is all he needs.
4. Instruct the phlebotomist to collect a new sample for cortisol at 8:00 a.m. today and then collect a second sample tonight at 8:00 p.m.

The first three choices for appropriate course of action are incorrect. Cortisol shows diurnal variation, as does ACTH. Highest levels are seen in the morning, while late in the evening the cortisol levels fall to their lowest levels. The doctor needs a morning and an evening specimen taken about 12 hours apart to see if normal diurnal variation is present. The standard reference ranges that physicians use to assess for diseases of the adrenal cortex typically are set for 8:00 a.m. and 8:00 p.m. samples. Therefore, the CLS should instruct the phlebotomist to collect a new sample for cortisol at 8:00 a.m. today and then collect a second sample tonight at 8:00 p.m. ●

CASE SCENARIO 11-2

Addison's Disease: The Man With Noticeable Pigments

The laboratory technologist was asked to help collect blood samples from patients in the emergency department since the other phlebotomists were otherwise busy. Since most of the lab requests were for tests in the Clinical Chemistry section, she agreed to assist in collection of blood samples from the patient, Mr. Brown. Mr. Brown was agreeable to the blood collection but appeared weak and not very responsive while the laboratory technologist performed the phlebotomy technique. She noticed that he was tanned but oddly enough had a darker tan under the arms, spots on the forehead, and dark lips. The preliminary diagnosis was dehydration, and a basic chemistry profile, complete blood cound (CBC), and urinalysis were the initial laboratory orders. The laboratory results were as follows:

Case Scenario 11-2 Addison's Disease: The Man With Noticeable Pigments *(continued)*

Test	Patient	Reference Range
Na$^+$ (mmol/L)	129	136–145
K$^+$ (mmol/L)	5.2	3.5–5.1
Cl$^-$ (mmol/L)	98	98–107
HCO$_3^-$ (mmol/L)	21	22–28
Anion gap (mmol/L)	10	5–10
Glucose (mg/dL)	49	74–100

Cortisol and other hormonal analyses will most likely be the next step for laboratory testing in this individual.

Cortisol Analysis

Cortisol analysis is dependent upon its chemical makeup and configuration, including hydroxylation of the 17th carbon atom. Most of the 17-hydroxycorticosteroid in the blood is cortisol that circulates bound to corticosteroid-binding protein due to its chemical makeup. This may also help to retain cortisol longer in circulation, slowing hepatic catabolism or urinary excretion. Historical cortisol methods of analysis were based upon general biochemical characteristics such as the Porter-Silber color reaction or sulfuric acid–induced fluorescence method. Chromatographic methods have the specificity to differentiate cortisol from other similar chemicals but are slow and labor intensive. Chromatography is not routinely used in clinical laboratory testing of cortisol for these reasons.

The most common method of analysis for cortisol in the clinical laboratory is immunoassay, such as an enzyme immunoassay (EIA) or fluorescence polarization immunoassay (FPIA). Serum or heparinized plasma can be used in analysis, with overnight refrigeration or freezing necessary if testing will not be performed within a few days. Reference ranges vary for cortisol depending upon time of collection. In general, the reference range for an 8:00 a.m. specimen in the adult is 5 to 23 μg/dL and at 4:00 p.m. in the adult it is 3 to 16 μg/dL. Although there is overlap in these ranges, in the individual, the 4:00 p.m. result is expected to be lower than the 8:00 a.m. result. Due to the overlap in ranges, the preferred evening sample time is 8:00 p.m. and the reference range in the adult is less than 5 μg/dL and less than 50% of the 8:00 a.m. sample.[1] However, due to convenience, the 4:00 p.m. sample and reference ranges are commonly used. Circadian rhythm is dependent upon sleeping, eating, and working cycles such that a person who sleeps during the day and works and eats at night most likely will have a reversal in these reference ranges.

Cortisol can be measured in a 24-hour urine specimen, in the free, unbound form. This measurement actually represents a more accurate picture of the active forms of cortisol, especially when excessive levels of cortisol are secreted. Urinary free cortisol (UFC) levels correlate well with signs and symptoms of Cushing's syndrome. During collection of the 24-hour urine, boric acid is added to the specimen to maintain pH below 7.5 and preserve the cortisol. Immunoassay methods, which are similar to plasma cortisol methods, are used for analysis of urinary free cortisol. An additional extraction step with an organic solvent is necessary to separate cortisol metabolites from UFC prior to addition of the specific antibody. This step helps to ensure specificity of the reaction with UFC. The reference range for UFC in the 24-hour specimen is highly method dependent. For example, in the traditional radioimmunoassay method described in Test Methodology 11–1, UFC is 20 to 90 μg/day in the adult.[5]

TEST METHODOLOGY 11-1.   CORTISOL BY IMMUNOASSAY

The Reaction Principle

This procedure is an automated heterogeneous enzyme immunoassay that utilizes radial partition for its separation phase. Serum cortisol is freed from its binding proteins by the addition of a sulfonic acid reagent. For urinary free cortisol levels, urine is extracted first to removed metabolites or conjugates that would cross-react with the antibody. Alkaline phosphatase–labeled cortisol is then added to compete with patient cortisol for specific antibody binding sites on a borosilicate paper matrix. A washing step elutes unbound substances radially (in a circular motion). After the addition of substrate, the enzyme-labeled bound cortisol forms measurable product with an inverse relationship between the amount of reaction and the amount of patient cortisol present in the reaction.

The Specimen

Serum or heparinized plasma may be used. If not tested within a few hours, the sample should be stored overnight under refrigeration or frozen for storage. Urine is generally a 24-hour specimen, maintained with a boric acid preservative and stored under refrigeration until collection is complete.

Reference Ranges

Urine, 24-hr free cortisol	20–90 μg/day
Serum, 0800 hr total cortisol	5–23 μg/dL
1600 hr total cortisol	3–16 μg/dL

Hypocortisolism

idiopathic - without a recognizable cause

atrophy - decrease in size or function

tubercular granuloma - a mass or nodule of chronically inflamed tissue with granulations that is usually associated with an infective process

Underfunctioning of the adrenal cortex is a chronic progressive disease, commonly due to **idiopathic atrophy** of the adrenal cortex. Primary hypocortisolism resides in the cortex of the adrenal gland, the primary endocrine organ. It is associated with increased levels of ACTH and decreased cortisol and UFC levels. Hypocortisolism is also called Addison's disease. Adrenal atrophy, or primary adrenal insufficiency, may be caused by autoimmune destruction, but destruction from neoplasm, **tubercular granuloma**, or metabolic defects may also cause adrenal gland failure, as may long-term use of certain medications such as ketoconozole, an antifungal medication. In the adult, this disease is characterized by insulin sensitivity; hypoglycemia; imbalances in carbohydrate, fat, and protein metabolism; and weakness. Other characteristics of hypocortisolism include increased urinary excretion of sodium, electrolyte imbalance, hypotension, dehydration, and potential for circulatory shock and cardiac weakness. Overstimulation of the pituitary by low circulating levels of cortisol accounts for increased ACTH output but also causes melanocyte-stimulating activity with resulting hyperpigmentation of skin and mucous membranes. Excessive melanin deposits in the skin and concentrates in certain areas, such as the elbows and knees and the inside of the mouth.[7]

Measurement of ACTH can determine if primary adrenal insufficiency is present as opposed to secondary or tertiary causes.[6] ACTH stimulation tests, using cosyntropin, synthetic ACTH, will differentiate primary from secondary causes of adrenal insufficiency. Specifically, synthetic ACTH will not cause the adrenal gland to respond in primary adrenal insufficiency if it is due to autoimmune or other glandular destruction. There will be a characteristic rise in cortisol levels following ACTH stimulation if the cause of adrenal atrophy is from medications or from secondary, pituitary failure.

Primary adrenal insufficiency is caused by destruction or defects in the adrenal gland, which result in decreased or absent secretion of adrenal hormones. Plasma and urinary cortisol and plasma aldosterone levels are decreased while plasma ACTH levels are increased. Cosyntropin, a normal stimulant for ACTH production, generally causes no rise in cortisol levels in primary adrenal insufficiency.

Secondary hypocortisolism is associated with both decreased ACTH and cortisol levels Symptoms are similar to those of Cushing's syndrome due to primary hypocortisolism, but it is generally of pituitary origin. Causes of pituitary failure include surgical removal of the pituitary (**hypophysectomy**) or pituitary failure, such as following head trauma or cerebral vascular accident or in obstetric complications. Additional tests can be performed to determine if the pituitary is underfunctioning, including the use of metyrapone to stimulate the pituitary gland. **Metyrapone**, also known as metapirone, is a hormone that inhibits biosynthesis of cortisol and corticosterone. If the pituitary gland is able to respond normally to metyrapone, plasma 11-deoxycortisol levels are greater than 7 μg/dL following overnight administration. If there is pituitary disease, the plasma 11-deoxycortisol levels remain less than 7 μg/dL. Similarly if the disease arises in the hypothalamus, the plasma 11-deoxycortisol levels remain less than 7 μg/dL. This stimulation test should only be performed after primary disease is ruled out as this test further stresses the individual with primary adrenal insufficiency.[5]

Tertiary hypocortisolism, although rare, usually arises in the hypothalamus. It has laboratory findings similar to those of adrenal insufficiency of pituitary origins, including a moderate cortisol rise following ACTH stimulation and lack of 11-deoxycortisol and ACTH elevations following metyrapone administration. A somewhat rare test protocol is the CRH stimulation test. In this procedure, synthetic CRH is given and plasma ACTH and cortisol levels are assessed at timed intervals up to 3 hours postdosage. Plasma ACTH and cortisol levels remains low if the disease is pituitary in origin. If the pituitary is able to respond, the disease is of tertiary or hypothalamic origin, and cortisol and ACTH levels rise following CRH stimulation.[5]

SUMMARY OF ADRENAL CORTEX DISORDERS

Table 11–3 summarizes adrenal cortex disorders such as Addison's and Cushing's syndromes by comparing and contrasting ACTH and cortisol levels, including stimulation and suppression tests.

> **Case Scenario 11-2** Addison's Disease: The Man With Noticeable Pigments
>
> **Follow-Up**
>
> The laboratory technologist was asked to help collect blood samples from patients in the emergency department. She noticed that one particular patient appeared weak and less responsive, was tanned, but oddly enough had a darker tan under the arms, spots on the forehead, and dark lips. The preliminary

continued

CLINICAL CORRELATION
Addison's disease is marked by deficient adrenocortical secretion and characterized by extreme weakness, loss of weight, low blood pressure, gastrointestinal disturbances, and brownish pigmentation of the skin and mucous membranes. The insufficiency may have primary or adrenal origin, or secondary or pituitary origin. Tertiary adrenal insufficiency most likely originates in the hypothalamus.

hypophysectomy - resection or removal of the pituitary

metyrapone - metabolic hormone that inhibits biosynthesis of cortisol and corticosterone and is used to test for normal functioning of the pituitary gland; also known as metapyrone

THE TEAM APPROACH
Assessment of adrenal disorders often requires administration of synthetic hormones. These unique testing protocols will involve laboratory staff, pharmacists, nurses, physicians, and possibly physician assistants. The laboratory technologist, particularly in a supervisory role, may be required to directly communicate with the patient's physician or nursing staff to ensure proper timing of blood collection following these challenge tests.

> **Case Scenario 11-2 Addison's Disease: The Man With Noticeable Pigments** *(continued)*
>
> diagnosis was dehydration. A basic chemistry profile, CBC, and urinalysis were the initial laboratory orders. The laboratory results showed decreased serum sodium, bicarbonate, and glucose compared with reference ranges, and increased potassium.
>
> The results indicate hypoglycemia, **hyponatremia**, and **hyperkalemia**. The physician ordered cortisol, ACTH, and aldosterone tests next. Cortisol 0800 hr was 3 μg/dL (reference range, 5 to 23 μg/dL) and 1600 hr was 2 μg/dL (3 to 16 μg/dL). Aldosterone 0800 hr (supine) was 2 mg/dL (3 to 16 mg/dL). These results indicate adrenal insufficiency and correlate with the symptoms of weakness, hypoglycemia, electrolyte imbalance, and dehydration. The ACTH levels were elevated, indicating primary adrenal insufficiency. A dose of 0.25 mg of cosyntropin (synthetic ACTH) was given and timed collection of plasma for cortisol was obtained at 0, 60, 120, and 180 minutes postdosage. The serum cortisol levels remained well below 7 μg/dL, confirming adrenal insufficiency. Further imaging and autoimmune testing will continue with this patient to determine the cause of the adrenal gland insufficiency. ●

hyponatremia - decreased sodium in blood plasma

hyperkalemia - increased potassium in blood plasma

ROLE OF ALDOSTERONE

zona glomerulosa - outermost of the three layers of the adrenal cortex that consists of round masses of granular epithelial cells that stain deeply

Aldosterone is another steroid synthesized by the **zona glomerulosa** of the adrenal gland but under stimulus of angiotensin II. It is made from cholesterol-based compounds such as pregnenolone in a biosynthetic pathway similar to that of cortisol. However, aldosterone and its immediate precursors, corticosterone and 11-deoxycorticosterone, are not 17-hydroxycorticosteroids. Figure 11–7 presents a simplified biosynthetic pathway for aldosterone. Secretion of aldosterone precur-

TABLE 11-3

Adrenal Gland Disorders

Condition	Cortisol and Urinary Free Cortisol	ACTH	Blood Pressure	Dexamethasone Suppression of Cortisol	Prone to Hyperglycemia
Primary hypercortisolism	Increased	Decreased	High	No, cortisol remains high	Yes
Secondary hypercortisolism	Increased	Increased		Yes, if benign pituitary adenoma. No, if ectopic ACTH-producing tumor.	Yes
Primary hypocortisolism	Decreased	Increased	Low	Not needed	No
Secondary hypocortisolism	Decreased	Decreased	Low	Not needed	No

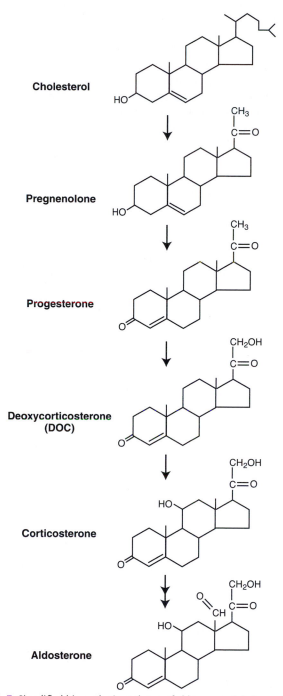

Cholesterol

Pregnenolone

Progesterone

Deoxycorticosterone (DOC)

Corticosterone

Aldosterone

Figure 11–7. Simplified biosynthetic pathway of aldosterone (cholesterol to aldosterone).

sors may also occur from ACTH stimulation or when potassium levels are elevated.[5] The main role of aldosterone is in mineral regulation by its impact on the distal tubules of the kidney to enhance reabsorption of sodium and some chloride in exchange for potassium. Thus, aldosterone is termed a *mineralcorticoid*, which describes its overall chemical makeup and its main principle of action. Aldosterone is regulated by the renin-angiotensin system.

Renin is a proteolytic enzyme synthesized and stored in the juxtaglomerulary cells of the renal glomeruli. When stimulated by low plasma volume pressure and hyponatremia, the juxtaglomerular cells release renin into circulation, where it hydrolyzes angiotensinogen, made by the liver, to angiotensin I. Renin release also may be stimulated due to the presence of other hormones and prostaglandins. Angiotensin I is rapidly converted to angiotensin II by circulating angiotensin-converting enzyme produced in the lungs. Angiotensin II stimulates the adrenal cortex to produce aldosterone and acts as a potent vasoconstrictor, raising blood pressure.[6]

Disorders Involving Aldosterone

hyperplasia - increase in cell mass, often with increased function

Hyperaldosteronism results from **hyperplasia** or adenoma of one adrenal gland, known as Conn's syndrome, from carcinoma, or from Cushing's syndrome. Hyperaldosteronism may also result from renin-secreting tumors, congenital adrenal hyperplasia, and other conditions including excessive ingestion of licorice. The main signs and symptoms of hyperaldosteronism are high blood pressure, low serum potassium, and high plasma aldosterone levels, and the patient may experience other electrolyte and acid-base disturbances. Plasma sodium levels remain normal since water is reabsorbed along with sodium. In contrast, hypoaldosteronism results from undersecretion of aldosterone. This is generally due to diffuse atrophy of the adrenal cortex as in Addison's disease, or after surgical treatment of adenoma, enzymatic deficiencies in the blood in conversion of precursors to aldosterone, after prolonged heparin therapy, or secondary to renal defects causing receptor defect or low renin output. Table 11–4 summarizes hyperaldosteronism and hypoaldosteronism.[6]

Testing aldosterone and renin requires collection at particular times of the day as aldosterone exhibits a circadian rhythm, as does cortisol. Routine analysis uses an immunoassay technique similar to that for cortisol but with antibody having specificity to the aldosterone molecule.[8] Plasma renin activity is often measured to assess the conversion of angiotensinogen to angiotensin I. Factors that affect renin release include upright posture, sodium in the diet, and various medications, including diuretics. These factors are often controlled for prior to testing aldosterone and renin activity.

The case scenarios of Cushing's syndrome and Addison's disease discussed the roles of the adrenal gland, the pituitary, and the hypothalamus and their interac-

TABLE 11-4

Hyperaldosteronism and Hypoaldosteronism

Condition	Aldosterone	Renin Activity	Blood Pressure	Serum Potassium
Primary hyper-aldosteronism	Increased	Decreased	High	Low
Secondary hyper-aldosteronism	Increased	Increased	Generally high except in edematous disorder	Low or low-normal
Primary hypo-aldosteronism	Decreased	Increased	Low	High

tion. A variety of tissues other than the adrenal glands synthesize and secrete hormones, such as the intestines, kidneys, heart, pancreas, and gonads. Some of these hormones are small molecules, such as peptides composed of only a few amino acids, while others are larger, more complicated molecules such as proteins or glycoproteins. The antigenic nature of polypeptides and proteins are utilized in the analysis for these hormones by immunoassay. These highly sensitive and specific assay methods provide reliable protein and polypeptide hormone results. Tables 11–5 and 11–6 provide a summary of important peptide and protein hormones, their sources, and their main actions within the body.

GROWTH HORMONE

Growth hormone (GH), a polypeptide hormone synthesized in abundance in the anterior pituitary, stimulates growth in cartilage and soft tissues in bone and muscle. Specifically, protein synthesis is induced along with a positive nitrogen and

TABLE 11-5

Peptide Hormones, Their Actions, and Their Sources

Hormone	Gland or Tissue Source	Action
Antidiuretic hormone (vasopressin)	Posterior pituitary	Water reabsorption and blood pressure elevation
Atrial natriuretic factor	Heart	Regulates blood pressure and volume in vascular and renal tissue
Cholecystokinin	Intestines	Contraction of gallbladder and pancreatic secretion
Corticotropin	Anterior pituitary	Stimulation of adrenocorticotropic hormone (ACTH) formation and secretion
Corticotropin-releasing hormone (CRH)	Hypothalamus	Stimulation of anterior pituitary to release ACTH
Gastrin	Intestines	Secretion of gastric acid by stomach
Glucagon	Pancreas	Glycogenolysis by the liver
Gonadotropin-releasing hormone (Gn-RH)	Hypothalamus	Release of luteinizing hormone (LH) and follicle-stimulating hormone (FSH) by anterior pituitary
Growth hormone-releasing hormone (GHRH)	Hypothalamus	Release of growth hormone (GH) by anterior pituitary
Insulin	Pancreas	Regulation of carbohydrate and fat metabolism by most cells
Melanocyte-stimulating hormone	Anterior pituitary	Darkening of skin and spread of pigment granules
Oxytocin	Posterior pituitary	Uterine and breast tissue contraction
Parathormone (parathyroid hormone)	Parathyroid gland	Regulation of calcium and phosphorus metabolism by bone, gastrointestinal tract, and kidney
Thyrotropin-releasing hormone (TRH)	Hypothalamus	Release of thyroid-stimulating hormone (TSH) and prolactin

TABLE 11-6

Protein Hormones, Their Actions, and Their Sources

Protein Hormone	Source	Action
Chorionic gonadotropin (hCG)	Placenta	Prolongs corpus luteum; possible steroidogenesis
Erythropoietin	Kidney	Red cell formation in bone marrow
Follicle-stimulating hormone (FSH)	Anterior pituitary	Growth of ovarian follicles and spermatogenesis
Growth hormone (GH)	Anterior pituitary	Growth of muscle and bone
Luteinizing hormone (LH)	Anterior pituitary	Ovulation, secretion of estrogens and progesterone; stimulation of testicular tissue and secretion of androgens
Prolactin	Anterior pituitary	Growth of mammary tissue and milk secretion

phosphorus balance and uptake of ions within growing tissues. Other hormones play a role in growth and work in conjunction with or under the influence of growth hormone. Secretion of GH typically surges a few hours after a meal or exercise or during sleep following hypothalamic release of growth hormone–releasing hormone (GHRH). Stress-related factors such as hypoglycemia, high levels of thyroxine, and significant exercise also stimulate GH secretion, which can lead to anabolism and tissue repair as needed. Other factors, such as high levels of glucocorticoids (including cortisol), suppress GH release. Growth-inhibiting hormones from the hypothalamus and gastrointestinal tract cause decline of GH levels needed to maintain homeostasis of growth.[5]

Disorders of Growth Hormone Secretion

Disorders of hypersecretion or hyposecretion of GH are rare and should be discussed based on occurrence before adolescence or after the bones have fused in adulthood, since the consequences are quite different. Hyposecretion of GH throughout childhood results in pituitary dwarfism whether due to congenital defects or acquired disorders of the pituitary. This condition is characterized by failure to grow normally. There are many causes of failure to grow, including nutritional or other endocrine disorders, such as hypothyroidism. Growth hormone deficiency is actually a rare cause of growth retardation. Hyposecretion in the adult is of little clinical significance and typically results from large nonsecreting pituitary adenomas.[5]

Hypersecretion due to pituitary adenoma in childhood, before long-bone growth is complete, results in gigantism, with proportionate excess growth in all or most skeletal bones and muscles. Continued hypersecretion will produce changes in the face and extremities and potentially early death from cardiac or neurological consequences. Hypersecretion of GH from the pituitary in the adult is termed *acromegaly*, meaning the patient has elongated extremities. It may be associated with normal serum levels of GH but, when the patient is given a dose of oral glucose, there is suppression of GH.[9]

CASE SCENARIO 11-3

Pheochromocytoma: A Red-Haired Woman With a Taste for Bananas

The note on the chart stated, "Explain diet restrictions for these tests fully. Previous results unreliable." The laboratory technologist looked at the previous laboratory tests. A 24-hour urine specimen had been ordered for metanephrines and vanillylmandelic acid (VMA). The results were high:

Test	Patient	Reference Range
Metanephrines (μg/day)	1500	74–297
VMA (mg/day)	13	1.4–6.5

The laboratory technologist explained the restrictions again. The patient, Gayle Campton, a slight, freckled, red-haired, 33-year-old woman, assured the technologist that she was almost following the dietary guidelines and was not taking any of the medications that were restricted. Upon further discussion, the patient noted that she had eaten a banana during the last hour of the period that she collected the urine. The laboratory technologist admonished her to refrain from eating anything that was restricted before and during the urine collection.

The patient was asked to follow the restrictions of the diet for 2 to 3 days before the start of the 24-hour urine collection and to continue the restrictions during the collection. The diet excluded the following items:

- Caffeine (found in coffee, tea, cocoa, and chocolate)
- Amines (found in bananas, walnuts, avocados, fava beans, cheese, beer, and red wine)
- Vanilla (in foods or fluids)
- Licorice
- Nicotine (4 hours before collection of urine and during the urine collection), alcohol (ethanol), and cocaine

She was also reminded to discontinue specific medications, including ephedrine, aspirin, levodopa, nitroglycerin, tricyclic antidepressants, tetracycline, theophylline, clonidine, methyldopa, guanethidine, bromocriptine, cimetidine, reserpine, and blood pressure medications.

Finally, the laboratory technologist reminded the patient that factors such as strenuous physical exercise or extreme physical or emotional stress can interfere with VMA and metanephrine tests and affect the accuracy of the results.

The results of testing the second 24-hour urine were similar to the first:

Test	Patient	Reference Range
Metanephrines (μg/day)	1450	74–297
VMA (mg/day)	12	1.4–6.5

Mrs. Campton had been experiencing headaches, sweating, **tachycardia**, and bouts of severe anxiety. She was severely hypertensive, although her high blood pressure appeared to be intermittent. The physician considered renal, vascular, endocrine, and drug-induced causes of **hypertension**. Among many explanations for the hypertension, the physician suspected an adrenal medullary hormone abnormality. The laboratory results indicated that his suspicions may be well founded.

tachycardia - racing heart rate

hypertension - in adults, blood pressure higher than 140 mm Hg systolic or 90 mm Hg diastolic on three separate readings recorded several weeks apart

ADRENAL MEDULLARY HORMONES

The adrenal medulla is a functional extension of the sympathetic nervous system, a division of the autonomic nervous system, which accelerates heartbeat, increases blood sugar, slows digestion, and dilates arteries. The medulla is composed of chromaffin cells, specialized sympathetic ganglia that are the site of catecholamine synthesis and secretion. The chromaffin cells are true neuroendocrine cells, providing a direct interface between the nervous and endocrine systems. Sympathetic, cholinergic stimulation of the cells results in secretion of **catecholamines** from the adrenal medulla.

The sites of catecholamine synthesis in the body are the central nervous system, postganglionic sympathetic neurons, and the adrenal medulla. The adrenal medulla is the major site of epinephrine production. Eighty percent of the catecholamine secretion of the medulla is in the form of epinephrine. In the blood, catecholamines circulate 50% bound to albumin.

The medullary hormones, epinephrine (also know as adrenaline), norepinephrine, and dopamine, have the same effects on target organs as direct stimulation by sympathetic nerves, although their effects are longer lasting and circulating hormones may cause effects in cells and tissues that are not directly innervated. The adrenal glands produce large amounts of catecholamines as a reaction to stress. Catecholamines are synthesized from the amino acid tyrosine through reactions that are catalyzed by the enzymes catechol-*O*-methyltransferase (COMT) and monoamine oxidase (MAO). They break down into the **catecholamine metabolites** vanillylmandelic acid (VMA) and metanephrine, which are passed in the urine (Fig. 11–8).

As amine hormones, epinephrine and norepinephrine, affect the biochemistry of the target cell by binding cell receptors. Binding of hormones to alpha receptors increases free calcium and decreases cyclic AMP (cAMP). Hormone-binding to beta receptors increases cAMP. Each type of receptor has its own unique pattern of distribution throughout the body. The relative number of each receptor type in each target organ aids in the determination of the nature of the response of the organ to the catecholamines. In general, alpha receptors stimulate contractile events, while beta receptors enhance relaxation. Catecholamines generally affect all tissues. However, the most pronounced effects are on heart, liver, skeletal muscle,

catecholamines - biogenic amines that contain an aromatic catechol and an aliphatic amine (e.g., epinephrine, norepinephrine, dopamine)

catecholamine metabolites - products of catecholamine metabolism (e.g., vanillylmandelic acid, homovanillic acid, metanephrine, normetanephrine)

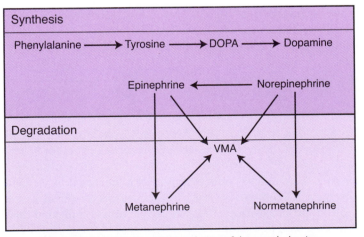

Figure 11–8. Synthesis and degradation of the catecholamines.

adipocytes, vascular smooth muscle, and bronchial smooth muscle. The physiological effects of the sympathetic response, called the "fight or flight" response, result when hormone binding of the alpha and beta receptors cause reactions within target tissue cells.

The major effects mediated by epinephrine and norepinephrine are

- Increased rate and force of contraction of the heart muscle, affected though epinephrine binding beta receptors.
- Vasoconstriction, which results in increased resistance and increased arterial blood pressure.
- Dilation of bronchioles.
- Increased glycogenolysis for energy production.
- Stimulation of lipolysis in fat cells, with more sustained energy production in many tissues than glycolysis.
- Increased metabolic rate, resulting in increased oxygen consumption and heat production.

DISORDERS OF ADRENAL MEDULLARY HORMONES

The diagnosis of disorders of the adrenal medulla is aided by laboratory measurement of hormone levels. Disorders of the adrenal medulla include pheochromocytomas and neuroblastomas.

Pheochromocytomas

Pheochromocytomas are tumors that produce excess catecholamines. The majority of pheochromocytomas arise from the adrenal medulla. The classic symptoms of pheochomocytomas are those attributable to excess hormone production, which include recurring episodes of sweating, headache, and a feeling of heightened anxiety. Although the disease is rare, any patient with hypertension that is difficult to control should be assessed for pheochromocytoma. The peak incidence for the disorder is in the third to fifth decades of life.

Pheochromocytoma is often referred to as the "ten percent tumor" because many characteristics of the disease occur about 10% of the time.[10–13]

- 10% of pheochromocytomas are malignant (90% are benign).
- 10% of those found on adrenal glands are present on both adrenals glands (90% are present on one adrenal gland).
- 10% are extra-adrenal (found within nervous tissue outside of the adrenal glands).
- 10% are diagnosed in children (90% in adults).
- 10% will recur in 5 to 10 years.
- 10% are associated with multiple endocrine neoplasia.
- 10% of patients present with a stroke (10% of pheochromocytomas are found after the patient has a stroke).

The diagnosis of pheochromocytoma hinges on the results of 24-hour urinary catecholamines and metanephrines and plasma catecholamines:

- 24-Hour Urinary Catacholamines and Metanephrines: Metabolites of the catecholamines are excreted in the urine as waste products. This test measures the catecholamines (epinephrine, norepinephrine, dopamine) as well as the breakdown products of these compounds that the liver and kidney have degraded.

- Plasma Catecholamines: Measurement of catecholamines in the blood is not as sensitive a test for pheochromocytoma as the 24-hour urine test. The urine test measures concentration levels over a 24-hour period, while the plasma test measures levels at a single point in time. Plasma levels are affected by physiological factors, such as position of the patient. Epinephrine in blood drawn when the patient is standing may be twice the level in blood drawn when the patient is supine.

adrenergic - pertaining to the adrenal gland, especially the neuroendocrine tissues of the medulla

Pheochromocytomas should be removed surgically. The use of combined alpha- and beta-**adrenergic** blockers or calcium antagonists has been shown to be effective in the control of blood pressure and symptoms of pheochromocytoma.[14] The most common sites of metastatic disease include lymph nodes, bones, liver, and lungs. If the tumor is successfully removed, long-term survival may be achieved; however, careful monitoring for recurrent disease by laboratory assessment and other findings will be necessary indefinitely.[15]

Neuroblastomas

Neuroblastoma occurs most often in children; 70% to 90% of neuroblastomas occur in children under the age of 5 years. Neuroblastoma can arise anywhere along the sympathetic nervous system chain; however, it most commonly arises from the adrenal medulla. Some of the symptoms associated with neuroblastoma, such as high blood pressure, rapid heartbeat, and diarrhea, are directly due to the effects of increased catecholamine secretion by the adrenal medulla. By the time the disease is diagnosed, the tumor has often spread to the lymph nodes, liver, lungs, bones, or bone marrow.

The diagnosis of neuroblastomas is achieved by a combination of distinguishing factors, which include immunohistochemistry identification of a tissue biopsy sample, finding of cancer cells in a bone marrow sample, and increased blood or urine levels of catecholamines or their metabolites. The urinary catecholamine metabolic end products, VMA and homovanillic acid (HVA), are measured more often than blood catecholamines.

Neuroblastomas are treated with surgery, radiation therapy, chemotherapy, and bone marrow transplantation.

Several imaging techniques aid in the diagnosis, staging, and assessment of the gland:

- *X-rays:* A standard chest x-ray is done if physicians suspect that a tumor has invaded the chest.
- *Computed tomography (CT; also called computed axial tomography [CAT]):* The CT scan is an x-ray procedure that produces detailed cross-sectional images of the body.
- *Magnetic resonance imaging (MRI):* MRI uses radio waves and strong magnets instead of x-rays. The energy from the radio waves is absorbed and then released in a pattern formed by the type of tissue and by certain diseases.
- *Positron emission tomography (PET):* PET scans use glucose that contains a radioactive atom. Cancer cells absorb high amounts of the radioactive glucose because of their high rate of metabolism.

- *Ultrasound:* Ultrasound uses sound waves, whose echoes produce a picture of internal organs or masses. The sound wave echoes are picked up by the transducer and converted by a computer into an image, which is displayed on a computer screen.

LABORATORY TESTING FOR ADRENAL MEDULLARY DISORDERS

A test for catecholamines measures the amount of epinephrine, norepinephrine, and dopamine produced by nerve tissue (including the brain) and the adrenal medullary glands. Both serum and urine may be tested for catecholamines. High levels of catecholamines, VMA, metanephrine, or HVA can indicate an adrenal gland tumor or another type of tumor that produces catecholamines. A person with a pheochromocytoma generally has blood catecholamine levels greater than 2000 ng/L and urine VMA levels greater than 11 mg/24 hr. However, high levels may also be seen with any significant stress, such as burns, systemic infection, surgery, and trauma. Lower than normal blood catecholamine values are rarely clinically significant.

The diagnosis of pheochromocytoma is established by the demonstration of elevated 24-hour urinary excretion of free catecholamines or catecholamine metabolites (VMA and total metanephrines). The measurement of plasma catecholamines can also be of value in the diagnosis of pheochromocytoma. However, the measurement of plasma catecholamines has limited sensitivity and specificity. Plasma metanephrines have been reported to be more sensitive than plasma catecholamines. When 52 patients with pheochromocytoma were studied, every patient was found to have elevated plasma levels of metanephrines, but 8 had normal levels of plasma catecholamines.[16] Quantification of urine metanephrine and normetanephrine (collectively referred to as "metanephrines") is commonly requested in the diagnosis and follow-up of patients with pheochromocytoma and related neurogenic tumors.[17]

Pharmacological testing with an agent such as clonidine is rarely required to make the diagnosis.[18] The clonidine suppression test is used to determine whether the high blood pressure is caused by an adrenal gland tumor or by other factors. Plasma catecholamine levels are measured before and after a small dose of clonidine is taken. If a tumor is present, catecholamine levels will not change. If the high blood pressure is due to other factors, catecholamine levels will usually decrease.

The diagnosis of neuroblastomas is aided by demonstration of increased blood or urine levels of catecholamines, increased VMA (the metabolite of norepinephrine) and increased HVA, the metabolite of dopamine.

Methodological development over the past 50 years has seen a progression of sophistication from the wet chemistry methods of the 1950s to the radioenzymatic assays of the 1980s and thence to high-performance liquid chromatography (HPLC) with electrochemistry detection and various immunoassay methods. Chromatography methods, including gas chromatography with mass spectrometry detection (GC-MS) and HPLC with electrochemical detection, are generally time consuming and technically demanding.[19–23] The use of radioactive substances constitutes a disadvantage, not offering an attractive substitute for existing chromatographic methods. Test Methodologies 11–2 through 11–5 describe analysis of plasma catecholamines, VMA, metanephrines, and HVA using HPLC.[24]

THE TEAM APPROACH
Health professionals who perform imaging, such as radiological technicians and technologists, are partners in the assessment of the adrenal gland by providing images of the body looking for evidence of disease, including tumors. This information is used along with clinical laboratory tests to help in diagnosis.

TEST METHODOLOGY 11-2.   PLASMA CATECHOLAMINES

Both free and conjugated catecholamines circulate in the blood. High sensitivity is required for assays for plasma catecholamines to measure the low concentration of free, active forms of catecholamines in the blood of normal individuals.

The Reaction Principle

The specimen is purified by extraction of the catechol group through selective absorption with borate affinity gel. The extracted amines are separated by HPLC. Amperometry or coulometry is used to detect and measure catecholamines. Both amperometry and coulometry measure current that is produced by oxidation of catecholamines.

The Specimen

Patient preparation must be standardized to the method used to obtain the reference range. The patient should be counseled to fast and refrain from using tobacco for 4 hours before blood collection. Drugs should be allowed to leave the system before blood collection; if possible, the patient should discontinue drug use for 3–7 days before the draw. A heparinized, anticoagulated blood specimen should be collected from the patient, who should be calm and/or in a supine position for 30 minutes prior to collection. The specimen should be chilled in ice water immediately after collection and the plasma separated as soon as possible. The specimen must be frozen immediately. Specimens are stable at −70°C for 6–8 months, but the analytes are unstable at ambient temperature, or 4°C.

Reference Ranges (in Supine Adult)

Epinephrine	<50 pg/ml
Norepinephrine	110–410 pg/ml
Dopamine	<87 pg/ml

TEST METHODOLOGY 11-3.   VANILLYLMANDELIC ACID

Vanillylmandelic acid is the major metabolite of epinephrine and norepinephrine.

Chemical Methodology

Amines in urine are separated by HPLC, using anion-exchange resin resolution. Amperometry or coulometry is used to detect and measure catecholamines.

The Specimen

Patient Preparation

A diet that restricts amines should be followed for 2–3 days before and during the urine collection. Nicotine must be restricted. If possible, medications, especially hypertensive medications, should be restricted for 3–7 days before the collection and during the collection.

Collection

A 24-hour urine specimen is recommended. The specimen must be refrigerated immediately after collection. Sample preservation can be maintained with the addition of 6N hydrochloric acid. Six milliliters of 6N HCl will be satisfactory in maintaining pH for adult collections. Acid preservation should be adjusted for volume in pediatric specimen collection. The pH must not fall below 2.

continued

TEST METHODOLOGY 11-3.   VANILLYLMANDELIC ACID *(continued)*

Reference Range

Adult   1.4–6.5 mg/day

The VMA-to-creatinine ratio will be reported if the patient is under 18 years old or the urine volume is less than 400 mL/24 hr. VMA/creatinine ratios are used for the diagnosis of pediatric patients.

TEST METHODOLOGY 11-4.   METANEPHRINES

Metanephrines (metanephrine and normetanephrine) appear in the urine as both free metabolites and conjugated molecules.

The Reaction Principle

The specimen is first hydrolyzed to purify all metanephrines to the free, unconjugated state. Amines are resolved by application to cation-exchange and anion-exchange resins, and separated by reversed-phase HPLC. The eluted amines are detected electrochemically.

The Specimen

A 24-hour urine specimen is required. Acidification and refrigeration are recommended during collection.

Reference Range (Adults)

Metanephrine   74–297 µg/day
Normetanephrine   105–354 µg/day

Reference ranges are age dependent and are expressed as a ratio to creatinine for pediatric patients.

TEST METHODOLOGY 11-5.   HOMOVANILLIC ACID

Homovanillic acid (HVA) is the major metabolite of dopamine and important in the clinical diagnosis and monitoring of neuroblastomas in pediatric patients. Neuroendocrine tumors are typically present with HVA elevations greater than 10 times the reference limit.

The Reaction Principle

Amines in urine are separated by HPLC, using anion-exchange resin resolution. HVA may be detected by amperometry or coulometry, simultaneously with other metabolites, or may be detected separately by ultraviolet or fluorescence spectrophotometry.

The Specimen

A 24-hour urine specimen is recommended. Acidification and refrigeration is recommended during collection.

Reference Range

Adult   1.4–8.8 mg/day

HVA-to-creatinine ratio will be reported if the patient is under 18 years old or the urine volume is less than 400 mL/24 hr.

Immunoassays, which are more suitable for highly sensitive and specific screening of large numbers of samples, have been described in the literature for catecholamine analysis. Enzyme immunoassay kits, based on microtiter plate technology, for the quantitative determination of urinary metanephrines have become commercially available. These kits offer an opportunity to replace chromatographic techniques for methods accessible to common routine clinical laboratories. Enzyme immunoassay methods are applicable in the quantification of urinary metanephrines as compared with methods using isotope dilution mass spectrometry. Immunoassay methods are qualified methods with sensitivity and specificity rates capable of aiding in the diagnosis of pheochromocytoma. These relatively simple methods can be performed in any clinical laboratory and may replace the present, more complicated, chromatographic techniques.[25] A fast, competitive enzyme immunoassay for measuring HVA in human urine samples has been developed using a monoclonal antibody with acetylcholinesterase as an enzyme label.[26] Monoclonal antibodies for HVA and VMA have been previously described[27] but have not been used to measure these metabolites in urine due to poor affinity and specificity. A fluorescence polarization immunoassay (FPIA) of urinary VMA with clinical applications and new strategies for polyclonal anti-HVA antibody production has been described.[28] Enzyme-linked immunosorbent assay (ELISA) kits are an acceptable alternative to HPLC.[29] An enzyme immunoassay for urinary VMA using polyclonal antiserum and VMA-acetylcholinesterase conjugate as enzymatic tracer has also shown good correlation with HPLC analysis in normal and pathological human urine samples.[30]

Case Scenario 11-3 Pheochromocytoma: A Red-Haired Woman With a Taste for Bananas

Follow-Up

The results of biochemical assessment and radiological imaging helped the physician diagnose a pheochromocytoma, found to be localized to one adrenal gland. An adrenalectomy was performed and no extra-adrenal disease was found. Repeat biochemical assays for catecholamines and metabolites were performed postoperatively to confirm that all functioning pheochromocytoma was removed.[31]

This case illustrates the importance of preanalytical factors. Although the banana eaten by the patient during the last hour of the 24-hour urine collection probably did not affect the results to a great extent, the need for recollection delayed diagnosis for several days. ●

CASE SCENARIO 11-4

Neonatal Hypothyroidism: Repeat Thyroid Testing on a Baby

The medical technologist was new to the section of the clinical chemistry laboratory where thyroid testing was performed. She first checked the neonatal samples, which were filter papers containing dried blood spots for proper amount and appearance of blood along with identification names, numbers, and dates, and matched them with the requisition forms. She also noted from the requisition forms that the samples were collected at least 24 hours after

Case Scenario 11-4 **Neonatal Hypothyroidism: Repeat Thyroid Testing on a Baby** *(continued)*

date of birth. One sample was unique in that it was named "Mary B. Jones" and was from a baby 1 week old. The specimen was sent from the physician's office. The test requisition indicated repeat testing due to poor feeding in the hospital. After verifying that all samples were acceptable, the medical technologist began setting up the tubes for extracting the dried blood samples for thyroxine testing.

ROLE OF ENDOCRINE GLANDS IN THYROID FUNCTION

Thyroid hormones are secreted based on a complex interaction of the hypothalamus, the adenohypophysis, and the thyroid gland. The hypothalamus has thyroid hormone receptors within many of its cells. It provides a tertiary level of control and stimulation of the thyroid gland by secreting thyrotropin-releasing hormone (TRH; also known as thyrotropin-releasing factor [TRF]), a peptide hormone, in response to lower than normal levels of thyroid hormone. Thyrotropin-releasing hormone may have many functions, but the primary function is to stimulate the adenohypophysis. The adenohypophysis, also known as the anterior pituitary, provides the secondary level of control and stimulation. It produces and secretes thyroid-stimulating hormone (TSH), or thyrotropin, a glycoprotein hormone. The main function of TSH is to stimulate the thyroid gland in hormonal production.

Figure 11–9 depicts the hypothalamic response to subnormal levels of circulating free **triiodothyronine (T_3)** and **thyroxine (T_4)**, releasing TRH. TRH stimulates the anterior pituitary to release thyrotropin (TSH), which in turn stimulates the thyroid to release T_4 and T_3. When T_3 and T_4 exceed normal levels, through

triiodothyronine (T_3) - more potent thyroid hormone, also known as 3,5,3'-triiodothyronine

thyroxine (T_4) - main hormone synthesized in the thyroid gland, also known as 3,5,3'5'-tetraiodothyronine

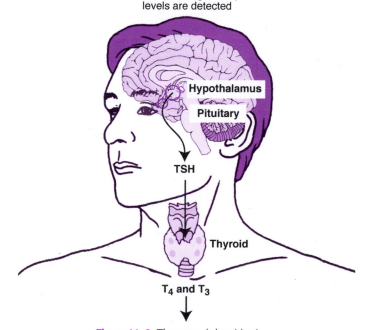

Figure 11–9. The normal thyroid axis.

negative feedback they influence the hypothalamus and pituitary gland to discontinue release of TRF and TSH. This cycle continues so that thyroid hormones are maintained at optimum steady-state levels.

Thyroid-Stimulating Hormone: Pituitary Hormone

Thyrotropin, or TSH, is a glycoprotein hormone composed of two polypeptide alpha and beta chains. The alpha chain of TSH is identical to that of other pituitary hormones such as luteinizing hormone and follicle-stimulating hormone. It is produced in the anterior pituitary, also known as the adenohypophysis, arising from inactive prehormone and prohormone. The hormone has a short half-life of minutes to a few hours when compared with other hormones such as steroids. TSH binds to a specific TSH receptor found in the cytoplasmic membrane of thyroid cells. It releases second messengers that activate cAMP and protein kinase and stimulate further biochemical cascades. Thyrotropin is transported free, not bound to a protein carrier, in body fluids. It is metabolized to active states from pre- and prohormones when active TSH is needed, in part from TRH stimulation.

The thyroid gland, a butterfly-shaped endocrine gland located in the neck, is the primary organ in this endocrine system. In response to TSH and to other adrenergic neuropeptides binding to cytoplasmic membrane receptors, the thyroid gland secretes the hormones T_4 and T_3.[8] These thyroid hormones are derived from tyrosine and iodine. When released into circulation, they ultimately produce a diverse systemic organic and metabolic response.

Thyroid Hormone Metabolism

The active thyroid hormones are made in the follicle, the fundamental structural unit of the thyroid gland, from tyrosine and iodine in the presence of peroxidase. Synthesis of triiodothyronine occurs in association with thyroglobulin, which contains iodine-trapping mechanisms forming the precursors mono-iodotyrosine (MIT) and di-iodotyrosine (DIT), and it is considered the prohormone to thyroxine. Some triiodothyronine (3,5,3′-triiodothyronine) is made from combining DIT and MIT, while thyroxine (or 3,5,3′,5′-tetraiodothyronine) is made from the combination of two DIT molecules. Around 80% of T_3 is formed in peripheral cells from enzymatic conversion of T_4, with the remaining amount formed from MIT and DIT coupling in the thyroid gland. Another thyroid hormone, reverse T_3 (3,3,5′-triiodothyronine), is made in smaller amounts as the inactive form of T_3. Significantly more reverse T_3 is formed during chronic illness.[8]

Triiodothyronine is more physiologically active than T_4. Greater than 99% of circulating T_4 is *in*active since it is protein bound, and 99.9% of T_3 is protein bound and inactive. However, circulating levels of T_3 and T_4 are not equal since there is much more T_4 circulating. Triiodothyronine is analyzed less frequently than other thyroid hormones. However, the test is ordered when a clinician suspects subclinical hyperthyroidism when free T_4 is normal. Triiodothyronine is typically elevated in hyperthyroidism. It is also typically decreased in situations of chronic illness due to stress and nonthyroid factors, so T_3 levels are not useful in differential diagnosis of hypothyroidism.

Hormones can gain entry to a cell based on chemical makeup, solubility, and ability to bind specifically to receptors. Thyroid hormones, considered the first

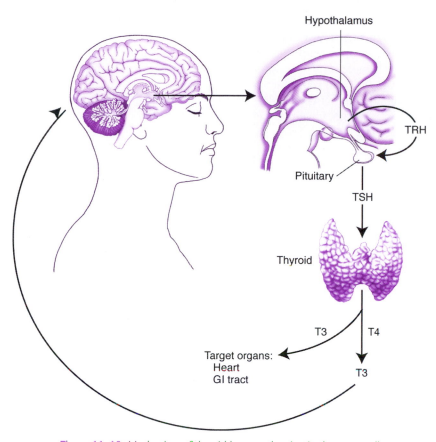

Figure 11–10. Mechanism of thyroid hormonal action in the target cell.

messenger, bind to cellular receptors based on structural specificity. This initiates release of second messengers and subsequent cellular responses. TSH binds to cytoplasmic cellular receptors in the thyroid gland, which initiates the secondary messenger response. Figure 11–10 illustrates the mechanism for TSH hormonal action in the thyroid gland. Thyroid hormones function in a manner similar to steroid hormones since thyroxine receptors are found in diverse number of cells and are intranuclear. Figure 11–10 illustrates this relationship. Thyroid hormones diffuse through the cytoplasmic and nuclear membranes and bind directly to specific receptors on the DNA of target cells. The result is regulation of nucleic acid activity, which ultimately produces many systemic effects.

Thyroid hormones are involved in growth and maturation of bones and other tissues of the skeletal system and of nerves in the central nervous system, and in regulation of growth hormones. They are also involved in body temperature regulation and generation of heat. Metabolic functions of thyroid hormones include regulating **basal metabolic rate** and fat, protein, and carbohydrate metabolism, including gluconeogenesis, glycogenolysis, lipolysis, and degradation of cholesterol and triglycerides. Thyroid hormones regulate cardiac output as determined by heart rate and respiration rate. Thyroid hormones influence mood and behavior also. Clinicians can assess thyroid function using clinical signs and symptoms such as body temperature, respiratory rate, and pulse. High levels of thyroid hormones

basal metabolic rate -
baseline rate of metabolism based on gender and weight (in kcal/24 hr)

will increase body temperature; increase basal metabolic rate, cardiac output, cardiac rate, and respiratory rate; and influence mood and behavior. Thyroid hormone levels also impact upon fetal development, particularly neurological development. Inadequate levels of thyroid hormone during fetal or infant development will impair growth and reproductive and mental development.

The thyroid gland also contains parafollicular cells that produce calcitonin and other similar peptides. Calcitonin is a polypeptide hormone is secreted in response to rising free calcium ion levels for the purpose of maintaining homeostasis and balancing the response of parathyroid hormone. This is discussed further in conjunction with parathyroid function later in this chapter.

Hypothyroidism

There are conditions in which the thyroid gland is underfunctioning, due to either congenital defect or illness that arises later in life. Primary hypothyroidism is named such because the disease resides in the thyroid gland. This disorder is associated with increased levels of TSH and decreased free T_4 levels. If hypothyroidism is due to autoimmunity, such as Hashimoto's thyroiditis, anti-microsomal antibodies or anti-thyroid antibodies are present. These autoantibodies are correlated with gradual destruction of thyroid function. Hashimoto's thyroiditis usually presents during the hypothyroid state following thyroid atrophy but may present as **euthyroid** with **goiter** due to the inflammatory state. Other possible causes of hypothyroidism in the adult include thyroidectomy, anti-thyroid drugs, and radioiodine therapy. Hypothyroidism in the adult is characterized by **myxedema**, the characteristic reaction to thyroid hormone deficiency, including puffiness in the face and surrounding the eyes due to accumulation of mucopolysaccharides and chondroitin sulfate. Other characteristics of hypothyroidism include cold intolerance, dry hair and skin, weight gain, personality change, and memory impairment.[6]

Neonatal primary hypothyroidism may be caused by a congenitally absent, atrophic, or dysfunctional thyroid gland, a disorder that occurs once in every 3500 live births.[32] As mentioned earlier, thyroid function is necessary for neurological development; therefore, untreated neonatal hypothyroidism results in profound impairment of growth and mental development. This disorder was formerly termed **cretinism**. In the United States, neonates are screened with total T_4 levels in order to determine if asymptomatic congenital hypothyroidism is present so that treatment can begin before irreversible neurological damage results. Treatment involves thyroid hormone replacement, such as levothyroxine, within the first week of life and continuing throughout adulthood, with care taken not to overtreat and create hyperthyroidism. Early treatment has been reported to promote normal mental development and linear growth in children, with congenital hypothyroidism studies reporting normal final adult height in patients.[33–35] Recent studies have also shown evidence that children with lifelong treatment of L-thyroxine have a higher incidence of obesity, which may make them prone to obesity-related illnesses.[36]

Secondary hypothyroidism is associated with both decreased TSH and free T_4. Symptoms are similar to those of primary hypothyroidism in the adult. It is generally of pituitary origin secondary to surgical removal of the pituitary or pituitary failure, such as following head trauma, cerebral vascular accident, or obstetric complications.

euthyroid - showing normal clinical signs and normal thyroid function status despite the indications of dysfunction in some thyroid test results

goiter - enlarged, usually hyperactive thyroid gland due to a variety of causes

myxedema - puffiness in the face and surrounding the eyes

cretinism - growth deficiency and mental retardation

Case Scenario 11-4 Neonatal Hypothyroidism: Repeat Thyroid Testing on a Baby

Follow-Up

The medical technologist was performing neonatal thyroid testing to include a repeat thyroid test on Mary B. Jones, age 1 week old, that was sent from the physician's office. The test requisition stated repeat testing was needed due to poor feeding in the hospital. The earlier thyroxine level on Baby Jones was 5.5 μg/dL (>7.5 μg/dL newborn screen). After verifying that all samples were acceptable, the medical technologist began setting up the dried blood extraction tubes for thyroxine testing. She noted that usually the thyroxine screening test in newborns was performed while the babies were still in the hospital prior to discharge. The common recommendation for neonatal testing is that specimens are collected when the newborn is at least 3 days old and after 24 hours of protein feeding in order to adequately supply nutrients to produce thyroid hormones. Given the common practice of dismissing mother and newborn baby within 48 hours of the mother's admission, it is likely that thyroxine levels may occasionally fall below normal reference ranges due to inadequate protein feeding rather than congenital hypothyroidism. Those situations call for a repeat thyroxine level performed during the first week, possibly at a clinic visit to the pediatrician, to ensure that the level reflects the patient's true thyroid status. If repeat thyroxine levels are found to be decreased, the next step is to analyze TSH to verify if primary hypothyroidism is present, as indicated by a TSH greater than 39 mU/L (reference range at 1 to 13 days, 1.0 to 38.9 mU/L). ●

THE TEAM APPROACH

Neonatal nurses or physician assistants in office settings may collect blood from neonates by heel stick for laboratory analysis.

Neonatal thyroxine levels are generally elevated at birth when compared to adults, such as 11.8 to 22.6 μg/dL for ages 1 to 3 days, due to maternal estrogen-induced thyroid-binding globulin (TBG) levels. The medical decision limit for detecting neonatal hypothyroidism is less than 7.5 μg/dL.[5] However, synthesis of thyroid hormones require adequate intake of proteins, so the thyroid screen should occur after adequate feedings. In preterm infants, thyroxine level is also lower and tends to rise up to typical reference ranges when term birth weight is reached. Thyroxine levels gradually decline to the adult reference range by age 10, with some fluctuations in the values at onset of puberty. Free thyroxine is generally near adult levels but generally is tested only after repeat thyroxine levels and TSH are determined to be abnormal.

CASE SCENARIO 11-5

Graves Disease: The Woman With Prominent Eyeballs

Laboratory testing for a 70-year-old female patient showed TSH of 0.03 μU/mL (reference range, 0.4 to 4.2 μU/mL in an adult <55 years old), free T_4 of 5.2 ng/dL (0.8 to 2.7 ng/dL). A request was made for assays of thyroid-stimulating immunoglobulins (TSI) and anti-thyroid microsomal antibodies (TMAbs), which require sending a specimen and requisitions to a reference laboratory. Further testing included an ultrasound of the thyroid, which confirmed the presence of a 0.94 × 0.87 × 0.94-cm left thyroid nodule.

TESTING FOR THYROID DISORDERS

The American Thyroid Association recommends a testing decision pathway for thyroid disorders in adult patients. Total thyroxine hormone levels should not be assessed in healthy or asymptomatic patients. In other words, total thyroxine level should not be used as a screening test to investigate for thyroid disease. If signs and symptoms of thyroid disorder are clear, the first laboratory test that should be ordered is TSH.[37] If the results are abnormal compared to age- and gender-adjusted reference ranges, thyroid disease is likely present. For example, if TSH is less than 0.1 μU/mL in the adult, primary hyperthyroidism is most likely present.[5] Free T_4 (or free T_4 index) can be analyzed if TSH results do not correlate with symptoms. However, due to the severe consequences of untreated thyroid disease in the neonate, particularly hypothyroidism, asymptomatic neonates are typically screened for T_4 (total thyroxine) and followed up with TSH testing if abnormal results are obtained.

Thyroid Function Testing

Analysis of thyroxine is best achieved by immunoassay of plasma and serum samples, such as enzyme immunoassay or fluorescent immunoassay, as described in Test Methodologies 11–6 and 11–7. Table 11–7 compares the reaction principles of various immunoassays used in hormone testing. The principle of enzyme immunoassay involves the use of enzyme-labeled antibody. For total thyroxine assays, since over 99% of the hormone is bound to protein, the first step in the reaction involves displacing the thyroxine from the binding proteins. Monoclonal or polyclonal antibody that is highly specific to thyroxine binds with the hormone. Enzyme-labeled hormone, when used instead of enzyme-labeled antibody, competes with the endogenous thyroxine. Substances that did not bind to antibody are removed from the system. Specific substrate is then added that reacts with the enzyme label, and product is formed that can be measured spectrophotometrically. Examples of enzyme immunoassays include microparticle capture enzyme immunoassay (MEIA) and enzyme-multiplied immunoassay technique (EMIT).

TEST METHODOLOGY 11-6.   TOTAL THYROXINE (T_4) BY EMIT

The Reaction Principle

Antibody that has specificity to thyroxine is added to the patient sample along with enzyme-labeled thyroxine (labeled with glucose-6-phosphate dehydrogenase). The binding of the antibody to the enzyme-labeled thyroxine inhibits the enzyme activity by interfering with the enzyme's active site for the substrate. When substrate (glucose 6-phosphate and NAD) is added to the system, it is catalyzed by any (leftover) unbound enzyme-labeled thyroxine to form product and NADH. This reaction is measured spectrophotometrically at 340 nm. The rate of product formation is directly proportional to the concentration of thyroxine in the patient sample. For example, if the patient sample contains a low amount of thyroxine, there will be a low amount of leftover enzyme-labeled thyroxine to react with the substrate and form the product. When there is low concentration of patient hormone, the majority of the antibody has been bound with the enzyme-labeled thyroxine.

TEST METHODOLOGY 11-6. TOTAL THYROXINE (T₄) BY EMIT (*continued*)

Interferences

Preanalytical errors: Repeated freezing and thawing of the serum or plasma sample or grossly hemolyzed or lipemic samples should be avoided. Use of the wrong type of anticoagulant, failing to store specimens older than 24 hours under refrigeration, or not allowing whole blood samples to fill the filter paper spot are also likely problems, particularly from samples collected from distant sites and sent to a referral laboratory. Generally thyroid hormone is quite stable, but sample handling requires analysis within 10 days of storage at refrigeration temperatures and within 30 days if frozen.

Analytical errors: These include moderate to gross hemolysis or lipemia. Enzyme immunoassay is quite sensitive for quantification of thyroid hormone due to the type of antibody utilized. Some other forms of enzyme immunoassay, including MEIA and CEDIA, may have higher levels of sensitivity than EMIT. Precision levels of at least 8% can be achieved by this method.

The Specimen

Serum or dried whole blood but heparinized or EDTA plasma samples may be used with some instrumentation. To avoid preanalytical errors, puncture must take place in the appropriate place on the disinfected, dry heel, collecting free-flowing drops of blood that can fully saturate two 0.5-inch circles, and the filter paper must be properly labeled with the patient's name and date of birth, and the date and time of collection. The blood drops must dry thoroughly in a cool, dry area before being placed in a transport bag with the test requisition form. Plasma or serum can be held up to 1 day at room temperature, up to 7 days at 2°–4°C, and up to 30 days if frozen. Dried whole blood is stable for up to 1 week. Proper collection, handling, and storage of samples for thyroxine testing is necessary in order to avoid preanalytical errors.

Reference Range

T₄ total, adult female   5.5–11.0 µg/dL
adult male   4.6–10.5 µg/dL

Analysis of thyroid-stimulating hormone is typically achieved by immunoassay techniques. Although radioimunoassay or immunoradiometric assay were historically used because of high specificity and sensitivity, the need for nuclear waste disposal has made them less desirable. Nonradioactive labels in immunosassay techniques are currently more common, including enzyme or fluorescent immunoassays. Fluorescent substrate–labeled inhibition immunoassay is one common method and is described in Test Methodology 11–7.

TEST METHODOLOGY 11-7. THYROTROPIN (TSH) FLUORESCENT SUBSTRATE–LABELED INHIBITION IMMUNOASSAY

The Reaction Principle

Fluorogenic substrate–labeled TSH is competing with patient TSH for antibody in this homogeneous assay. Only unbound (leftover) labeled TSH reacts with the enzyme to form fluorescent product. There is a direct relationship between fluorescence and the amount of TSH present in the test sample. In other words, the highest fluorescence is emitted by the sample or standard with the highest levels of TSH.

continued

TEST METHODOLOGY 11-7.   THYROTROPIN (TSH) FLUORESCENT SUBSTRATE–LABELED INHIBITION IMMUNOASSAY *(continued)*

Interferences

This method exhibits good sensitivity and specificity, and no nuclear waste disposal is required. Sensitivity requirements for TSH testing are less than 0.1 mU/L since this is the medical decision limit for primary hyperthyroidism. Lipemia, hemolysis, and icterus may provide spectrophotometric interference.

The Specimen

Serum or plasma free from lipemia, hemolysis, and icterus. Specimens are stable for up to 5 days at 2°–8°C and up to 30 days when stored at –20°C.

Reference Range (Adult)

<55 years of age	0.4–4.2 μU/mL
≥55 years of age	0.5–8.9 μU/mL

In serum, the protein-bound forms of T_4 and T_3 predominate, being transported by thyroid-binding globulin (TBG), thyroid-binding albumin (TBA), and prealbumin, also know as transthyretin. The protein-bound aspect of thyroid hormones affects activity as previously discussed, as well as methods of analysis. Total T_4 levels reflect the protein-bound thyroxine and are affected by TBG, TBA, and thyroid-binding prealbumin levels. Measuring the free sites on the TBG or unsaturated thyroid-binding globulin (UTBG) levels can relate to total and free thyroid hormone levels and was used extensively in the past. This type of testing has become nearly obsolete now that free thyroxine levels can be easily measured.

TABLE 11-7

Immunoassay Methods for Thyroxine Testing

Method	Description	Characteristics
Fluorescent Polarization Immunoassay (FPIA)	Competitive reaction: fluorophore-labeled thyroxine competes with patient thyroxine for antibody in homogeneous system. Antibody-bound labeled thyroxine rotates slowly, emitting lower energy polarized light. Highest polarized light emitted by sample or standard with no thyroxine.	Good sensitivity and specificity; moderate complexity; fewer safety regulations to follow compared with radioimmunoassay (RIA).
Fluorescent Substrate-Labeled Inhibition Immunoassay	Competitive reaction: fluorogenic substrate–labeled thyroxine competing with patient T_4 for antibody in a homogeneous assay. Only unbound, leftover labeled T_4 reacts with enzyme to form fluorescent product. Highest fluorescence emitted by sample or standard with highest levels of T_4.	Good sensitivity and specificity and no nuclear safety regulations required.

TABLE 11-7 (continued)

Immunoassay Methods for Thyroxine Testing

Method	Description	Characteristics
Chemilumine-scence	Peroxidase-labeled antibody binds with patient hormone (antigen) to form complex (similar to ELISA). Addition of luminol or acridium esters substrate forms an oxidized product that emits light for short time measured by a luminometer.	Substrate reacts with enzyme label to form fluorescent product.
Microparticle Enzyme Immu-noassay (MEIA)	MEIA is similar to enzyme-linked immunosorbent assay (ELISA) in that there is a double-antibody system that forms a "sandwich" with the hormone.	Sensitivity may be better than other immunoassay methods; highly automated; quick turnaround time and no nuclear safety regulations are required.

Enzyme-Multiplied Immunoassay Technique (EMIT)

EMIT is a homogeneous competitive immunoassay. Homogeneous means that wash steps are not required to separate antibody-bound hormone from nonbound substances or labeled from unlabeled hormone. A competitive immunoassay is often more sensitive than a noncompetitive assay and requires competition of patient hormone and (reagent) labeled hormone for specific antibody. The labeled hormone is involved in the detection process.

Historical Methods of Thyroid Testing

Since it was difficult to measure free thyroxine in the past, indirect methods were historically used, including thyroid update or thyroid hormone binding ratio (THBR) levels. Measuring the amount of unoccupied binding sites on TBG or other proteins was used to determine THBR for estimation of free thyroid hormone level. Methods that estimate the amount of protein binding to thyroid hormones include THBR, thyroid uptake (T uptake), or T_3 uptake, the classic test. T_3 uptake is the historical method that uses ^{125}I-labeled T_3 to measure thyroid-binding proteins. This method measured the number of available binding sites that could accept the labeled T_3. Due to the confusion of patient's T_3 level with results of the T_3 uptake test (often abbreviated as T_3U), it was recommended by the American Thyroid Association that the term *thyroid hormone binding ratio* be used.[5] Some physicians may continue to order total thyroxine and THBR in order to get a calculated free T_4 index along with TSH. There is an increased total T_4, increased THBR, and increased calculated free T_4 index in primary hyperthyroidism.

In general, THBR levels, no matter how they are determined in the procedure, are inversely related to TBG levels. Increased THBR indicates low levels of TBG.

Because TSH and free T_4 levels more adequately indicate thyroid function, experts currently recommend not using THBR for routine thyroid testing. However, these historical tests are still available with some instrumentation and clinicians may be inclined to order these tests. The typical reference range for free T_4 index in the adult is 4.2 to 13.0 μg/dL, if the THBR method is used.[5]

Thyroid-binding protein levels fluctuate with various conditions other than thyroid function. For example, conditions that decrease the amount of TBG, transthyretin, and the like, such as nephrotic syndrome or liver failure, will also cause the total T_4 level to be decreased. Increased TBG and transthyretin levels are found in pregnancy and oral estrogen usage and cause increased total T_4 but normal free T_4 (and normal free thyroxine index [FTI]). Acute hepatitis and some drug therapy can also increase TBG levels.

Free T_4 levels typically are measured with an immunoassay methodology. A major component of this procedure involves separating the trace amounts of free T_4 from protein-bound T_4. Separation is typically achieved by ultracentrifugation using a Millipore filter prior to analysis with immunoassay. Fluorescent or chemiluminescent immunoassays are popular methods to analyze free T_4 levels. The typical reference range for free T_4 in the adult is 0.8 to 2.7 ng/dL.[5]

HYPERTHYROIDISM

Thyroid disorders occur more frequently in women than in men, occurring in up to 10% of all women. Tests for levels of TSH, free thyroxine, and free triiodothyronine are need by clinicians to make the diagnosis. Generally, high TSH values suggest primary hypothyroidism, while suppressed levels indicate primary hyperthyroidism. Signs and symptoms of hyperthyroidism include goiter (enlarged thyroid gland), optic changes including **exophthalmos**, proximal muscle weakness, tachycardia, atrial fibrillation, **hyperthermia**, and weight loss or inability to gain weight. Among women, the most common etiology of thyroid disease is thyroid autoimmunity, with Graves' disease more common than Hashimoto's thyroiditis. Other causes of primary hyperthyroidism include thyroid adenoma, toxic multinodular goiter, and thyroid carcinoma. Table 11–8 summarizes the typical laboratory findings in thyroid diseases.

Thyroxine or free thyroxine levels are not always necessary for diagnosis if hyperthyroid symptoms of increased respiratory rate and pulse, weight loss, enlarged thyroid gland, fatigue, sweating, and exophthalmos are present and if TSH is less than 0.1 mU/L (reference range of 0.4 to 4.2 mU/L in an adult <55 years old).

exophthalmos - protrusion of eyeballs due to accumulation of fluid and metabolic products

hyperthermia - heat intolerance and higher than normal body temperature

TABLE 11-8				
Diagnostic Indicators of Thyroid Disease				
Disease	TSH	T_4 (total)	FT_4	T_3
Primary hyperthyroidism	Decreased	Increased	Increased	Increased
Secondary hyperthyroidism	Increased	Increased	Increased	Increased
Primary hypothyroidism	Increased	Decreased	Decreased	Decreased
Secondary hypothyroidism	Decreased	Decreased	Decreased	Decreased

Hyperthyroidism is common in both young women and older women. Particularly in young women, subtle symptoms may be dismissed and go undiagnosed until pregnancy. Determining that thyroid dysfunction is present during pregnancy requires understanding of thyroid metabolism. For example, concentrations of both total T_4 and total T_3 increase in early pregnancy as the result of an increased TBG and a reduced peripheral TBG degradation rate. In spite of these changes in total hormone concentration, the free T_4 and T_3, which are the active forms, typically remain within normal limits. Serum levels of TSH tend to decrease in the first trimester of pregnancy but by the second trimester return to normal. This suppression in serum TSH values in the first trimester is due to negative feedback from elevated levels of human chorionic gonadotropin (hCG), which binds to thyroid gland TSH receptors.[38] The rise in hCG may cause high elevations of free T_4 concentrations, as seen is **thyrotoxicosis**. The thyroid gland enlarges slightly in normal pregnancy, but usually is not associated with clinical goiter due to adequate iodination of water and salt. The pathological finding of the presence of a goiter during pregnancy, along with continued decreased in TSH, indicates the likelihood of hyperthyroidism during pregnancy.[39]

Graves' disease is characterized as a toxic diffuse goiter (an enlarged, hyperactive thyroid gland) with an immunologic origin. Patients with Grave's disease have circulating thyroid-stimulating antibodies (TSAb). This is most likely due to a defect in suppressor T lymphocytes, which allows for antigenic stimulation by thyroid antigens and production of immunoglobulins. Some of these antibodies (formerly known as long-acting thyroid stimulators) can bind with the TSH receptor and stimulate the thyroid gland to oversecrete. This condition is more common in young adults, particularly women. Treatment generally involves antithyroid agents that impair the iodine coupling reactions. Surgical removal of the thyroid or radioactive sodium iodine treatments are also used in many circumstances. If untreated or complicated by secondary conditions such as severe infection, trauma, toxemia of pregnancy, or diabetic ketoacidosis, a life-threatening condition known as *thyroid storm* can result. This is characterized by abrupt onset of fever, muscle weakness and wasting, emotional disturbances, and possible coma.

Toxic multinodular goiter, also known as Plummer's disease, is a more common cause of hyperthyroidism in older adults. The cause of hyperactive nodes in the thyroid is unknown, but it is generally thought that it is not immunologic. There is typically increased T_3 but an absence of anti-thyroid antibodies or symptoms of exophthalmos. Surgical or radionuclear removal of the nodule is the effective treatment for multi- or single-nodular goiter.

Secondary hyperthyroidism correlates with increased levels of TSH and increased levels of free T_4. The symptoms are typically the same as in primary hyperthyroidism except there is no indication of autoimmunity. The disease usually has its origin in the pituitary gland, such as from a secreting adenoma, inflammatory disease causing **ectopic** thyrotoxicosis, or trophoblastic tumors.

Toxic goiter is an enlarged thyroid gland containing multiple nodules that hypersecrete while other areas are nonsecreting. This is usually nonimmunologic in origin. Thyroid carcinoma is a very rare malignancy of the follicles of the thyroid gland, prone to metastasis.

Other conditions are associated with abnormal thyroid diagnostic indicators such as chronically ill patients and those with hyperproteinemia. These patients have normal thyroid function but abnormal TBG levels. Table 11–9 depicts diagnostic indicators for various thyroid disorders.

thyrotoxicosis - acute illness due to hyperthyroidism

■■ CLINICAL CORRELATION
Graves' disease is the most common cause of primary hyperthyroidism, most likely due to autoimmunity due to TSI antibodies (formerly called long-acting thyroid stimulator). Thyroid adenoma is a single nodule in the thyroid gland causing hypersecretion of thyroid hormones. Thyroiditis is the inflammation of the thyroid gland arising from autoimmunity or possible infections.

ectopic - occurring outside the expected location

TABLE 11-9

Thyroid Disorders and Diagnostic Indicators

Disease	TSH	Free T_4	TSI	TMAb	TR Ab	Clinical Signs and Symptoms
Graves' disease	Decreased	Increased	Positive	Positive		Exophthalmia, thin, increased heart rate, increased body temperature
Hashimoto's thyroiditis	Decreased early on but increased late in illness	Increased early on but decreased late in illness		Positive		Positive anti-thyroglobulin Ab; positive anti-thyroid peroxidase Ab
Chronic ill euthyroid		Normal				Decreased T_4 and TBG; increased rT_3
Hyperpro-teinemic*		Normal				Increased T_4 and TBG; normal rT_3

Case Scenario 11-5 Graves Disease: The Woman With Prominent Eyeballs

Follow-Up

Laboratory testing for the 70-year-old female patient showed decreased TSH and increased free T_4, and an ultrasound of the thyroid confirmed the presence of a left thyroid nodule. Since the TSH level was low and the free thyroxine levels was elevated, primary hyperthyroidism was suggested. A request for thyroid-stimulating immunoglobulins (TSI) was sent to a reference laboratory. The TSI level was found to be 122% (reference range, 0% to 130%), and anti-thyroid microsomal antibodies (TMAb) were present at a high titer. This strongly indicates that the patient has Grave's disease and will most likely require radioiodine irradiation or surgical removal of the thyroid gland. ●

CASE SCENARIO 11-6

Diabetes Insipidus: A Patient With Very Dilute Urine

A patient in the intensive care unit with a diagnosis of head trauma, receiving intravenous fluids, has had normal random urinalysis with the exception of sustained urine specific gravity of 1.002 to 1.006 over the past 18 hours. Serum electrolytes and random glucose have been within reference ranges. After reviewing the blood and urine laboratory test results, his physician ordered a serum-to-urine osmolality ratio.

Secretion of antidiuretic hormone (ADH) helps to regulate the osmolality of the blood using the kidneys' ability to conserve water at the collecting ducts and electrolytes at the loop of Henle. Osmoreceptors in the hypothalamic region of the brain respond readily to changes in plasma osmolality and blood volume, such that when osmolality and blood volume increase, the posterior pituitary releases ADH. The plasma osmolality threshold for ADH is around 280 mOsm/Kg. Other stimuli for ADH release include stress and chemical agents such as barbiturates, nicotine, opiates, and anesthetics. Thirst is also regulated by similar mechanisms, which causes the person to desire water and helps replenish the water balance. Often in a normal individual, the urine osmolality is one to three times that of serum osmolality. When the normal individual is deprived of water, the ratio of urine to serum osmolality increases up to 4.5. Negative feedback, meaning cessation of ADH release, is generally due to atrial natriuretic peptide or other substances such as glucocorticoids, phenytoin, or alcohol. Unlike many hormones, ADH secretion is from the posterior pituitary after synthesis in the hypothalamus.[5]

DISORDERS OF WATER BALANCE

Polyuric states are those in which excessive urine output occurs unrelated to fluid, alcohol, or caffeine intake, originating in the kidneys or hypothalamic-pituitary region. The term **diabetes insipidus** reflects lack of ADH release or lack of renal response to ADH. For example, diabetes insipidus from lack of ADH secretion will cause less conservation of water by the renal collecting ducts. Excessive urinary output is dilute. Polyuria can be induced from drinking large amounts of fluid. Urine output is dependent on fluid intake but typically is less than 2.5 L/24 hr. Excessive output, such as 15 to 20 L/24 hr, almost always indicates total lack of ADH release, inducing **polydipsia** or excessive thirst. If replacement fluids are maintained through intake or intravenous fluids, plasma electrolyte levels and osmolality can remain essentially normal. If the individual does not have access to sufficient replacement fluids, such as in infants, the elderly, or confined individuals, hypertonic plasma can result and electrolytes become imbalanced. **Hypernatremia** would be the most common result. Despite the stimulus of hypertonic plasma, ADH cannot be released if hypothalamic or pituitary insufficiency exists. In those circumstances, the urine osmolality becomes even more dilute than the serum osmolality. Nephrogenic diabetes insipidus results when the kidneys are unable to respond to ADH, such as in chronic renal failure, polycystic disease, metabolic disorders, or drug exposure.[5]

Osmotic diuresis and psychogenic polydipsia can also cause polyuria. In osmotic diuresis, **hypertonicity** of plasma is usually the cause, such as in diabetes mellitus with hyperglycemia and ketosis. Thus diabetes mellitus can cause polyuria and polydipsia, but the serum and urine are hyperosmolar due to excessive glucose and ketones. In psychogenic polydipsia, the psychological disorder induces the patient to have chronic excessive fluid intake, which induces polyuria. In either of these conditions, the polyuria is not due to ADH defects.

Diabetes insipidus can arise from cranial or renal origins. Hypothalmic diabetes insipidus (DI), also known as central or cranial DI, is due to destruction of the ADH-producing region of the hypothalamus and posterior pituitary secondary to trauma, cerebral vascular accident or aneurysm, neoplastic destruction, or autoim-

polyuric - exhibiting excessive urine output (>2.5 L/24 hr)

diabetes insipidus - lack of antidiuretic hormone output or response causing polyuria and potential dehydration

polydipsia - excessive thirst

hypernatremia - increased sodium in blood plasma

CLINICAL CORRELATION

Urine and plasma osmolality tests, along with dehydration and saline infusion challenges, are helpful in diagnosis of DI. Overnight deprivation of water induces dehydration, causing urine osmolality to remain less than 1.5 times plasma osmolality.

hypertonicity - increased concentration of a body fluids due to increased solute compared to water in the solution

CLINICAL CORRELATION

Diabetes mellitus is due to lack of release or response to insulin. It also causes polyuria but due to osmotic diuresis from hyperglycemia and ketonemia. It is associated with hyperosmolar urine and serum, unlike diabetes insipidus, which is associated with hypo-osmolar urine and often normal serum osmolality.

hypo-osmolality - decreased concentration (tonicity) of a body fluid due to decreased solute compared to water in the solution

hypernatriuric - exhibiting increased urinary sodium

■■   **CLINICAL CORRELATION**

Secretion of inappropriate antidiuretic hormone is due to excessive secretion of ADH secondary to a variety of conditions or drugs. It is associated with urinary sodium levels >60 mmol/L, urine-to-serum osmolality ratio >3.0 with no fluid restrictions, and urine osmolality >100 mOsm/Kg following water-loading test.

munity. Nephrogenic diabetes insipidus is due to lack of renal response to ADH. It is caused by a variety of renal disorders including rare congenital or X-linked recessive disorder or, more commonly, renal tubular defect associated with arterial stenosis (acute tubular necrosis). Other causes include hypokalemia secondary to endocrine disturbances and hypercalcemia from hyperparathyroidism, and it may be drug induced, from demeclocycline or lithium toxicity. Serum or urinary ADH levels, which would be elevated, can distinguish nephrogenic from hypothalamic DI but generally are not needed for differential diagnosis. Following 12-hour water deprivation and ADH administration, the patient continues to exhibit polyuria and **hypo-osmolality** of the urine, indicating nephrogenic DI.[5]

Hyperosmolar, **hypernatriuric** urine is associated with many conditions, including secretion of excessive ADH, or syndrome of inappropriate antidiuretic hormone secretion (SIADH). Coupled with unrestricted fluid intake, the urinary output may be normal in SIADH, but fluid restrictions can cause oliguria and hypo-osmotic plasma, including hyponatremia. This relatively common syndrome results from a variety of causes including malignancy, pulmonary or chronic central nervous system disorders, and drug toxicity. Hypo-osmotic plasma and hyponatremia are common to many disorders, including congestive heart failure, nephrotic syndrome, cirrhosis, renal insufficiency, and to SIADH, so a differential diagnosis is important. In SIADH, urinary sodium levels often are elevated, urine-to-serum osmolality ratio is slightly greater than 1.0, and serum osmolality is usually less than 270 mOsm/Kg. Unlike in SIADH, urinary sodium levels are generally normal in congestive heart failure, cirrhosis, or other hemodilution disorders. A water loading test can be performed to aid in diagnosis of SIADH. In the water loading test protocol, urine and serum osmolality are measured before and after approximately 1 L of fluid is ingested over a 30-minute period. In the normal individual, urine osmolality should drop to 100 mOsm/kg, but it remains elevated in the patient with SIADH. Also in SIADH, urine output remains relatively low despite intake of fluid.[5]

◗ **Case Scenario 11-6** Diabetes Insipidus: A Patient With Very Dilute Urine

Follow-Up

A patient with head trauma has had normal random urinalysis results with the exception of sustained urine specific gravity of 1.002 to 1.006 over the past 18 hours. These values are lower than usual. Serum electrolytes and random glucose were within reference ranges. His physician ordered a serum/urine osmolality ratio. The following results were obtained: serum osmolality, 296 mOsm/Kg (reference range, 275 to 295 mOsm/kg); urine osmolality, 236 mOsm/Kg (60 to 1200 mOsm/kg); urine/serum osmolality ratio, 0.8 (reference range, 1 to 3); and 12-hr fluid-restricted urine/serum osmolality ratio, 0.6 (3 to 4.7). The urine/serum osmolality ratio was decreased and continued to be decreased even with fluid restriction. Urinary output was increased at 19 L/day (reference range, 0.5 to 2.5 L/day), and cranial, hypothalamic diabetes insipidus was suspected secondary to head trauma. The patient's urine osmolality increased by more than 10% and output decreased 60 minutes after subcutaneous aqueous ADH (vaspopressin) was given. These findings indicate that the patient indeed has hypothalamic diabetes insipidus, a condition in which he is lacking ADH but is capable of responding physiologically when given treatments of ADH. ◗

CASE SCENARIO 11-7

Hyperparathyroidism: The Patient With Elevated Calcium Levels

A medical technologist was overseeing the specimen referral area. He was preparing specimens from one patient to be sent to the reference laboratory for 25-hydroxy vitamin D, parathyroid hormone, and calcitriol. The referral laboratory provided specific instructions for the correct labeling of samples, packaging, dry ice preparation, and requisitions. The requisition required listing the patient's preliminary diagnosis, and serum and urinary calcium, phosphorus, and alkaline phosphatase levels. The 45-year-old female patient's diagnosis was osteoporosis and hypercalcemia. Her laboratory values were calcium, 12.1 mg/dL (reference range, 8.6 to 10.2 mg/dL); ionized calcium, 1.56 mmol/L (1.15 to 1.33 mmol/L); phosphate, 2.2 mg/dL (2.5 to 4.5 mg/dL); alkaline phosphatase, 60 IU/L (42 to 98 IU/L); and 24-hour urinary calcium, 167 mg (100 to 250 mg).

MINERAL METABOLISM

Calcium is a common mineral found in bones, teeth, and plasma. Within blood, calcium is mainly found in plasma as opposed to intracellular spaces. Bone can remodel, a combination of depositing new bone and breaking down old bone. Hormones and vitamins play a role in regulation of bone growth and absorption of old bone, known as **resorption**, and cause the release of calcium into body fluids, including plasma. Resorption occurs in the **osteoclasts**, cells that break down bone. Thus bone contributes calcium, phosphorus, and other minerals to body fluids and body fluids contribute calcium and other minerals to bone.[6]

Approximately 50% of the plasma calcium is active in the form of free ions, while the remaining half is bound to albumin. Thus ionized calcium levelsare roughly one half of total serum calcium levels. pH plays a role in formation of protein-bound calcium in that alkaline conditions provide more anionic protein and enhance binding of cationic calcium, while acidic conditions encourage less cationic binding to protein, maintaining more Ca^{++}. This occurs at a concentration predicted by pH units.[5]

Intracellular calcium, although found in small amounts, plays a major role in muscle contraction, glycogen metabolism, hormone secretion, blood hemostasis, enzyme activation, and a variety of other physiological functions. Intracellular calcium is concentrated in mitochondria and endoplasmic reticula. It is an important intracellular second messenger, activating enzymes such as phosphorylase kinase via proteins or directly activating enzymes such as adenylate cyclase.

Within bone, calcium is found in hydroxyapatite crystals of calcium and phosphate providing strength to bone. Bone is continually remade (remodeled) as a balance of formation and breakdown. **Osteogenesis** is the process of producing or forming bone, which incorporates phosphates and calcium into the hydroxyapatite. Bone also contains collagen and other protein molecules such as osteocalcin that provide strength and support and most likely play a role in mineral deposition.[5] The hormones that regulate bone **remodeling** are calcitonin, parathyroid hormone, and vitamin D, a hormone-like steroid.

Parathyroid hormone (PTH) is a single-chain polypeptide with an amine and a carboxyl terminus, produced by the parathyroid glands located in front of and surrounding the thyroid gland. The parathyroid gland releases PTH when ionized

resorption - to soak up or take in again

osteoclasts - phagocytic cells in bone responsive to parathyroid hormone in bone breakdown

osteogenesis - production or formation of bone

remodeling - the overall effect of depositing and absorbing bone to remake new bone

calcium falls below normal levels in the extracellular fluids, including plasma. PTH has many functions, including action upon bone, intestines, and kidneys. Renal responses to PTH include promotion of the active form od vitamin D (1,25-hydroxylation), increasing tubular reabsorption of calcium, and decreasing tubular reabsorption of phosphates. Bone response to PTH is rapid resorption, or breakdown, with resulting release of calcium and phosphates into the plasma. Intestinal response is to work concurrently with vitamin D in absorbing calcium from food-stuffs. In normal situations, PTH works along with vitamin D and calcitonin to maintain normal amounts of calcium in bone and plasma such that excretion of urinary calcium matches dietary and bone contribution of calcium to the plasma.

Calcitonin is produced by the parafollicular cells of the thyroid gland and is secreted in response to hypercalcemia. It helps to counterbalance PTH responses to raise plasma calcium, excrete phosphorus, and resorb bone. The main function of calcitonin is to inhibit osteoclastic bone activity, thus helping to conserve bone and lower plasma calcium levels. Deficiencies in this hormone can result from thyroid disease or can occur secondary to thyroid removal. Exogenous calcitonin can be given to help control calcium levels and restore homeostasis.

Active vitamin D (1,25-dihydroxycholecalciferol) is also known as calcitriol. It is derived from 7-dehydrocholesterol, its provitamin form found in skin. The provitamin is transformed at ultraviolet (UV) wavelengths to form previtamin D in the skin. From there, it is bound to carrier proteins and circulates to the liver, where it is converted to 25-hydroxycholecalciferol. This compound then enters the circulation; when it reaches the kidney, and dependent on PTH regulation and low calcium levels, final hydroxylation occurs yielding active calcitriol. Figure 11–11 shows

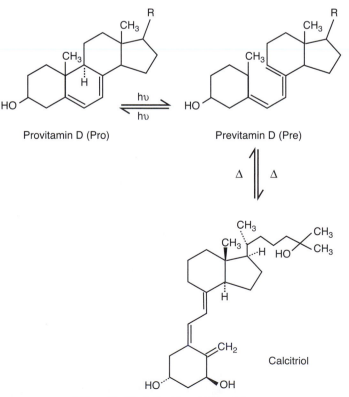

Provitamin D (Pro)   Previtamin D (Pre)

Calcitriol

Figure 11–11. Active Vitamin D and its precursors.

the conversion of provitamin D to its intermediate steps and finally to its active form, calcitriol. Dietary supplements may provide previtamin D forms, bypassing the need for UV activation.[6] Calcitriol, although referred to as vitamin D, functions as a steroid by promoting intestinal absorption of calcium and phosphorus, mobilizing bone, and restoring calcium and phosphorus levels to normal. Deficiencies or lack of response to this hormone can cause muscular and bone abnormalities, particularly lack of mineralization and remodeling with resulting softening and weaknesses. *Rickets* is the term that generally describes calcitriol deficiencies in infants and children with resulting bone deformities.[6]

Hypercalcemia is defined as total serum calcium greater than 11.0 mg/dL (reference range, 8.6 to 10.2 mg/dL) or ionized calcium greater than 1.50 mmol/L (1.15 to 1.33 mmol/L). Hypercalciuria is defined as total urine calcium greater than 300 mg/day in the adult male.[6] Symptoms of hypercalcemia tend to be vague but may include gastrointestinal symptoms, neurologic changes, or, in extreme cases, coma. Hypercalcemia can be a sign of serious disease and is one of the most commonly diagnosed metabolic disorders. The most frequent cause of hypercalcemia is primary hyperparathyroidism. Other causes of hypercalcemia include malignancy, sarcoidosis, hypervitaminosis of vitamin D, and immobilization.[5]

Hypercalcemia can commonly result from primary hyperparathyroidism. Additional laboratory indications of primary hyperparathyroidism include hypophosphatemia, elevated urinary phosphate and calcium levels, elevated parathormone levels, and serum magnesium on the low side of normal.[6] Primary hyperparathyroidism results from parathyroid adenoma with hypercellular parathyroid tissue, hyperplasia of the parathyroid glands, or multiple endocrine neoplasia, or occurs secondary to neck irradiation.[40] If primary hyperparathyroidism does not present with straightforward indicators, a calcium challenge can be performed in which serum PTH levels should be suppressed in the normal individual following intravenous calcium infusion, whereas those with secreting adenomas of the parathyroid gland will continue to secrete PTH. This challenge can also be performed following parathyroidectomy to determine the success of the surgery.[5] Secondary hyperparathyroidism is a result of hypocalcemia secondary to renal insufficiency or intestinal malabsorption. In those conditions, calcium loss from the kidneys or gastrointestinal tract stimulates parathyroid secretion of PTH. An overactive parathyroid gland can release enough PTH to counteract the calcium loss, with normal to low-normal plasma calcium levels resulting.[6]

The specificity and sensitivity of immunoassay methods for PTH have been greatly improved in recent years, making it a much more reliable test for primary hyperparathyroidism. The current assay helps to differentiate primary hyperparathyroidism from the other non-PTH causes of hypercalcemia in which the circulatory PTH level is suppressed.[5]

Primary hyperparathyroidism is generally caused by an adenoma. Parathyroid carcinoma is a rare disease, comprising between 0.5% and 4% of all cases of primary hyperparathyroidism. It affects both genders equally and occurs predominantly during the fourth to sixth decades of life, although a wide age range is seen. Markedly elevated serum calcium levels (>14 mg/dL), very high serum PTH levels, a palpable neck mass, and laryngeal nerve palsy are clinical hints to the diagnosis of parathyroid carcinoma. Often the patient returns with recurrent or metastatic disease, sometimes many years after the initial diagnosis.[41,42] This emphasizes the need for lifetime monitoring of serum calcium levels in the patient who has undergone resection of a parathyroid adenoma. Complications of untreated primary hyperparathyroidism include recurrent **nephrolithiasis** and

CLINICAL CORRELATION
Multiple endocrine neoplasia is a condition in which hypersecretion of multiple hormones occurs, including islet cell, parathyroid, pituitary, and sometimes thyroid and adrenal hormones. It is associated with hyperparathyroidism, gastrin-secreting tumors, and acromegaly from pituitary adenomas.

nephrolithiasis - presence of calculi in the urinary tract; urate nephrolithiasis indicates the presence of uric acid in the stone

osteopenia - decreased bone mass, or loss of bone density

tetany - neuromotor irritability accompanied by muscular twitching and eventual convulsions; generally due to low calcium levels

spasms - twitching of muscles, which may accompany muscle ache

✓ **Common Sense Check**
Since anticoagulants other than heparin are not acceptable because they remove calcium, check that plasma doesn't contain sodium citrate or EDTA, which are commonly used in hematology testing.

✓ **Common Sense Check**
If total serum calcium is decreased, check to see if serum albumin is also decreased. If not, ionized calcium may be a better test of calcium status. It should be roughly equal to half of the total serum calcium level.

osteopenia.[43] *Nephrolithiasis* is the term for kidney stones or calculi occurring in the urinary tract.

The second most common cause of hypercalcemia is hypercalcemia of malignancy. a condition associated with increased mortality.[41] Up to 58% of hospitalized patients with hypercalcemia have an associated cancer.[44] Hypercalcemia is usually seen in squamous cell cancers, lymphomas, and bone and breast cancers and only rarely with skin cancers. In these malignancies, substances secreted by the tumors often cause release of calcium from the bone, acting in a manner similar to PTH. Multiple myeloma, or malignancy of the bone marrow, causes hypercalcemia from several additional factors. Total serum calcium is elevated due to increased protein binding and from proteolytic lesions of the bone in multiple myeloma.

Hypercalcemia is associated with renal diseases such as postrenal acute renal failure, occurs as a sequela to nephrolithiasis, or is due to sarcoidosis. Postrenal acute renal failure has been discussed thoroughly in Chapter 6 (Assessment of Renal Function). The term describes conditions that cause renal failure due to problems with urine flow and output such as constriction or blockage due to calculi. There are many causes of renal calculi, but hypercalcemia from hyperparathyroidism can cause inorganic calcium oxalate or calcium citrate precipitation resulting in obstruction of urinary flow.

Sarcoidosis is a systemic disorder with unknown cause that can affect multiple organs, including the kidneys. Renal impairment is usually due to an overproduction of 1,25-dihydroxy vitamin D, leading to hypercalciuria with or without hypercalcemia. These imbalances can result in nephrocalcinosis and renal failure. There is an increase in the circulating immune complexes, particularly immunoglobulin A immune complexes, in sarcoidosis, and it typically runs a benign course and has a spontaneous remission.[6]

Hypercalcemia can also arise from hypervitaminosis of vitamin D (calcitriol). Excessive levels of vitamin D cause increased intestinal absorption and excessive bone resorption. The resulting hypercalcemia caused by elevated vitamin D typically suppresses PTH levels.

Hypocalcemia occurs when total serum calcium is less than 8.8 mg/dL in the presence of normal serum proteins. Causes of hypocalcemia include hypoparathyroidism, pseudohypoparathyroidism, vitamin D deficiency, renal tubular diseases, acute renal failure, gastrointestinal malabsorption, and acute pancreatitis. Signs and symptoms of hypocalcemia are generally subtle unless profound hypocalcemia exists, in which case **tetany**, **spasms**, and convulsions can result. Neonatal hypocalcemia can result from prematurity or exchange transfusions without adequate replacement and has serious neuromuscular consequences from resulting tetany.

Pseudohypoparathyroidism is a condition in which the parathyroid secretes adequate amounts of PTH but bone and/or kidneys are not responsive. This is a rare hereditary condition that often results in abnormal calcitriol activation and abnormal bone development. Calcium levels may be low-normal, but response to PTH does not result in the typical excretion of urinary phosphates.

Hypocalcemia can result from a variety of renal diseases, including renal insufficiency or renal tubular disease. Renal insufficiency (acute renal failure) as described earlier, is caused by a variety of situations, is associated with electrolyte and mineral imbalances, and, depending on the cause, may result in hypocalcemia. Acute renal failure causes sodium and calcium loss and plasma potassium, magnesium, and phosphate elevations. It is also associated with subnormal levels of calcitriol due to inability to activate precursors to vitamin D. Acute renal failure can be prerenal, due to decreased circulation, low blood volume, or decreased fluid volume reaching the kidney. It can also be renal, due to tubular necrosis, or postrenal, due to obstructions to the flow of urine out of the kidney. Renal tubular disease can be a result of congenital or hereditary conditions or acquired secondary to drug or heavy metal toxicity. Renal tubular acidosis is an example of renal tubular disease with resulting electrolyte and mineral imbalances. Fanconi's syndrome is another renal tubular disease associated with mineral and electrolyte disturbances, including profound hypocalcemia, hypophosphatemia, and acidosis. Hypocalcemia tends to stimulate parathyroid secretion, resulting in secondary hyperparathyroidism in an attempt to normalize the calcium levels.

Gastrointestinal malabsorption of fats can be due to generalized intestinal diseases or secondary to pancreatitis with loss of lipase secretion. The result is steatorrhea, fat malabsorption, and increased fecal fat with mineral loss. Hypocalcemia and hypomagnesemia are complications of gastrointestinal malabsorption.

Total calcium is measured by a variety of methods but most commonly by dye-binding methods such as *o*-Cresolphthalein Complexone or asenazo III. In these methods, absorbance due to the production of chromagen relates directly to the concentration of total serum calcium once protein-bound forms are released. This is described in Test Methodology 11–8. Titrimetric, fluorometric methods have been phased out due to the ease of automation when performing spectrophotometric methods. The reference method is by atomic absorption spectroscopy while ion-selective electrode technology is used to measure ionized calcium. Free calcium is the ionized form and is typically measured by ion-selective electrode methods such as that described in Test Methodology 11–9.

TEST METHODOLOGY 11-8.   TOTAL CALCIUM BY *O*-CRESOLPHTHALEIN COMPLEXONE

The Reaction Principle

Ortho-Creosolphthalein Complexone (3',3"-bis[[bis-{carboxymethyl}amino]-methyl]-5',5"-dimethlyphenolphthalein) dye forms a red chromagen with calcium in an alkaline solution, after being first released from protein in an acid solution. Absorbance is measured at 580 nm. Magnesium is removed by 8-hydroxyquinoline buffered at pH 12.

Interferences

Temperature and pH of the reagents are critical for good reaction. Nonlinearity at low concentrations may be likely. Hemolysis, lipemia, and icterus can interfere with some methods. Hemolysis can cause variable results due to increased absorbance from hemoglobin at 580 nm but decreased effect due to dilution.

The Specimen

Serum is preferred. Heparinized plasma may be used, but reference ranges are slightly higher than in serum. Other anticoagulants are not acceptable because they remove calcium. The sample is stable for 1 week at 2°–4°C and several months at –20°C.

Urine specimens should be acidified to prevent mineral precipitation.

Reference Ranges (Adult)

Serum	8.6–10.2 mg/dL
Urine	50–150 mg/24 hr (diet dependent)

TEST METHODOLOGY 11-9.   IONIZED CALCIUM BY ION-SELECTIVE ELECTRODES

The Reaction Principle

An electrode with a calcium-selective membrane, a reference electrode, and a reference solution are used to measure calcium ion activity. The membrane often is composed of a neutral carrier in polyvinyl chloride. The inner reference solution is a calcium chloride and saturated silver chloride solution, and the internal silver/silver chloride reference electrode measures the change in potential across the KCl salt bridge versus the external silver/silver chloride reference electrode due to the presence of Ca^{++} ions at the membrane. Calcium activity is converted to concentration using an activity coefficient based on the typical ionic strength in whole blood, serum, and plasma.

Interferences

There is minimal interference from other cations, such as H^+, Mg^{++}, Na^+, or K^+. Presence of erythrocytes in whole blood compared with plasma is minimized by flow-through technology, with changes made to the reference solution and salt bridge. Temperature is maintained at 37°C to maintain ionic strength.

The Specimen

Heparinized plasma may be used, but reference ranges are slightly higher than in serum. Other anticoagulants are not acceptable because they remove calcium. The sample is stable for 1 week at 2°–4°C and several months at –20°C.

Reference Ranges

Adult   1.15–1.33 mmol/L

Phosphates and magnesium are minerals similar to calcium in that they are found as inorganic forms in bone and teeth and in smaller amounts intracellularly or in plasma, bound to protein or ionized. Total phosphates are typically measured by a chemical reaction with ammonium molybdate. Test Methodology 11–10 describes this procedure in more detail.

Phosphates are also regulated by PTH and activated vitamin D (calcitriol), with the kidneys playing a major role in homeostasis as described earlier in this chapter. Phosphates are found in a variety of forms, but inorganic phosphate ions predominate intracellularly and in plasma and are the form measured. Hypophosphatemia is common and may indicate a disorder or a transient change such as following intake of a meal or insulin release. A low plasma phosphate level tends to signal clinically significant changes in other minerals such as calcium and magnesium, as with hyperparathyroidism, renal tubular defects, malabsorption or dietary deficiencies, and adrenal or thyroid hormonal imbalances. In acid-base disturbances, such as respiratory alkalosis or diabetic ketoacidosis, severe hypophosphatemia is common. Thus a decreased serum phosphate level is rare by itself but suggests the need for investigating further abnormalities. Hyperphosphatemia is commonly associated with renal insufficiency, accompanying a rise in plasma potassium and creatinine levels along with loss of sodium and calcium. It tends to trigger secondary hyperparathyroidism as discussed earlier.

Magnesium is found protein bound and as a divalent cation with an intracellular predominance compared with amounts in plasma. False increases in serum magnesium arise when erythrocytes are not separated from hemolyzed blood or serum

TEST METHODOLOGY 11-10.   TOTAL PHOSPHATES

The Reaction Principle

Ammonium molybdate, $(NH_4)_6Mo_7O_{24} \cdot 4 H_2O$, reacts with inorganic phosphates, forming colorless phosphomolybdate complexes that absorb maximally in UV light.

An alternative reaction is to reduce phosphomolybdate to molybdenum blue, which absorbs maximally at 600 nm. Ascorbic acid and ferrous sulfate are common reducing agents used in this second step since they create a stable product.[5]

Interferences

Hemolysis falsely increases phosphorus due to intracellular release. Citrate, oxalate, and EDTA anticoagulants interfere. Variations in phosphate levels can be caused by long-term storage in warm temperatures. Icterus, hemoglobin, and lipemia may interfere. Residual detergent in glassware or water causes false increase.

The Specimen

Serum. Heparinized plasma is 0.3 mg/dL lower than serum.

Reference Range

Adult   2.5–4.5 mg/dL

in a timely manner. Magnesium is measured by a dye-binding method such as described in Test Methodology 11–11.

As discussed with calcium and phosphates, renal control, acid-base balance, and intestinal absorption are the chief regulators of magnesium levels. Parathyroid hor-

TEST METHODOLOGY 11-11.   TOTAL MAGNESIUM BY METALLOCHROMIC INDICATOR METHOD

The Reaction Principle

Calmagite (1-[1-hydroxy-4-methyl-2-phenylazo]-2-naphthol-4-sulfonic acid) forms a colored complex in an alkaline solution with magnesium to be measured spectrophotometrically at around 540 nm. Additional substances such as potassium cyanide, a calcium chelating agent, and surfactants are added to minimize interference from calcium, heavy metals, lipemia, or proteins.[5]

Interferences

Hemolysis or delayed separation of serum from blood cells should be avoided since either can provide intracellular magnesium. Lipemia and icteric specimens may have interference, depending on methodology and ability to provide a specimen blank or bichromatic measurements.

The Specimen

Serum or heparinized plasma. Other anticoagulants can't be used since they chelate out magnesium.

Urine specimens should be acidified to prevent mineral precipitation.

Reference Ranges (Adult)

Serum   1.6–2.6 mg/dL
Urine   3.0–5.0 mmol/24 hr

mone may play a minor role, with a direct relationship between PTH secretion and plasma magnesium response as with calcium, versus the indirect relationship with plasma phosphates. Diet is the main source of magnesium, as evident in starvation, poor diet in chronic alcoholism, long-term parenteral feeding, or gastrointestinal malabsorption and steatorrhea, which may result in hypomagnesemia. Hypoparathyroidism, especially secondary to surgical removal of the parathyroid glands, and renal or acid-base disorders also are causes of hypomagnesemia. Neonatal hypomagnesemia and hypocalcemia result from prematurity, acid-base disturbances, or exchange transfusions, with serious consequences. Mineral replacement therapy may be needed for magnesium and calcium in those situations. Hypermagnesemia can result from renal insufficiency and/or excessive treatment with antacids or other magnesium-containing medications. Cardiac and neuromuscular changes occur similar to those with hyperkalemia, and treatment with diuretics and calcium may be helpful.

Case Scenario 11-7 Hyperparathyroidism: The Patient With Elevated Calcium Levels

Follow-Up

The referral laboratory received the samples in acceptable condition and analyzed 25-hydroxy vitamin D, parathyroid hormone, calcitriol, and osteocalcin. The results were as follows: osteocalcin, 18.7 ng/mL (reference range, 0.4 to 8.2 ng/mL); 25-hydroxy vitamin D, 67 ng/mL (10 to 55 ng/mL); PTH, 69 pg/mL (10 to 65 pg/mL); and calcitriol, 32 pg/mL (15 to 60 pg/mL). Thus osteocalcin, vitamin D, and PTH were all elevated and the calcitriol was normal. The patient's complaint was of chronic muscle pain, fatigue, and twitching, and she has a previous diagnosis of osteoporosis. She had repeated elevated levels of serum calcium, ranging from 11.3 to 12.1 mg/dL (compared to the reference range of 8.6 to 10.2 mg/dL); other laboratory results were phosphate, 2.2 mg/dL (2.5 to 4.5 mg/dL); alkaline phosphatase, 60 IU/L (42 to 98 IU/L); 24-hour urinary calcium, 167 mg (100 to 250 mg); and magnesium, 1.7 mg/dL (1.6 to 2.6 mg/dL). After parathyroidectomy, the PTH level dropped significantly (68%) to 10 pg/mL, and the serum calcium level was normal, ranging from 8.2 to 9.6 mg/dL. The surgical specimen revealed excessive number of cells in the parathyroid tissue in most of the parathyroid glands. The postoperative drop in PTH level close to 70% favors a diagnosis of primary hyperparathyroidism.[41] The patient had clinical improvement and increased energy, and she no longer complained of muscle pain or twitching. Therapy included hormone replacements, multivitamins, and 1500 mg of calcium daily added to her dietary program. ●

PREANALYTICAL VARIATIONS IN HORMONE TESTING

Some unusual hormonal testing may be necessary to help the clinician make a differential diagnosis. Nonroutine testing may require sending the specimens out to a referral laboratory for testing. Adherence to acceptable specimen collection, handling, and storage protocols will be necessary in order to avoid preanalytical errors and provide the best specimens for laboratory testing. All specimen handling requirements for endocrine testing must be met. For example, ACTH and ADH are quite unstable and easily oxidized, so care is needed to keep the samples in ice water or frozen if not analyzed immediately. Some of the hormones require extensive patient preparation, such as avoidance of specific foods or medications. Catecholamines, and in particular epinephrine and norepinephrine, will typically elevate in response to the stress of the venipuncture procedure, so insertion of a venous catheter 30 minutes prior to collection of blood samples is recommended to provide better results. Tables 11–10, 11–11, and 11–12 summarize some of the key information for specimen collection and storage of protein hormones and steroid hormones. As usual, care must be taken to properly identify the patient prior to collection and to properly label the specimens obtained, making certain the information matches that on the test requisition forms.

TABLE 11-10

Protein Hormone Testing: Special Instructions[5]

Hormone	Instructions for Specimen Collection and Handling
ACTH	Time of collection for ACTH is important. ACTH is easily oxidized, degraded by proteolysis during freezing and thawing, and adsorbed to glass: store prechilled EDTA specimen, iced and centrifuged, at 4°C; store supernatant at –20°C prior to analysis, with possible antioxidants such as mercaptoethanol added.
LH and FSH	Day of the monthly cycle is important for collection or use of serial testing. Serum must be free from hemolysis, lipemia, or icterus due to spectrophotometric or fluorometric detection of label; stability is maintained for longer than 2 weeks at –20°C. Urine may be tested from preservative-free samples maintained at –20°C prior to testing.
Thyrotropin (TSH)	Serum or plasma must be free from lipemia, hemolysis, and icterus. Specimens are stable for up to 5 days at 2°–8°C and up to 30 days when stored at –20°C.
Antidiuretic hormone or oxytocin	Easily oxidized, degraded by proteolysis during freezing and thawing, and adsorbed to glass: store prechilled EDTA specimen, iced and centrifuged, at 4°C; store supernatant at –20°C prior to analysis.

TABLE 11-11

Amino Acid Hormone Testing: Special Instructions[5]

Hormone	Instructions for Specimen Collection and Handling
Thyroxine (T_4) and free thyroxine	Serum, heparinized or EDTA plasma free from gross hemolysis; stable up to 7 days at 2°–8°C and up to 30 days when stored at –20°C. Avoid repeat freezing and thawing. For the neonatal screen, dried capillary blood obtained 3–7 days after 24 hours of complete protein feeding has begun. Blood is placed on clean filter paper, allowed to soak through on two $1/2$-inch circles, and allowed to air-dry before transport; avoid heat, light, and contact before and during transport.

continued

TABLE 11-11 *(continued)*

Amino Acid Hormone Testing: Special Instructions[5]

Hormone	Instructions for Specimen Collection and Handling
Triiodothyronine (T_3), free T_3, and reverse T_3 (rT_3)	Serum, heparinized or EDTA plasma free from gross hemolysis; stable up to 7 days at 2°–8°C and up to 30 days when stored at –20°C. Avoid repeat freezing and thawing.
Vanillylmandelic acid	24-hr urine is preserved with 10 mL of 6 mol/L HCl with refrigeration during the collection process and stored at –20°C if not analyzed immediately.
	Intake of chocolate, coffee, bananas, vanilla, citrus fruits, antihypertensive drugs, or aspirin may cause interference with some methods.
Catecholamines	Early a.m. collection in the fasting patient after remaining recumbent for at least 30 minutes after venous line is inserted. The patient should also avoid coffee, tea, and tobacco products for 4 hours and antihypertensive medications for 2 days prior to collection.
	Specimens are collected in prechilled heparinized tubes, maintained in ice water, and centrifuged at 4°C; supernatant is stored at –70°C prior to analysis.
	24-hr urine is preserved with 10 mL of 6 mol/L HCl with refrigeration during the collection process and stored at –20°C if not analyzed immediately.

TABLE 11-12

Steroid Hormone Testing: Special Instructions[5]

Hormone	Instructions for Specimen Collection and Handling
Cortisol and free cortisol	Time of collection is important; 8:00 a.m. specimen is generally 50% higher than 8:00 p.m.
	Serum or heparinized plasma; stored overnight at 2°–8°C or for up to 30 days at –20°C.
	24-hour urine is preserved with 10 g boric acid, refrigerated during collection and prior to testing.
Aldosterone	Heparinized or EDTA plasma is collected in prechilled tubes, centrifuged at 4°C, and stored at –20°C for up to 30 days. Varies with positioning of patient at time of collection; upright for 2 hours prior to collection or supine as indicated on test requisitions.
	24-hr urine is preserved with boric acid to achieve pH of 2.0–4.0; refrigerated during the collection process and stored at –20°C if not analyzed immediately.
Renin	EDTA plasma, free from hemolysis, is obtained from a patient (upright and ambulatory at least 30 minutes), centrifuged at room temperature, and stored at –20°C if not analyzed immediately.
	Time of day, posture, salt intake, and medication use, particularly diuretics, should be noted.
	24-hr urine sodium and creatinine are collected prior to renin activity assay.

SUMMARY

This chapter emphasized synthesis of hormones by glandular tissue, sites of synthesis and distribution, and roles of hormones within the body. Imbalances in homeostasis were discussed, including problems with growth and development and even life-threatening metabolic problems. Cushing's syndrome, Addison's disease, pheochromotocytoma, thyroid and parathyroid disorders, and diabetes insipidus were described through seven case scenarios that illustrated the role of laboratory testing in diagnosis, treatment, and monitoring of patients with endocrine disorders.

EXERCISES

As you consider the scenarios presented in this chapter, answer the following questions:

1. Describe three main types of hormones in terms of whether they require a carrier molecule when circulating in the bloodstream and where their receptor is located in the target cell.

2. Discuss the biologically active forms of steroid and thyroid hormones.

3. Describe the typical abnormal laboratory findings and physical characteristics of Graves' disease.

4. Describe the typical abnormal laboratory findings and physical characteristics of Hashimoto's thyroiditis.

5. Discuss the typical TSH and thyroxine findings in neonatal hypothyroidism.

6. Compare and contrast the typical abnormal laboratory findings and physical characteristics of Cushing's syndrome versus Addison's disease.

7. Describe the typical abnormal laboratory findings and physical characteristics of pheochromocytoma.

8. Discuss the advantages and disadvantages of measuring urine metabolites versus blood hormones for adrenal medullary disorders.

9. Compare and contrast chromatography and immunoassay methods for assessing adrenal medullary disorders.

References

1. Griffin J, Ojeda S (eds): *Textbook of Endocrine Physiology*, ed 5. Oxford, UK: Oxford University Press, 2004.
2. Stumvoll M, Goldstein BJ, Van Haefton TW: Type 2 diabetes: principles of pathogenesis and therapy. *Lancet* 2005; 365:1333–1346.
3. Gaw A, et al: *Clinical Biochemistry: An Illustrated Coulour Text*. Edinburgh: Churchill Livingstone, 1995.
4. Hoshiro M, et al: Comprehensive study of urinary cortisol metabolites in hyperthyroid and hypothyroid patients. *Clin Endocrinol (Oxf)* 2006; 64:37–45.
5. Fauci A, et al (eds): *Harrison's Principle of Internal Medicine*, ed 14. New York: McGraw-Hill, 1998.
6. Beers M, Berkow R: *The Merck Manual of Diagnosis and Therapy*, ed 17. Rahway, NJ: Merck & Co., 1999.
7. Esperon PS: Hyponatremic coma as a manifestation of Addison's disease. *J Pediatr (Rio J)* 2001; 77:337–342.

8. Hanquez C, et al: A competitive microtitre plate enzyme immunoassay for plasma aldosterone using a monoclonal antibody. *J Steroid Biochem* 1988; 31:939–945, 1988.

9. Daughaday WH, Cryer PE: Growth hormone hypersecretion and acromegaly. *Hosp Pract* 1978; 13:75–80.

10. Whalen RK, Althausen AF, Daniels GH: Extra-adrenal pheochromocytoma. *J Urol* 1992; 147:1–10.

11. Norton JA, Le HN: Adrenal tumors. In DeVita VT Jr, Hellman S, Rosenberg SA (eds): *Cancer: Principles and Practice of Oncology*, ed 6. Philadelphia: Lippincott Williams & Wilkins, 2001, pp 1770–1787.

12. Young JB, Landsberg L: Catecholamines and the adrenal medulla: pheochromocytoma. In Wilson JD, et al. (eds): *Williams Textbook of Endocrinology*, ed 9. Philadelphia: WB Saunders, 1998, pp 705–716.

13. Bravo EL, Gifford RW Jr: Current concepts. Pheochromocytoma: diagnosis, localization and management. *N Engl J Med* 1984; 311:1298–1303.

14. Bravo EL: Evolving concepts in the pathophysiology, diagnosis, and treatment of pheochromocytoma. *Endocr Rev* 1994; 15:356–368.

15. Brennan MF, Keiser HR: Persistent and recurrent pheochromocytoma: the role of surgery. *World J Surg* 1982; 6:397–402.

16. Lenders JW, et al: Plasma metanephrines in the diagnosis of pheochromocytoma. *Ann Intern Med* 1995; 123:101–109.

17. Rosano TG, Swift TA, Hayes LW: Advances in catecholamine and metabolite measurements for diagnosis of pheochromocytoma. *Clin Chem* 1991; 37(10 Pt 2):1854–1867.

18. Sjoberg RJ, Simcic KJ, Kidd GS: The clonidine suppression test for pheochromocytoma: a review of its utility and pitfalls. *Arch Intern Med* 1992; 152:1193–1197.

19. Kagedal B, Goldstein DS: Catecholamines and their metabolites. *J Chromatogr* 1988; 429:177–233.

20. Dale G, et al: Urinary excretion of HMMA and HVA in infants. *Ann Clin Biochem* 1988; 25(Pt 3):233–236.

21. Davis BA, Durden DA, Boulton AA: Simultaneous analysis of twelve biogenic amine metabolites in plasma, cerebrospinal fluid and urine by capillary column gas chromatography–high resolution mass spectrometry with selected-ion monitoring. *J Chromatogr* 1986; 374:227–238.

22. Kinoshita Y, et al: Determination of vanillylmandelic acid, vanillactic acid, and homovanillic acid in dried urine on filter-paper discs by high-performance liquid chromatography with coulometric electrochemical detection for neuroblastoma screening. *Clin Chem* 1988; 34:2228–2230.

23. Leung PY, Tsao CS: Preparation of an optimum mobile phase for the simultaneous determination of neurochemicals in mouse brain tissues by high-performance liquid chromatography with electrochemical detection. *J Chromatogr* 1992; 576: 245–254.

24. Rosano TG, Whitley RJ: Catecholamines and serotonin. In Burtis CA, Ashwood ER (eds): *Tietz Textbook of Clinical Chemistry*, ed 3. Philadelphia: WB Saunders, 1999, pp 1570–1600.

25. Wolthers BG, et al: Evaluation of urinary metanephrine and normetanephrine enzyme immunoassay (ELISA) kits by comparison with isotope dilution mass spectrometry. *Clin Chem* 1997; 43:114–120.

26. Taran F, et al: Competitive enzyme immunoassay with monoclonal antibody for homovanillic acid measurement in human urine samples. *Clin Chem* 1997; 43:363–368.

27. Mellor GW, Gallacher G, Landon J: Production and characterisation of antibodies to vanillylmandelic acid. *J Immunol Methods* 1989; 118:101–107.

28. Mellor GW, Gallacher G: Fluorescence polarization immunoassay of urinary vanillylmandelic acid. *Clin Chem* 1990; 36:110–112.

29. Creces J, Appleton C: Catecholamines and Their Metabolites: Evaluation of a Commercial ELISA. Brisbane, Australia: QML Pathology, 2005.

30. Taran F, et al: Competitive enzyme immunoassay for urinary vanillylmandelic acid. *Clin Chim Acta* 1997; 264:177–192.

31. Young JB, Landsberg L: Catecholamines and the adrenal medulla: pheochromocytoma. In Wilson JD, et al (eds): *Williams Textbook of Endocrinology*, ed 9. Philadelphia: WB Saunders, 1998, pp 705–716.

32. Fisher DA, Foley BL: Early treatment of congenital hypothyroidism. *Pediatrics* 1989; 83:785–789.

33. Fisher DA: The importance of early management in optimizing IQ in infants with congenital hypothyroidism. *J Pediatr* 2000; 136:273–274.

34. Salerno M, et al: Longitudinal growth, sexual maturation and final height in patients with congenital hypothyroidism detected by neonatal screening. *Eur J Endocrinol* 2001; 145:377–383.

35. Morin A, et al: Linear growth in children with congenital hypothyroidism detected by neonatal screening and treated early: a longitudinal study. *J Paediatr Endocrinol Metab* 2002; 15:973–977.

36. Wong SC, Ng SM, Didi M: Children with congenital hypothyroidism are at risk of adult obesity due to early adiposity rebound. *Clin Endocrinol (Oxf)* 2004; 61:441–446.

37. Ladenson PW, et al: American Thyroid Association guidelines for detection of thyroid dysfunction. *Arch Intern Med* 2000; 160:1573–1575.

38. Mestman JH, Goodwin TM, Montoro M: Thyroid disorders in pregnancy. *Endocrinol Metab Clin North Am* 1995; 24:41–71.

39. Mestman JH: Perinatal thyroid dysfunction: prenatal diagnosis and treatment. Medscape General Medicine, posted July 17, 1997. Available at *www.medscape.com.*

40. Bilezikian JP, Potts JT, Fuleihan Gel-H: Summary statement from a workshop on asymptomatic primary hyperparathyroidism: a perspective for the 21st century. *J Clin Endocrinol Metab* 2002; 87:5353–5361.

41. Busaidy NL, Jimenez C, Habra MA: Parathyroid carcinoma: a 22-year experience. *Head Neck* 2004; 26:716–726.

42. Chow E, et al: Parathyroid carcinoma—the Princess Margaret Hospital experience. *Int J Radiat Oncol Biol Phys* 1998; 41:569–572.

43. Kearns AE, Thompson AG: Medical and surgical management of hyperparathyroidism. *Mayo Clin Proc* 2002; 77:87–91.

44. Grau AM, Hoff AO, Lee JE: Carcinoma of the parathyroid glands. In Pellitteri PK, McCaffrey TV (eds): *Endocrine Surgery of the Head and Neck.* New York: Delmar Learning, 2003, pp 429–440.

12

The clinical laboratory provides objective criteria for the assessment of reproductive and fetal disorders.

Reproductive Endocrinology and Fetal Testing

Wendy Arneson and Jean Brickell

The laboratory provides vital information regarding reproductive endocrinology, pregnancy, and fetal testing for physicians and other health-care providers. This chapter will focus on fertility, pregnancy, and fetal well-being assessment. Laboratory tests for reproduction, pregnancy, and fetal assessment and procedures of analysis will be discussed in the context of six scenarios. These will illustrate the importance of providing quality laboratory results and correlating laboratory values with disorders such as complications of pregnancy, infertility, premature birth, assessment of lung maturity, hemolytic disease of the newborn, and neural tube defects. The importance of recognizing and minimizing preanalytical, analytical, and postanalytical errors will also be discussed throughout the chapter. Although there are many tests for fetal assessment and many reproductive hormones are analyzed in the clinical laboratory, detailed test methods will be provided for the most commonly measured analytes. As members of the health-care team, laboratory technologists work with many health-care professionals as they care for the mother and fetus, particularly those physicians and nurses in labor and delivery, neonatology, and emergency medicine. The side boxes in this chapter provide common sense tips, definitions of terms, brief descriptions of pathophysiology, and clinical correlations as well as reminders of the team approach in health care. Text boxes within the chapter outline methodology for laboratory assessment of nutrition and digestive function.

OBJECTIVES

Upon completion of this chapter, the student will have the ability to

- Describe the typical finding in hCG levels over a 48-hour period in normal pregnancy, ectopic pregnancy, and threatened spontaneous abortion.
- Differentiate qualitative and quantitative hCG in terms of principle of method, uses, and where testing is generally performed.
- Describe the diagnostic value of monitoring LH, FSH, and estradiol levels in women and LH, FSH, and testosterone levels and semen analysis in male fertility testing.
- Describe the cause of hemolytic disease of the newborn and give an example of the testing methodology that is used to assess this disease.
- Correlate changes in concentration of phospholipids in the developing fetal lung with testing methodology for fetal lung maturity.
- Explain the typical specimen collection and handling of amniotic fluid, including special steps needed for preservation of substances to be tested.

CASE SCENARIO 12-1

Pregnancy Testing: Yes or No?

Ms. Garcia left her urine specimen in the physician's office laboratory for a pregnancy test. It was properly labeled and she said to the technologist, "I think I am pregnant but the test I did last night at home said 'not pregnant'."

PREGNANCY

A typical uncomplicated pregnancy lasts 40 weeks calculated from the first day of the last menstrual period (LMP). In a typical menstrual cycle, the first 13 days lead up to **ovulation** or release of the **oocyte** from the ovary. **Sperm cells** reach the oocyte by traveling up the vagina, into the **uterus**, and out of the fallopian tubes to the region next to the ovary. **Fertilization** is the union of the oocyte and sperm cell forming a **zygote**, and it occurs in the first few days following ovulation. For the sake of determining gestational age, fertilization is thought to occur on day 14 of the cycle. The zygote travels down the fallopian tube toward the uterus, begins dividing, and forms a ball of cells known as the **morula**. At around day 19 following the LMP or day five or six after conception, the morula enters the uterus and differentiates into a **blastocyst** that consists of a hollow, fluid-filled ball of cells with an inner cell mass at one end and surrounded by an outer cell layer. The blastocyst implants in the uterus on days six to eight. This signifies the true beginning of pregnancy, which can be verified with clinical signs and symptoms.[1]

As the pregnancy progresses, the inner cells of the blastocyst further divide, forming the yolk sac, amniotic cavity, and **embryo**. The amniotic cavity will hold the developing embryo suspended in the **amniotic fluid**. The yolk sac provides nutrition support cells for the embryo and a portion of the umbilical cord. The outer cell layer of the blastocyst will form the embryonic chorionic villi and, with the uterine lining, will form the placenta. The placenta provides for the exchange of gases, nutrients, and waste products between the developing embryo and the mother.

In the embryo, rapid cell division continues with organs developing from specialized cells and tissues. By 10 weeks after the LMP, the embryo contains most of the organs and is referred to as a **fetus**. By 25 weeks, the fetus has grown to approximately 700 g and 30 cm in length.[1] Organs complete growth and maturation until approximately 40 weeks' gestation when, at birth, the fetus becomes separated from the placenta and begins autonomous life as a newborn baby or neonate.[2] Figure 12–1 depicts the stages of development of the human embryo.

Markers of Pregnancy

The placenta produces several hormones that help to sustain the pregnancy, including **human chorionic gonadotropin (hCG)**, **human placental lactogen (hPL)**, and **progesterone**. Chorionic gonadotropin is a glycoprotein hormone with two nonidentical subunits (alpha and beta polypeptide chains). It has structural similarities to other hormones such as luteinizing hormone (LH) and follicle-stimulating hormone (FSH), particularly in the alpha chain, while the beta chain is unique to hCG. This hormone is produced by chorionic villi of the implanted blastocyst and triggers the **corpus luteum** to release progesterone and estrogen. hCG

ovulation - cyclic release of an oocyte by the ovary

oocyte - female reproductive cell; ovum

■ **CLINICAL CORRELATION**
Ultrasound imaging, performed by an ultrasound technician, is also used to verify pregnancy and later to verify fetal age based on femur length or size of cranium and pelvic girdle.

sperm cell - male germinal cell

uterus - hollow muscular organ located in the pelvic cavity of the woman in which the blastocyst implants and the fetus develops

fertilization - union of two gametes: male (sperm cell) and female (oocyte)

zygote - single cell formed from fertilization of the oocyte and sperm cell

morula - differentiated zygote that develops a cavity forming the blastocyst

blastocyst - spherical shell enclosing fluid-filled cavity with the inner cell mass that will become the embryo at one pole and an outer layer of cells that will form the embryonic placenta

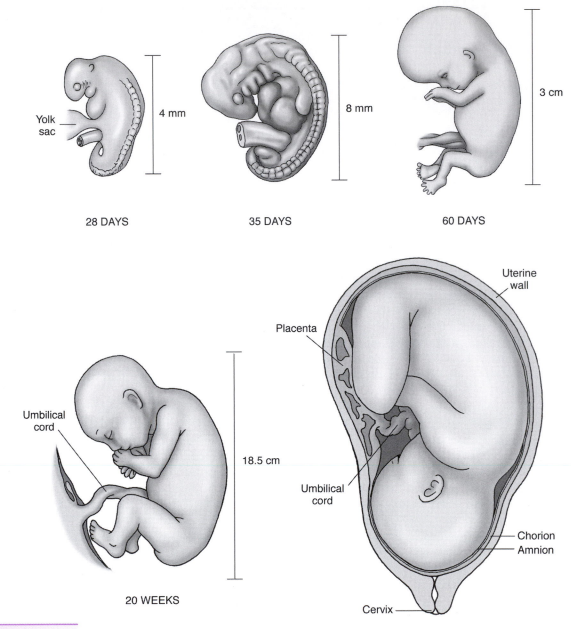

Figure 12–1. Stages of development of human embryo, including mature fetus.

embryo - rapidly growing and developing human organism before the 10th week of gestation

amniotic fluid - liquid that surrounds the fetus in the amniotic cavity

fetus - unborn but recognizable human organism between 10 weeks' and 40 weeks' gestation

helps maintain the uterine lining, the **endometrium**, with an adequate uterine blood supply until placental synthesis of progesterone begins. Detectable levels of hCG begin at about 22 days from the LMP, which is approximately 8 to 11 days from conception. Initially, hCG levels raise exponentially, more than doubling each week during the first weeks in normal pregnancies.[3] Figure 12–2 depicts typical hCG levels over time during pregnancy. Once progesterone is produced by the placenta to maintain uterine function, hCG is no longer needed and the amount levels off and declines by approximately 12 to 14 weeks' gestation.

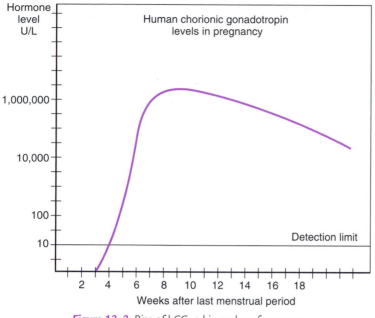

Figure 12–2. Rise of hCG, a biomarker of pregnancy.

human chorionic gonadotropin (hCG) - classic hormone marker of pregnancy produced by the placenta after the fertilized ooctye implants

human placental lactogen (hPL) - hormone produced by the placenta and involved in maternal glucose and fat metabolism and mammary gland function

progesterone - steroid hormone produced by the corpus luteum and placenta that prepares the endometrium for blastocyst implantation and maintains pregnancy

corpus luteum - yellow glandular mass that develops from an ovarian follicle following the release of a mature oocyte and secretes progesterone

endometrium - lining of the uterus

estriol - 18-carbon steroid molecule that is the main estrogen found in pregnant women

follicle - sac produced by the ovary containing an oocyte

estrone - 18-carbon steroid molecule that is less active than other estrogens

✓ **Common Sense Check**
When analyzed in a laboratory setting, patient urine must be collected in a clean container, labeled properly with the correct patient information, and stored in a refrigerator if not analyzed within a few hours.

▪▪ **CLINICAL CORRELATION**
The patient's history of first day of the last menstrual period is used to correlate with pregnancy test results and help to determine gestational age.

Human placental lactogen is a single polypeptide chain with similarities in structure to growth hormone. Along with other hormones at the end of pregnancy, it helps to prepare the mammary glands for lactation. Early in pregnancy, the most likely role for this hormone is in regulating metabolism of maternal fats and glucose, inhibiting maternal insulin, and sparing glucose for fetal metabolism.[1]

Progesterone and **estriol** are important steroids produced during pregnancy. Progesterone, a steroid with 21 carbons, is made by the placenta from maternal cholesterol. Progesterone helps to maintain the endometrium, the uterine tissue lining, by promoting growth and thickening of mucosal cells and an adequate uterine blood supply. When progesterone levels are not adequate, fetal demise occurs because of poor uterine blood supply and resulting endometrial sloughing. Progesterone also inhibits further ovarian **follicle** development. Estriol is the major estrogen produced by the placenta during pregnancy[4] but **estrone** and **estradiol** are also produced from androgen precursors such as **dehydroepiandrosterone** sulfate (DHEAS), which is produced by the maternal and fetal adrenal glands.

Chorionic gonadotropin is the most commonly measured of these three hormones, especially as an early indication of pregnancy and in some cases even before the first missed menstrual period. Test Methodology 12–1 depicts qualitative pregnancy testing with hCG, and Test Methodology 12–2 describes quantitative testing. All three of these important hormones can be used to assess adequate placental function during the early stages of pregnancy.

Problems in Early Pregnancy

Difficulty with pregnancies in early stages may include ectopic pregnancies and failure to maintain the pregnancy in the uterus, leading to **miscarriage**. *Ectopic pregnancy* means that the fertilized ovum is unable to implant in the uterus because it remains in the fallopian tubes or another displaced location such as the ovary or

estradiol - 18-carbon steroid molecule that is the main estrogen found in nonpregnant women

dehydroepiandrosterone - 19-carbon molecule found in small amounts as a precursor to some estrogens in women and as a precursor to male sex steroids in men

miscarriage - sudden unplanned evacuation of the uterus, ending pregnancy

TEST METHODOLOGY 12-1.   QUALITATIVE HUMAN CHORIONIC GONADOTROPIN BY IMMUNOASSAY

Qualitative tests provide results that are either positive or negative for the substance to be tested, while quantitative tests provide numerical values as results. In the case of qualitative hCG, a positive test result means the patient is most likely pregnant and a negative result indicates the patient is most likely not pregnant. This test, performed using a urine specimen, is usually less sensitive than a quantitative test but also is a simpler to perform and less expensive. This type of test, used in satellite laboratories or physician office laboratories, is categorized as waived testing under federal regulations and is available for patients as a home test kit. The test requires only a few steps and the results are read within a few minutes by color change reaction. The result will be positive when the hCG concentration is at least 30 IU/L, which is often only a day or two after the first missed menstrual period. In terms of gestational age, this is around day 30 of the last menstrual period.

The Reaction Principle

Antibody specific to whole molecule hCG or the beta polypeptide chain is bound to a nitrocellulose filter paper and reacts with patient hCG from the urine sample. Unbound materials are washed away with the flow of urine sample over the filter paper while peroxidase-labeled antibody that is specific to the hCG–anti-hCG complex flows into the area. In this step, the patient hCG becomes sandwiched between the two antibodies. A benzedrine substrate and buffers are then added, and an insoluble colored product forms on the filter paper to indicate the presence of patient hCG.

Interferences

False-positive results occur because of interference from some proteins, drugs, bacteria, or erythrocytes or leukocytes in the urine. Using centrifuged urine can eliminate interference from particles. Positive hCG results should correlate with the patient's history and physical examination. Negative results may be due to a very dilute urine or urine that has been exposed to heat. Generally a negative result indicates a need to retest the patient urine in a few days if menses do not begin.

The Specimen

The first morning urine, centrifuged if necessary to remove cells and particulates, is used. The specimen should be stored at refrigeration temperature if not tested within a few hours or frozen if not tested within 24 hours.

Reference Range

Negative for the nonpregnant woman.

CLINICAL CORRELATION

A diagnosis of ectopic pregnancy is determined from patient history with reported pain and bleeding, physical examination (possibly including imaging showing a pelvic mass), and often hCG levels that are abnormally low and have a slow rate of increase.

ultrasound - imaging technique that uses high-frequency sound waves to create images of internal organs, tissue, and blood vessels

ovarian ligaments. This condition appears to be on the increase but is most likely reported more frequently due to improved diagnostic tools. Ectopic pregnancy remains one of the most common causes of maternal death during the first trimester, typically characterized by severe pain and hemorrhage as with clotting disorders, a more severe complication that may lead to death. The cause of ectopic pregnancy is most likely scarred or obstructed fallopian tubes secondary to sexually transmitted disease or repeated pelvic inflammatory disease.[6]

The ectopic pregnancy can be visualized with **ultrasound** by about 6 weeks after the LMP when hCG levels are 1500 IU/L or higher.[7] Ultrasound imaging is generally used to verify the presence of ectopic pregnancy, and surgical intervention is usually required to stop the bleeding and repair the site.[7]

TEST METHODOLOGY 12-2.   QUANTITATIVE hCG BY ENZYME IMMUNOMETRIC ASSAY

Quantitative hCG tests are more sensitive than qualitative tests, detecting hCG levels at 5 to 10 IU/L, and are necessary when ruling out pregnancy before the first menstrual period. This information regarding very early pregnancy is helpful prior to surgery or other potentially harmful medical interventions. Quantitative hCG tests require an automated instrument to read results, often by some labeled immunoassay method, and standard solutions of hCG for instrument calibration and calculation of results. Serial hCG levels are helpful to rule out abnormalities in the pregnancy; however, for accurate interpretation of test results, such testing is best performed by the same laboratory using the same methodology.[5] In a healthy pregnancy, hCG will double about every 2 days during weeks 2 to 5, while in abnormal pregnancies such as ectopic pregnancies or in impending miscarriage, the hCG levels do not double as quickly or may even decline. Measurement of hCG at 16 to 20 weeks' gestation is used in combination with other tests (e.g., chromosomal tests) for prediction of Down syndrome, in which the hCG is generally higher than the reference range.

The Reaction Principle

This is a double-antibody technique in which first antibody to hCG is bound to the whole molecule, followed by an enzyme-labeled antibody specific to the beta polypeptide chain (anti-hCG:anti-hCG beta sandwich). Following addition of substrate and buffers, the colored product forms in proportion to the patient's hCG level and is measured photometrically.

Interferences

Hemolysis, lipemia, or turbidity may account for interfering absorbances.

The Specimen

Fresh serum free from hemolysis, lipemia, or turbidity should be tested within a few hours or stored at –20°C until testing can occur.

Reference Ranges

Not Pregnant	<5 IU/L
4 Weeks' gestation after LMP	5–100 IU/L
5 Weeks' gestation after LMP	200–3000 IU/L
6 Weeks' gestation after LMP	10,000–80,000 IU/L
15–26 Weeks after LMP	5000–80,000 IU/L

Spontaneous abortion, more commonly referred to as miscarriage, is failure to maintain the pregnancy to full term or until a viable baby can be delivered. This sudden, unplanned disruption in the pregnancy is associated with vaginal bleeding, cramping pain, a previous positive hCG test, and decreasing hCG levels over a 48-hour period. History, physical examination, and possibly imaging techniques are often necessary to rule out ectopic pregnancy.[8] A normally progressing pregnancy will result in a doubling of hCG in 2 to 3 days. Likewise, an intrauterine pregnancy can usually be visualized accurately with ultrasound by about 5 to 6 weeks after the LMP, when hCG levels are 6500 IU/L or higher.[1] Newer ultrasound techniques may detect pregnancies at earlier stages,[7] but there are higher false-positive and false-negative rates.[1] There are many causes of miscarriage, but the most common is an abnormally developing blastocyst or embryo. Over half of the spontaneous abortions that occur in the first trimester result from an abnormality in the fetus, such as chromosomal abnormalities incompatible with life.[9] Miscarriage can also result from hormonal fluctuations, including inadequate levels of progesterone or estrogens that are necessary for maintenance of the uterine lining. A sudden drop in progesterone levels will cause the endometrium to slough, evacuating the embryo and causing menstruation to begin. This may happen early before pregnancy is suspected and, if it occurs repeatedly, may be the cause of infertility.[1,10]

Trophoblastic Neoplasm

Trophoblastic neoplasm results in a tumor growth in the uterus rather than a fetus. This type of neoplasm, or new and abnormal growth, results from an intrauterine or ectopic pregnancy and is quite rare, particularly in the malignant forms. There are several types, including hydatiform mole, invasive hydatiform mole, and choriocarcinoma. In hydatiform mole, the pregnancy becomes nonviable and the chorionic villi grow abnormally, resulting in edema and grapelike clusters of watery sacs in the uterus that are visible by ultrasound. Invasive hydatiform mole is similar to hydatiform mole but the chorionic villi grow to invade the uterine smooth muscles. Choriocarcinoma, also called metastatic trophoblastic disease, is a malignancy in which the chorionic villi not only invade the uterus but spread to surrounding organs. The latter is a carcinoma arising from the trophoblast. In contrast, hydatiform mole is a benign growth of the trophoblast.[2] Quantitative levels of hCG, which are very high in these neoplasms, are helpful in monitoring treatment and progression of neoplastic disease since levels correlate with the amount of tumor present. For example, a patient with hCG of 400,000 IU/L or higher would be expected to have a poor prognosis even with treatment. Within 24 hours of successful removal of the tumor, the hCG level should drop by half considering half-life and correlation with amount of tumor.[11]

Multiple Fetuses and Pregnancy Hormones

Multiple fetuses in the pregnancy, including twins, will also affect the quantity of hormone detected in urine and serum. With a twin pregnancy, the level of hCG in the mother's serum is close to double the range for a single-fetus pregnancy. This is important to consider when correlating hCG levels with early abnormal pregnancies and with midterm diagnostic procedures that include hCG. The use of hCG and other maternal serum tests for fetal assessment are discussed later in this chapter. Detecting twins or higher order multiple pregnancies relies on using ultrasound techniques, illustrating the need for several diagnostic tools for management of pregnancy by health-care providers.[1]

Case Scenario 12-1 Pregnancy Testing: Yes or No?

Follow-Up

Ms. Garcia left her urine specimen in the physician's office laboratory for a pregnancy test. The laboratory staff performed a qualitative pregnancy test with her urine sample with a positive result. The history and physical

Case Scenario 12-1 Pregnancy Testing: Yes or No? *(continued)*

examination correlated with these results, and Ms. Garcia was found to be 5 weeks pregnant based on her last menstrual period. ●

PREGNANCY TESTS AND EARLY MARKERS OF PROBLEMS

Questions that were considered in Case Scenario 12–1 will serve to summarize this portion of the chapter:

1. *What is the main urinary marker for pregnancy?* Human chorionic gonadotropin is the main marker.
2. *What is the difference in methodology and clinical value of qualitative and quantitative pregnancy tests?* Qualitative tests provide positive or negative hCG results to help determine if the patient is pregnant or not pregnant. These are usually simple immunoassay tests performed on a urine specimen and having one or few steps in analysis. Qualitative tests are less sensitive than a quantitative test but they have the advantages of being faster and easier to perform and, because they do not require an instrument to read the results, they are less expensive. Qualitative testing can generally detect pregnancy within a few days after the first missed menstrual period. A quantitative pregnancy test, which is generally performed using serum, is more sensitive in that hCG can be detected even before the first missed menstrual period (e.g., by day 21 to 27 from the last menstrual period). Quantitative hCG tests are labeled immunoassay methods that require automated instrumentation. This more sensitive testing is useful for detecting pregnancy prior to surgery or other invasive techniques or to measure in a series to monitor for healthy progression of pregnancy or rule out abnormal pregnancy.
3. *What other markers are there for pregnancy, and how do they correlate with uncomplicated simple pregnancy?* Other hormones are produced during pregnancy, including estriol and hPL, which tend to rise at a predictable rate. Another estrogen, estradiol, is higher in the nonpregnant women, while estriol is the main estrogen found in pregnant women. Additional markers of pregnancy include physical signs of pregnancy and ultrasound imaging of the uterus by 6 weeks of gestation.
4. *What early markers are there for problem pregnancies such as ectopic, trophoblastic, or multiple pregnancies or threatened miscarriages?*

Quantitative hCG tests are used in conjunction with history, physical examination, and ultrasound for detecting abnormal pregnancy, such as ectopic pregnancy, or miscarriage. There is an exponential increase in hCG early in a normal pregnancy. In ectopic or misplaced pregnancy, the hCG value may continue to increase but not to a level as high as that for a normal pregnancy, while fetal demise and impending miscarriage are indicated by leveling off or falling of hCG levels. Trophoblastic diseases such as hydatiform mole result from the demise of the fetus but with an abnormal growth of remaining trophoblastic cells causing higher than normal levels of hCG. Ultrasound and other imaging techniques will indicate grapelike clusters of watery sacs instead of a fetus. Multiple fetuses, including twins, will result in hCG levels higher than those expected for a single fetus or for the gestational age. Ultrasound can be used to verify the presence of multiple fetuses.

CASE SCENARIO 12-2

Infertility and Polycystic Ovarian Disease: "String of Pearls" in a Bearded Lady

The special chemistry section received laboratory requests for the following hormones: total testosterone, free testosterone, FSH, midfollicular LH, midfollicular prolactin, androstenedione, DHEAS, dihydrotestosterone, androstandiol glucuronide, and sex hormone–binding globulin. Many of these laboratory tests were to be sent to a reference laboratory. The referral database was consulted so that the correct type of specimen was collected and proper storage and handling conditions were met prior to performing the tests at the reference laboratory. The patient was a 23-year-old African-American female with a preliminary diagnosis of hirsutism and infertility. Previous laboratory results showed a slightly elevated 8:00 a.m. plasma cortisol level but a low-dose dexamethasone test showed normal cortisol suppression. The following laboratory results were obtained initially from the special chemistry section:

Test	Result	Reference Range
Testosterone, total (ng/dL)	65	15–70
FSH, midcycle (mIU/mL)	3	0.2–17.2
LH, midcycle (mIU/mL)	19	21.9–56.6
Estradiol, midcycle (pg/mL)	151	150–750
Prolactin (ng/mL)	14	<20 in nonpregnant women
DHEAS (μg/mL)	3.0	0.36–3.2

SEX STEROIDS

Estrogens and androgens are reproductive hormones. They are steroid hormones, derived from cholesterol. Due to their lipid chemical makeup, these hormones are water insoluble. Therefore, these hormones are bound to a carrier molecule, such as sex hormone–binding globulin, which is protein in nature when in circulation.

Steroid hormones have relatively long plasma half-lives, usually ranging from 1 to 2 hours. These hormones travel to their site of action and diffuse through the lipid bilayer cell membrane to reach the specific intracellular receptor. Examples include the estrogens, such as estradiol and estrone, and androgens such as testosterone.

The metabolic pathway for production of estrone (E_1) and estradiol (E_2), the two main estrogen hormones found in the nonpregnant woman, is depicted in Figure 12–3. Estradiol is the most potent female hormone and can be used to evaluate ovarian function and reproduction.[4] The biochemical pathway for the production of testosterone and other androgens is depicted in Figure 12–4. This information is helpful for understanding some disorders in which biosynthetic enzymes are absent, resulting in a deficiency of some hormones and an overabundance of others.

Protein and Peptide Reproductive Hormones

Other important reproductive hormones include glycoprotein hormones made by the pituitary gland, such as luteinizing hormone (LH) and follicle-stimulating hormone (FSH). Protein hormones are composed of amino acids in specific sequences

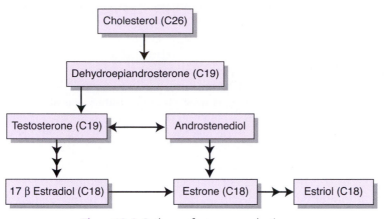

Figure 12–3. Pathway of estrogen production.

bonded with peptide bonds. During the processes of synthesis, these particular proteins have additional chemical groups added, including carbohydrates, which form more complex proteins know as glycoproteins and contain secondary and tertiary bonds that provide unique configurations. Gonadotropin-releasing hormone (Gn-RH), a hypothalamic hormone, is a peptide. Protein hormones, such as LH, FSH, and Gn-RH, combine with specific cellular receptors on the plasma membrane before initiating their cellular response. The half-life of these peptide and glycoprotein hormones is much shorter than the steroid hormones, with a typical plasma half-life of a few minutes to up to 1 hour.

Inhibin is a peptide hormone with two forms, A and B. Inhibin is secreted by the ovary for the purpose of inhibiting pituitary release of FSH and stimulating one dominant follicle. Inhibin B is found only in females. Inhibin A is produced by the follicle prior to ovulation and later by the corpus luteum. Inhibin A is also found in males and is secreted by the **Sertoli cells** of the testes to regulate FSH and sperm production. It exhibits negative feedback on the anterior pituitary to shut down production of FSH, which will shut down testosterone production in the testes.

Sertoli cells - specialized cells in the seminiferous tubules of the testis that produce inhibin and factors that help sperm maturation

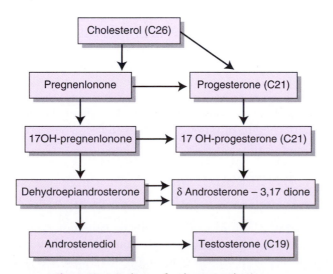

Figure 12–4. Pathway of androgen production.

ENDOCRINE GLANDS INVOLVED IN REPRODUCTION

The hypothalamus is derived from neuroendocrine tissue in the mesencephalon, or middle section of the brain. It provides the tertiary level of control and stimulation of hormone secretion. The hypothalamus makes releasing hormones such as thyroid-releasing hormone (TRH) and Gn-RH, both peptide in nature. The primary function of these hormones is to stimulate pituitary secretion of secondary hormones such as LH and FSH. However, these hormones also respond to other hormones in a positive and negative feedback system such that a highly coordinated monthly cycle occurs in the mature female. There is a similar coordinated cycle in the mature male that spans a 24-hour cycle. Other hypothalamic hormones that play a role in sexual development and reproduction include TRH and cortisol-releasing hormone (CRH), which have the ability to stimulate secondary endocrine glands.[4]

The pituitary gland is composed of two unique glandular tissues, the neurohypophysis and the adenohypophysis, which secrete a variety of hormones. The neurohypophysis or posterior pituitary stores and releases two main hormones produced in the hypothalamus, antidiuretic hormone (ADH) and oxytocin. The main function of ADH is in maintaining water balance and that of oxytocin is stimulation of uterine contractions during labor and breast milk ejection during lactation. The adenohypophysis or anterior pituitary provides a secondary level of control and stimulation of reproductive hormones through release of LH and FSH. Other pituitary hormones also may play a role in reproduction, including thyroid-stimulating hormone (TSH), growth hormone, and adrenocorticotropic hormone (ACTH). Thyroid-releasing hormone binds to plasma membrane receptors of cells in the pituitary gland to stimulate production and release of TSH, which in turn binds to receptors in cells of the thyroid gland to initiate secretion of thyroid hormones. These hormones play a role in the development of secondary sex characteristics, including distribution of body fat, muscles, and hair. Hypothalamic CRH binds to specific receptors in cells of the pituitary gland to stimulate production and release of ACTH. ACTH binds to receptors in cells of the adrenal cortex and stimulates production of steroid hormones, including 1-hydroxypregnenolone and 17-hydroxyprogesterone, precursors to estrogen and androgen. In the **prepubescent** child and in postmenopausal women, the adrenal gland continues to secrete the majority of sex steroids since the **gonads** are relatively inactive.[4]

The primary reproductive organs, the ovaries in females and the testes in males, contain cells that respond to the binding of LH and FSH to specific cellular receptors, causing the secretion of hormones such as estrogen and testosterone. These steroid hormones produce diverse organic and metabolic responses. Other consequences of testicular and ovarian hormonal response include release of the mature **gametocytes**, or oocytes (ovary), and sperm cells (testes) and responsiveness to other hormones such as estradiol and inhibin. Details of the highly coordinated process of ovulation and fertilization are discussed in the next section.

OVERVIEW OF NORMAL FEMALE REPRODUCTIVE PHYSIOLOGY

Females are born with all of their ovarian follicles containing oocytes. In the sexually mature female, usually only one follicle matures, and therefore only a single oocyte is released, each month. The maturation of a follicle and release of a mature

prepubescent - before sexual maturity

gonads - reproductive organs: the testes in the male and ovaries in the female

gametocyte - sperm cell or oocyte

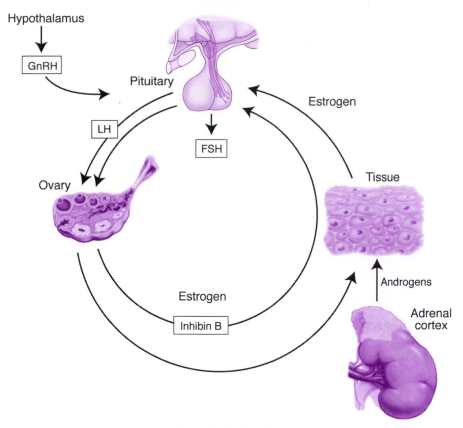

Figure 12–5. Ovulation.

oocyte occurs midway in the menstrual cycle in the process known as ovulation. This process is coordinated by a highly ordered series of hormonal signals. These hormonal signals include hypothalamic stimulation of the pituitary by Gn-RH, resulting in periodic secretion of LH and FSH by the pituitary gland. Figure 12–5 depicts the relationship of the reproductive glands and hormones secreted in reproduction.

After the onset of puberty, the hormonal signals begin with episodes of FSH secretion over a monthly cycle, which stimulates a small group of follicles to prepare for ovulation. As the FSH concentration rises at the beginning of each cycle, one dominant follicle is the most responsive to FSH and LH. This follicle participates in the process of ovulation, or separation from the ovary and release of the oocyte next to the fallopian tube. Cells in the follicular lining are further stimulated by other hormones, including LH, to develop a lipid-rich mass surrounding the oocyte, called the corpus luteum. The corpus luteum is further stimulated by LH and initiates the production of progesterone, which plays a major role in maintaining the endometrial lining.[12]

The fate of the corpus luteum is quite varied depending on the presence or absence of sperm cells. If sperm cells are not present to fertilize the released oocyte, the corpus luteum degenerates and dies after about 10 days, resulting in a drop in progesterone levels. If sperm cells travel up from the vagina to the fallopian tubes and fertilize an oocyte, a zygote results. The zygote travels down the fallopian tube, where it begins the process of rapid division. Pregnancy begins with implantation of the blastocyst in the endometrium of the uterus. The blastocyst produces hGC, which stimulates the corpus luteum to continue production of hormones for 10 to 12 weeks until the placenta functions in that capacity. Occasionally more than one follicle is stimulated and fertilized, which can result in fraternal twins or higher order multiple births.[12]

The Role of Inhibins

follicular phase - first half of the female menstrual cycle leading up to maturity of one follicle and release of an oocyte

Inhibins, protein hormones secreted by the ovary and corpus luteum, are involved in reproduction as previously mentioned. Inhibin A has a suppressive effect on FSH levels following ovulation. Inhibin B levels rise early in the **follicular phase** and most likely play an important role in ensuring that only one follicle is released during ovulation. Inhibin A levels decline with the degeneration of the corpus luteum when fertilization does not take place, while inhibin B levels remain elevated. Since the patterns of inhibin A and B secretion vary during the phases of the menstrual cycle, it is quite likely that they play different reproductive roles.[13,14]

THE FEMALE REPRODUCTIVE CYCLE

Day one of the female reproductive cycle is counted from the first day of menses. The reproductive or menstrual cycle is divided into two main phases over an average of 28 days: the follicular phase and the **luteal phase**. The early stage of a monthly cycle is termed *follicular* since the maturation of the follicle and its ability to secrete hormones is a key event and because the hormone FSH plays a key role. Early in this phase, LH levels begin to rise as well, and together FSH and LH bind to the specific receptors of one dominant follicle.

luteal phase - second half of the female menstrual cycle following ovulation and the dominance of the corpus luteum

Pituitary secretion of FSH occurs in response to hypothalamic secretion of Gn-RH. The pituitary also responds to the negative feedback control of low levels of circulating estradiol and progesterone that occur with the demise of the corpus luteum from the previous cycle. In other words, in the previous cycle, if the oocyte is not fertilized within a few days of ovulation, it dies and estradiol levels fall off. The corpus luteum also dies and progesterone levels fall off. When these hormone levels drop to below a threshold level, the pituitary is then stimulated to begin secretion of FSH and LH for the next monthly cycle. The ovaries also regulate FSH secretion by production of inhibin A and B. As LH and FSH levels rise, the follicles within the ovaries produce estrogen, especially estradiol. Increasing levels of estradiol in the later days of the follicular phase trigger Gn-RH secretion, followed by more LH secretion at midcycle. In addition, estradiol promotes thickening of the endometrial lining.

■■
■■ **CLINICAL CORRELATION**
The surge of LH and FSH that mark ovulation also cause various clinical signs and symptoms that can be used to predict ovulation, including thickening of cervical mucus and a slight rise in body temperature, measured in the morning before rising.

Ovulation occurs at around day 14 of a 28-day menstrual cycle, but the events that surround ovulation occur between days 10 and 16. At the time of ovulation, the highest levels of LH, FSH, and inhibin A exist in the sexually mature female. Figure 12–5 shows the relative hormonal levels at the time of ovulation.

After ovulation there is a shift into the luteal phase. This is so named because of the development of the corpus luteum from the lining cells of the mature follicle. The transition between the end of the luteal phase in one monthly cycle and the follicular phase of the next monthly cycle is marked by menses. Menses, or sloughing of the uterine lining, results if pregnancy did not occur and the corpus luteum died. Hormonal changes triggers this event, including the drop of progesterone production and estradiol levels due to the destruction of the corpus luteum. The first few days of menses are signaled by very low levels of the reproductive hor-

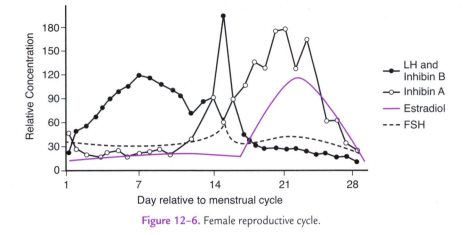

Figure 12–6. Female reproductive cycle.

mones, with FSH and LH levels beginning to rise again in the first few days of the new monthly cycle. Figure 12–6 shows the relative levels of FSH, LH, and estradiol during the phases of the female reproductive cycle.[12] Test Methodology 12–3 describes the method for estradiol analysis.

TEST METHODOLOGY 12-3.   ESTRADIOL BY IMMUNOASSAY

A direct immunoassay for estradiol is the most common method of analysis for women of reproductive age. Although there are several types of estrogens, estradiol is the most common estrogen found in the nonpregnant female and is used to assess ovulatory status. Estradiol is bound to binding globulin in serum and must be displaced prior to analysis by one of a variety of methods.

The Reaction Principle

In a heterogeneous reaction, estradiol is first displaced from binding globulins with 8-anilino-1-naphthalene sulfonic acid. Free estradiol reacts with anti-estradiol antibody that has been bound to a filter paper. Excess unbound substances are washed away and a second alkaline phosphatase–labeled antibody is added. Unbound antibody is washed away, followed by addition of substrate. Colored product forms in proportion to the amount of patient estradiol and is measured spectrophotometrically.

Interferences

Free fatty acids can interfere, as well as estrogens from oral contraceptives or estrogen replacement therapy.

The Specimen

Fresh serum or heparinized plasma free from turbidity should be tested within a few hours or stored at –20°C until testing can occur.

Reference Ranges (Adult Women)

Early follicular phase	20–150 pg/mL
Midcycle	150–750 pg/mL
Luteal phase	30–450 pg/mL
Postmenopausal	<20 pg/mL

NORMAL MALE REPRODUCTIVE PHYSIOLOGY

Because reproductive problems may affect men as well as women, a brief review of the normal male reproductive physiology is warranted. Men continually produce mature sperm cells in the seminiferous tubules of the testes, with the highest numbers around 72 hours after the last **ejaculation**. Sperm production occurs under the complex interaction of hormonal signals similar to the female reproductive cycle. After the onset of puberty, a daily circadian rhythm of FSH begins involving the testicular Sertoli cells, which secrete inhibin B, and the seminiferous tubules, which produce mature sperm cells. Inhibin B helps regulate spermatogenesis and exhibits negative feedback on FSH secretion by the anterior pituitary. The testes are further stimulated by other hormones, including LH, which assists **Leydig cells** in production of testosterone. Among other roles, testosterone helps to maintain **libido**.

ejaculation - ejection of sperm cells and seminal fluid at orgasm

Leydig cells - specialized interstitial cells of the testes surrounding the tubules that produce testosterone

libido - sexual desire

HORMONAL CHANGES IN MENOPAUSE

Menopause is defined as cessation of menstruation and fewer remaining follicles causing infertility, generally at around 50 years of age. Perimenopause, the period of time leading into the menopause in women, is often characterized by irregularity in length of the menstrual cycle. Perimenopause is marked by dramatic changes in the hypothalamic-pituitary-ovarian axis. An early finding is a rise in circulating FSH levels unaccompanied by a rise in LH. It has been suggested that there is a decreased secretion of ovarian inhibin along with the decreasing follicular pool, which may be the primary cause of the rise in FSH. The resultant ovarian changes include short follicular phases with early ovulation, and ovarian insufficiency characterized by lower levels of estrogen and progesterone secreted for shorter periods of time compared with the luteal phase of younger women. The major significant endocrine event in women in the early perimenopausal phase is a fall in the circulating levels of inhibin B with no significant change in inhibin A or estradiol. Early onset of menopause, also known as premature ovarian failure, may be a cause of infertility in women greater than 30 years of age.[15,16]

FEMALE INFERTILITY

Infertility can result from ovulatory or uterine problems; mechanical problems, including obstruction of the fallopian tubes; male fertility factors; or multiple factors in either sex or combined female and male factors. Ovulatory problems are the most common cause of female infertility. Polycystic ovarian syndrome (PCOS) affects up to 5% of reproductive-age women. It is the most common cause of ovulatory infertility. PCOS is a condition characterized by multiple ovarian cysts, often found in a row, resembling a "string of pearls." Ovarian cysts are fluid-filled sacs arising from follicles swollen with fluid that are prevented from producing mature oocytes. Patients with PCOS also have hormonal imbalances, including decreased levels of LH, FSH, and progesterone and increased androgen production, including excess testosterone and DHEAS causing hirsutism or male facial patterns of hair growth. Insulin resistance is a common associated condition. PCOS is generally diagnosed when two of the following three criteria are present and other possible causes can be ruled out: clinical or laboratory results showing excess androgen secretion, decreased or absence of ovulation, and ovaries found by imaging techniques such as ultrasound to contain many cysts. Although the exact etiology of the problem is still unknown, genetic factors may be involved.[17]

Around the time of menopause, impairment of ovulation may cause infertility with adverse effect on follicle size and oocyte quality despite regular ovulation and normal gonadotropin levels. These factors are considered when treating older women with infertility. Serum levels of LH, FSH, and inhibin A and B may be helpful in assessing infertility and treatment options.[18,19] Infertility diagnostic testing is as varied as treatment options. The patient workup for infertility includes a careful, detailed history, which can help to limit the number of laboratory tests required. Availability of tests varies from center to center, so availability is one of the considerations for infertility testing. Typical laboratory tests ordered are FSH on day three of the ovulatory cycle, LH, estradiol, prolactin, and TSH levels. Measurement of ovarian and adrenal androgens such as testosterone and DHEAS should be decided on the basis of ovulatory status of the patient and the clinical picture.

Treatment for Infertility

In the past 25 years, treatment for infertility has changed significantly and is dependent on whether the origin is within the reproductive organs, hormonal, or a combination of several factors. In vitro fertilization (IVF) has become commonplace. This technique involves using agents to induce ovulation, stimulating the ovaries to produce several mature follicles, removing multiple oocytes, and allowing fertilization to occur outside of the body in a controlled in vitro environment. The zygote undergoes divisions in the laboratory, and the blastocyst (or earlier state embryo) is then transferred to the woman's uterus for implantation and, hopefully, a resulting pregnancy. Initially, IVF was performed without giving medication to simulate the ovaries to develop multiple follicles. New medication options make the IVF procedure much more efficient, some improving uterine blood flow and endometrial development, and pregnancy rates have continued to increase.[20,21]

Case Scenario 12-2 Infertility and Polycystic Ovarian Disease: "String of Pearls" in a Bearded Lady

Follow-Up

The special chemistry section had received laboratory requests for several hormone levels on a 23-year-old African-American female with a preliminary diagnosis of hirsutism and infertility. Previously laboratory results showed a slightly elevated 8:00 a.m. plasma cortisol level, but a low-dose overnight dexamethasone test showed normal cortisol suppression. This corresponds with mild hypercortisolism typical of obesity. The patient was found to be 70 pounds overweight. The initial laboratory results obtained from the special chemistry section showed slightly elevated LH at midfollicular cycle; normal FSH, prolactin, and estradiol at midcycle; and normal initial results for the androgens testosterone and DHEAS.

continued

Case Scenario 12-2 Infertility and Polycystic Ovarian Disease: "String of Pearls" in a Bearded Lady *(continued)*

Test	Result	Reference Range
Testosterone, total (ng/dL)	65	15–70
FSH, midcycle (mIU/mL)	3	0.2–17.2
LH, midcycle (mIU/mL)	19	21.9–56.6
Estradiol, midcycle (pg/mL)	151	150–750
Prolactin (ng/mL)	14	< 20 in nonpregnant women
DHEAS (µg/mL)	3.0	0.36–3.2

Results from the reference laboratory showed increased free testosterone of 11.5 pg/mL (reference range, 1.1 to 6.3 pg/mL), increased androstenedione of 315 ng/dL (85 to 175 ng/dL), increased androstandiol glucuronide of 540 ng/dL (60 to 300 ng/dL), and decreased sex hormone–binding globulin level. An ultrasound revealed a normal-sized uterus and multicystic ovaries with "string of pearls" appearance. A diagnosis of polycystic ovarian disease was made and treatment was begun. The tumors produced increased amounts of male hormones, which stimulated an elevated LH level and lowered production of sex hormone–binding globulin. Progesterone values are often abnormal in these cases. This condition and the resulting male hormone levels are one of the more common causes of ovarian infertility. It is associated with male pattern hair distribution in women. ●

Infertility of Multiple Causes

Around 15% of all couples in the United States experience infertility, with roughly half of cases due to a male factor. Analysis of semen is one of the first steps in assessing infertility and in treatment strategies. Semen analysis involves sperm concentration (number per milliliter) and vitality, morphology and motility testing, and viscosity and volume of seminal fluid. Obtaining a semen sample is less invasive than many of the procedures for assessing male fertility and is necessary at some point to help determine the type of medical intervention needed to assist in reproduction. Infection and anatomic problems can be common causes of male infertility, affecting the sperm cells or seminal fluid. Generally these conditions can be easily treated.[22] Endocrine and immunologic parameters are measured in both male and female infertility to determine cause and direct treatment.[4] Hormone treatments or surgeries, when indicated, can also be used to address male fertility factors, including sperm motility and seminal fluid viscosity.

CASE SCENARIO 12-3

Preanalytical Error in Reproductive Testing: How Important Is the Timing?

Serum samples from a 34-year-old female patient were sent to a fertility reference laboratory to test for FSH, LH, and estradiol levels. Specimens were collected at the OB/GYN clinic and were labeled as midfollicular samples.

Case Scenario 12-3 **Preanalytical Error in Reproductive Testing: How Important Is the Timing?** *(continued)*

Specimens were collected and transported in the proper manner, were labeled, and matched the test requisition forms. The following results were obtained:

Test	Result	Reference Range
LH (mIU/mL)	1.8	21.9–56.6
FSH (mIU/mL)	4.9	0.2–17.2
E_2 (pg/mL)	135	150–750

QUALITY ASSESSMENT

As described earlier in this chapter, FSH, LH, and estradiol levels fluctuate dramatically during the ovulatory cycle of a normal adult female. In an average 28-day cycle, FSH levels begin to rise by day three, stimulating the ovary to release estradiol and the pituitary to release LH. These hormones stimulate ovulation at midcycle and development of the corpus luteum for potential fertilization. Usually at midcycle, there is a peak of circulating FSH, LH, and estradiol concentrations as well as increased clinical signs of ovulation, such as a slight increase in basal body temperature and cervical mucus production. It is generally a complex interaction of hormones and physical changes that allow for ovulation and then fertilization of an oocyte by sperm. Fertility testing involves assessing many of these aspects. Test Methodologies 12–4 and 12–5 describe methods of analysis for LH and FSH, respectively.

TEST METHODOLOGY 12-4.   LH BY TWO-SITE IMMUNOMETRIC ASSAY

The Reaction Principle

Patient sample containing LH is mixed with antibody to LH attached to glass-fiber paper. A second labeled antibody is added after a wash step and incubated. Following a second wash step, buffer and reagents are added to enhance the signal, which is detected by the photometer.

Antibody specificities have greatly improved, with minimal cross reaction with FSH, hCG, and other similar molecules.[23]

The Specimen

Fresh serum free from hemolysis, lipemia, or turbidity should be tested within a few hours or stored at –20°C until testing can occur.

Reference Ranges (Adult Women)

Early follicular phase	1.7–15.0 mIU/mL
Midcycle	21.9–56.6 mIU/mL
Luteal phase	0.6–16.3 mIU/mL
Postmenopausal	14.2–52.3 mIU/mL

Reference Range (Adult Men)

1.2–7.8 IU/L

TEST METHODOLOGY 12-5.   FSH BY IMMUNOASSAY

The Reaction Principle

Patient sample containing FSH is mixed with antibody to FSH attached to glass-fiber paper. A second labeled antibody is added after a wash step and incubated. Following a second wash step, buffer and reagents are added to enhance the signal, which is detected by the photometer.

Antibody specificities have greatly improved, minimizing the likelihood of cross reaction with LH, hCG, and other similar chemicals.

The Specimen

Fresh serum free from hemolysis, lipemia, or turbidity should be tested within a few hours or stored at $-20°C$ until testing can occur.

Reference Ranges (Adult Women)

Early follicular phase	1.4–9.9 mIU/mL
Midcycle	0.2–17.2 mIU/mL
Luteal phase	1.1–9.2 mIU/mL
Postmenopausal	19.3–100.6 mIU/mL

Reference Range (Adult Men)

1.4–15.4 IU/L

Quality assessment of laboratory testing for fertility involves the same aspects discussed in previous chapters. Policies and procedures must be in place to prevent as many errors as possible before the testing has occurred, during analysis, and after the results are obtained. These factors are the preanalytical, analytical, and postanalytical variations of laboratory testing.

Preanalytical Errors

If the patient specimen identification is not matched correctly to the patient, a serious preanalytical error has occurred. Laboratory results obtained from the wrong patient will not provide useful information to the physician who is attempting to diagnose or treat a fertility problem. This identification process includes the correct identification of secondary tubes or cups in which samples of the specimen are placed, since sample mix-up can also occur at the bench where testing will occur. The use of barcode labels or accession numbers can help with identification. Specimen collection and handling must be processed within guidelines that include the use of the correct anticoagulant, prompt separation of serum or plasma from the cells when required, and storage at the correct temperature prior to testing. Many laboratory tests require patient preparation or careful timing for specimen collection. Fertility hormone levels fluctuate significantly from day to day, so collecting the specimens on the correct day and labeling them with the day of the ovulatory cycle is important. For example, day three, midcyle (around day 14), and sometimes late cycle (or day 21) are common days that LH, FSH, and estradiol values are requested to assess fertility in a female patient. Males can also have LH and FSH levels measured to assess fertility, but the timing within a month is not critical. The use of well-written procedures and training of personnel for proper collection, handling, and transport of specimens is vital, particularly when specimens need to be transported to a distant site for analysis, adding a layer of separation by distance, which hampers communication.

Analytical Factors

Using well-written procedures and quality control policies can help to minimize analytical errors as well. Quality control practices include the use of quality control samples, which are analyzed in conjunction with patient samples at least once in a 24-hour period, and then use of specific rules for acceptance and rejection of analytical runs. Analytical errors are minimized when highly accurate and precise methods of analysis are chosen. Choosing methods that minimize analytical interference from common chemicals such as proteins, lipids, or other hormones is important in accurate fertility testing. For example, since LH, FSH, TSH, and hCG have virtually identical alpha polypeptide chains but unique beta polypeptide chains in their chemical makeup, assays now are specific to the whole molecule or the beta polypeptide to provide specificity for the hormone of choice. Performing daily and periodic maintenance of equipment and instruments helps to retain optimal operating conditions for instrumentation. A critical factor in the analysis of LH and FSH is the use of calibrators of different strengths. Calibrator concentration and makeup vary from method to method and can be kit dependent, so that serial changes in a patient's gonadotropin levels should be monitored from the same laboratory using the same methodology to minimize analytical changes due to calibration.[24]

Postanalytical Factors

Postanalytical variables include reporting the patient results in a timely manner and in an accepted format that can be understood and correctly interpreted by the health-care providers. Maintaining and monitoring records of patient results can sustain quality assessment practices.

Case Scenario 12-3 **Preanalytical Error in Reproductive Testing: How Important Is the Timing?**

Follow-Up

A patient in the OB/GYN clinic had a presumptive diagnosis of infertility. The physician noticed while interpreting the patient's LH, FSH, and estradiol results that all were all well below reference ranges for midcycle hormones: LH, 1.8 mIU/mL (reference range, 21.9 to 56.6 mIU/mL); FSH, 4.9 mIU/mL (6.2 to 17.2 mIU/mL); and E_2, 135 pg/mL (150 to 750 pg/mL). However, the patient provided basal body temperature records that indicated a slight peak on days 15 and 16 of her ovulatory cycle. In addition, the hormone results were within reference range for day three of the ovulatory cycle, and the dates on the specimens appeared to correspond to day three of her cycle rather than midcycle. After further discussion with the patient, the nurse determined that she had not returned at midcycle but at day three for specimen collection. Thus a preanalytical error occurred because the specimen for LH, FSH, and estradiol testing was not collected on the correct day that corresponds to the middle of her ovulatory cycle, giving falsely lower results than the presumed midcycle results. The patient was given clearer instructions for returning the next month for repeat testing of these hormones, and an appointment for collection on the correct day of her ovulatory cycle was set. ●

CASE SCENARIO 12-4

Fetal Assessment for Open Neural Tube Defects and Down Syndrome: MoM Testing for Baby's Health

A 36-year-old female had blood collected for alpha fetoprotein and other prenatal tests. The patient had a history of irregular menses, but it was determined by ultrasound and last menstrual period that she was 16 weeks pregnant. The following results were obtained: alpha fetoprotein, maternal serum at 16 weeks: 30.0 μg/L (34.8 μg/L **median**).

median - the middle value of a population

ALPHA FETOPROTEIN

Alpha fetoprotein (AFP) is the most significant protein found in the second trimester fetus. It is a transport protein produced by the fetal liver with a function similar to that of albumin in the infant or adult body fluids. Its main role is to bind and transport substances that are not very water soluble, such as steroid hormones, vitamins, lipids, and bilirubin. It is found in amniotic fluid and maternal circulation only in small amounts under normal circumstances due to its large molecular weight and inability to diffuse readily to maternal circulation from the fetoplacental circulation. AFP levels in maternal serum (MSAFP) correlate with some birth defects in the fetus. For example, MSAFP is found at lower than expected levels in Down syndrome and at higher than expected amounts in open neural tube defects.

Open Neural Tube Defects

Open neural tube defects in the fetus occur early in the first trimester as the spinal cord and brain are developing from an embryonic structure called the neural tube. These defects are termed *congenital disorders* because they are present at birth. Failure of the neural tube to fuse will lead to permanent defects in the brain and/or spinal cord to include spina bifida, **encephalocele**, and **anencephaly**. Spina bifida is also known as **meningomyocele**. It generally involves only problems with the spinal cord, resulting in progressive motor impairment. Encephalocele is a central nervous system defect involving the brain.

Encephalocele is a protrusion of brain tissue through an abnormal opening, while anencephaly is a condition in which the fetus does not develop a cerebrum. Folic acid deficiency is strongly linked to impairment in embryonic development, including neural tube defects. Open neural tube defects such as spina bifida occur in about 4 per 10,000 live births, considered frequent enough to screen in prenatal testing. It has been found that nearly 90% of fetuses with open neural tube defects provide the maternal serum with an increased amount of AFP, usually more than double the normal amount. It is likely that this transport protein leaks out into the amniotic fluid because of the anatomic deviation. Open neural tube defects of the fetus will be evident upon high-resolution ultrasound and are confirmed by an increased level of AFP in amniotic fluid.[1]

encephalocele - congenital opening in the skull with protrusion of brain tissue

anencephaly - a fatal congenital absence of or greatly reduced brain, particularly the cerebrum, resulting from failure of the neural tube to close during organ formation

meningomyocele - congenital opening in the spinal cord membranes through which the cord protrudes; also called spina bifida

Down Syndrome

Down syndrome occurs in about 1 in 800 live births, increasing in incidence in mothers over the age of 35 years. It is a serious congenital disorder of the autosomal chromosome 21 with either a **trisomy** (three copies) of the long arm, or translocations or mosaics of the long arm, generally in the q22.1 to q22.3 region. The baby with Down syndrome has serious physical and developmental problems, including congenital heart defects, growth and mental retardation, muscular weakness, flat facial profile with slanting eyes, broad short skull, broad hands with short fingers, and possible anatomic defects in the esophagus. Metabolic changes in the fetal liver and fetoplacental unit provide some biochemical markers for this syndrome in the unborn baby. A fetus with Down syndrome provides up to 25% less AFP to maternal serum, and significantly decreased amount of unconjugated estriol, but significantly increased amount of chorionic gonadotropin. These three changes in maternal serum are termed a *triple screen* for Down syndrome. An additional test, dimeric inhibin A (DIA), has been suggested, making this a quadruple screen. The definitive test for Down syndrome is fetal karyotyping from cells obtained in amniotic fluid at 18 to 20 weeks or from chorionic villi sampling at 10 weeks.[1]

trisomy - three copies of a chromosome instead of the normal two

Trisomy 18

Another profound chromosomal defect is trisomy 18 or **Edwards' syndrome**. It is rare in live births, but studies of spontaneous abortion conclude that this may be the most common cause of miscarriage and the most common chromosomal defect at conception. As the name suggests, there is an extra copy of chromosome 18, which results in open neural tube defects and death of the infant within a few months. The triple screen of maternal serum provides the same type of abnormal results as in Down syndrome, while fetal karyotyping is the definitive test and will differentiate trisomy 21 from 18.[1]

Edwards' syndrome - congenital and fatal defect of the fetus (trisomy 18) causing severe multiorgan defects, including mental deficiency

FETAL SCREENING

The occurrence of Down syndrome and open neural tube defects are frequent enough to warrant prenatal testing for these disorders. Likewise, some intervention can be performed **in utero** to correct some complications such as heart defects in Down syndrome or neural tube defects. Finally, prenatal counseling can begin early to prepare the family for a baby with one of these disorders.[25] Screening for fetal disorders such as Down syndrome or spina bifida can be done simply with maternal serum at 16 to 18 weeks of pregnancy. Like most screening tests, the medical decision limits are set so that they are sensitive for detecting the disorder and not likely to have a false negative, overlooking the presence of the disorder. Thus a negative or normal result generally indicates the fetus does not have the disorder in question. Screening tests are not definitive and require additional tests such as high-resolution ultrasound and amniocentesis to rule out false-positive results and provide a more definite result.[25] Interpretation of the screening tests depends on which disorder is being considered. For example, looking at MSAFP alone, levels are increased in open neural tube defects and decreased in Down syndrome and trisomy 18. Maternal serum AFP is also decreased if gestational age is lower than presumed or if fetal demise has occurred. IT is increased if gestational age is higher than presumed or if multiple fetuses are present. Maternal race and weight play a role in MSAFP levels as well.[1]

in utero - within the uterus

Between 16 and 20 weeks of pregnancy, the fetus is growing rapidly and many biochemical markers of disease, such as AFP levels, change significantly within 1 week. Thus timing of the test and matching it to the gestational age is very important. Since high-resolution ultrasound is not always available to more accurately assess fetal age, time since LMP is often used as an estimate. Table 12–1 lists the typical reference median values for MSAFP, according to weeks of gestation, for immunoassay methods. Use of weeks of gestation from LMP can introduce the error of falsely over- or underestimating fetal age. Likewise, multiple pregnancies can affect the interpretation of results as two fetuses can nearly double the amount of AFP found in maternal circulation. High-resolution ultrasound, when used, is the best assessment of fetal age, condition, and number of fetuses to correspond with MSAFP and other biochemical markers of fetal disease. Multiples of the median (MoM) is a statistical application of a biochemical marker that is used to normalize values for reference ranges that change readily with age or other factors. Using MoM values for MSAFP helps the physician to interpret the result compared with gestational age and estimate a reference range.[1]

MULTIPLES OF THE MEDIAN

Multiples of the median is a calculation that is used to assist in a determining a medical decision limit when values change readily and variation due to different methods and laboratory instruments is high. The calculation helps to individualize a biochemical marker's reference range and provides the most useful information to the physician for interpretation. For example, the test result for MSAFP is divided by the median for that week of gestation to give a risk factor for the disorder. Since some analytes, such as AFP, vary based on maternal race or weight, the medians can be set based on those factors as well. Thus a risk factor using MSAFP can take into account age of gestation, maternal weight, and race to give the best interpretive value. As an example, in open neural tube defects, the MSAFP is generally twice as high as the usual reference range considering gestational age, race, twins or higher order multiples, and maternal weight, so the MoM is generally 2.0.[26] Some laboratories used 2.5 as the MoM cutoff for MSAFP.[1]

Example Calculation of MoM

Studies at University Hospital found that the medians for alpha fetoprotein were lower than found in published reference books, possibly due to the method of

TABLE 12-1

Median MSAFP Versus Weeks of Gestation After LMP

Weeks of Gestation After LMP	Median MSAFP (in µg/L)
14	25.6
15	29.9
16	34.8
17	40.6
18	47.3
19	55.1
20	64.3
21	74.9

TABLE 12-2

Unconjugated Estriol (uE$_3$) Reference Ranges Versus Weeks of Gestation After LMP

Weeks of Gestation After LMP	uE$_3$ Reference Ranges (in ng/mL)
16	0.30–1.05
18	0.63–2.30

analysis used and the predominance of white patients in their population. Ms. Jones' MoM for MSAFP was calculated as follows:

Ms. Jones' MSAFP at 16 weeks' gestation since LMP was 47.0 µg/L.
MSAFP median at 16 weeks' gestation at University Hospital was 31.8 µg/L.

MoM calculation = patient MSAFP/median MSAFP = 47.0/31.8 = 1.48

Given that the common MoM medical decision limit for MSAFP is 2.0, this result of 1.48 is not considered a positive screening result for open neural tube defects, including spina bifida.

Amniocentesis is generally performed following maternal serum screening tests that fall outside of the normal reference ranges. Amniotic AFP levels help to confirm or rule out abnormalities in the maternal serum levels. The definitive test for open neural tube defects is, however, high-resolution ultrasound imaging. The definitive test for chromosomal defects is karyotyping of chorionic villi or fetal cells in amniotic fluid. There is generally a waiting period of a couple of weeks before amniocentesis can be scheduled, and it is often set for 20 weeks' gestation. This waiting period can bring considerable anxiety to the patient, particularly if counseling has not taken place. Due to false-positive results and the anxiety and expense of additional testing, some women elect to not have maternal serum screening in subsequent pregnancies. Communication with the patient about risks and benefits of prenatal testing, including causes of false-positive results, may help to alleviate some of this anxiety.[27]

Median values for unconjugated estriol and chorionic gonadotropin also change rapidly based on weeks of gestation. Therefore, the correct reference median should be used for proper interpretation of the patient's results. Tables 12–2 and 12–3 list the typical reference medians for unconjugated estriol and dimeric

THE TEAM APPROACH

The obstetrician correlates information obtained from the patient history with ultrasound and other clinical findings to determine gestational age. This is important when interpreting fetal assessment tests such as alpha fetoprotein levels. The laboratory must provide fetal age-specific reference ranges or medians for alpha fetoprotein since values change quickly in the first and second trimester fetus.

TABLE 12-3

Median Dimeric Inhibin A (DIA) Levels Versus Weeks of Gestation After LMP

Weeks of Gestation After LMP	Median DIA (in ng/L)
15	174
16	170
17	173
18	182
19	198
20	222

inhibin A versus weeks of gestation from LMP. Test Methodology 12–2 gives typical reference ranges for chorionic gonadotropin based on gestational weeks.

Case Scenario 12-4 Fetal Assessment for Open Neural Tube Defects and Down Syndrome: MoM Testing for Baby's Health

Follow-Up

A 36-year-old female had blood collected for alpha fetoprotein and other prenatal tests. The patient had a history of irregular menses, but it was determined by ultrasound and reported last menstrual period that she was 16 weeks pregnant. Alpha fetoprotein level from maternal serum at 16 weeks was 30.0 μg/L (34.8 μg/L median).

MoM calculation = patient MSAFP/median MSAFP = 30.0/34.8 = 0.86

Given that the common MoM medical decision limit for MSAFP is 2.0, this result of 0.86 is not considered a positive screening result for open neural tube defects, including spina bifida. This value appears to be lower than the reference range. ●

Alpha Fetoprotein Levels and Fetal Disorders

These questions were considered in Case Scenario 12–4:

1. *What are the causes of decreased maternal serum alpha fetoprotein levels?* Down syndrome and trisomy 18 can cause as much as a 25% decrease in MSAFP. However, other factors need to be considered, such as condition of the fetus, maternal race and age, and laboratory-to-laboratory variation in reference ranges. Misjudging the fetal age even by 1 week can influence which reference range should be considered. For example, if the patient in Case Scenario 12–4 were in fact 15 weeks pregnant, the median reference would be 29.9 μg/L.

2. *What are the causes of increased maternal serum alpha fetoprotein levels?* Open neural tube defects such as spina bifida and anencephaly can typically increase MSAFP by double or more. Twins or multiple pregnancies can also increase the result. If the fetal age is more than presumed, the wrong reference range may be used. For example, if the patient in Case Scenario 12–4 were 17 weeks pregnant, the median reference would be 40.6 μg/L.

3. *Are there additional tests that can be performed to confirm or rule out these fetal disorders?* Quantitative hCG, unconjugated estriol, and dimeric inhibin A (DIA) levels, along with AFP, can be used to predict the likelihood of these fetal disorders. This is called the quadruple screen. Using age-adjusted reference ranges is important, and substituting a median value based on gestational age and performing the multiples of the median (MoM) calculation to compare with a medical decision limit can improve the interpretation. The definitive test for Down syndrome and trisomy 18 is karyotyping of fetal cells from amniotic fluid. Amniotic fluid AFP levels can be used to confirm MSAFP interpretation, along with visualization of the fetus with high-resolution imaging techniques.

OTHER SIGNIFICANT BIRTH DEFECTS AND INBORN ERRORS OF METABOLISM

Several birth defects causing inborn errors of metabolism occur frequently enough that neonatal screening is fairly common. These inborn errors of metabolism include phenylketonuria, galactosemia, branched-chain amino acid metabolic disorders, and tyrosinemia. Galactosemia was discussed in Chapter 4 (Diabetes and Other Carbohydrate Disorders).

Phenylketonuria (PKU) occurs in 1 of every 25,000 live births. It results from a congenital absence of the enzyme phenylalanine hydroxylase, which converts phenylalanine into tyrosine.

Branched-chain amino acid disorders occur less frequently than PKU, and one common form is called maple syrup urine disease (MSUD). Maple syrup urine disease was so named because one of the early indications of its presence is that the urine of a newborn with this condition has a sweet odor. It is a disease in which branched-chain ketoacid dehydrogenase complex is lacking, resulting in an accumulation of valine, leucine, and isoleucine in blood and the associated metabolites in urine. The untreated disorder results in poor growth, poor muscle tone, and brain toxicity in the neonate. Homocystinuria occurs at about the same frequency as MSUD but is due to an enzyme defect in cystathionine beta-synthase causing skeletal abnormalities and mental developmental delays.

Tyrosinemia is also less common than PKU, but also has profound effects in the neonate if undetected and untreated. Infantile tyrosinemia (type I) is generally due to absence of fumarylacetoacetase, which causes multiple problems including liver and kidney disease that results in nodular replacement of normal functional tissue. If left untreated, tyrosinemia is generally fatal within the first 12 months of life, usually from liver failure. There are other types and causes of tyrosinemia as well, but infantile tyrosinemia is the main one detected in neonatal testing.

Table 12–4 summarizes common metabolic testing in newborns to detect inborn errors of metabolism. Complex confirmatory testing is now available, including enzyme assays and definitive amino acid quantification using liquid chromatography with mass spectrometry. Some gene testing is available.[28]

CLINICAL CORRELATION
As a result of PKU, phenylalanine accumulates in the blood and body fluids and seriously impairs nerve development in the newborn. Since phenylalanine is not produced in the body but only supplied by diet, this disease can be controlled by a special diet to prevent accumulation of phenylalanine.

✓ **Common Sense Check**
Neonatal testing is often performed before a baby is named, so identification is listed with the mother's last name. For example, the baby of Ms. Doe would be named "Baby Doe" but would be given his or her own identification number. It is important to verify the identification number as well as the name for neonatal testing.

TABLE 12-4

Neonatal Metabolic Testing of PKU, MSUD, and other Inborn Errors of Metabolism

Disorders	Lab Testing	Inborn Error
PKU	Excess phenylalanine in serum, excess phenylpyruvic acid in urine	Absence of phenylalanine hydroxylase
MSUD	Valine, leucine, and isoleucine in urine	Absence of branched-chain ketoacid dehydrogenase
Galactosemia	Excess galactose and galactose 1-phosphate in serum and urine	Galactose-1-phosphate uridyltransferase
Homocystinuria	Excess homocysteine and methionine in serum and urine	Cystathionine beta-synthase
Tyrosinemia	Excess tyrosine in serum and urine	Absence of fumarylacetoacetase

TABLE 12-5

Physiological Differences in Neonates Compared to Adults

Analytes	Reference Ranges in Neonates	Reference Ranges in Adults
Bilirubin	2.0–6.0 mg/dL (0–1 day) 6.0–10.0 mg/dL (1–2 day)	0–2.0 mg/dL
Creatinine	0.3–1.0 mg/dL (2–4 day) 0.2–0.4 mg/dL (1 wk–2 yr)	0.9–1.3 mg/dL
Glucose	40–60 mg/dL (1 day) 50–80 mg/dL (2 day–2 yr)	74–100 mg/dL
Oxygen (PO_2)	8–24 mm Hg (at birth) 33–75 mm Hg (5–10 min) 55–80 mm Hg (1 hr) 54–95 mm Hg (1 day)	83–108 mm Hg
Potassium	3.7–5.9 mmol/L (newborn) 4.1–5.3 mmol/L (1 wk–2 yr)	3.5–4.5 mmol/L
Thyroxine, total	11.8–22.6 μg/dL (1–3 day) 9.9–16.6 μg/dL (1–2 wk) 7.2–14.4 μg/dL (1–4 mo) 7.8–16.5 μg/dL (4–12 mo) 7.3–15.0 μg/dL (1–5 yr)	4.6–10.5 μg/dL
TSH	1.0–39.0 μIU/mL (0–4 day) 1.7–9.1 μIU/mL (2–20 wk) 0.7–64.0 μIU/mL (21 wk–20 yr)	0.4–4.2 μIU/mL

REFERENCE RANGES IN NEONATES

There are some physiological differences between neonates and older children or adults, as indicated by laboratory results. As mentioned in an earlier chapter, newborn babies have slower renal and hepatic functions in the first few days of life affecting many biochemical substances, including carbohydrates and waste products. Therapeutic drug levels may have different therapeutic ranges for neonates and children than for adults. Examples of these differences are illustrated in Tables 12–5 and 12–6. Physiological changes due to pregnancy from fetal and maternal hormones also result in changes in reference ranges for some analytes.

TABLE 12-6

Physiological Differences in Children Compared to Adults

Analytes	Reference Ranges in Children	Reference Ranges in Adults
Alkaline phosphatase	54–369 U/L (4–15 yr)	53–128 U/L
Creatinine	0.3–0.7 mg/dL (2–12 yr) 0.5–1.0 mg/dL (adolescent)	0.9–1.3 mg/dL
Glucose	60–100 mg/dL	74–100 mg/dL
Lead	0–10 μg/dL	0–25 μg/dL
Potassium	3.4–4.7 mmol/L	3.5–4.5 mmol/L
Thyroxine, total	6.4–13.3 μg/dL (5–10 yr) 5.6–11.7 μg/dL (10–15 yr)	4.6–10.5 μg/dL

TABLE 12-7

Physiological Changes in Normal Pregnancy[1]

Analyte	Third Trimester Pregnancy Compared to Nonpregnant State
Urea nitrogen	Decreased by 25%
Creatinine	Decreased by 20%
Bilirubin	Decreased by 20%
Albumin	Decreased by 20%
PTH	Increased by 35%
Alkaline phosphatase	Nearly quadrupled
Transferrin	Nearly doubled
Cholesterol and LDL-cholesterol	Increased by 50%
HDL-cholesterol	Increased by 30%
Fasting triglycerides	Nearly quadrupled
Ferritin	Decreased by 50%
TSH	Increased by 40%
Cortisol	Nearly tripled
Fibrinogen	Increased by 50%

Typical changes in common laboratory results in a pregnant woman are indicated in Table 12–7.

CASE SCENARIO 12-5

Hemolytic Disease of the Newborn: Two Rh-Negative Mothers

Betty Martin and Lisa Johnson were both waiting for the results of amniotic fluid analyses. Both women had Rh-negative blood types and the fathers of their unborn children had Rh-positive blood types. Both women had been pregnant before and were now in the 34th week of gestation. Prenatal antibody studies showed that both mothers had developed antibodies to Rh factor. Betty Martin had a low **antibody titer** and Lisa Johnson had a high antibody titer. Ultrasound imaging suggested there was fluid accumulation in fetal tissue of both pregnant women, but results were not conclusive. The physician was concerned about risk for development of erythroblastosis fetalis, or hemolytic disease of the newborn, in both fetuses.

antibody titer - measure of the amount of antibody against a particular antigen present in the blood

DEVELOPMENT OF HEMOLYTIC DISEASE OF THE NEWBORN

Hemolytic disease of the newborn, or erythroblastosis fetalis, is a condition that occurs when there is an incompatibility between the expressed blood groups of the mother and the fetus. The disease process develops when the blood cells of the mother come in contact with incompatible cells. Such contact may occur when the mother's cells come in contact with incompatible cells through transfusion or through contact with an infant's blood during pregnancy. The mother's immune system recognizes the incompatible cells as foreign and develops antibodies against them. The mother becomes sensitized to these cells. If the immune process is begun when an infant is delivered, the antibodies will not affect that infant. However, antibody may be directed against blood cells of a subsequent pregnancy of a fetus with incompatible blood.

Antibodies may cross the placenta, destroying the red blood cells of the fetus. If the destruction process is directed against the fetus, the disease is called *erythroblastosis fetalis*. If the disease develops in the newborn, the disease is called *hemolytic disease of the newborn*. Rh, or D, antigens are the most common antigens associated with the incompatibility that will require intervention. However, other blood group antigens have been linked to the disease.[23,29]

Antibody attack on the fetus or newborn red blood cells lyses the cell membranes. The fetus or newborn reacts to this hemolytic process by producing new red blood cells quickly and releasing them into the peripheral blood. Some of the cells that are released are immature blast forms of the erythrocyte blood cell series, thus the term *erythroblastosis fetalis*.

The lysed cells release hemoglobin, which is converted to bilirubin in the spleen, liver, and bone marrow. As a fat-insoluble substance, the excess bilirubin is deposited in lipid-rich tissues of the skin as yellow coloration, known as jaundice. The symptoms of hemolytic disease can range in severity. Mild hyperbilirubinemia may be cleared by the placenta and detoxified by the maternal liver. As the hemolysis increases, the liver of the fetus becomes enlarged with the efforts of clearing cell remnants. In the fetus, fluid accumulates within the tissues and **hydrops fetalis** develops. In hyperbilirubinemia of severe hemolytic disease of the newborn, bilirubin infiltrates may be deposited in the brain. This accumulation is called **kernicterus**. Kernicterus may lead to brain damage and death of the newborn.

Diagnosis of erythroblastosis fetalis or hemolytic disease of the newborn is based on sequential investigation of the disease process. First, the mother's blood is tested for antibodies. Antibody studies are routine testing procedures for Rh-negative mothers. Testing includes analysis for $Rh_o(D)$ antibody and for other antibody systems. Ultrasound imaging may follow the discovery of presence of antibody. Ultrasound may be used to identify fetal liver or spleen enlargement and to assess fluid buildup in fetal tissues. Positive findings on ultrasound imaging may lead to amniocentesis. Through this procedure, the amniotic fluid that surrounds fetus is sampled for analysis. The severity of fetal hemolysis may be determined through assessing the bilirubin concentration of the amniotic fluid.[30] The procedure for testing bilirubin in amniotic fluid is discussed in Test Methodology 12–6. The Liley chart (Fig. 12–7) is used to interpret the spectral scan of amniotic fluid for bilirubin.[31]

hydrops fetalis - stasis of fluids in tissue spaces, secondary to loss of albumin, leading to a condition in infants of hepatosplenomegaly and respiratory and circulatory distress

kernicterus - yellow staining of the lipid-rich meninges of the brain and spinal cord due to bilirubin infiltrates

TEST METHODOLOGY 12-6.   BILIRUBIN SCAN IN AMNIOTIC FLUID

The amniotic fluid bilirubin scan is used to evaluate fetal hemolysis, which helps determine the presence and severity of hemolytic disease of the newborn. The degree of hemolysis is assessed by a spectrophotometric method at an optical density of 450 nm. This spectrophotometric method measures the change in absorbance of bilirubin from amniotic fluid and alerts the physician when intervention may be necessary.

The Reaction Principle

The specimen is scanned by a spectrophotometer from 350-nm to 550-nm wavelengths of light. A change in absorbance (ΔA) at 450 nm corresponds to the amount of bilirubin present. Change in absorbance is plotted on a Liley chart (see Fig. 12-7, ΔA vs. gestational age), and the degree of severity is evaluated by a zone method.

continued

TEST METHODOLOGY 12-6. **BILIRUBIN SCAN IN AMNIOTIC FLUID** *(continued)*

Interpretation of the Liley chart is as follows:

Zone 1: no intervention necessary
Zone 2: monitor for development of disease
Zone 3: severe disease

Interferences

Excessive exposure to light, grossly bloody specimens, or specimens contaminated with meconium (fetal feces) may interfere with test results.

The Specimen

Amniotic fluid after the first 2 or 3 mL of the specimen, which are discarded, is stored in an amber-colored conical centrifuge tube and protected from light. The specimen will be centrifuged or filtered before analysis.

Reference Range

Zone 1 in Liley chart is considered low risk.

At birth, the newborn fetal umbilical cord blood may be tested for bilirubin, blood type, and presence of antibody. Sequential testing of newborn blood will assess the extent of bilirubinemia and the change over time of bilirubin concentration.

Treatment for erythroblastosis fetalis or hemolytic disease of the newborn is based on the extent of hyperbilirubinemia and anemia, the age of the infant, whether the infant was born close to full term or not, and the general health of the

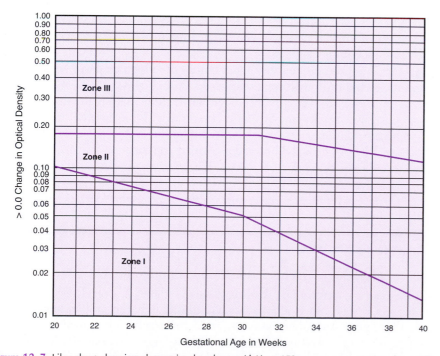

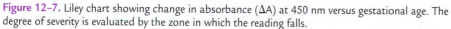
Figure 12–7. Liley chart showing change in absorbance (ΔA) at 450 nm versus gestational age. The degree of severity is evaluated by the zone in which the reading falls.

infant. Treatment during pregnancy may include intrauterine blood transfusion of the fetus. Intrauterine blood transfusion may be necessary if the hemolytic process causes severe anemia. If testing of the amniotic fluid shows that the fetus has mature lungs, early delivery may be induced to prevent influx of additional maternal antibody. After birth, hyperbilirubinemia may be treated with **phototherapy**. Exchange transfusion is accomplished by withdrawing damaged blood and replacing it with donor blood in small amounts. Exchange transfusion of the newborn's blood may be considered if the bilirubin level approaches 16 to 20 mg/dL to prevent kernicterus.

Hemolytic disease of the newborn may be prevented with early prenatal care. If the Rh-negative mother is identified early in her first pregnancy, the probability for developing **sensitization** to incompatible antigens may be lessened. The Rh-negative mother may be given $Rh_o(D)$ immune globulin, which prevents maternal sensitization to fetal $Rh_o(D)$-positive cells. The Rh-negative mother should receive the first dose of the immune globulin at the 28th week of gestation and the second dose within 72 hours after birth of the child.

phototherapy - exposure to sunlight or artificial ultraviolet light for therapeutic purposes, such as treating neonatal hyperbilirubinemia

sensitization - production of antibody as a response to antigen exposure

---

Case Scenario 12-5 Hemolytic Disease of the Newborn: Two Rh-Negative Mothers

Follow-Up

The results of the bilirubin scans on amniotic fluid were as follows:

Test	Betty Martin	Lisa Johnson
Optical density units	0.02	0.2
Zone interpretation	1	3

The interpretation of the spectrophotometry scan at 450 nm showed that Betty Martin's fetus is mildly affected by the hemolytic process of antibody destruction. Ms. Martin will be monitored at 2-week intervals to assess the development of further hemolysis. Antibody titer, ultrasound imaging for size of the fetus, and amniocentesis for bilirubin scan will be performed. If these test results do not change toward higher zones, the pregnancy will be allowed to continue to full term with spontaneous delivery.

The interpretation of Lisa Johnson's amniotic fluid analysis shows that her fetus requires much more immediate treatment. Ms. Johnson's fetus is severely affected by the hemolytic process as indicated by the higher zone with the Liley chart. The physician will consider treating the fetus or delivering the child before more destruction can occur. This situation is discussed in the next case scenario. ●

CASE SCENARIO 12-6

Fetal Lung Maturity: Is This Baby Mature Enough for Early Delivery?

The physician has determined that Ms. Johnson's fetus is severely affected by hemolysis as a result of blood type incompatibility between mother and fetus. The concern now is whether the fetus can be delivered soon to avoid further damage from hemolysis. First, fetal lung maturity must be assessed. The physician requests fetal lung maturity tests on the amniotic fluid.

FETAL LUNG MATURITY

In Case Scenario 12–6, the physician may consider using **glucocorticoids** for improving fetal lung maturity. Steroid drugs will cause premature liberation of **surfactant** from the **alveoli** and the possibility for increasing synthesis of lung surfactant. **Pneumocytes**, two cell types that form the alveoli of the lung, are involved in fetal lung function. Type I pneumocytes are simple squamous epithelial cells that provide gaseous exchange; type II pneumocytes produce surfactant. Steroid drugs will cross the placenta and, at 34 weeks' gestation, can assist type II pneumocytes to release surfactant.[32–34] The physician may also consider intrauterine transfusion to transfer intact red blood cells into the fetus to replace fetal red blood cells that have been lysed by antibody.

However, at 34 weeks of gestation, the physician will also consider delivering the baby prematurely to prevent further red blood cell destruction. The question to consider for this procedure is, "Is this baby mature enough for early delivery?" If the baby is delivered before the lungs have had time to fully mature, neonatal **respiratory distress syndrome** (RDS; also called hyaline membrane disease) may result. Respiratory distress syndrome is caused by the inability of immature lungs to produce pulmonary surfactant, the lipid conjugate that reduces surface tension in the lungs and promotes inflation of the lungs.

Laboratory testing for lung maturity is important in management of hemolytic disease of the newborn and in other conditions in which the fetus may be delivered prematurely, such as **premature labor, premature rupture of membranes, preeclampsia**, and **eclampsia**. The results of these tests are used to determine whether to attempt to suppress labor or to induce delivery.

Pre-eclampsia usually appears during the second half of pregnancy, generally after the 20th week. Also referred to as *toxemia of pregnancy*, pre-eclampsia is a condition that pregnant women can develop. It is marked by specific symptoms including water retention (with swelling particularly in the feet, legs, and hands), high blood pressure, and protein in the urine. All three symptoms must be present at the same time for a diagnosis of pre-eclampsia.

In the mature fetus, pulmonary surfactant is rich in phosphatidylcholine (lecithin) and phosphatidylglycerol (PG). The production of these phospholipids may be measured as an absolute concentration or as a ratio with another lipid, sphingomyelin, a nonpulmonary lipid whose concentration is relatively constant in amniotic fluid. Assessment of the ratio allows for variations of concentrations of lipids inherent in the collection of amniotic fluid by amniocentesis. A lecithin-to-sphingomyelin ratio, or L/S ratio, of greater than 2 suggests lung maturity. An L/S ratio of less than 2 would indicate a need to delay delivery as long as possible to allow time for lecithin production.

Case Scenario 12-6 Fetal Lung Maturity: Is This Baby Mature Enough for Early Delivery?

Lung Maturity Testing in Ms. Johnson's Fetus

At the physician's request, the laboratory tested Ms. Johnson's amniotic fluid for phosphatidylglycerol (PG). The semiquantitative immunologic agglutination test was reported as positive. A positive PG test correlates well with the presence of this phospholipid by thin-layer chromatography and with the absence of subsequent respiratory distress syndrome.

---

glucocorticoids - adrenal cortical hormones primarily active in protecting against stress and affecting protein and carbohydrate metabolism

surfactant - a substance that reduces the surface tension of the moist surfaces of solid tissue

alveoli - sacs at the end of air ducts in the lungs and in contact with capillaries that allow gases to diffuse in or out (singular: alveolus)

pneumocytes - two types (I and II) of cells that form the alveoli of the lungs

respiratory distress syndrome (RDS) - severe impairment of respiratory function in a preterm newborn due to immaturity of the enzymatic system essential for pulmonary surfactant production

premature labor - labor that begins between 20 and 38 weeks' gestation

premature rupture of membranes - rupture of amniotic membrane prior to the time labor is expected

pre-eclampsia - a complication of pregnancy characterized by increasing hypertension, proteinuria, and edema

THE TEAM APPROACH

Disease of the mother and child in pregnancy must be assessed from an interdisciplinary approach. The laboratory must collaborate to provide the physician with information about the clinical chemistry of the disease, the blood cell assessment, and the immunohematology results.

eclampsia - coma and convulsive seizures of the mother between week 20 of pregnancy and the end of the first week after birth

AMNIOTIC FLUID COLLECTION

The primary function of amniotic fluid is to provide a protective cushion for the fetus, allow for movement, and regulate temperature. Amniocentesis is the fluid collection procedure in which a sample of the amniotic fluid surrounding a fetus is removed by means of a fine needle inserted through the abdomen and into the uterus of the pregnant woman.

Amniocentesis is commonly performed for women whose pregnancies may be high risk. These risk factors include age of the mother over 35 years, diabetic mothers, mothers who have other children who have a genetic problem, mothers who have had an abnormal serum triple screen test (AFP, estriol, and hCG) and mothers who are Rh sensitized. Laboratory testing of amniotic fluid involves analysis of bilirubin, AFP, and a variety of tests for fetal lung maturity (FLM). Prenatal testing of several fetal disorders using amniotic fluid first occurs between 14 and 20 weeks' gestation. Fetal cells in the fluid can be tested in the laboratory and studied to detect the presence of certain genetic disorders or physical abnormalities, and examined to determine the gender of the fetus. During the third trimester of pregnancy but less than 35 to 36 weeks' gestation, fluid collected from the amniocentesis procedure is analyzed to evaluate FLM.

Ultrasound examination is always performed before an amniocentesis to determine the location of the fetus during the procedure. The use of the ultrasound image can determine gestational age and the placement of the fetus and placenta, and evaluate if enough amniotic fluid is present. Amniocentesis can be considered when enough amniotic fluid is present, starting at about 14 weeks' gestation.

Exchanges of water and chemicals take place between the fluid, the fetus, and the maternal circulation. After the first trimester, the amniotic fluid is composed mainly of fetal urine and is the major contributor to the fluid volume. Fetal swallowing of the amniotic fluid regulates the increase in amniotic fluid from the fetal urine. Therefore, amniotic fluid is representative of fetal metabolism.

A maximum of 30 mL of fluid can be collected. The first 2 or 3 mL should be discarded because they may contain maternal blood, tissue fluid, and maternal cells. Sterile plastic syringes and conical centrifuge tubes should be used for the collection and transportation of the amniotic fluid. Specimens for cytogenetic studies are maintained at 25° to 37°C incubation prior to analysis to prolong the life of the cells needed for analysis. Specimens should not be frozen, refrigerated, or centrifuged. Specimens for FLM tests should be placed in ice for delivery to the laboratory and refrigerated prior to testing. The specimen will be centrifuged or filtered before analysis. Specimens for bilirubin analysis in cases of hemolytic disease of the newborn must be protected from light. The sample should be collected in an amber-colored tube. The appearance of the amniotic fluid can indicate the presence of certain chemicals. For example, degree of redness indicates presence of hemoglobin. Table 12–8 correlates various colors of amniotic fluid with presence of chemicals and associated disease states.

✓ **Common Sense Check**
Any specimen that will be tested for bilirubin should be protected from light.

Visual Inspection

During the first and second trimesters, amniotic fluid is yellow and clear. It becomes colorless in the third trimester. By 33 to 34 weeks' gestation, cloudiness and woolly aggregates are noted, and, as term approaches, turbidity appears. Amniotic fluid with obvious turbidity will usually have a mature L/S ratio.

TABLE 12-8

Significance of Amniotic Fluid Color

Color	Significance
Colorless	Normal
Blood-streaked	Traumatic tap, abdominal trauma, intra-amniotic hemorrhage
Yellow	Hemolytic disease of the newborn (HDN), bilirubin
Dark green	Meconium (first bowel movement)
Dark red-brown	Fetal death

TESTS FOR FETAL LUNG MATURITY

Surfactant Test

An FLM test checks the development of an unborn baby's lungs to see if the baby will be able to breathe on his or her own after birth. The test is performed on amniotic fluid. Fetal lung maturity testing is performed when early delivery of the baby may be likely or necessary. The results of the test assess surfactant, a surface-active lipoprotein mixture that coats the fetal alveoli and prevents collapse of the lungs by reducing the surface tension of pulmonary fluids. Some of this secreted surfactant reaches the amniotic fluid, which allows laboratory assessment of FLM. Two compounds, lecithin and PG, are surfactants present in 10% and 70% of total phospholipid concentration, respectively, and can be measured by the laboratory. In high enough levels, these surfactants allow contraction and expansion of the neonatal alveoli.[35] Test Methodologies 12–7 through 12–10 describe laboratory tests for the evaluation of fetal lung maturity.

TEST METHODOLOGY 12-7.   MEASUREMENT OF SURFACTANT FUNCTION: FOAM STABILITY INDEX

This test appears to be a reliable predictor of fetal lung maturity. Subsequent respiratory distress syndrome (RDS) is very unlikely with a foam stability index (FSI) value of 47 or higher. The methodology is simple, and the test can be performed at any time of day by persons who have had only minimal instruction. The assay appears to be extremely sensitive, with a high proportion of immature results being associated with RDS, as well as moderately specific, with a high proportion of mature results predicting the absence of RDS.

The Reaction Principle

The test is based on the manual FSI, a variation of the amniotic fluid "shaken" test. The kit currently available contains test wells with a predispensed volume of ethanol. The addition of 0.5 mL of amniotic fluid to each test well in the kit produces final ethanol volumes of 44% to 50%. A control well contains sufficient surfactant in 50% ethanol to produce an example of the stable foam endpoint.

The amniotic fluid–ethanol mixture is first shaken, and then the FSI value is read as the highest value well in which a ring of stable foam persists.

continued

TEST METHODOLOGY 12-7.   MEASUREMENT OF SURFACTANT FUNCTION: FOAM STABILITY INDEX (continued)

Interferences

Contamination of the amniotic fluid specimen by blood or meconium invalidates the FSI results. The FSI can function well as a screening test.

The Specimen

Amniotic fluid after the first 2 or 3 mL, which are discarded, is collected in a sterile plastic syringe and placed in a conical centrifuge tube. Amniotic fluid is transported in ice for delivery to the laboratory and refrigerated prior to testing. The specimen will be centrifuged or filtered before analysis.

Reference Range

Positive with fetal lung maturity.

TEST METHODOLOGY 12-8.   PHOSPHATIDYLGLYCEROL

Phosphatidylglycerol (PG) is a phospholipid produced by mature type II pneumocytes that reduces the surface tension of the moist surfaces of the alveolar tissue and prevents collapse during gaseous exchange.

The Reaction Principle

A rapid immunologic semiquantitative agglutination test (Amniostat-FLM) can be used to determine the presence of PG. The test can detect PG at a concentration >0.5 μg/mL. It takes 20 to 30 minutes to perform and requires only 1.5 mL of amniotic fluid. A positive Amniostat-FLM correlates well with the presence of PG by thin-layer chromatography and the absence of subsequent RDS. It can be applied to samples contaminated by blood and meconium.

The Specimen

Amniotic fluid after the first 2 or 3 mL, which are discarded, is collected in a sterile plastic syringe and placed in a conical centrifuge tube. Amniotic fluid is transported in ice for delivery to the laboratory and refrigerated prior to testing. The specimen will be centrifuged or filtered before analysis.

Reference Ranges

Positive with fetal lung maturity.

TEST METHODOLOGY 12-9.   FLUORESCENT POLARIZATION FLM/TDx® TEST

As the fetus matures, the surfactant lipid increases and the fluorescent polarization (FP) decreases. A ratio of 50 to 70 mg surfactant per gram of albumin is considered a sign of mature fetal lungs. Fluorescent dye is added to the sample and reacts with surfactant phospholipids and albumin found in the amniotic fluid.

continued

TEST METHODOLOGY 12-9. FLUORESCENT POLARIZATION

FLM/TDx® TEST (continued)

The Reaction Principle

The Abbott TDx analyzer is an automated fluorescence polarimeter used to determine surfactant/albumin ratio. The test requires 1 mL of amniotic fluid and can be run in less than 1 hour. The results are quantitative, and changes in the results indicate changes in the risk of RDS. The procedure runs on an automated platform and is based on the partitioning of a fluorescent dye between surfactant phospholipid (low polarization) and albumin (high polarization). The TDx test correlates well with the L/S ratio and has few falsely mature results, making it an excellent screening test. However, hemolysis may interfere with testing.[32,36,37]

The Specimen

Amniotic fluid after the first 2 or 3 mL, which are discarded, is collected in a sterile plastic syringe and placed in a conical centrifuge tube. Amniotic fluid is transported in ice for delivery to the laboratory and refrigerated prior to testing. The specimen will be centrifuged or filtered before analysis.

Reference Range

Fetal lung maturity: ratio of milligrams of surfactant per gram of albumin of 50/1 to 70/1.

TEST METHODOLOGY 12-10. OPTICAL DENSITY OF AMNIOTIC FLUID

The optical density (OD) of amniotic fluid can relate to the amount of surfactants present, which is related to fetal lung maturity. Optical density is another term for light absorbance.

The Reaction Principle

This method is thought to evaluate the turbidity changes in amniotic fluid that are dependent on the total amniotic fluid phospholipid concentration. An OD of 0.15 or greater at a wavelength of 650 nm correlates extremely well with a mature L/S ratio and the absence of RDS. Contamination with blood or meconium invalidates the results.

The Specimen

Amniotic fluid after the first 2 or 3 mL, which are discarded, is collected in a sterile plastic syringe and placed in a conical centrifuge tube. Amniotic fluid is transported in ice for delivery to the laboratory and refrigerated prior to testing. The specimen will be centrifuged or filtered before analysis.

Reference Range

Positive for amniotic fluid fetal lung surfactants.

Other Fetal Lung Maturity Tests

Other tests for the evaluation of fetal lung maturity include lamellar body counts and the L/S ratio. Lamellar bodies are the storage form of surfactant and are similar in size to normal platelets. Thus they can be counted on a cell counter similar to a hematology analyzer. A count of these bodies estimates the amount of surfactant present. The test requires less than 1 mL of amniotic fluid and takes 15 minutes to perform. A lamellar body count greater than 30,000/μL is highly predictive of pulmonary maturity, while a count less than 10,000/μL suggests a risk for RDS. Neither meconium nor lysed blood has an effect on the lamellar body count. The lamellar body cell count provides an accurate estimate of surfactant in diabetic women, who may have elevated lipid concentrations as a result of diabetic pathology. The lamellar body count method has been shown to be faster and less technique dependent than traditional phospholipid analysis. This technique has a sensitivity that is comparable to analysis of phospholipids and a specificity that is slightly lower than more traditional methods.[32,38–40]

Historically, the L/S ratio has been the most valuable assay for the assessment of fetal pulmonary maturity. From 18 to 32 weeks, levels of lecithing and sphingomyelin are equal to each other and the L/S ratio remains 1.0. Lecithin then rises rapidly, and an L/S ratio of 2.0 is observed at 35 weeks. A ratio of 2.0 or greater has repeatedly been associated with pulmonary maturity. The thin-layer chromatography method is labor intensive (taking 3 to 5 hours to perform) and is a complex, poorly reproducible procedure. Most laboratories should send this test out to a reference laboratory.

A mature L/S ratio of 2.0 predicts the absence of RDS in 98% of neonates. With a ratio of 1.5 to 1.9, approximately 50% of infants will develop RDS. Below 1.5, the risk of subsequent RDS increases to 73%. Thus the L/S ratio, like most indices of fetal pulmonary maturation, rarely errs when predicting fetal pulmonary maturity but is frequently incorrect when predicting subsequent RDS. Many neonates with an immature L/S ratio will not develop RDS.

Case Scenario 12-6 Fetal Lung Maturity: Is This Baby Mature Enough for Early Delivery?

Follow-Up

On the basis of the PG test in an amniotic fluid specimen, Ms. Johnson's fetus appeared to have adequate lung maturity, and labor was induced to prevent influx of additional maternal antibody because of erythroblastosis fetalis. Ms. Johnson delivered a small baby girl. After birth, the baby's hyperbilirubinemia was treated with phototherapy. Since bilirubin levels approached 16 mg/dL, exchange transfusion was accomplished by withdrawing damaged blood and replacing it with donor blood in small amounts. Although the newborn did not develop respiratory distress syndrome, she was also monitored closely for adequate oxygenation during the first 3 days of her life. ●

SUMMARY

The laboratory provides qualitative and quantitative data to help the health-care provider make decisions about treatment for the pregnant woman and unborn child. An understanding of the developing physiology of the fetus is used to predict outcome by assessing chemical changes in the mother and fetus. In assessing the mother and fetus, a team approach within the laboratory is necessary. Hematologic and immunohematologic changes must be correlated with clinical chemistry changes of body fluid analysis.

EXERCISES

As you consider the scenarios presented in this chapter, answer the following questions:

1. Describe human chorionic gonadotropin in terms of typical amounts found in serum or urine in normal pregnancy, ectopic pregnancy, and threatened spontaneous abortion.

2. Describe the chemical makeup of hCG, FSH, LH, and estradiol as they relate to principles of analysis using specific antibody.

3. Differentiate qualitative and quantitative hCG in terms of principle of method and uses.

4. List the main causes of hemolytic disease of the newborn.

5. Diagram the testing algorithm that may be used to assess erythroblastosis fetalis of the fetus.

6. Describe the methodology that is used to measure increased bilirubin in amniotic fluid.

7. Describe chemical changes that occur in the developing fetal lung.

8. Explain how the knowledge of the chemical changes that occur in the developing fetal lung is used to assess fetal lung maturity.

References

1. Red-Horse K, et al: Trophoblast differentiation during embryo implantation and formation of the maternal-fetal interface. *J Clin Invest* 2004; 114:744–754.
2. Carr BR, Bradshaw KD: Disorders of the ovary and female reproductive tract. In Fauci A, et al (eds): *Harrison's Principle of Internal Medicine*, ed 14. New York: McGraw-Hill, 1998.
3. Barnhart KT, et al: Symptomatic patients with an early viable intrauterine pregnancy: hCG curves redefined. *Obstet Gynecol* 2004; 104:50–55.
4. Haymond S, Gronowski AM: Reproductive related disorders. In Burtis CA, Ashwood ER, Bruns DE (eds): *Tietz Textbook of Clinical Chemistry and Molecular Diagnostics*. Philadelphia: WB Saunders, 2006.
5. Higgins TN, et al: Measurment of inaccuracy and imprecision of HCG methods using dilutions of WHO 4th IS-HCG standard and a pregnant patient's serum. *Clin Biochem* 2004; 37:152–154.
6. Tenore JL: Ectopic pregnancy. *Am Fam Physician* 2000; 62:000–000.
7. Wenk RE: Laboratory aspects of gestation management. In Henry JB (ed): *Clinical Diagnosis and Management by Laboratory Methods*, ed 20. Philadelphia: WB Saunders, 2001.
8. Barnhart K, et al: Decline of serum human chorionic gonadotropin and spontaneous complete abortion: defining the normal curve. *Obstet Gynecol* 2004; 104:975–981.
9. Beers M, Berkow R: *The Merck Manual of Diagnosis and Therapy*, ed 17. Rahway, NJ: Merck & Co., 1999.
10. Murray H, et al: Diagnosis and treatment of ectopic pregnancy. *CMAJ* 2005; 173:1503.
11. Young RC: Gynecologic malignancies. In Fauci A, et al (eds): *Harrison's Principle of Internal Medicine*, ed 14. New York: McGraw-Hill, 1998.
12. Smyth CD, et al: Ovarian thecal interstitial androgen synthesis is enhanced by a FSH-stimulated mechanism. *Endocrinology* 1993; 133:1532–1538.
13. Groome NP, et al: Measurement of dimeric inhibin-B throughout the human menstrual cycle. *J Clin Endocrinol Metab* 1996; 81:1401–1405.
14. Welt CK, et al: Frequency modulation of follicle-stimulating hormone (FSH) during the luteal-follicular transition: evidence for FSH control of inhibin B in normal women. *J Clin Endocrinol Metab* 1997; 82:2645–2652.

15. Klein NA, et al: Reproductive aging: accelerated ovarian follicular development associated with a monotropic FSH rise in normal women. *J Clin Endocrinol Metab* 1996; 81:1038–1045.

16. Danforth DR, et al: Dimeric inhibin: a direct marker of ovarian aging. *Fertil Steril* 1998; 70:119–123.

17. Rossing MA, et al: Ovarian tumors in a cohort of infertile women. *N Engl J Med* 1994; 331:771–776.

18. Jenkins JM, et al: Comparison of "poor" responders with "good" responders using a standard baseline/HMG regime for IVF. *Hum Reprod* 1991; 6:918–921.

19. Van Rysselberge M, et al: Fertility prognosis in IVF treatment of patients with cancelled cycles. *Hum Reprod* 1989; 4:663–666.

20. Sher G, Fisch JD: Vaginal sildenafil (*Viagra*): a preliminary report of a novel method to improve uterine artery blood flow and endometrial development in patients undergoing IVF. *Hum Reprod* 2000; 15:806–809.

21. Sher G, Fisch JD: Effect of vaginal sildenafil on the outcome of in vitro fertilization (IVF) after multiple IVF failures attributed to poor endometrial development. *Fertil Steril* 2002; 78:1073–1076.

22. Sarkar S, Henry JB: Andrology laboratory and fertility assessment. In Henry JB (ed): *Clinical Diagnosis and Management by Laboratory Methods*, ed 20. Philadelphia: WB Saunders, 2001.

23. Bevis DA: Blood pigments in haemolytic disease of the newborn. *J Obstet Gynaecol Br Emp* 1956; 63:68–75.

24. Demers LM, Vance ML: Pituitary function. In Burtis CA, Ashwood ER, Bruns DE (eds): *Tietz Textbook of Clinical Chemistry and Molecular Diagnostics*. Philadelphia: WB Saunders, 2006.

25. Delzell JE: What can we do to prepare patients for test results during pregnancy? *West J Med* 2000; 173:183–184.

26. O'Brien JE, et al: Maternal serum alpha-fetoprotein screening: the need to use race/ethnic specific medians in Asians. *Fetal Diagn Ther* 1993; 8:367–370.

27. Rausch DJ, Lambert-Messerlian GM, Canick JA: Participation in maternal serum screening for Down syndrome defects, and trisomy 18 following screen-positive results in a pregnancy. *West J Med* 2000; 173:180–183.

28. Chace DH, Kalas TA, Naylor EW: Use of tandem mass spectrophotometry for multianalyte screening of dried blood specimens for newborns. *Clin Chem* 2003; 49:1797–1817.

29. Merck Manual of Diagnosis and Therapy Online. Rahway, NJ: Merck & Co., revised 2005. Available at *www.merck.com/mrkshared/mmanual/section19/chapter260/260b.jsp*

30. Harmening DM: *Modern Blood Banking & Transfusion Practices*, ed 5. Philadelphia: FA Davis Co, 2005, p. 388.

31. Liley AW: Liquor amnii analysis in the management of the pregnancy complicated by rhesus sensitization. *Am J Obstet Gynecol* 1961; 82:1359–1370.

32. Purandare CN: Fetal lung maturity. *Obstet Gynecol India* 2005; 55:215–217.

33. Liggins G, Howie R: A controlled trial of antepartum glucocorticoid treatment for the prevention of the respiratory distress syndrome in premature infants. *Pediatrics* 1972; 50:515–525.

34. Royal College of Obstetricians and Gynaecologists: *Antenatal Corticosteroids to Prevent RDS*. Guideline Number 7. London: Royal College of Obstetricians and Gynaecologists, 1996.

35. Ashwood ER: Standards of laboratory practice: evaluation of fetal lung maturity. *Clin Chem* 1997; 43:211–214.

36. Grenache DG, Parvon CA, Gronowski AM: Preanalytical factors that influence the Abbott TDx Fetal Lung Maturity II Assay. *Clin Chem* 2003; 49:935–939.

37. Fant CR, et al: Assessment of the diagnostic accuracy of the TDx-FLM II to predict fetal lung maturity. *Clin Chem* 2002; 48:761–765.

38. DeRoche ME, et al: The use of lamellar body counts to predict fetal lung maturity in pregnancies complicated by diabetes mellitus. *Am J Obstet Gyncol* 2002; 187:908–912.

49. Neerhof MG, et al: Lamellar body counts compared with traditional phospholipids analysis as an assay for evaluating fetal lung maturity. *Obstet Gynecol* 2001; 97:305–309.

40. Beinlich A, et al: Lamellar body counts in amniotic fluid for prediction of fetal lung maturity. *Arch Gynecol Obstet* 1999; 262(3-4):173–180.

The clinical laboratory is an important partner in the assessment of malignant disorders.

Malignancy Disorders and Testing

Michelle Kanuth, Camellia St. John, and Wendy Arneson

Tumor markers, by broad definition, are biochemical analytes that are useful for cancer detection, tumor growth prediction, or progression of the illness. They are most commonly used in diagnosis of lymphoma, leukemia, and colorectal, pulmonary, gastric, pancreatic, breast, liver, or prostatic carcinomas. Tumors are rapidly dividing cells, often unresponsive to normal physiological stimuli, and may appear in the wrong place. The center of a tumor is typically dead or dying cells that exude substances that can be analyzed and are therefore a marker for presence of tumor. Other types of tumor markers arise from cellular products, receptors, or genetic markers. Different terms are used to discuss unusual cell growth, including neoplasia, anaplasia, carcinoma, adenoma, and metastases. These terms and other information about tumor markers and tests to detect them will be discussed further in this chapter. This chapter describes the role of the laboratory in assessing and monitoring for malignancy diseases. The chapter explores the assessment of specific malignancies, including multiple myeloma, breast cancer, prostatic cancer, oat cell carcinoma of the lung, and pancreatic cancer, including methods of analysis with a focus on quality assurance of laboratory results. There is also a discussion about the determination of medical decision limits for tumor marker levels taking into consideration the diagnostic and analytical sensitivity and specificity of the analyte in question. The student is referred to Chapter 2 (Quality Assessment) for a discussion of medical decision limits and calculations of positive and negative predictive values. The side boxes in this chapter provide common sense tips, definitions of terms, brief descriptions of pathophysiology, and clinical correlations as well as reminders of the team approach in health care. Text boxes within the chapter outline methodology for laboratory assessment of nutrition and digestive function.

OBJECTIVES

Upon completion of this chapter, the student will have the ability to:

- Explain the meaning of each of the following terms, listing specific examples when applicable: malignancy, tumor, cancer, benign, neoplasm, tumor marker, diagnostic sensitivity, diagnostic specificity, positive predictive value, negative predictive value, receiver operating characteristic (ROC) curve, medical decision limit (cutoff), and tumor load.
- Categorize tumor markers based on a logical classification system, relating to chemical makeup and general methodology of analysis.
- Discuss the differences between screening for cancer in an asymptomatic general population, in symptomatic patients within high-risk groups, in diagnostic or confirmatory tests, and in monitoring for success of treatment or recurrence of malignancy based on tumor marker levels, citing specific examples.
- Explain the value of specific tumor markers for diagnosis and treatment of patients with gastrointestinal, breast, prostatic, uterine, testicular, and leukemic malignancies.
- Calculate diagnostic sensitivity, diagnostic specificity, positive predictive value, and negative predictive value, when given appropriate data.

Antigenic tumor markers have become a very important part of measuring treatment efficacy for cancers diagnosed primarily by other means. Tumor markers can also help the physician in monitoring for recurrences of malignancy and spreading tumors or metastases in the patient. Most tumor markers are not good analytes for screening tests, as in general they are not specific to malignancies. They can also be found in abnormal concentrations in conditions other than malignancies. However, once a diagnosis of a particular malignancy is made, these antigens can be very helpful in determining whether or not treatment is effectively reducing the tumor mass. Once the presence of a tumor is detected, the oncologist will order a baseline tumor marker measurement. Which marker is assayed will depend on the tumor's primary location. Then, during treatment, serial assays will be done to determine whether or not the treatment is working. Effective treatment will drop the level of the tumor marker precipitously and the level will remain within the reference range. Rising levels after treatment are often associated with recurrence or metastases.

Neoplasia is a general term for accelerated growth of tissue, which could be benign or malignant. Malignant growth is completely unrestricted and tends toward **metastasis**, or spreading past normal tissue boundaries into distant organs or sites. **Anaplasia** is a general term for loss of cell differentiation and change in cell and tissue structure from typical or normal. Other terms that relate to the origin or type of tumor include *carcinoma* and *adenoma*. A carcinoma is a malignant growth arising from skin or organ tissue epithelium, while an adenoma is a benign growth arising from glandular epithelium.[1]

LABORATORY TESTS TO SCREEN FOR DISEASE

Laboratory tests in the past have been used to screen for early stages of disease in the asymptomatic population. On the surface this seems like an ideal test system for serious and potentially fatal diseases such as malignancies. However, many laboratory tests are not suitable for screening asymptomatic people because of issues with test specificity and sensitivity. For example, pronouncing a patient "negative" for cancer when the laboratory test was not able to detect the lowest levels of the tumor marker could have serious consequences. Analytical sensitivity relates to the lowest concentration of a substance that can be detected in a test system. Likewise, **diagnostic sensitivity** is similar in regard to detecting a low concentration of a biochemical substance that relates to the disease in its early stages. Diagnostic sensitivity and analytical sensitivity both relate to the **false-negative** rate. That is, the false-negative rate determines whether a test result is truly negative or, in fact, the test should be positive but the disease has undetectably low levels of tumor marker.

Analytical specificity is another important issue in laboratory testing, particularly in regard to tumor marker tests. It would not be desirable to make the diagnosis of "positive" for cancer and begin complicated treatment strategies on the basis of one flawed test, particularly one that detected several chemicals along with or in place of the desired tumor marker. Analytical specificity refers to the ability to detect only the chemical desired with little or no interference from other chemicals. **Diagnostic specificity** is similar in that a diagnosis of malignancy based on a tumor marker should relate only to the presence of the tumor marker and not to interfering substances. For example, if the presence or increased amounts of a tumor marker in the patient's body fluid may indicate **malignant** *or* nonmalignant disease, this is not desirable.[2]

There are several categories of **tumor markers** based on their chemical makeup or general nature in the human body. Some of the oldest biochemical tests used

neoplasia - accelerated new growth, either benign or malignant

metastasis - tumor appearance in a different body site than the primary tumor of the same cell line

anaplasia - loss of cell differentiation and change in structure

diagnostic sensitivity - the likelihood that, given the presence of disease, an abnormal test result predicts the disease

false negative - result below the decision limit in a patient who has the disease

diagnostic specificity - the likelihood that, given the absence of disease, a normal test result excludes disease

malignant - characterized by completely unrestricted cell growth with a tendency to spread

tumor markers - surface molecules on tissue or proteins in serum that, in higher than normal quantities, are associated with the presence of malignancies

TABLE 13-1

Categories, Examples, and Locations of Tumor Markers

Categories	Example: Location of Cancer
Enzymes	Alkaline phosphatase: bone, liver, sarcoma
	Amylase: pancreatic
	Creatine kinase 1 (CK-1): prostate, small cell lung
	Lactate dehydrogenase: liver, lymphoma
	Prostatic acid phosphatase: prostate
	Prostate specific antigen: prostate
Hormones	ACTH: Cushing's syndrome, small cell lung
	ADH: small cell lung, adrenal cortex
	Calcitonin: medullary thyroid
	Chorionic gonadotropin: choriocarcinoma, testicular
	Growth hormone: pituitary adenoma, lung
Oncofetal antigens	Alpha fetoprotein: liver, germ cell
	Carcinoembryonic antigen: colorectal, GI, lung
Carbohydrate antigens	CA 15-3: breast, ovarian
	CA 125: ovarian, endometrial
	CA 19-5: GI, pancreatic, ovarian
	CA 19-9: pancreatic, GI, liver
Proteins	Monoclonal paraproteins (MC): myeloma
	Nuclear matrix protein 22: transitional cell carcinoma of urinary tract
	Bladder tumor-associated antigen: bladder
Receptors	Estrogen receptor: breast
	Progesterone receptor: breast
Genes	n-*ras* mutation: acute myeloid leukemia
	k-*ras* mutation: leukemia, lymphoma
	c-*myc* translocation: lymphoma, small cell lung
	c-*erb* B-2 amplification: breast, ovarian, GI

as tumor markers are proteins, enzymes, and hormones. The role and clinical significance of all three biochemical tests are described in Chapter 1 (Overview of Clinical Chemistry). Newer laboratory techniques have yielded additional types of tumor marker testing such as carbohydrate markers, blood group antigens, receptors, and genetic markers. Table 13–1 lists seven main types of tumor markers, specific examples of each type, and the location of common types of cancer that they indicate. Table 13–2 describes the most common tumor markers, the tissues and type of cancer they are associated with, and nonmalignant causes for elevations in those tumor markers.

TUMOR MARKERS FOR COLORECTAL CANCER

As mentioned earlier, tumor marker testing should not be used to screen asymptomatic or low-risk patients for cancer because of concerns for poor diagnostic sensitivity and specificity. An example of a test with a high **false-positive** rate is the fecal occult blood test for colorectal cancer. Colorectal cancer does correlate with fecal occult blood, but there are many other causes of blood in the feces as well. Some noncancerous causes of fecal blood include gastrointestinal (GI) bleeding

false positive - result at or above the decision limit in a patient who does not have the disease

TABLE 13-2
Common Tumor Markers[3]

Tumor Marker	CA 125 (Cancer Antigen 125)	CA 15-3 (Cancer Antigen 15-3)	CA 19-9 (Cancer Antigen 19-9)	CEA (Carcinoembryonic Antigen)	AFP (Alpha Fetoprotein)	PSA (Prostate Specific Antigen)	β-hCG (Beta Human Chorionic Gonadotropin)
Cancer in which it is useful	**Ovarian** (also, to a lesser extent, breast, lung, and GI tract)	**Breast** (also, to a lesser extent, ovarian, lung, pancreatic, colon, and liver)	**GI tract (including hepatobiliary, hepatocellular, gastric, pancreatic, and colorectal)**	**Colon** (also other GI, lung, pancreatic, breast ovary, and uterine)	**Primary hepatocellular, testicular, ovarian, epithelial GI tumors**	**Prostate**	**Trophoblastic tumors, germ cell malignancies**
Nonmalignant conditions in which elevations are also seen and false positive reactions	Female genital tract conditions (endometriosis, normal pregnancy, pelvic inflammatory disease, uterine fibroids), hepatitis, pancreatitis, and cirrhosis	Systemic lupus erythematosus (SLE), sarcoidosis, tuberculosis, hepatitis, and cirrhosis	Pancreatitis, any inflammatory gastrointestinal disorders	Liver diseases Note: smokers have slightly high levels	Viral hepatitis, cirrhosis Normally seen in fetal life and small amounts in adult GI tract	Benign prostatic hyperplasia (BPH), prostatitis	Pregnancy

polyp - small tumor common to rectum or other vascular areas

such as from aspirin or other medications, hemorrhoids, **polyps**, or GI ulcers. These conditions would all cause a poor diagnostic specificity of the fecal occult blood test for colorectal cancer but fairly good diagnostic specificity for GI bleeding. The fecal occult blood test by the guaiac method also yields positive results due to presence of chemicals other than blood, such as myoglobin or peroxidase activity. Analytical false-positive results can be due to recent intake of foods such as red meat containing animal myoglobin or radishes, turnips, or other foods that contain perioxidase. These foods would cause poor diagnostic specificity for GI bleeding and for colorectal cancer. Thus, a high false-positive rate due to poor analytical specificity can have an impact on diagnostic specificity as well.

Clinicians often use several diagnostic indicators along with tumor marker tests, such as history and physical examination, in order to improve the diagnostic specificity for a diagnosis of malignancy. For example, since colorectal cancer is quite common and there is an increase in likelihood with age, guidelines have been set up to suggest screening everyone age 50 years and older with fecal occult blood testing. However, care must be taken prior to testing to limit medications and food that can induce a false-positive result. Screening and early detection recommendations also include flexible **sigmoidoscopy** every 5 years with a **digital rectal examination**. If fecal occult blood is positive, or if **adenomatous** or cancerous polyps smaller than 1 cm or any polyps larger than 1 cm are found on sigmoidoscopy, either a **colonoscopy** or double-contrast barium enema is performed. Thus the fecal occult blood test serves as the first line of testing and, if positive results are obtained, it indicates the need for more expensive and invasive testing for colorectal cancer.[4]

sigmoidoscopy - examination of the lower portion of the colon (sigmoid portion) with an instrument

digital rectal examination - palpation of the prostate gland with a gloved finger inserted into the rectum

adenomatous - referring to neoplasm of glandular cells

colonoscopy - examination of the upper portion of the rectum with an instrument

Changes in other clinical chemistry analytes can also be associated with tumors. These analytes are not specific enough to be called tumor markers but do provide additional information for the clinician in making a differential diagnosis. For example, calcium is elevated in malignancy, but elevated levels are also associated with a variety of other disorders, including hyperparathyroidism. Chapter 11 (Endocrine Disorders and Testing) provides more details about hypercalcemia. The second most common cause of hypercalcemia is malignancy. This is termed *hypercalcemia of malignancy* (HM), a condition associated with increased mortality in patients with malignancy. Hypercalcemia is not a rare circumstance in malignancy in that up to 58% of hospitalized patients with hypercalcemia have an associated cancer. Hypercalcemia is usually seen in squamous cell cancers and bone and breast cancers and only rarely with skin cancers. Increased parathyroid-related protein is the hallmark of HM and may be one of the main causes of hypercalcemia.[5]

CASE SCENARIO 13-1

Multiple Myeloma: An Unusual Band in Protein Electrophoresis

In a small hospital, the laboratory technologist was viewing the report for the basic metabolic chemistry profile on Mr. Rice and noticed a decreased serum albumin of 3.1 g/dL (reference range, 3.5 to 5.2 g/dL) and an decreased albumin/globulin (A/G) ratio along with an elevated total serum protein of 8.8 g/dL (6.0 to 8.0 g/dL). The complete blood count (CBC) showed decreased red blood cells (RBCs), white blood cells (WBCs), and hemoglobin. The urinalysis showed 3+ proteinuria and 10 to 15 hyaline casts per low-power field (LPF), but there was no hematuria or hemoglobinuria. The physician reviewed the results and, based on symptoms and laboratory results, she ordered a

Case Scenario 13-1 Multiple Myeloma: An Unusual Band in Protein
Electrophoresis *(continued)*

serum protein electrophoresis, which was sent to a referral laboratory. Fecal
occult blood was tested three times but came back negative each time, ruling
out the source of decreased RBC count as gastrointestinal blood loss. When
the results of the serum protein electrophoresis came back, there was a slight
decrease in albumin and a small amount of **M protein** in the gamma globulin
region. The protein electrophoresis results of this patient are shown below;
total serum protein was 8.8 g/dL.

Protein Fraction	Result (%)	Result (g/dL)	Reference Ranges (g/dL)
Albumin	35.2	3.1	3.5–5.2
Alpha$_1$ globulin	3.4	0.3	0.2–0.4
Alpha$_2$ globulin	6.8	0.6	0.4–0.8
Beta globulin	8.0	0.7	0.5–1.1
Gamma globulin	46.6	4.1	0.6–1.3

Protein fraction (g/dL) = fraction % × total serum protein (g/dL)
Albumin = 35.2% × 8.8 g/dL = 3.1 g/dL

Six months later, when Mr. Rice returned for the follow-up laboratory tests,
the laboratory technologist noticed that he had difficulty in settling comfort-
ably in the phlebotomy chair. He looked well-nourished but pale. The CBC
results were essentially the same but there was a slightly lower RBC count, and
the urinalysis was unchanged with 3+ proteinuria. The total serum protein
was higher at 9.4 g/dL (reference range, 6.0 to 8.0 g/dL), which prompted a
second serum protein electrophoresis to be ordered and sent to the referral
laboratory.

The second serum protein electrophoresis showed a more pronounced M
protein level. The protein electrophoresis results are shown below; total serum
protein was 9.4 g/dL.

Protein Fraction	Result (%)	Result (g/dL)	Reference Ranges (g/dL)
Albumin	34.0	3.2	3.5–5.2
Alpha$_1$ globulin	3.2	0.3	0.2–0.4
Alpha$_2$ globulin	6.4	0.6	0.4–0.8
Beta globulin	9.6	0.9	0.5–1.1
Gamma globulin	46.8	4.4	0.6–1.3

The laboratory technologist called the physician when the results arrived,
and the physician ordered an immunoelectrophoresis (IEP). The technologist
suggested that an immunofixation electrophoresis (IFE) should be ordered
instead. IEP has been replaced by this test, which is easier to interpret and less
vulnerable to technical error. Figure 13–1A shows the results of Mr. Rice's second serum protein electrophoresis and his IFE, which depicts an immunoglobulin G (IgG) κ (kappa) protein band. Compared to the normal pattern shown
in Figure 13–1B, Mr. Rice's results are significantly increased. Mr. Rice's
physician ordered a bone marrow aspirate and biopsy to make a final diagnosis
of multiple myeloma.

M protein - paraprotein visible in protein electrophoresis
causing a tall peak in the densitometry pattern, also called
an M spike

■■ **CLINICAL CORRELATION**
The fecal occult blood test
measures hidden blood in
feces. When visible blood is
present in feces, it is not
referred to as occult blood
since it is not hidden. Occult
blood is detected by a colorimetric test in which the peroxidase activity of the blood
hemoglobin reacts with guaiac
reagents to form a color.
Occult blood is one of the most
common tests for detecting a
bleeding ulcer or malignancy in
the gastrointestinal tract. Fecal
occult blood also could result
from trace amounts of blood
excreted from hemorrhoids.

continued

Case Scenario 13-1 **Multiple Myeloma: An Unusual Band in Protein Electrophoresis** *(continued)*

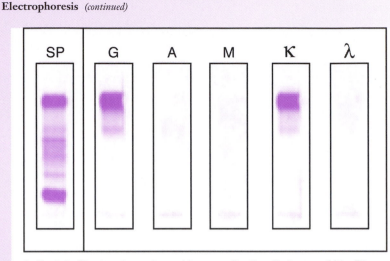

A. Protein Electrophoresis and Immunofixation Patterns of Mr. Rice

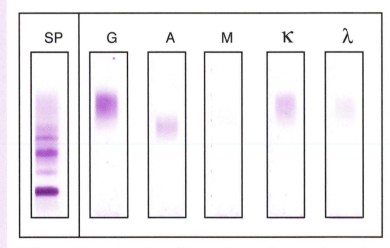

B. Protein Electrophoresis and Immunofixation Patterns of normal serum

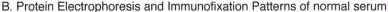

Figure 13–1. Protein electrophoresis pattern of *(A)* Mr. Rice and *(B)* normal control.

Source: From Protein Electrophoresis and Immunofixation: Interpretive Guide (CD module). Beaumont, TX: Helena Laboratories, 2006; reprinted with permission.

CLINICAL CORRELATION

In monoclonal gammopathy, there is growth of one lymphocyte or plasma cell line at a faster rate than normal causing an increased production of a particular type of paraprotein immunoglobulin. Monoclonal gammopathies represent a group of related disorders with secretion of a single type of immunoglobulin or its components.[6]

PROTEIN ELECTROPHORESIS

Total serum protein is made up of hundreds of proteins produced in the liver and immunoglobulins produced by plasma cells in the bone marrow. Refer to the basic structure of an immunoglobulin in Chapter 3. Under the influence of an electrophoretic field, various immunoglobulins migrate over a broad distance within the gamma globulin region because of their differences in isoelectric point. Refer to the principle of electrophoresis as described in Chapter 3 (Laboratory Techniques and Instrumentation).

Monoclonal gammopathy is often recognized by an immunoglobulin peak in the serum or urine electrophoresis pattern. Diagnosis, staging, and treatment of monoclonal gammopathies are based upon the presence, level, and type of immunoglobulin.[7] There are generally six main types of monoclonal gammopathies with unique characteristics to be discussed: multiple myeloma, Waldenström's **macroglobulinemia**, heavy chain disease, **amyloidosis**, monoclonal gammopathy of undetermined significance (MGUS), and solitary plasmacytoma. These will be discussed in more detail. Rarely a protein electrophoretic peak, or M spike, in the gamma globulin region is due to serious infection.[8] The malignant or abnormal plasma cells in these disorders may produce an intact immunoglobulin, free light chains without heavy chains, and rarely only heavy chains. The cells may produce immunoglobulins with usual or missing amino acids, or immunoglobulins with two or more heavy chain classes. However, each abnormal plasma cell line produces only a kappa chain or a lambda chain, never both.[9]

MULTIPLE MYELOMA

Muliple myeloma is a generalized disease of malignant plasma cells that affects approximately 1300 older people in the United States each year. The median age at diagnosis is 65 years, and only 15% of patients are younger than 50 years. The typical survival is 3 years, but approximately 10% of patients live more than 10 years. Most patients have hyperproteinemia due to a monoclonal protein (M protein) causing a tall peak in the **densitometry** pattern, also called an M spike, in serum, urine, or both. The majority of these patients also have bone involvement. The diagnosis of multiple myeloma is most often reached after they develop symptoms of severe back pain and an elevated serum protein level, mild anemia, proteinuria, or **lytic** bone lesion. Renal failure is a common complication, correlated with increasing proteinuria and attributed to hypercalcemia or advanced disease when excessive light chains of **paraproteins** are produced and excreted into the urine. These free light chains, known as **Bence Jones proteins**, tend to overwhelm the renal system and become filtered into urine despite their large molecular mass. Hyperproteinemia is a key indication of multiple myeloma, when the total plasma protein exceeds 8.5 g/dL. When the paraprotein immunoglobulin levels alone exceed 6 g/dL, **hyperviscosity** of the plasma occurs causing **rouleaux** erythrocytes and other further complications.[5] Generally there is a single abnormal clone of a plasma cell or B lymphocyte. However, in some cases, more than one clone may produce monoclonal gammopathies. These cases are usually **biclonal** and very rarely **triclonal**.[6,7]

The main tumor markers in serum and urine for multiple myeloma are paraprotein immunoglobulins. Serum and urine protein electrophoresis provide the initial screen for paraproteins. In this technique, the carbonyl groups of the proteins are charged anionic due to the presence of excess hydroxyl ions from the alkaline pH buffer diluent. The serum sample containing the charged protein groups is applied to a small well within an agarose gel medium. The gel is introduced into an electrophoretic cell containing a cathode and anode. A constant voltage is applied to the electrophoretic cell. Albumin is the most anionic of all the serum proteins and migrates closest to the anode when a constant voltage is applied, while the immunoglobulins are the least anionic and migrate furthest from the anode. The method of protein electrophoresis is based on this principle and is described in more detail in Chapter 3. The principle and specific aspects of protein electrophoresis are described in Test Methodology 13–1.

---

monoclonal - arising from one cell line

gammopathy - any disease in which serum immunoglobulins are increased

macroglobulinemia - disease of plasma cells marked by excess production of immunoglobulin M (IgM)

amyloidosis - metabolic disorder with starch accumulation in organs and tissues

densitometry - using colorimetry to determine the quantity of a dense region, such as in protein electrophoresis densitometry

lytic - rupturing or breaking down cell membranes

■■ CLINICAL CORRELATION

Multiple myeloma is a tumor arising in the bone marrow associated with multiple organ system involvement, including bone lesions, decreased blood cell production, and possible kidney disease.

paraprotein - an abnormal plasma protein, such as a macroglobulin, cryoglobulin, or immunoglobulin

Bence Jones protein - free light chains of the immunoglobulin molecule

hyperviscosity - gelatinous nature or excessive viscosity

rouleaux - stickiness of erythrocytes causing a stacked coin appearance

biclonal - arising from two cell lines

triclonal - composed of three clones of plasma cell lines that each produce one type of identical antibody

TEST METHODOLOGY 13-1.   PROTEIN ELECTROPHORESIS

The Reaction Principle

Patient's serum or concentrated urine or cerebrospinal fluid (CSF) is placed into a sample trough within agarose gel, which is placed in an alkaline buffer solution, and a standardized voltage is applied to allow separation of the major protein groups by electrophoresis. The result is six or more fractions of separated proteins, including the main fractions of albumin and alpha$_1$, alpha$_2$, beta$_1$, beta$_2$, and gamma globulins, from anode to cathode. Following electrophoresis, the agarose gel is processed in acetic acid and alcohol washes to fix the proteins in the agarose. Following a wash step, the protein fractions are stained with Coumassie Brilliant Blue protein stain. After a second wash, fixed protein bands can be visualized and quantified with densitometry.

Interferences

Hemolysis in the serum causes an increase in the beta globulin fraction due to free hemoglobin or in the alpha$_2$ globulin region due to haptoglobin-hemoglobin complexes. Fibrinogen is generally not present since serum is used. If centrifugation occurs before complete clotting of the whole blood, serum may contain fibrinogen, a beta globulin of around 0.3 g/dL. This may be especially associated with the point of sample origin on the gel. The reference ranges for total serum protein and the beta globulin region are not set to include fibrinogen or hemoglobin, so their accidental presence causes confusion in interpretation.

Bacterial growth impedes separation of proteins, which can be overcome by using fresh buffer and keeping it refrigerated between uses. Excess heat and friction can cause poor separation and resolution of bands, which can be overcome by using freshly made buffer of the correct ionic strength and using the buffer while it is still cold. Distortions in the protein fractions may be due to a bent or dirty pipette tip or to drying of the support medium. Care should be taken to use a clean, unbent pipette tip that does not gouge into the gel. The gel should be kept covered to prevent dehydration during processing. Overloading the gel with sample can cause distortion due to excess albumin.

The Calculations

$$\% \text{ protein fraction} \times \text{total protein (g/dL)} = \text{protein fraction (g/dL)}$$

The Specimen

Fresh serum without hemolysis or fibrin strands is recommended. Serum can be used if stored for up to 5 days at 2° to 8°C. Frozen serum can be used if gently thawed and thoroughly mixed prior to use.

Urine can also be tested but must be concentrated to a protein content of at least 3 g/dL using a concentration filter device, such as the device made by Amicon Corporation. It requires up to 5 mL of urine sample.

Cerebrospinal fluid may also be analyzed, again after concentrating the CSF in a concentrating chamber device. Concurrent CSF and serum must be collected with the same 6-hour period and, if analysis is delayed, samples should be frozen, rethawed, and mixed thoroughly prior to analysis.

Reference Ranges

Serum

Albumin (g/dL)	3.5–5.2
Alpha$_1$ globulin (g/dL)	0.2–0.4
Alpha$_2$ globulin (g/dL0	0.4–0.8
Beta globulin (g/dL)	0.5–1.1
Gamma globulin (g/dL)	0.6–1.3

continued

TEST METHODOLOGY 13-1. **PROTEIN ELECTROPHORESIS** *(continued)*

Urine, 24-Hour

Albumin (%)	1.4–2.3 g/dL
Alpha₁ globulin (%)	0.9–1.6 g/dL
Alpha₂ globulin (%)	0.6–1.2 g/dL
Beta globulin (%)	0.3–0.5 g/dL
Gamma globulin (%)	0.1–0.2 g/dL

After the protein fractions are separated by electrophoresis and quantified with densitometry, the results are evaluated. Paraprotein immunoglobulins are usually present in the gamma globulin region but may be found in the beta and even alpha globulin region due to their abnormal chemical makeup. If paraproteins are noted in the protein electrophoretic pattern, it is useful to identify the type of heavy chain and light chain present in the immunoglobulin. This is achieved with immunoelectrophoresis as described in Test Methodology 13–2.[10]

TEST METHODOLOGY 13-2. **SERUM IMMUNOFIXATION ELECTROPHORESIS**

The Reaction Principle

Patient's serum diluted in alkaline buffer is placed into six separate wells within agarose gel, which is placed in an electrophoretic chamber, and a standardized voltage is applied to allow separation of the major protein groups by electrophoresis. The result is six identical tracks of separated proteins. One of the tracks is treated with a protein fixative and becomes the reference track. The remaining tracks are treated with specific heavy chain and light chain antisera that react with specific immunoglobulins in the separated protein tracks, causing them to be immunofixed in the agarose. All proteins not reactive with the antisera in the five treated tracks are removed in a wash step, followed by staining with Coumassie Brilliant Blue protein stain. After a second wash, fixed protein bands can be observed and compared with the bands found in the reference track, in order to identify the type of immunoglobulin by its heavy chain and light chain. Paraproteins often show as a distinct, sharply defined precipitin band with one heavy chain and one light chain. This information, coupled with the high-resolution protein electrophoresis and immunoglobulin quantitation, is helpful in characterization of gammopathies.

Interferences

Antigen excess occurs when the sample contains excessive amounts of protein that overwhelm the antibody. This is generally overcome by beginning with a more dilute sample based on the total protein and gamma globulin protein levels obtained with serum protein electrophoresis. Likewise, antibody excess occurs when the total serum protein and gamma globulin protein levels are lower than the equivalence point with the antibody. Both cause poor resolution of protein bands. Using a less dilute sample can overcome this problem.

The Specimen

Fresh serum without hemolysis or fibrin strands is recommended. Serum can be used if stored for up to 5 days at 2° to 8°C. Frozen serum can be used if gently thawed and thoroughly mixed prior to use.

continued

TEST METHODOLOGY 13-2.   SERUM IMMUNOFIXATION

ELECTROPHORESIS (*continued*)

Urine and CSF can also be tested but must be concentrated to a protein content of at least 5 g/dL using a concentration filter device.

Reference Ranges

Normal serum generally lacks the presence of sharply defined precipitin bands in the gamma globulin region. The fixed total serum protein track should act as a reference for the immunoglobulin tracks. Sharply defined precipitin bands indicate monoclonal proteins (M spike) associated with malignant and nonmalignant lymphocyte disorders.

choroid plexus - cavities in the cerebrum lined with thin membranes and blood vessels

ultrafiltrate - filtrate formed under pressure, such as found in the choroid plexus

multiple sclerosis - a progressive neurodegenerative disease affecting the axons of nerves in the area surrounding the ventricles of the brain but not the peripheral nerves

oligoclonal - showing small discrete bands in the cerebrospinal fluid electrophoresis indicating local production of immunoglobulin G (IgG)

Cerebrospinal fluid (CSF) is created under pressure as plasma diffuses through thin, vascular membranes within the ventricles of the brain. This region is called the **choroid plexus**. Spinal fluid is reabsorbed into the blood vessels in the choroid plexus, causing it to contain only low molecular weight molecules and no cells and to appear clear and colorless. Therefore, CSF is called an **ultrafiltrate**. CSF contains proteins but in different proportions than in serum or plasma. The most noticeable feature of proteins within the CSF is that there is a predominant prealbumin protein and an extra type of transferrin. This extra transferrin form is called tau protein, which is chemically different than regular transferrin, causing a unique migration within an electrophoretic field. Chapter 2 (Quality Assessment) describes collection and handling of CSF, including a figure depicting the collection process.

Analysis of CSF protein levels through quantification and electrophoresis is requested primarily to detect increased permeability of the blood-CSF barrier to plasma proteins or increased synthesis of immunoglobulins in the brain or spinal cord. The blood-CSF barrier is breached in central nervous system disorders such as hemorrhage, inflammation, or tumors of the spinal cord. Increased synthesis of IgG at the site of nerve axon damage, such as in **multiple sclerosis**, is associated with unusual CSF protein electrophoretic patterns and **oligoclonal** immunoglobulin bands.[11]

Figure 13–2 shows several patterns to illustrate normal and abnormal serum protein electrophoresis (SPE) and IFE findings in gammopathies, such as IgG κ, immunoglobulin M (IgM) κ, and immunoglobulin A (IgA) λ bands. Figure 13–3 shows the SPE and IFE patterns of urine that contains free light chains.

Pathology of Multiple Myeloma

Major clinical features include pain, anemia, fatigue, increased infections, and possible progression to renal failure. The severe localized back pain is caused by pathological fractures of the vertebrae or ribs; such breaks in bone arise in the absence of force or trauma. These patients fatigue easily due to severe anemia. Polyuria is a feature of this illness, usually due to hypercalcemia secondary to bone lysis and bone malignancy. Severe renal failure can result, especially as monoclonal immunoglobulins overwhelm the renal system and are increasingly excreted into urine. Recurrent infections are also common due to multiple factors, including a marked depression of uninvolved immunoglobulins. The presence of a lytic bone lesion, serum myeloma protein levels greater than 3.0 g/dL, IgG or IgA myeloma

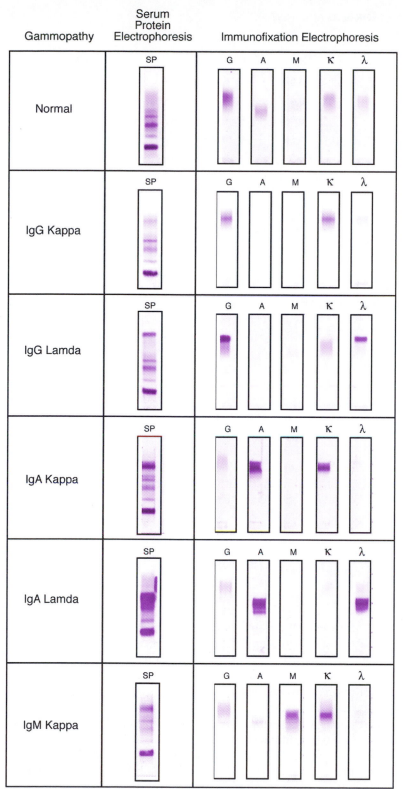

SP: serum protein electrophoresis
IFE: Immunofixation electrophoresis

Figure 13–2. Normal and abnormal serum protein electrophoresis and immunofixation electrophoresis findings in gammopathies, such as IgG κ, IgM κ, and IgA λ bands. *Source: From Protein Electrophoresis and Immunofixation: Interpretive Guide* (CD module). Beaumont, TX: Helena Laboratories, 2006: reprinted with permission.

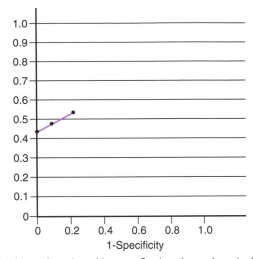

Figure 13–3. Urine protein electrophoresis and immunofixation electrophoresis showing free light chains. *Source: From Protein Electrophoresis and Immunofixation: Interpretive Guide (CD module). Beaumont, TX: Helena Laboratories, 2006; reprinted with permission.*

prognosis - prediction of the course and end of a disease and estimate of chance for recovery

cluster of differentiation (CD) - cell membrane molecules used to classify leukocyte subsets

protein, Bence Jones protein levels greater than 50 mg/dL, or abnormalities of the spine with earlier progression of the disease indicate a poor **prognosis**. Symptomatic patients experience sheets of plasma cells present in a lytic bone lesion or contiguous soft tissue mass, often in 10% or more of marrow plasma cells. The malignant plasma cells can be characterized by unique cell markers that help in differentiating them from other cell lines. They generally express CD38 and CD56 antigen, but usually do not express other B-cell antigens, such as CD19, CD20, and CD23.[5] (CD stands for **cluster of differentiation**.)

NEW TECHNIQUES TO HELP DIAGNOSIS OF MONOCLONAL GAMMOPATHIES

High-resolution electrophoresis and quantification of M proteins are newer techniques that are helpful in characterizing monoclonal gammopathies. High-resolution electrophoresis is named such because it gives better resolution of serum, urine, and CSF proteins than standard electrophoresis. It separates several other fractions beyond albumin and the four globulin fractions, often totaling 10 to 12 fractions. Also, high-resolution electrophoresis permits better detection of low-concentration M proteins migrating in the α_2, β, or γ regions of the gel. Using densitometry to quantify the M proteins can be helpful in assessing the tumor load and in determining whether the disease is progressing. Historically, nephelometric and turbidimetric immunoassays of M proteins are the most common methods for quantifying immunoglobulins. Those techniques are highly automated, providing ease and reproducibility of results. However, specificity to monoclonal immunoglobulins is limited since the reagents used in nephelometry are developed for a variety of normal immunoglobulins. Thus the concentration of M components is often under- or overestimated. Newer adaptations to electrophoresis and densitometry allow for quantification of M proteins. Because of these peculiar immunologic properties of nephelometry, the best way to assess the concentration of a high-concentration M component is now by densitometry.[7]

OTHER DISORDERS OF LYMPHOCYTES

In addition to multiple myeloma, there are other disorders of the lymphocytes that cause gammopathies, including Waldenström's macroglobulinemia, heavy chain disease, amyloidosis, and monoclonal gammopathy of undetermined significance. The term *heavy chain diseases* refer to a family of rare, lymphoma-like clinical disorders that produce a monoclonal but incomplete immunoglobulin component without the associated light chains.

Waldenström's Macroglobulinemia

In Waldenström's macroglobulinemia, there is malignancy of mature lymphocytes that produce a monoclonal IgM globulin. This disease affects about 3000 people in the United States each year. The average age at onset of the disease is 65, with a survival rate of 5 years. The disease usually presents with anemia and bleeding when tumor growth spreads to lymph nodes, spleen, and bone marrow. Some patients may have complications from the IgM, such as hyperviscosity syndrome, **cryoglobulinemia** with **Raynaud's syndrome**, and many other complications of blood vessels and nerves. An abnormal protein level of at least 3.0 g/dL usually indicates a serious situation.[5]

cryoglobulinemia - presence in the blood of an abnormal protein that forms gels at low temperatures

Raynaud's syndrome - disease of small arteries and arterioles of unknown cause with exaggerated vasomotor response to cold or emotion

Amyloidosis

Amyloidosis is a disorder of plasma cells or lymphocytes that produce a monoclonal immunoglobulin, such as lambda light chains. A majority of these patients have a small monoclonal immunoglobin on serum or urine electrophoresis. The condition leads to fibrous protein and starch deposits in multiple organs, and approximately 20% of patients also have overt evidence of multiple myeloma or Waldenström's disease.[5]

Monoclonal Gammopathy of Undetermined Significance

Sometimes a monoclonal protein is determined in an asymptomatic patient but the disorder never progresses to a malignant disorder. This lymphocyte disorder has been termed *monoclonal gammopathy of undetermined significance* (MGUS). MGUS is found in approximately 1% of otherwise healthy persons over the age of 50 years, and the frequency is 3% among those over 70. People with MGUS usually have a monoclonal peak of IgG, IgA, or IgM type of less than or equal to 2.5 g/dL, the number of marrow plasma cells is less than or equal to 10%, and there are no bone lesions and no Bence Jones protein. Some patients with prolonged and mild stages of multiple myeloma present similarly to those with MGUS. They have no symptoms but have a small amount of monoclonal protein on serum electrophoresis. However, the number of marrow plasma cells is greater than 10% and serum monoclonal protein is greater than 2.5 g/dL. This distinguishes multiple myeloma, in the asymptomatic stage, from MGUS.[5]

Case Scenario 13-1 Multiple Myeloma: An Unusual Band in Protein Electrophoresis

Follow-Up

Mr. Rice had usually high total serum protein and an unexpected band found in the electrophoretic pattern. This was 2.6 g/dL of IgG κ M protein that was determined by high-resolution protein electrophoresis and densitometry. His routine testing revealed a total serum protein of 9.4 g/dL and 4.4 g/dL gamma globulin proteins as determined by electrophoresis. Bone marrow aspirate and biopsy revealed 25% plasma lymphocytes, and lytic bone lesions found with x-ray helping the physician to make a final diagnosis of multiple myeloma. The physician discussed treatment options with the patient given his age, physical condition, and prognosis after consultation with **oncologists**. Since the patient will be predisposed to superinfection, pathological fractures, anemia, and other complications, frequent clinic visits will be required. Serum and urine protein electrophoresis will be periodically requested to observe for Bence Jones proteins, free light chains that increase the likelihood of renal disease. ●

CASE SCENARIO 13-2

Medical Decision-Making for Malignancy: Correlating Tumor Marker Results with Likely Disease

The Oncology Department of the University Laboratory wants to offer CA 125 testing. The laboratory will need to collect good data in order to determine the medical decision level for proper interpretation of CA 125 in regard to ovarian cancer.

The technologist reviewed recent literature and found a study of women with ovarian cancer that was confirmed with surgical techniques. At the chosen **medical decision limit**, CA 125 had a diagnostic sensitivity of 65% and specificity of 88% for predicting ovarian cancer. Positive predictive value for serum CA 125 was 98%, whereas the negative predictive value was 23%. This indicated a high false-negative rate when CA 125 values were used without consideration of other diagnostic tests. Newer imaging techniques were helpful in predicting tumor recurrence along with serial measurements of CA 125.[12,13] A commonly used medical decision limit for CA 125 is 35 U/mL.[14]

medical decision limit - the value for a test result that is used in making the diagnosis

CA 125

CA-125 is a **mucin**-type carbohydrate marker associated with ovarian and endometrial carcinomas. It is associated with normal ductal tissue but rarely is detected except in carcinomas including bladder cancer. Under some circumstances this tumor marker is elevated in patients with pericarditis, cirrhosis, endometriosis, pregnancy or ovarian cysts. Thus, determining the proper medical decision limit is helpful in improving the diagnostic sensitivity and specificity of CA-125 as a tumor marker.[14]

mucin - a glycoprotein found in mucus, formed from mucigen and soluble in water

MEDICAL DECISION LIMITS

One important aspect of setting a medical decision limit is the diagnostic specificity of a laboratory test. This is the ability of the laboratory test to predict the absence of disease when the test result is outside of that decision limit. For example, with a tumor marker such as CA 125, the diagnostic specificity would be close to 100% if the medical decision limit was set to a point at which, below that value, there was a high likelihood that the patient did not have ovarian cancer. Similarly, the negative predictive value of a test is defined by the number of patients with a negative result, or one below the medical decision limit, who don't have the disease or tumor. These is also sometimes referred to as the true-negative (TN) test result, while a false-negative (FN) test result is one that is negative based on the decision limit despite the presence of the disease in the patient. The predictive value of a negative result is the number of true negatives out of the total negative test results, including true-negative and false-negative results. The true-negative rate is another way to define diagnostic specificity, which is the ratio of the true-negative test results to the total number of negative test results, including those falsely positive that should have tested as negative.

The diagnostic sensitivity predicts the presence of a disease such as a tumor using a tumor marker test. Thus the diagnostic sensitivity of CA 125 predicts the likelihood of ovarian cancer given a certain medical decision limit. Diagnostic sensitivity relates to the positive predictive value of a test: the percentage of patients with a positive result above the medical decision limit who actually have the tumor. This is sometimes referred to as a true-positive (TP) result. Diagnostic sensitivity also relates to the false-positive (FP) rate, which is equal to the percent specificity subtracted from 100%. Refer to the following formulas for calculating these values:

$$\text{Predictive value of negative result} = \text{TN}/(\text{TN} + \text{FN}) \times 100\%$$
$$\text{Predictive value of positive result} = \text{TP}/(\text{TP} + \text{FP}) \times 100\%$$
$$\text{False-positive rate} = 100\% - \% \text{ specificity}$$
$$\text{True-negative rate} = \text{diagnostic specificity} = \text{TN}/(\text{TN} + \text{FP}) \times 100\%$$
$$\text{True-positive rate} = \text{diagnostic sensitivity} = \text{TP}/(\text{TP} + \text{FN}) \times 100\%$$

Let us practice using these formulas with the specific example of CA 125 and its ability to predict ovarian cancer in women. In this example, the medical decision limit of 20.0 U/mL was chosen and 113 women were studied. Of these 113 women, 70 women were found to have ovarian cancer as determined by imaging techniques and biopsy, while 43 women had no evidence of ovarian cancer. A positive test result means the CA 125 is greater than or equal to 20.0 U/L and a negative result is below 20.0 U/L. Of the 113 patients, 33 had ovarian cancer and a positive CA 125 test. Therefore, these 33 patients had a **true-positive** CA 125. There were also 37 patients with ovarian cancer but a CA 125 of less than 20.0 U/L, a negative test result. These 37 patients had false-negative results. The 33 true-positive and 37 false-negative test results account for the total of 70 women who did have ovarian cancer. Likewise, there were 4 patients without ovarian cancer but a CA 125 greater than or equal to 20.0 U/L. These positive test results were falsely positive. The remaining 39 patients had true-negative test results since they did not have ovarian cancer and also had negative results (CA 125 less than or equal to 20.0 U/L). These data are presented in Table 13–3.

Using the equations presented earlier, the calculation for the predictive value of a negative result is $39/(39 + 37) \times 100\% = 51\%$. The calculation of the sensi-

true positive - result at or above the decision limit in a patient who has the disease

TABLE 13-3

Example of Specific CA-125 Levels and Presence of Ovarian Cancer

Ovarian Cancer Status (N = 113)	CA 125 Level	
	>20.0 U/L, Positive Test	≤20.0 U/L, Negative Test
No, negative for disease	4, false positive	39, true negative
Yes, positive for disease	33, true positive	37, false negative

tivity, or true-positive rate, is 33/(33 + 37) × 100% = 47%. The specificity, or true-negative rate, is calculated as 39/(39 + 4) × 100% = 91%. Therefore, the false-positive rate, or % specificity subtracted from 100%, is 9% or 0.09 (1 − 0.91 = 0.09). This value will be used in a ROC curve later.

These values are helpful in determining the usefulness of a laboratory test, such as a tumor marker, at a specific medical decision limit. By changing the medical decision limit up or down, these values will change. For example, if one wanted to increase the predictive value of a positive result for a tumor marker, one could increase the medical decision limit concentration, such as increasing the decision limit for CA 125 to a value higher than 20.0 U/L. However, this would be at the expense of the negative predictive value and false-positive rate. In other words, there would likely be patients in the earlier stages of ovarian cancer who are not detected because of the increase in the medical decision limit. In fact, the diagnostic specificity and sensitivity rates tend to be inversely related. The best medical decision limit is one having both the highest diagnostic specificity *and* sensitivity, keeping the false-positive *and* false-negative results at a minimum. A **receiver operating characteristic (ROC) curve** is used to determine the best medical decision limit.

receiver operating characteristic (ROC) curve - a plot of the diagnostic specificity versus sensitivity of a test

Increasing the Medical Decision Limit

These rates would all typically change if the medical decision limit changes because the parameters of false and true positive are defined by the medical decision limit. So let us observe what results are obtained with different medical decision limits for the same patient results given a particular CA 125. Using 50.0 U/L as an example for the same 113 patient results, the number of patients with ovarian cancer and a positive CA 125 result changes to 30. You will notice that the number of true-positive results decreased and yet the number of patients with ovarian cancer (70) didn't change. By changing the parameters for the limit of CA 125 being classified as positive, the true-positive rate and sensitivity changed slightly. In fact, the sensitivity would be 30/70 or 43% with this change in the decision limit. Notice that 3 more patients with ovarian cancer, probably in its earlier stages, were not detected by the higher medical decision limit. Thus the false-negative rate increased. The change is even more noticeable in the true-negative rate. Of the 43 patients who did not have ovarian cancer, all 43 had a CA 125 less than 50.0 U/L, giving them a negative classification of the test value. Thus an improvement in specificity occurs, with 43/43 or 100% specificity, with a decrease in sensitivity to 43% for early detection of the disease. So the true-positive rate decreased but the true-negative rate increased. These data can be represented by a table such as Table 13–4.

The calculation for the negative predictive value of the result is 43/(43 + 40) × 100% = 52%. The calculation of the sensitivity or true-positive rate is 30/(30 + 40) × 100% = 43%, while the specificity is 43/(43 + 0) × 100% = 100%. There-

TABLE 13-4

Increasing the Medical Decision Limit: Example CA-125 Levels and Ovarian Cancer Status

Ovarian Cancer Status (N = 113)	CA 125 Level	
	>50.0 U/L, Positive Test	≤50.0 U/L, Negative Test
No, negative for disease	0, false positive	43, true negative
Yes, positive for disease	30, true positive	40, false negative

fore, the false-positive rate, or % specificity subtracted from 100%, is 0% or 0.0. This value will be used in a ROC curve in order to visualize the impact of diagnostic sensitivity on specificity.

Decreasing the Medical Decision Limit

Given the decrease in diagnostic sensitivity when the medical decision limit is increased, it is valuable to consider the improvement in sensitivity when lowering the medical decision limit. In the example of our study of 113 women, 70 of whom have ovarian cancer, it was decided to consider a medical decision limit between 20.0 and 50.0 U/L. In that case, 38 of the 70 women with ovarian cancer had a positive test result at 40 U/L while 34 of the 43 women without ovarian cancer had a negative test results. Let us calculate the diagnostic data to see how the percentages changed. Refer to Table 13–5 to view the data.

The calculation for sensitivity, or true-positive rate, is $38/(38 + 32) \times 100\% = 54\%$, while the calculation for specificity $= 34/(34 + 9) \times 100\% = 79\% = 0.79$. Therefore, the specificity subtracted from 100% is $1.0 - 0.79 = 0.21$. This value will be used in a ROC curve later. The calculation for the predictive value of a negative result is $34/(34 + 32) \times 100\% = 52\%$, while the predictive value of a positive result is $38/(38 + 9) \times 100\% = 81\%$. Thus, by decreasing the medical decision limit from 150.0 to 125.0 U/L, the sensitivity of the test improved but the specificity decreased from 100% to 79%.

How Can the Best Medical Decision Limit Be Determined?

Continuing to adjust the medical decision limit will change the classification of a CA 125 test result as positive or negative, while obviously not changing the true cancer status of the patient. A few more observations regarding the data and calculations

TABLE 13-5

Decreasing the Medical Decision Limit: Example of CA-125 Levels and Ovarian Cancer Status

Ovarian Cancer Status (N = 113)	CA 125 Level	
	>40.0 U/L, Positive Test	≤40.0 U/L, Negative Test
No, negative for disease	9, false positive	34, true negative
Yes, positive for disease	38, true positive	32, false negative

TABLE 13-6

CA 125 Study in 113 Women: Specificity and Sensitivity at Different Medical Decision Limits

Decision Limit for CA 125 (U/L)	1 – Diagnostic Specificity	Diagnostic Sensitivity
20.0	0.09	0.47
40.0	0.21	0.54
50.0	0	0.43

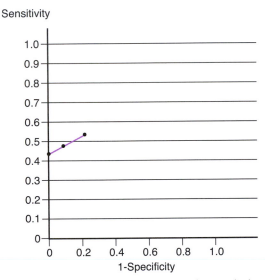

Figure 13–4. ROC curve of CA-125 for sample data.

can arrive at the best balance of diagnostic specificity and sensitivity. Also, a ROC plot of 1 – diagnostic specificity, versus the dependent factor, sensitivity, can help to visualize the best balance. When three or more data points are plotted, a curve is produced in which the point closest to the upper left corner indicates the best medical decision limit from the study data. Table 13–6 and Figure 13–4 present the comparative date and the ROC curve obtained in the ovarian cancer example.

Case Scenario 13-2 Medical Decision-Making for Malignancy: Correlating Tumor Marker Results with Likely Disease

Follow-Up

The desire to offer testing for CA 125 as a tumor marker for ovarian cancer and determining the medical decision level for proper interpretation of CA 125 involved clinical laboratory scientists, managers, and the laboratory director, a pathologist. Data were collected from the medical records department and permission was granted to obtain or use previously preserved serum samples from patients who were undergoing diagnostic studies for ovarian cancer. After a review of literature and the creation of a ROC curve from the

Case Scenario 13-2 Medical Decision-Making for Malignancy: Correlating Tumor Marker Results with Likely Disease *(continued)*

collected data, it was decided to set the medical decision limit for CA 125 at 40 U/L. This limit was highly accurate in predicting the recurrence of ovarian cancer after treatment and, when coupled with high-resolution imaging techniques such as ultrasound and magnetic resonance imaging, it had a relatively high positive predictive value for initial occurrence of ovarian cancer. ●

CASE SCENARIO 13-3

Ruling In or Ruling Out Breast Cancer: A Frightened Young Woman Has a Breast Lump

The clinical laboratory scientist (CLS) student was learning the test procedures at the tumor marker area. The CLS mentor first described the patient. The 24-year-old woman had had a breast biopsy that was positive for stage II breast carcinoma. Now the physician has ordered a CA 15-3 test to determine whether this tumor marker was elevated and could be used as a measure of treatment efficacy. The breast tissue was also to be assessed for the presence or absence of HER2/neu to determine whether or not the tumor would respond to Herceptin (trastuzumab) therapy.

The primary technique used for CA 15-3 testing is **chemiluminescence** immunoassay, as described in Test Methodology 13–3. However, there are

chemiluminescence - light emitted by a chemical reaction

TEST METHODOLOGY 13-3.   CHEMILUMINESCENCE IMMUNOASSAY FOR CA 15-3

The Reaction Principle

The principle of chemiluminescence immunoassay is identical to that of any other immunoassay with a chemiluminescent compound as an enhancer to the enzyme-substrate detection system. A chemical with luminescent properties, such as luminol, is oxidized by the enzyme reaction and excited. This excited reaction decays to the ground state by emitting light. This photon reaction is then measured in a luminometer, a type of photomultiplier.

Interferences

Interferences with the reaction may occur due to low-affinity antibodies to CA 15-3 being used in the reaction system and from inadequate washing between steps of the procedure. Nonspecific interactions may also occur, giving a high background count, and must be blocked with a protein such as bovine serum albumin, milk powder, or 1% serum lacking the ligand being assayed.

The Specimen

200 microliters of serum or plasma is required. Acceptable anticoagulants include sodium heparin and EDTA.

Reference Ranges

Reference ranges are dependent on methodology and reagents. The reference range for one chemiluminescent enzyme-linked immunosorbent assay (ELISA) for CA 15-3 is 0 to 31 U/mL

continued

many different methods for assaying CA 15-3, and levels obtained using different kits or methods cannot be compared with each other.[15,16] Refer to the Immunoassay section of Chapter 3 (Laboratory Techniques and Instrumentation) to review the principles of immunoassay methods.

The CLS student had to prepare the tissue sample for transport to a reference molecular diagnostics laboratory by taking it to the histology laboratory for embedding in paraffin. HER2 protein is elevated in some particularly aggressive breast carcinomas and possibly other cancers. Interest in this protein was amplified by discovery of a drug for treatment of HER2-positive cancers called Herceptin (trastuzumab). Evaluation of HER2 status currently has two clinical functions: as a predictive marker for response to Herceptin and as a prognostic marker. It was discovered that fluorescent in situ hybridization (FISH), which detects copies of HER2 DNA, was a more objective and accurate method of predicting response to Herceptin than immunohistochemistry. FISH is now being done in some clinical settings, primarily in reference laboratories. Test Methodology 13–4 describes this technique.

THE TEAM APPROACH

HER2 testing is done in the molecular diagnostics laboratory by FISH. FISH started as a research tool, but is now being done in some clinical settings, primarily in reference laboratories. Communication with clerical staff, nursing staff, and scientists at the reference laboratory may be necessary in order to collect, process, and transport acceptable specimens.

TEST METHODOLOGY 13-4.   FISH METHODOLOGY FOR HER2 DNA

The Reaction Principle

Cells from the submitted tissue are treated with heat and formamide to separate the DNA strands. Specific sequences of short areas of unique HER2 DNA, called probes, are prepared and a colored fluorescent reagent is attached to the probes. The probes are added to the reaction chamber and allowed to *anneal* to the DNA in the patient's cells. *Hybridization* will only occur if the probe is the exact compliment to the DNA sequence in the cell. If this hybridization occurs, the cell will fluoresce when viewed under a fluorescent microscope.[17-19]

The Specimen

Tumor cells from a biopsy sample are used. Metaphase or interphase cells will react in the test system. Paraffin-embedded, formalin-fixed tissue is used.

Reference Range

This test is reported as amplified or nonamplified based on 20 interphase cells. Nonamplified means that the tumor is HER2 negative.

THE CELL CYCLE

The cell cycle is an ordered sequence of events in which a single cell duplicates its chromosomes and divides into two cells. Figure 13–5 depicts this cell cycle. The entire cycle takes approximately 24 hours During this cycle, the cell proceeds from a resting, quiescent state to an actively dividing state through the processes of chromosomal (DNA) replication, RNA synthesis (transcription), and protein synthesis (translation), all of which direct the morphological changes that occur when a cell

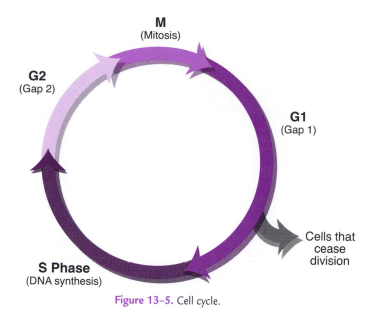

Figure 13–5. Cell cycle.

divides. The cell cycle is divided into four phases: G_0, G_1, S, G_2 and M (G_0 is a non-dividing, quiescent state). Stimulation by cytokines causes the cell to move into G_1, or gap 1, the state prior to the start of DNA synthesis. G_1 takes about 11 hours. Then the cell enters the S (synthesis) phase where DNA replication occurs, which requires about 8 hours. G_2, or gap 2, occurs after DNA synthesis, and the cell remains in this phase for 4 hours. All portions of the cell cycle other than the M phase are collectively referred to as interphase. The M phase (mitosis), where cell division occurs, is quite short, only requiring about 1 hour. Most cells, after fetal life is completed, remain for long periods in the G_0 state as nongrowing, nondividing cells. Appropriate stimulation of such cells induces them to return to G_1 and resume growth and division when necessary.[20–22]

When a malignancy occurs, the cell cycle is sped up and almost constant cell division occurs. Cells that should be in G_0 do not even go into that phase, and instead cycle continuously, producing daughter cells at a constant and massively overproductive rate. This change occurs gradually, as several mutations in the DNA build up and add to the overproduction. Most of the problem occurs from disorders of cell cycle regulation. Normally, the cell cycle can be stopped in G_1 if there is DNA damage, and this allows time for the DNA to be repaired. Then the cell cycle can be completed with repaired DNA being replicated. When this stoppage in G_1 does not occur, usually due to a problem with a regulatory protein called p53, the damaged DNA is replicated. More DNA damage occurs each cycle and builds up until the cell never stops cycling. Eventually, the cells do not respond to any of the normal "stop" signals, nor do they undergo apoptosis, and they become immortal.

MOLECULAR DIAGNOSTICS

Molecular diagnostics laboratories perform testing that detects the DNA of specific organisms that codes for specific proteins, or a specific sequence of DNA in

polymerase - an enzyme that catalyzes the addition of nucleotides to the DNA chain

THE TEAM APPROACH

A nurse calls from the oncologist's office wanting a patient's HER2 and CA 15-3 result STAT. Neither of these tests can be performed in an urgent manner, because each requires several hours to complete. The student CLS is given the task of explaining this to the nurse. The nurse is frustrated, stating that the doctor needs this information right away to help the frightened patient, who calls the office every few hours. The CLS explained the time frame for doing each test by giving the nurse a simplified overview of the length of each incubation period and the number of steps for each test, then totaling up the time required. This allowed the nurse, in turn, to explain the delay to the oncologist and the patient.

primer - short piece of DNA that is a known sequence for DNA that is being replicated

order to allow detection of small amounts of viruses, a mutant gene sequence, or DNA that codes for an abnormal protein. The major testing done by these laboratories involves **polymerase** chain reaction (PCR), reverse transcriptase–PCR (RT-PCR), and FISH. We have already discussed FISH in relation to the HER2/neu test.

PCR is a method for taking a very small amount of sample DNA, making more of it, and then detecting the DNA. The test system consists of the four building block nucleotides of DNA, sample DNA (patient sample), a heat-stable polymerase, and **primers**. The first step is to heat the sample DNA to separate the two strands. Then the primers are added and the mixture is allowed to cool. At the lower temperature, the primers will hybridize to the complimentary sequence on the sample DNA and the DNA polymerase and the nucleotides are added. The temperature is raised again to allow the best function of the polymerase enzyme and the polymerase adds nucleotides in the appropriate order to compliment the sample sequence.[23]

RT-PCR begins with messenger RNA (mRNA) in the patient sample. This test measures the DNA that is actually being expressed in the patient, because it has been transcribed. The mRNA is "reverse transcribed" back to DNA by an enzyme called reverse transcriptase. Once this step is completed, the procedure is the same as PCR.

Microarrays are a method for detecting several DNA sequences at once. A chip is impregnated with spots of different DNA sequences. The mRNAs from the patient sample are reverse transcribed into DNA, then the sample DNAs are fluorescent-tagged, added to the microarray, and allowed to anneal, if complimentary to the chip DNA sequences. The DNA that is complimentary to any spot DNA on the microarray chip is detected after annealing by the fluorescent tag.[24] Tissue microarrays have recently been developed to target gene amplifications in breast cancer, including the HER2/neu gene. In these microarrays, the tissue from many breast cancer sufferers is placed on the microarray chip and analyzed by FISH.[25,26] This method allows analysis of up to 1000 tissue samples at a time.

Case Scenario 13-3 Ruling In or Ruling Out Breast Cancer: A Frightened Young Woman Has a Breast Lump

Follow-Up

The CA 15-3 result on the young woman came back elevated at 324 U/mL, indicating that CA 15-3 monitoring would be of use during therapy. Her tumor was HER2/neu nonamplified; therefore, Herceptin therapy would not be useful. When the result for the CA 15-3 was ready, the CLS student called the nurse, asked for her by name, and provided the result as soon as it was confirmed. She did the same the next day when the HER2/neu result was received from the reference laboratory, cementing the relationship.

The patient followed up by having testing for breast cancer gene mutations 1 and 2 (*BRCA1* and *BRCA2*), since her mother had died of breast cancer at age 53 and her maternal aunt had been diagnosed with breast cancer at age 47. She possessed the *BRCA1* mutation, and was seeking genetic counseling. ●

CASE SCENARIO 13-4

Screening for Prostate Cancer: What Was the Current PSA?

While entering prostate specific antigen (PSA) results into the tumor marker database, a clinical laboratory scientist noted that James Braun, age 58, had previous results at yearly intervals since age 55. The values had remained stable in the range of 3.2 to 3.4 ng/mL (reference range, 2.0 to 4.0 ng/mL) until this past year, when a value of 4.2 ng/mL was determined 6 months ago. The CLS recalled that generally PSA is analyzed every 12 months. "Did his current PSA of 4.2 ng/mL indicate prostatic cancer?" she wondered.

PROSTATE CANCER

The prostate is a doughnut-shaped glandular organ found surrounding the urethra in men. Its function is to secrete seminal fluids. Prostatic cancer is common in males, and the second most common cause of cancer death among males, with increasing chance of developing this cancer over time. Risk factors for prostatic cancer in males include age over 40 years. For example, the incidence of prostatic cancer increases with age such that more than 50% of males over the age of 70 years have cancer of the prostate. Prostate cancer may be asymptomatic or may present with symptoms of generalized **prostatism**.

Benign prostate cell growth is generally responsive to little or no treatment. Detection of prostate cancer is achieved by a combination of physical examination, biochemical testing, and imaging techniques. Physical examination by digital rectal examination of the prostate will also provide valuable information but should generally be performed after the blood sample has been drawn since biochemical markers and tumor-associated antigens can be quickly released even with mild tissue trauma from the physical examination.[27]

Tumor Markers for the Prostate

Prostate specific antigen (PSA) is a tumor marker for prostatic carcinoma. The perfect tumor marker would be highly specific to a particular tumor within a specific tissue, be released into blood or urine for ease of analysis, provide body fluid levels that correlate with amount of tumor cells or malignancy, have potential for detection prior to overt symptoms or in early stages, have a short half-life so that changes reflect response to therapy, and have the ability to be assessed with near 100% sensitivity and specificity. Prostatic acid phosphatase (PAP) meets some of those requirements but falls short in sensitivity. Prostate specific antigen meets nearly all these requirements in detecting prostatic cancer.[28] However, it is also released into blood and body fluids when the prostate is inflamed and enlarged, the condition known as prostatism. Prostatic specific antigen and prostatic acid phosphatase are tumor markers that are best utilized if the patient has certain risk factors for cancer of the prostate. As with other tumor marker tests, these tests are not valuable as a cancer screening tests in the general population since both are present normally in small amounts in body fluids.[29]

Tumor markers for the prostate provide valuable information that, along with physical examination, aid in diagnosis of prostatic cancer when elevated above the reference range. In particular, when the plasma or serum value doubles within 12

CLINICAL CORRELATION
Prostatism is the condition of partial or complete blockage of the urethra due to an enlarged prostate gland. It is associated with increased frequency of urination but difficulty in fully emptying the bladder and may be caused by benign or cancerous tumors in the prostate.

prostatism - the condition of partial or complete blockage of the urethra due to an enlarged prostate gland

benign - cell growth that doesn't spread and is cured with removal

months or less, it is a strong indication of risk for prostatic cancer and indicates the need for more invasive tests such as biopsy.[30] The problem lies in establishing a consensus for a reference range and setting a useful upper limit to make a medical decision. Many clinicians interpret PSA and PAP tumor marker results by testing middle-aged males annually in conjunction with physical examination and medical history findings.[31] Specifically, one model considers age and results of digital rectal examination and serum PSA in order to predict prostatic cancer in men.[32] While some clinicians feel that the value of PSA for screening for prostatic cancer in older males is currently not as valuable as it once was, others note that mortality from this type of cancer has declined since PSA screening became common. Probably the most important factor in improving the positive predictive value of tumor markers is the medical decision limit.[30] The medical decision limit is outside of the normal reference range and is the cutoff point when the laboratory result begins to indicate a particular disease. For example, with a tumor marker, it is often a certain value that, when met or exceeded, indicates a high likelihood of a particular cancer.[2]

Prostate Specific Antigen

Prostatic specific antigen is a single-polypeptide tumor-associated antigen. It is a glycoprotein that is most likely produced in the rough endoplasmic reticulum and granules of columnar **acinar** prostate cells. It is a protease with trypsin-like enzymatic activity and functions to liquefy seminal fluid. Given its biochemical make-up, PSA is highly antigenic and readily measured by immunoassay techniques. The first techniques for analysis of PSA were various types of immunoradiometric assay (IRMA).[25]

Prostate specific antigen levels may not provide enough information for staging of cancer. However, these tumor markers generally provide useful information in follow-up to treatment.[33] For example, in a longitudinal study following patients undergoing treatment for prostatic cancer, very low PSA levels after 5 years indicated a high likelihood for long-term remission.[34] Since so many older men are having PSA levels assessed frequently, there is a wealth of data concerning PSA, benign prostatic hyperplasia (BPH), and prostatic cancer. A recent study that involved data collected over a 20-year period concluded that recent findings show that serum PSA is statistically related only to prostate tumor size, whereas serum PSA was related more significantly to prostate cancer 20 years ago. In the last 5 years, serum PSA has only been related to BPH. There is an urgent need for serum markers that reflect the size and grade of this ubiquitous cancer.[29]

PSA levels have improved diagnostic sensitivity for detection of prostatic cancer when compared to PAP but are better in detecting prostate cancer in men over the age of 62. PSA suffers from somewhat poor diagnostic specificity due to false-positive results in men with a noncancerous inflammatory condition of the prostate termed *benign prostatic hyperplasia*. BPH is a much more common condition than prostatic cancer, and some cases do progress to develop prostatic cancer. False-positive results can also arise from digital rectal examination of the prostate, so it is recommended that blood samples be obtained prior to this physical examination.[25] As mentioned earlier, a small amount of PSA is normally present in the serum of men, so determining the level that is considered abnormal is important for the diagnosis of prostatic disease. Various decision levels have been suggested, including 2.0, 3.0, or 4.0 ng/mL according to the age of the male. Reference ranges may need to be race adjusted before prediction of prostatic cancer is improved, since African-American males seem to have higher PSA levels. One suggestion is to provide age-adjusted reference ranges, with 0 to 2.0 ng/mL suggestive of prostatic dis-

acinar - granular tissue that makes up a gland such as the pancreas or prostate

ease in white men younger than 62 years of age.[35] A decision tree has been suggested using 4.0 ng/mL as the decision point to perform a more invasive but definitive test for prostatic cancer, a tissue biopsy. The recommendation is that PSA levels of 0 to 3.9 ng/mL are considered in the normal reference range and there is no need for a biopsy, while 4.0 ng/mL and higher indicates the need for biopsy. At PSA levels greater than 10 ng/mL, a biopsy is highly recommended and there is a greater than 50% probability that prostate cancer will be detected.[12]

Assay methodology makes a difference as well, in terms of whether total or free PSA is measured. The classic total PSA assay was measured by immunoassay, first by radioimmunoassay and now using chemiluminescent or microcapture enzyme immunoassay. Test Methodology 13–5 presents a common method of analysis for PSA. Ordinarily, 35% of total PSA is free, with the remainder complexed with protease inhibitors.[36] Reporting the free and total PSA levels can help to improve the diagnostic specificity of PSA for prostatic cancer since men with prostate cancer are more likely to have less free PSA than those with BPH. Thus the use of assays capable of measuring free or complexed fractions of PSA have helped to reduce the number of unnecessary biopsies.[37,38]

Prostatic Acid Phosphatase

One of the earliest tests for prostate cancer was acid phosphatase. Acid phosphatase, prostatic fraction (PAP), is an endogenous enzyme similar to alkaline

---

TEST METHODOLOGY 13-5.   PSA BY MICROPARTICLE ENZYME IMMUNOASSAY

The Reaction Principle

The sample is introduced into the reaction cell containing anti-PSA–coated microparticles suspended in assay diluent. During the incubation period, the PSA binds to the anti-PSA–coated microparticles, forming an antibody-antigen complex. An aliquot of the reaction mixture is transferred to the glass-fiber matrix, which causes irreversible binding of the antibody-antigen complex to the glass-fiber matrix. Following a wash step to remove unbound substances, anti-PSA alkaline phosphatase conjugate is added and incubated. A second wash step removes unbound materials, followed by addition of 4-methylumbelliferyl phosphate substrate. The fluorescent product is measured by the optical assembly with a direct relationship of fluorescence and sample PSA.

Interferences

Human anti-mouse antibodies from patients who have received preparations of mouse monoclonal antibodies (for diagnosis or therapy) will give variable results. Prostatic manipulative procedures, including biopsy and digital rectal examination, may release transient amounts of PSA, giving erroneous results. Hormonal therapy may also cause discrepant results.

The Specimen

Serum stored at 2° to 8°C prior to testing; frozen if delay in testing of over 24 hours. Frozen samples should be mixed thoroughly after thawing with avoidance of repeated thawing and refreezing.

Reference Range

Adult male   0–4.0 ng/mL
Abbott Laboratories; Diagnostic Division. Abbott Park, IL.

phosphatase. Acid phosphatase (ACP) is found in the lysosomes of many cells, including prostate, liver, spleen, and bone marrow and other organelles of erythrocytes. The majority of serum ACP arises from erythrocytes and prostatic tissues in males. Historically ACP was analyzed by kinetic reaction using enzyme kinetics and repeating the analysis with addition of tartrate ions in order to analyze PAP. The prostatic portions of the enzyme are inhibited when tartrate is added. This allowed for determining the percentage of prostate fraction of the total ACP activity. However, due to the extreme instability of the enzyme in serum and some lack of specificity in the analysis, other methods of analysis were explored for PAP. Currently, it is more common to analyze PAP by immunoassay, which relies on its antigenic reactivity in the immunoassay. This method for analysis of PAP recognizes all molecules of the enzyme, including those that are catalytically inactive. It has improved analytical sensitivity over the kinetic methods, but the diagnostic sensitivity and specificity of PAP are somewhat poor for prostatic cancer in its earliest treatable stages. When alternative tumor markers became available, PAP was utilized less frequently.[30]

Other Prostate Tumor Markers

Other prostatic cancer tumor markers have been utilized in the past, including total acid phosphatase activity, total alkaline phosphatase activity, and bone fraction of alkaline phosphatase activity. These enzymes have varying degrees of tissue specificity to the prostate gland, with bone alkaline phosphatase more specific than acid phosphatase activity, which is more specific than total alkaline phosphatase activity.[25] Recently developed prostatic cancer tumor markers include proPSA, which is a precursor to active PSA, and prostate specific membrane antigen (PSMA). Serum concentrations of these two markers are elevated in prostate cancer and have strong ability to discriminates between cancer and BPH or no disease. Two surprising prostatic cancer tumor markers are **insulin-like growth factor**-1 (IGF-1) and **insulin-like growth factor binding protein**-3 (IGFBP-3), which are associated with increased risk for prostate cancer.[39] There are also gene-based and cell-based biomarkers that are useful for characterizing carcinoma cells from biopsied prostatic tissue. None of these recently developed tumor marker tests is used as commonly as free and total PSA levels, but their use may become more widespread in the future.

THE TEAM APPROACH

When an unusual test request comes to the laboratory, such as for IGF-1 or IGFBP-3, the test often is sent to a reference laboratory. It is important that the correct specimen is collected, and that it is handled and packaged correctly to keep it preserved prior to testing. Often these specimens are sent some distance, so specimens may require packing in dry ice. The process requires communication between laboratory staff responsible for sending the specimens and the nurse, medical assistant, or physician assistant who may be collecting the sample to ensure that no errors occur.

insulin-like growth factor - peptide similar in chemical structure and activity to insulin

insulin-like growth factor binding protein - a soluble protein that binds insulin-like growth factors and affects them at the cellular level

Case Scenario 13-4 Screening for Prostate Cancer: What Was the Current PSA?

Follow-Up

As was discussed, most clinicians recognize that BPH, a condition that may not require treatment, and prostatic cancer can both cause elevated PSA levels. Likewise, if a digital rectal examination was performed prior to the sample collection, there could be some release of PSA due to the medical examination. It is unusual for a second PSA to be ordered within a 12-month period unless symptoms of prostatism or other evidence of enlarged prostate is found by the clinician. Given that the second PSA level greater than 4.0 ng/mL for this patient, the clinician will most likely follow up with an ultrasonogram of the prostate and possibly a needle biopsy sample. Thus the serum tumor marker test can be helpful to decide if further, more invasive and/or more expensive testing is necessary to aid in the diagnosis of cancer. ●

CASE SCENARIO 13-5

Ectopic Hormone Production due to Oat Cell Carcinoma: Is Hyperosmolar Urine due to SIADH?

The medical technology student was performing electrolyte and osmolality testing in her second week of clinical chemistry internship and noticed that a patient result had an elevated urine osmolality and decreased serum osmolality as compared with reference ranges. The plasma sodium was 125 mmol/L (reference range, 136 to 145 mmol/L), nearing the critical value set by the laboratory. The supervising instructor helped the student to verify results. They noted that the patient is an 88-year-old female, admitted through the emergency department with a preliminary diagnosis of hypertension, vomiting, and lethargy. After results were reported, the instructing technologist suggested that the student review causes for these findings of hyperosmolar urine and hyponatremia.

SODIUM AND WATER BALANCE

Sodium and water balance have been discussed in Chapter 6 (Assessment of Renal Function), relating the role of the kidneys in maintenance of electrolyte and water balance through reabsorption and secretion. Most of the sodium regulation occurs in the proximal convoluted tubules under the influence of a sodium threshold and active transport, while water levels are controlled primarily through osmosis. Some hormonal influence, including from antidiuretic hormone (ADH) and aldosterone, is also exerted in the renal system. Antidiuretic hormone, also known as vasopressin, is secreted by the posterior pituitary in response to osmoreceptors in the brain. It stimulates the renal collecting ducts to reabsorb water, thus conserving more water in times of water deprivation. Aldosterone, secreted by the adrenal cortex, induces the distal convoluted tubules to reabsorb sodium and chloride in exchange for potassium. Since these hormones function in an integrated fashion, they help to maintain homeostasis of water and electrolytes by finishing the reabsorption and secretion phase within the kidney. Excessive secretion of these hormones can cause water and electrolyte imbalances.[40]

Conditions also exist that cause insufficient secretion of ADH, which also affects water balance. The general term for lack of diuretic hormone is *diabetes insidipidus*. This condition is discussed in more details in Chapter 11 (Endocrine Disorders and Testing). Insufficient output of ADH is usually a result of renal disease, but hypothalamic malignancy can cause destruction of cells that produce or secrete ADH. Thus, although diabetes insipidus is generally considered an endocrine disease often secondary to renal disorders, it may result from neoplastic destruction of the glands that secrete the hormone.

✓ Common Sense Check
After verification that a critical low result is not due to preanalytical or analytical error, it is important to report the result verbally and in writing as soon as possible according to the policy of the laboratory or hospital. Critical lab results are indications that the patient needs immediate attention and treatment so that further complications don't occur.

Hyponatremia

The patient in Case Scenario 13–5 has hyponatremia. Hyponatremia may be caused by renal conditions such as salt-losing nephritis, renal tubular acidosis, chronic renal failure, or nephrotic syndrome. Increased urine sodium levels usually indicate renal sodium loss such as from salt-losing nephritis or from diuretics. There are nonrenal causes of hyponatremia also, including syndrome of inappropriate ADH

psychogenic - of mental origin, such as compulsive drinking of water in psychogenic water overload

secretion (SIADH), diuretics such as thiazine, **psychogenic** water overload, cellular shift changes from acidosis, and edema secondary to cirrhosis or congestive heart failure. Urine sodium levels are usually normal or decreased in hyponatremia due to edema. Thus urinary sodium levels and physical examination assist the clinician in determining the cause of hyponatremia and hyperosmolar urine.

Ectopic Hormone Production

Hypersecretion of hormones can occur in a variety of disorders, as discussed in Chapter 11. Hypersecretion of ADH refers to production and release of the hormone in the absence of the usual stimuli of hyperosmolar plasma. Even when the plasma becomes hypo-osmolar, ADH can continue to be released in cases of SIADH. This condition can be due to nonmalignant diseases of the central nervous system or pulmonary system or can occur as a side effect from certain drug therapies. SIADH can also result from adenocarcinoma of the lung. Any one of these serious conditions requires consideration, differential diagnosis, and specific treatment.

Lung Pathology

ectopic hormone secretion - production of hormones by nonendocrine cells

Lung tissue is composed of several types, including bronchial epithelial, squamous, undifferentiated large cell, and undifferentiated small cell types. Lymphoid tissue also resides in the lungs. Malignancies can arise in any one of these cell types, with bronchogenic carcinoma, associated with cigarette smoke, comprising the majority. Most lung cancers are associated with persistent cough that may include wheezing and other breathing problems. Hypercalcemia and **ectopic hormone secretion** may be the first sign of some types of lung cancer, including small cell carcinoma. Hormones that can be secreted include ADH, adrenocorticotropic hormone (ACTH), somatostatin, and parathyroid-related peptide. Other diagnostic indicators are needed, including imaging techniques. Chest x-ray and computed tomography (CT) scanning are valuable in visualizing and staging the tumor, including lymph node involvement.[1]

> **Case Scenario 13-5** Ectopic Hormone Production due to Oat Cell Carcinoma: Is Hyperosmolar Urine due to SIADH?
>
> **Follow-Up**
>
> The patient was admitted to the hospital to investigate the cause of her hyperosmolar urine, since medications were ruled out. Addison's disease due to adrenal failure was ruled out since cortisol and aldosterone levels were within normal reference ranges. Thyroid hormone levels were within normal reference ranges as well. Immediate treatment for the patient involved withdrawal of fluids in order to allow the sodium and water levels to attempt to stabilize. The patient's history revealed a 40-year history of cigarette smoking and surgical removal of the left kidney due to renal carcinoma several years ago. The diagnosis of oat cell carcinoma was made based on CT of the chest and biopsy of the right lung. The patient and her family were instructed as to their treatment options given the stage and type of lung cancer and the patient's physical condition. ●

CASE SCENARIO 13-6

Pancreatic Cancer: Searching for the Cause of High Amylase Levels

Amylase and lipase tests were ordered on Ms. Jameson, a 57-year-old white woman with a diagnosis of jaundice, diabetes mellitus, and pancreatitis. The medical technologist made a manual dilution for the lipase test since it exceeded linearity of the instrument. The instrument would make a $1/2$ dilution prior to reporting and since the method was linear to 400 U/L, this indicated that lipase was greater than 800 U/L. In this instance the procedure called for a $1/4$ dilution in bovine albumin diluent prior to analysis and noted that dilution of more than $1/4$ would cause technical problems. The technologist noted that amylase was 104 U/L (reference range, 45 to 113 U/L) and bilirubin was 6.7 mg/dL (0.2 to 1.3 mg/dL). Other laboratory results from the same specimen were abnormal, including cholesterol at 383 mg/dL (reference range, less than 200 mg/dL), triglycerides at 420 mg/dL (less than 250 mg/dL), alkaline phosphatase at 213 U/L (35 to 100 U/L), and lactate dehydrogenase at 293 U/L (100 to 250 U/L). CBC, CA 19.9, and CA 19-5 were also ordered.

> ✓ **Common Sense Check**
>
> It is important to be familiar with the upper limit linearity of test procedures, how the automated instrument indicates that a result exceeded linearity, and whether the sample is automatically diluted and retested or if a manual dilution is required. This information is found in the manufacturer's test procedure and should also be found in the laboratory procedure. It is good practice to refer to these procedures when linearity is exceeded.

PANCREATIC CANCER

Pancreatic cancer is the fourth most common cause of cancer death in the United States. Of the 32,000 patients diagnosed with pancreatic carcinoma in the United States in 2004, approximately 40% presented with locally advanced disease.[42] Pancreatic cancer is difficult to diagnose until it is advanced and, thus, chemotherapy and radiation therapy haven't been very successful in curing or treating the disease. Because pancreatic cancer often presents with nonspecific symptoms until it reaches advanced stages, there is a need for good diagnostic indicators. Some indicators that have been used include serum enzymes such as amylase and lipase, ectopically produced hormones, and tumor-associated antigens such as CA 19-5. Those that provide the best diagnostic specificity and sensitivity include CA 19-5 and CA 19.9.[42,43]

The pancreas is composed of several types of cells, including glandular cells such as the alpha, delta, and beta islet cells that produce and secrete metabolic and digestive hormones. There are also acinar cells, granular cells that produce secretions such as the digestive fluids containing trypsin, lipase, and amylase. The pancreas also contains ductal cells that provide the tubes to allow passage of the pancreatic digestive secretions into the small intestine. Tumors can arise from any of these cell lines.[44]

Pathology of the Pancreas

Serum amylase and lipase levels are increased when compared to reference ranges in cases of acute or chronic inflammation of the pancreas. Amylase and lipase levels are not 100% specific to pancreatic disease but help to support clinical findings of pancreatitis. In general, serum amylase and lipase increase on the first day of the disorder and return to normal within a week. More details about acute and chronic inflammation of the pancreas are discussed in Chapter 10 (Assessment of Nutrition and Digestive Function).

Malignant tumors of the pancreas most often occur in the head of the pancreas from ductal epithelium, causing obstruction of the bile duct. Thus, biliary enzymes such as alkaline phosphatase and gamma-glutamyltransferase may be elevated to indicate bile duct obstruction due to malignancy of the head of the pancreas. Later, jaundice and elevated total and direct bilirubin become strong diagnostic indicators. One less commonly used but fairly promising enzyme marker of pancreatic carcinoma, due to its diagnostic sensitivity, is serum galactosyltransferase isoenzyme II.[44]

Pancreatic endocrine tumors do occur, although less frequently than ductal or acinar tumors. Occasionally insulinomas, or insulin-secreting tumors, occur, most frequently in the body and tail of the pancreas instead of the head. Most of these are adenomas, benign secreting tumors. Non-beta islet cell tumors are associated with excessive secretion of gastrin or secretin. Hypergastrinemia serves as a diagnostic indicator and also causes the complication of peptic ulcers and other clinical findings associated with Zollinger-Ellison syndrome. Hypersecretion of secretin by these tumors is associated with watery diarrhea, hypokalemia, and achlorhydria without excessive gastrin secretion or peptic ulcers. Vasoactive intestinal peptide (VIP) carcinoma, sometimes called VIPoma, is rare. VIPomas secrete excessive amounts of VIP that causes a special clinical syndrome characterized by secretory diarrhea, hypokalemia, and achlorhydria.[43]

Pancreatic Tumor Markers

Various tumor markers have been used to aid in diagnosis of pancreatic tumors. In one study, the tumor markers CA 195, CA 19.9, and some less commonly used markers (CA 242, CAM 43 and TPS) were compared for diagnostic specificity and sensitivity in detecting pancreatic cancers. TPS had the best sensitivity but the poorest specificity. TPS is a circulating marker of rapid cellular growth. Sensitivities were 98% for TPS, 79% for CA 19.9, 76% for CA 195, 57% for CA 242, and 60% for CAM 43. Values elevated above the medical decision limit for the tumor markers, however, did not appear until the second stage of cancer. Specificities calculated for the group with pancreatic diseases were 95% for CAM 43, 84% for CA 242, 60% for CA 19.9, 53% for CA 195, and 22% for TPS. This information is summarized in Table 13–7. Considering both sensitivity and specificity, CA 19.9 showed good sensitivity (79%) and high specificity (60% to 100%). It is recommended by some scientists that the other markers could be used alone or with CA 19.9.[42]

TABLE 13-7

Diagnostic Specificity and Sensitivity for Pancreatic Cancer Tumor Markers

Tumor Marker	Diagnostic Specificity	Diagnostic Sensitivity
CAM 43	95%	60%
CA 242	84%	57%
TPS	22%	98%
CA 195	53%	76%
CA 19.9	60%	79%

Case Scenario 13-6 Pancreatic Cancer: Searching for the Cause of High Amylase Levels

Follow-Up

Amylase and lipase were ordered on Ms. Jameson, a 57-year-old white woman with a diagnosis of jaundice, diabetes mellitus, and pancreatitis. CBC, CA 19.9, and CA 195 were also ordered. The lipase result determined from the $\frac{1}{4}$ dilution was 876 U/L ($219 \times 4/1 = 876$). This result is quite elevated above the reference range. Bilirubin, triglycerides, cholesterol, alkaline phosphatase, and lactate dehydrogenase were also elevated. Amylase was in the normal reference range. The CBC revealed 91% neutrophils with an increase in band neutrophils. The patient appeared jaundiced, correlating with the elevated serum bilirubin level. Cancer of the head of the pancreas was suspected given the history, physical examination, and clinical presentation, which is why tumor markers were also ordered. If they were elevated above the reference range, it would most likely indicate cancer of the head of the pancreas in stage 2 or later. Chemotherapy and radiation therapy would most likely be initiated. ●

SUMMARY

Tumor markers such as PSA, CA 125, CA 19.9, and other markers for colorectal, pulmonary, gastric, pancreatic, breast, liver, or prostatic carcinomas were discussed. Which marker is assayed will depend on the tumor's primary location. However, as indicated, most tumor markers are not good screening tests, because they tend to be nonspecific and can be elevated in conditions other than malignancies. Once the diagnosis is made, tumor markers are very helpful in determining whether or not treatment is reducing the tumor load or the cancer is recurring or metastatic. Once the presence of a tumor is detected, the oncologist will order a baseline tumor marker measurement and, during treatment, serial assays will be done to determine whether or not the treatment is working. Effective treatment will drop the level of the tumor marker precipitously and the level will remain within the reference range. Rising levels after treatment are often associated with recurrence or metastasis. These terms and other information about tumor markers and tests to detect them were discussed in this chapter.

EXERCISES

As you consider the scenarios presented in this chapter, answer the following questions:

1. Define tumor marker using prostate specific antigen as an example for both benign and malignant growths.

2. Write the formula for diagnostic sensitivity.

3. Explain CA 195 in terms of type of tumor marker and common associated malignancies.

4. Explain how enzymes can be tumor markers, listing two common examples, including their associated tissues of origin.

5. Discuss the reaction principle for analysis of two common breast cancer tumor markers.

6. Explain the value of M protein, a paraprotein immunoglobulin, for diagnosis and treatment of patients with monoclonal gammopathies.

7. Calculate diagnostic specificity, positive predictive value, and negative predictive value given the following PSA data: frequency of true negatives = 75, frequency of false negatives = 25, frequency of true positives = 85, and frequency of false positives = 15.

8. Explain the role of diagnostic specificity and sensitivity and receiver operating characteristic (ROC) curves in determining the best medical decision limit.

References

1. Fenton RG, Longo DL: Cell biology of cancer. In Fauci AS, et al (eds): *Harrison's Principles of Internal Medicine*, ed 14. New York: McGraw-Hill, 1998.
2. Crawford E: PSA testing: what is the use? *Lancet* 2005; 365:1447–1449.
3. See S: Cancer markers of the 1990s: comparison of the new generation of markers defined by monoclonal antibodies and oncogene probes to prototypic markers. *Clin Lab Med* 1990; 10:1–31.
4. Mandel JS, et al: Reducing mortality from colorectal cancer by screening for fecal occult blood. Minnesota Colon Cancer Control Study. *N Engl J Med* 1993; 328:1365–1371.
5. Cisneros G, et al: Humoral hypercalcemia of malignancy in squamous cell carcinoma of the skin: parathyroid hormone-related protein as a cause. *South Med J* 2001; 94: 329–331.
6. Longo DL: Plasma cell disorders. In Fauci AS, et al (eds): *Harrison's Principles of Internal Medicine*, ed 14. New York: McGraw-Hill, 1998.
7. Alexanian R, Weber D, Lui F: Differential diagnosis of monoclonal gammopathies. *Arch Pathol Lab Med* 1999; 123:108–113.
8. Goeken JA, Keren DF: Introduction to the Report of the Consensus Conference on Monoclonal Gammopathies. *Arch Pathol Lab Med* 1999; 123:104–105.
9. Attaelmannan M, Levinson SS: Understanding and identifying monoclonal gammopathies. *Clin Chem* 2000; 46(8B):1230–1238.
10. *Protein Electrophoresis and Immunofixation: Interpretive Guide* (CD module). Beaumont, TX: Helena Laboratories, Inc., 2006.
11. Hauser SL, Goodkin DE: Multiple sclerosis and other demyelinating diseases. In Fauci AS, et al (eds): *Harrison's Principles of Internal Medicine*, ed 14. New York: McGraw-Hill, 1998.
12. Low RN, et al: Treated ovarian cancer: MR imaging, laparotomy reassessment, and serum CA-125 values compared with clinical outcome at 1 year. *Radiology* 2005; 235:918–926.
13. Mano A, et al: CA-125/auc as a new prognostic factor for patients with ovarian cancer. *Gynecol Oncol* 2005; 97:529–534.
14. Jacobs I, Bast RC: The CA 125 tumor-associated antigen: a review of the literature. *Hum Reprod* 1989; 4:1–12.
15. Findeisen R, et al: Chemiluminescent determination of tissue polypeptide antigen (TPA), cancer antigen 15-3 (CA 15-3), carcinoembryonic antigen (CEA) in comparison with vascular epithelial growth factor (VEGF) in follow-up of breast cancer. *Luminescence* 2000; 15:283–289.
16. Horowitz GL, et al: Modular analytics: a new approach to automation in the clinical laboratory. *J Automated Methods Manage Chem* 2005; 1:8–25.
17. Prati R, et al: Histopathologic characteristics predicting HER2/neu amplification in breast cancer. *Breast J* 2005; 11:433–439.
18. Li-Ning TE, et al: Role of chromogenic in-situ hybridization (CISH) in the evaluation of HER2 status in breast carcinoma: comparison with immunohistochemistry and FISH. *Int J Surg Pathol* 2005; 13:343–351.

19. Mass RD, et al: Evaluation of clinical outcomes according to HER2 detection by fluorescence in-situ hybridization in women with metastatic breast cancer treated with trastuzumab. *Clin Breast Cancer* 2005; 6:240–246.

20. Tyson JJ, Csikasz-Nagy A, Novak B: The dynamics of cell regulation. *Bioassays* 2002; 1095–1099.

21. Tyson JJ, et al: Checkpoints in the cell cycle from a modeler's perspective. *Prog Cell Cycle Res* 1995; 1:1–8.

22. Nojima H: Cell cycle checkpoints, chromosome stability and the progression of cancer. *Hum Cell* 1997; 10:221–230.

23. Lonn U, et al: Demonstration of gene-amplification by PCR in archival paraffin-embedded breast cancer tissue. *Breast Cancer Res Treat* 1994; 30:147–152.

24. Ji, MJ, et al: Microarray-based method for genotyping of functional single nucleotide polymorphisms using dual-color fluorescence hybridization. *Mutat Res* 2004; 548: 97–105.

25. AL-Kuraya K, et al: Prognostic relevance of gene amplifications and coamplifications in breast cancer. *Cancer Res* 2004; 64:8534–8540.

26. Sauter G, Simon R, Hillan K: Tissue microarrays in drug discovery. *Nature Rev Drug Discovery* 2003; 2:962–972.

27. Armbruster DA: Prostate-specific antigen: biochemistry, analytical methods and clinical applications. *Clin Chem* 1993; 39:181–195.

28. Bernstein LH, et al: Medically significant concentrations of prostate-specific antigen in serum assessed. *Clin Chem* 1993; 39:896.

29. Stamey TA, et al: The prostate specific antigen era in the United States is over for prostate cancer: what happened in the last 20 years? *J Urol* 2005; 173:2205–2206.

30. Woeste S: Diagnosing prostate cancer. *Lab Med* 2004; 36:399–400.

31. Hernandez J, Thompson M: Prostate-specific antigen: a review of the validation of the most commonly used cancer biomarker. *Cancer* 2004; 101:894–904.

32. Karakiewicz PI, et al: Development and validation of a nomogram predicting the outcome of prostate biopsy based on patient age, digital rectal examination and serum prostate specific antigen. *J Urol* 2005; 173:1930–1934.

33. Cooperberg MR, et al: The University of California, San Francisco Cancer of the Prostate Risk Assessment score: a straightforward and reliable preoperative predictor of disease recurrence after radical prostatectomy. *J Urol* 2005; 173:1938–1942.

34. Low PSA levels at 5 years indicate low odds of relapse. *Lab Med* 2002; 33:911.

35. Datta MW, et al: Prostate cancer in patients with screening serum prostate specific antigen values less than 4.0 ng/dl: results from the Cooperative Prostate Cancer Tissue Resource. *J Urol* 2005; 173:1546–1551.

36. Lilja H: Significance of different molecular forms of serum PSA: the free, noncomplexed form of PSA versus that complexed to alpha 1-antichymotrypsin. *Urol Clin North Am* 1993; 20:681.

37. Catalona WJ, et al: Comparison of digital rectal examination and serum prostate specific antigen in the early detection of prostate cancer: results of a multicenter clinical trial of 6,630 men. *J Urol* 1994; 151:1283–1290.

38. Partin AW, et al: Complexed prostate specific antigen improves specificity for prostate cancer detection: results of a prospective multicenter clinical trial. *J Urol* 2003; 170: 1787–1791.

39. Tricoli JV, Schoenfeldt M, Conley BA: Detection of prostate cancer and predicting progression: current and future diagnostic markers. *Clin Cancer Res* 2004; 10:3943–3953.

40. Moses AM, Streeten DHP: Disorders of the neurohypophysis. In Fauci AS, et al (eds): *Harrison's Principles of Internal Medicine*, ed 14. New York: McGraw-Hill, 1998.

41. Willett CG, et al: Locally advanced pancreatic cancer. *J Clin Oncol* 2005; 23:4538–4544.

42. Kazmierczak SC, Catrou PG, Van Lente F: Diagnostic accuracy of pancreatic enzymes evaluated by use of multivariate data analysis. *Clin Chem* 1993; 39:1960–1965.

43. Banfi G, et al: Behavior of tumor markers CA19.9, CA195, CAM43, CA242, and TPS in the diagnosis and follow-up of pancreatic cancer. *Clin Chem* 1993; 39:420–423.

44. Mayer RJ: Pancreatic cancer. In Fauci AS, et al (eds): *Harrison's Principles of Internal Medicine*, ed 14. New York: McGraw-Hill, 1998.

The clinical laboratory is an important partner in the assessment of therapeutic drug monitoring and toxicology.

Therapeutic Drug Monitoring and Toxicology

Dean L. Arneson and Wendy Arneson

therapeutic drug monitoring - measuring serum levels of a drug to aid in adjusting drug dosage

toxicity - poisoning due to exposure to a toxin, including drugs, gases, heavy metals, and alcohols

alcohols - methanol (CH_3OH), isopropanol ((CH_3)$_2CHOH$), and ethylene glycol ((CH_2OH)$_2$), which are chemically similar to ethanol due to the –OH group

Medications are supposed to be helpful while poisons are obviously harmful. However, medications can reach harmful levels in the blood and the risk of taking the drug then outweighs its benefit. **Therapeutic drug monitoring** is performed in order to help determine adequate blood levels of medication when treating the underlying disorder. In addition, plasma levels of drugs are useful to assess degree of **toxicity** expected in patients. Acetaminophen and ethyl **alcohol** become toxic when taken at higher than recommended levels, while other substances such as methanol are toxic to people at any level. This chapter explores situations and problems involving laboratory personnel to illustrate the correlation of laboratory values with disorders. Methods of analysis, including chromatography and immunoassay, will be addressed in this chapter. The student will also become acquainted with the team effort in working with pharmacy and emergency department (ED) personnel. Paramount in the proper analysis of drugs and toxic substances are the following: acceptable specimen collection, handling, and transport; periodic quality control testing and instrument calibration; accurate specimen analysis; correctly evaluating the patient results; evaluating all aspects of quality assurance; and promptly communicating the laboratory results to the health-care personnel. The side boxes in this chapter provide common sense tips, definitions of terms, brief descriptions of pathophysiology, and clinical correlations as well as reminders of the team approach in health care. Text boxes within the chapter outline methodology for laboratory assessment of nutrition and digestive function.

OBJECTIVES

Upon completion of this chapter, the student will have the ability to

  ▪ List common preanalytical errors resulting from improper specimen collection and handling for therapeutic drugs, alcohol, and drugs of abuse.

  ▪ Discuss commonly encountered sources of analytical interference due to related chemicals, isopropanol, botanicals, and anticoagulants and from evaporation.

  ▪ Describe the principles of analyses for therapeutic drugs, drugs of abuse, and alcohol in terms of key reagents, their roles, and endpoint detection.

  ▪ Verify calculation of osmolality and osmolal gap when it is required.

  ▪ Evaluate patient sample collection and handling processes in terms of impact on the outcome to include communicating with other members of the health-care team.

  ▪ Compare and correlate alcohol and mercury results with expected previous findings and with pathology, suggesting appropriate course of action.

  ▪ Describe the correct method of recording patient therapeutic drug and drug of abuse results, including decimal place and unit.

  ▪ Discuss situations regarding acetaminophen and drugs of abuse in which it is important to communicate results to health-care providers.

Therapeutic Drug Monitoring

CASE SCENARIO 14-1

Therapeutic Ranges: Trouble for Baby Jones

The technologist analyzed gentamicin for Baby Jones, who was born 4 weeks prematurely. The diagnosis listed for Baby Jones was *Haemophilus influenza* meningitis. She had the following gentamicin results:

	Patient	Reference Range
Peak (µg/mL)	0.5	3–5
Trough (µg/mL)	5	<2

Before reporting these results, the technologist noted that they did not fall within therapeutic ranges. The technologist realized that the **peak** level should be higher than the **trough** level. What are some of the explanations for these results?

1. One or both were mislabeled specimens (i.e., from the wrong patient).
2. Incorrect time for collecting either sample was recorded in the chart by (nurse or physician assistant) nonlaboratory personnel.
3. Personnel collected one or both specimens at the incorrect times.
4. Some other type of preanalytical or analytical variations happened with one or both specimens.

After checking the label and condition of the specimen, the patient result should be compared with the **therapeutic range**. Peak level should be higher than the trough.

peak - the highest level of a particular drug found in the blood following administration of a dose

trough - the lowest level of a particular drug found in the blood following administration of a dose and just prior to the administration of the next dose, after a peak in drug level

therapeutic range - beneficial serum drug concentration levels, including a lower and an upper limit

THERAPEUTIC DRUG MONITORING

Therapeutic drug monitoring (TDM) came about in order to help improve the outcome of certain types of drug therapy. Some medications have toxic effects at blood levels only slightly higher than the upper limit of the therapeutic range (e.g., digoxin). Likewise, some medications even at therapeutic doses may give side effects that make patients less likely to comply with the prescribed therapy.

Toxicity may cause organ damage, such as to the liver or kidneys, which further affects the circulating levels of the drug or its by-products. **Nephrotoxicity** is very common and can lead to acute renal failure. Monitoring the blood level of these drugs is helpful to determine if the dosage amount or interval between doses is appropriate, particularly if the kidneys are failing since elimination of drug is decreased in kidney failure. Subsequent dosage adjustment will be used to maximize drug efficacy while minimizing toxicity. Although many medications do not cause toxicity when given in the usual doses and therefore don't require TDM, we will focus on general categories and some specific drugs that do.[1]

Patient drug levels are compared to a reference range called the therapeutic range. This range includes a lower value, which is the **minimum effective concentration**, and an upper value, just below the **minimum toxic concentration**. Blood levels of the drug fluctuate as it is handled by different organ systems within the body. Peak levels depend on how the drug is administered and the body's

nephrotoxicity - damage to the kidneys

minimum effective concentration - the lower limit of the therapeutic range

minimum toxic concentration - the lower limit of the toxicity range

half-life - time needed for the concentration of a drug to decrease by half.

steady state - condition in which the average drug concentration remains in equilibrium after multiple intervals of drug dosage

pharmacokinetics - the relationship of drug concentration to time

ability to absorb and distribute the drug. Trough drug levels depend on the body's ability to metabolize and eliminate the drug. The time frame for a drug concentration to decrease by half is termed the **half-life ($t\frac{1}{2}$)**. If a drug is given once per $t\frac{1}{2}$, an equilibrium termed **steady state** is reached after 4 to 5 half-lives.

As a rule of thumb, the effectiveness of therapeutic drugs should be monitored by the parameter that is easiest to measure. For example, with certain drugs usefulness may be determined as easing of symptoms. Blood pressure is the best measure of efficacy of furosemide or other blood pressure medication dosage. Periodic measuring of prothrombin time is useful for monitoring warfarin (Coumadin) and coagulation management. Tests to monitor the effectiveness of therapeutic drugs should be ordered for the correct time of day, and results should be evaluated carefully. In a study of hospitalized patients receiving cardioactive medications, 49% of the drug testing was performed for irrational indications and 36% of the drug results were not evaluated correctly. The study concluded that pharmacists should become more involved in monitoring drug assays for interpretation and follow-up.[2]

ROUTES OF DRUG ADMINISTRATION

There are various routes of drug administration. These include but are not limited to oral (per os, or PO), intravenous (IV), intramuscular (IM), on the skin, in the rectum or cheek, and inhalation and epidermal routes.[3] Each route of administration will result in a characteristic concentration versus time that can be depicted graphically. The relationship of drug concentration versus time is termed **pharmacokinetics**. For a drug given intravenously, the gastrointestinal (GI) system is bypassed and the drug is immediately distributed to the bloodstream. The graph of blood concentration of drug versus time illustrated in Figure 14–1 depicts this immediate absorption. In contrast, a drug taken orally must pass through the GI system before it is absorbed into the bloodstream. Figure 14–2 depicts the relationship of time versus blood concentration of drug following oral dosage.

Drugs are processed in the body through four main phases. *Absorption* is the process in which the drug enters the bloodstream from the GI tract with an oral dose, intramuscularly, via skin absorption, or from under the tongue (sublingually). Drugs taken intravenously enter directly into the bloodstream. Following the absorption phase, distribution occurs. *Distribution* is the spread of drug via the cir-

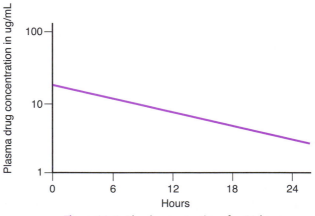

Figure 14–1. Blood concentration after IV dosage.

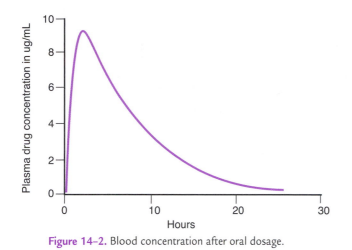

Figure 14–2. Blood concentration after oral dosage.

culatory system to organs and tissues throughout the body following the absorption phase. Distribution does depend on fluid volume and circulation. Drug binding occurs during this stage and, thus, not all of the drug dose becomes available to the tissues. *Metabolism* begins shortly after distribution and commences the elimination phase. Metabolism is the process in which the parent drug is transformed to a more easily excreted form, such as water insoluble. The metabolite may be pharmacologically active or inactive. *Elimination* is the process by which drugs are removed from the body by metabolism and excretion processes. Renal excretion is the prime method of eliminating water-soluble drugs and metabolites.

DRUG METABOLISM

Many drugs are metabolized by enzymes working in **first-order (metabolic) kinetics**. As the drug concentration increases, the rate of hepatic metabolism by enzymes increases to keep up with the amount of drug present. In other words, the velocity of drug metabolism by enzymes is proportional to the concentration of the substrate (drug). This type of drug clearance, generally represented by a skewed type of curve, is the typical response with most drugs after administration of only one dose. Patients taking drugs that continue to follow nonlinear kinetics must be monitored by TDM very closely.

Some drugs are absorbed by the liver during GI absorptive circulation and metabolized quickly before they have a chance to reach the systemic circulation. This is termed the *"first-pass effect."* Lidocaine, a cardioactive drug, exhibits first-pass metabolism. Therefore, it is retained in circulation longer if it is administered as an intramuscular injection rather than an oral dose.

Some drugs are metabolized by **zero-order kinetics** in which the metabolizing enzyme active sites are fully saturated with drug. The hepatic enzymes metabolize the drug at maximum velocity (V_{max}). Therefore, the concentration of the drug does not affect its metabolic rate, which is already at a maximum. **Ethanol**, phenytoin, and salicylates all follow zero-order kinetics at typical or therapeutic levels.

The kidneys eliminate water-soluble drugs through glomerular filtration. Only free drugs and water-soluble metabolites can pass through the kidney into the urine for elimination. Other routes of drug elimination are through elimination of bile

first-order (metabolic) kinetics - reaction in which the velocity of metabolism by enzymes is proportional to the concentration of substrate (drug)

zero-order kinetics - catalyzed reaction with all active sites of the enzyme filled with substrate so reaction occurs at its fastest rate; also called saturation kinetics

ethanol - ethyl alcohol, CH_3CH_2OH

and feces, especially for lipid-soluble drugs, and through gaseous expiration from the lungs. Due to the role of the kidney in elimination of many drugs, it is also prone to toxicity and possible failure. Effective elimination of drugs requires adequate renal function so, in situations of renal failure, circulating drug levels stay elevated longer than with normal renal function.

Drugs typically measured in TDM are classified into categories. There are seven common categories of drugs monitored by blood levels. These are antibiotics, cardioactive drugs (so-called antiarrhythmic drugs that control normal heart rhythm), antineoplastics (drugs to control cell growth), medications to control seizures (so-called antiepileptic drugs), bronchodilators (so-called antiasthmatic drugs), antipsychotics (drugs that control the mind and behavior, including depression), and immunosuppressive agents (drugs that inhibit immunity).

DRUG ACTION OF ANTIBIOTICS

Antibiotics are used to treat infectious illnesses by stopping the growth of pathogenic bacteria or by killing the bacteria outright. The drug action is often aimed at ribosomal translation or protein synthesis in the dividing bacteria. Inhibition of cell wall assembly is a common mechanism of antibiotics. Aminoglycosides such as gentamicin, tobramicin, streptomycin, and kanamycin are very effective in treating systemic infections from gram-negative bacteria such as *Pseudomonas*, *Proteus*, *Escherichia coli*, *Klebsiella*, *Enterobacter*, and *Serratia* as well as staphylococci. These aminoglycosides exhibit broad-spectrum bacterial action against aerobic gram-negative organisms by binding to their 30S ribosomes, which inhibits protein synthesis. Aminoglycosides are effective against bacteria that are resistant to less toxic drugs such as methicillin. Aminoglycosides can also be used in conjunction with other antibiotics for the treatment of *Listeria* and gram-positive coccal infections.[3]

Vancomycin and chloramphenicol also treat serious infections. Vancomycin is a glycopeptide active against gram-positive cocci, particularly those resistant to methicillin. It is especially useful in treatment of methicillin-resistant *Staphylococcus aureus* (MRSA) and *Corynebacterium* infections. Vancomycin is bactericidal (killing bacteria) against most gram-positive organisms but only bacteriostatic (stopping growth) against enterococci. The main mode of action is to inhibit cell wall synthesis. Chloramphenicol is bactericidal to gram-negative organisms such as *Neisseria meningitidis*, *Pseudomonas*, *Haemophilus influenzae*, *Salmonella typhi*, *Brucella*, *Bordatella pertussis*, *Vibrio cholerae*, *Shigella*, *E. coli*, *Chlamydia*, and *Mycoplasma*. Its mode of action is by binding to 50S ribosomes, which inhibits protein synthesis. Chloramphenicol and similar antibiotics, although they are used to treat life-threatening infections, can become toxic with high doses or long-term use.[3]

Therapeutic drug monitoring of antibiotics primarily includes aminoglycosides, vancomycin, and chloramphenicol. Most other antibiotics, such as tetracycline or erythromycin, are able to achieve and maintain therapeutic levels with standardized dosing intervals and are not prone to toxicity at typical doses. They have a wide therapeutic index, meaning there is only minimal risk of reaching the minimum toxic concentration. Aminoglycosides and chloramphenicol have a rather narrow therapeutic index and serious toxic consequences. Aminoglycosides in excess are associated with nephrotoxicity and **ototoxicity**. In addition, aminoglycosides such as gentamicin are poorly absorbed via the GI tract and require IV or IM administration.[4] Chloramphenicol toxicity is associated with aplastic anemia, a serious situation that calls for maintenance of drug level in the therapeutic range.

THE TEAM APPROACH
The nurse, physician assistant, or physician may request blood levels of a drug to be determined based on patient findings. These findings vary, but in the case of antibiotics could be indications of renal toxicity or hearing impairment. The laboratory technologist is a valued team member in TDM and toxicological assessment.

THE TEAM APPROACH
Since laboratory personnel may not collect a blood specimen, it is important that those who do have good information and training. Specific points when collecting therapeutic drug samples include proper labeling, choosing the correct collection tube, proper mixing, and quick transport to the laboratory.

ototoxicity - damage to the hearing of the patient

ANALYSIS OF ANTIBIOTICS

Gentamicin, tobramycin, and vancomycin are most commonly analyzed by a non-isotopic immunoassay such as fluorescence polarization immunoassay (FPIA). This method is highly sensitive and specific for these drugs, is highly automated, and requires only a moderate complexity of skill for performing the analysis.

A general rule of thumb for timing of TDM blood samples is that specimens for peak drug levels are drawn 1 hour after an oral dose is given and the trough drug level specimens are drawn at the t½ or just prior to giving the next dosage. This rule is not true for drugs such as phenobarbital, phenytoin, digoxin, lithium, and the aminoglycoside antibiotics or for pediatric or some elderly patients, whose fluid levels and metabolic and renal function are different than adults. Most dosing and timing information is derived from study of young healthy adults, but adaptations have been made for pediatric and geriatric patients, who tend to have a decreased drug clearance.

Specimen collection for analysis of antibiotics allows for serum and other types of body fluids. The specimen of choice for gentamicin and tobramycin is serum, but EDTA plasma can be used. Heparin has been shown to deactivate gentamicin by forming an inactive complex that interferes with some immunoassay procedures. Most vancomycin methods call for serum but allow heparinized and EDTA plasma. Often only vancomycin trough levels are monitored for therapeutic range due to the drug's long distribution phase.

The typical method of choice for analysis of chloramphenicol is by high-pressure liquid chromatography (HPLC) in order to differentiate parent drug from active metabolite. Immunoassay methods are now also available for chloramphenicol as for other antibiotics. You should always refer to manufacturer's information regarding specific sources of preanalytical and analytical interferences.

The specimen of choice for chloramphenicol testing is serum, but heparinized and EDTA plasma or cerebrospinal fluid can be analyzed. Typically the trough level is used to evaluate therapeutic effects and the peak level, drawn 1 to 2 hours postdose, is used to monitor toxic levels of chloramphenicol. Often a clotted blood sample is to be collected, but the container should not have gel separation barriers, which leach out some drugs. Likewise, some drugs such as lidocaine, propranolol, and tricyclic antidepressants are disturbed by the plasticizer found in some stoppers (TBEP), so special collection tubes may be required.[5]

Antibiotics are typically reported in whole numbers as micrograms per milliliter, with different expected ranges for samples drawn at peak and trough times. It is important to report these results in the standardized format in order to avoid confusion on the part of health-care providers when interpreting therapeutic drug levels. Typical reference ranges are listed in Table 14–1.

Case Scenario 14-1 **Therapeutic Ranges: Trouble for Baby Jones**

Follow-Up

The peak gentamicin level for Baby Jones was found to be lower than the trough level. In fact, the peak level matched the expected therapeutic range for a trough sample and the trough level was found to be within the expected therapeutic range for a peak sample. Quick inspection of the samples revealed that the patient identification information was correct but the terms *trough* and

continued

Case Scenario 14-1 **Therapeutic Ranges: Trouble for Baby Jones** *(continued)*

peak were switched on the labels based upon when the medication was given. The information was corrected before release into the hospital information system. The test results from the correct time frames revealed the following results, which were consistent with therapeutic ranges:

	Patient	Reference Range
Peak (μg/mL)	5	3–5
Trough (μg/mL)	0.5	<2 ●

CASE SCENARIO 14-2

Monitoring Digoxin Levels: A Confused Man in the ED

The laboratory technician was asked to draw blood from a 68-year-old male patient in the ED. The technician had to wait a few minutes until they completed the electrocardiogram (ECG) before beginning the blood draw. The patient was found to be confused but cooperative with the phlebotomy technique. The physician assistant continued questioning the patient while the technician finished labeling the specimens. It was discovered that the patient was unclear if he took double the dosage of digoxin or forgot to take the medication. The random digoxin was 2.4 ng/mL (reference range, 0.5 to 1.5 ng/mL).

DRUG ACTION OF CARDIOACTIVE AGENTS

Several types of medications are used to treat arrhythmias, including cardiac glycosides and other cardioactive agents. Digitalis plants (*Digitalis lanata*, or foxglove)

TABLE 14-1

Typical Adult Reference Ranges for Common Antibiotics[1]

Gentamicin (Garamycin®) and Tobramycin (Nebcin®)			
Reference Range	Gentamicin:	Peak: 5–8 μg/mL	Trough: <2 μg/mL
	Toxic:	Peak: >10 μg/mL	Trough: >2 μg/mL
	Tobramycin:	Peak: 5–8 μg/mL	Trough: <2 μg/mL
	Toxic:	Peak: >10 μg/mL	Trough: >2 μg/mL

Chloramphenicol (Chloromycetin®)
Reference Range
Therapeutic: 10–25 μg/mL
Toxic: >25 μg/mL

Vancomycin (Vancocin®)
Reference Range
Peak: 20–40 μg/mL
Trough: 5–10 μg/mL
Toxic: >80 μg/mL

provide a group of cardiac glycosides including digoxin and digitoxin. The basic mechanism of action is to regulate the rhythm of the heart by inhibition of Na^+ and K^+ transport within myocardial membranes at the level of the Na-K-ATPase pump. The resulting decreased transmembrane potential in the myocardium and influx of ionized calcium improves cardiac muscle contraction and rhythm.[3]

Other cardioactive drugs important in TDM include lidocaine and quinidine. Lidocaine affects the timing of contraction in ventricular myocardium and is used to treat premature ventricular contractions (PVCs). Quinidine is used to treat a variety of cardiac rhythm problems, including premature atrial contractions, PVCs, and ventricular tachycardia, by several mechanisms, including blocking sodium channels. Quinidine is also used in conjunction with digoxin or other medications to treat premature contraction of the atria. Procainamide is used to treat cardiac arrhythmias by affecting rate of cardiac muscle contractions. The parent drug, procainamide, and its hepatic metabolite, *N*-acetylprocainamide (NAPA), both have cardioactive affects.

TOXICITY OF CARDIOACTIVE DRUGS

Toxic effects of cardioactive drugs such as digoxin include changes in heart rate and contractions (including PVCs), nausea, visual distortion, central nervous system (CNS) depression, seizures, decreased blood pressure, and/or decreased cardiac output of blood. Toxic effects of excessive procainamide are similar and include slowing of heart muscle contractions and rate and changes in normal rhythm. Thus, it is noted that some of the symptoms of toxicity are the same as undertreatment of the underlying illness. In addition, if drug elimination is slowed due to impaired circulation, congestive heart failure, or impaired hepatic or renal function, the usual dosing interval of the drug may be too frequent and drug toxicity can result from higher than expected drug levels. Providing serum drug concentrations, as well as hepatic and renal function test results, may be necessary to determine the cause of the symptoms.

METHODS OF ANALYSIS FOR THERAPEUTIC DRUGS

There is no one method that can be used to measure all drugs and toxic compounds. However, since medications are usually only present in small amounts in the patient's body, as compared to glucose or urea, the method must be sensitive to these minute levels of drug. As mentioned earlier with antibiotic assays, one common type of immunoassay is fluorescent polarization immunoassay (FPIA). This method can also be used for quantification of drugs of abuse, hormones, and some toxins.[7] Refer to Chapter 3 (Laboratory Techniques and Instrumentation), which describes specific information about immunoassays.

When drug concentration is measured, the value reflects both the protein-bound and non–protein-bound or free drug. The free drug concentration will reflect the pharmacological response but, because the total and free drug concentrations are often similar, total drug concentration will be adequate for TDM. However, there are circumstances when the measurement of free drug levels would be of clinical value, such as when the free drug level is considerably less than total drug concentration or when two drugs compete for binding sites on albumin. In the latter circumstance, the drug with the lower affinity for albumin will reach higher free drug concentrations in the plasma, and the free drug level should be

> **THE TEAM APPROACH**
> Digoxin toxicity remains a common clinical problem despite continuing advances in understanding cardiac glycosides. Providing serum drug concentrations can aid physicians in decision-making and has been shown to reduce the incidence of digoxin toxicity.[4,6]

monitored for possible toxic effects. The amount of free drug in a patient sample is determined by analyzing a protein-free filtrate produced by a selective filtering membrane. The filtering membrane will allow only the non–protein-bound substances to pass through to be analyzed.

How Is Enzyme-Multiplied Immunoassay Used to Measure Digoxin?

In enzyme-multiplied immunoassay technique (EMIT), enzyme-labeled digoxin competes with digoxin in the patient sample for a limited amount of antibody specific to digoxin. Generally all the patient digoxin binds with antibody and there is plenty of antibody left over to react with the enzyme-labeled digoxin. When antibody binds to the enzyme-labeled digoxin, the enzyme is inhibited and won't react with its substrate, preventing formation of product. There is generally leftover free enzyme-labeled digoxin. This will react with the substrate to form a product that is measured spectrophotometrically. An increase in absorbance due to the product in the reaction is directly proportional to amount of patient drug. Test Methodology 14–1 describes in more detail the principle of digoxin analysis by enzyme immunoassay.

TEST METHODOLOGY 14-1.   DIGOXIN (LANOXIN)

The Reaction Principle

In enzyme-multiplied immunoassay by EMIT 2000, patient digoxin and enzyme-labeled digoxin can both bind with specific antibody. Glucose-6-phosphate dehydrogenase (G6PD)-labeled digoxin competes with patient digoxin for a limited amount of anti-digoxin antibody. Antibody binding to enzyme-labeled digoxin inhibits the G6PD from reacting with its substrate, preventing formation of product. Excess free enzyme-labeled digoxin reacts with substrate to form product, which is measured spectrophotometrically. An increase in absorbance by the product is directly proportional to amount of patient drug.

Characteristics

Antibody is capable of distinguishing digoxin from digitoxin. This method has satisfactory precision and accuracy for therapeutic drug monitoring purposes, a sensitivity of less than 0.1 μg/L, and very low likelihood of digoxin-like immunoreactive substance (DLIS) interference.

Interferences

Common oleander and foxglove extract may cross-react with immunoassay methods. Other herbal supplements that may cause immunoassay interference include borage leaves, *Bufo marinus,* and *Veratrum viride.* There is minimal interference from DLIS, common in autoimmune disorders.

The Specimen

Serum, heparinized, or EDTA plasma drawn 8 hours or more after the dose.

Therapeutic Range

0.5–1.5 ng/mL

Toxic Levels

Adult	>2.0 ng/mL
Child	>3.0 ng/mL

Complementary or Herbal Medicines' Effect on Therapeutic Drug Monitoring

Some chemical constituents of herbal food supplements or plant substances can produce toxic side effects when ingested that are similar to digoxin or digitoxin toxicity. Analytical interference with some immunoassays can occur due to cross-chemical reactions.[8,9] Common oleander, a flowering shrub, has been known to impart toxic reactions similar to cardiac glycosides and to cross-react with immunoassay methods. Other herbal supplements that cause similar toxic side effects and immunoassay interference include borage leaves, *Bufo marinus*, *Veratrum viride*, and foxglove extract.[8–10] Chromatographic methods can be used to differentiate toxicity due to digoxin from that due to herbal chemicals.[11,12]

> **Case Scenario 14-2** Monitoring Digoxin Levels: A Confused Man in the ED
>
> **Follow-Up**
>
> The elderly male patient in the ED with irregular heart rhythm was confused and unclear if he took double the dosage of digoxin or forgot to take the medication. The random digoxin was 2.4 ng/mL (reference range, 0.5 to 1.5 ng/mL), which indicates presence of a toxic high drug level. Renal and hepatic function for the patient was later found to be unimpaired based on normal creatinine and bilirubin results. There was no evidence of circulatory problems. Renal failure, declining hepatic function, or poor circulation could all prolong the elimination of a drug, causing it to maintain higher than expected levels, but they were ruled out. Likewise, changes in fluid levels can affect distribution of the drug to the tissues and cause it to remain longer in blood circulation. The patient's current dosage will need to be adjusted down and/or the dosing interval lengthened to provide a drug level within the therapeutic range for the immediate future. The pharmacist and physician will work together on this adjusted dosage schedule. Detailed instructions and clarifications should be given to the patient and caregivers by the health-care providers in order to aim for better medication dosing. Knowledge of some interfering food supplements, including certain botanicals, should also be discussed with the patient and caregivers if there are indications that the patient is taking certain herbal supplements. ●

> **CASE SCENARIO 14-3**
>
> **Antiepileptic Medication Testing: Why Is She Still Having Seizures?**
>
> An adult patient in the clinic with history of seizure is currently taking phenytoin and experiences a seizure during an electroencephalogram (EEG). The physician is considering administration of a new antiepileptic drug, levetiracetam, along with phenytoin (Dilantin) for seizure control. The patient's random Dilantin level is 19 μg/mL (reference range, 10 to 20 μg/mL). The health-care team will be considering these questions:
>
> 1. What type of seizures is phenytoin most effective in controlling?
> 2. What drug-drug interactions can be expected with a patient taking several antiepileptic drugs?

ANTIEPILEPTIC DRUGS

absence seizures - mild, brief attacks with altered consciousness, eyelid fluttering, and abrupt stopping of activity with no memory of the attack

tonic-clonic seizures - loss of consciousness and balance followed by contractions of the muscles of the extremities, trunk, and head, often with an uncontrolled outcry at the onset

partial seizures - motor, sensory, or psychomotor phenomena without loss of consciousness

partial-complex seizures - brief loss of contact with surroundings; may accompany staring, automatic purposeless movements, and unintelligible sounds followed by motor activity and short-term confusion

epilepsy - a recurrent disorder of cerebral function characterized by a variety of attacks caused by excessive discharge of cerebral neurons

Characteristics of antiepileptic drugs (AEDs; also known as anticonvulsants) include the type of seizures typically controlled, pharmacological effects, and toxic effects. Phenobarbital is one of the oldest prescribed medications in use. The parent drug, primidone, and its major metabolite, phenobarbital, have antiepileptic affects. Phenobarbital is a slow-acting barbiturate used to control all seizures except **absence seizures**. Toxic effects of phenobarbital include drowsiness, fatigue, depression, and decreased mental capacity. Primidone is used in treatment of **tonic-clonic seizures** and **partial seizures**. Toxic levels of primodone cause sedation, nausea, vomiting, diplopia, dizziness, and ataxia. Phenytoin is used in treatment of tonic-clonic seizures, partial or **partial-complex seizures**, and status epilepticus. Phenytoin is not effective for absence seizures. Toxic effects of phenytoin may cause nystagmus and ataxia and even increased seizure activity. Carbamazepine is used in treatment of generalized tonic-clonic, partial, and partial-complex seizures and in some specific types of nerve pain. It also has an antidiuretic effect, thus reducing concentrations of antidiuretic hormone. Valproic acid is used to treat absence seizures.[3] Table 14–2 lists drug and generic names for anticonvulsant medications.

Epilepsy is a recurrent disorder of cerebral function characterized by sudden, brief attacks of altered consciousness, motor activity, sensory phenomena, and/or inappropriate behavior caused by excessive discharge of cerebral neurons. It can be classified into many seizure disorders, including absence seizures, partial-complex or partial seizures, and tonic-clonic seizures. Absence seizures were formerly termed *petit mal seizures*, in which the patient experiences brief attacks with loss of consciousness and eyelid fluttering, as well as abruptly stopping activity with no memory of the attack. In partial-complex seizures, the patient loses contact with the surroundings for a short time, which may be manifested as staring, performing automatic purposeless movements, uttering unintelligible sounds, and resisting aid, followed by motor activity and short-term mental confusion. Partial seizures are characterized by motor, sensory, or psychomotor phenomena without loss of consciousness. Tonic-clonic seizures are typically associated with loss of consciousness and balance, followed by contractions of the muscles of the extremities, trunk, and head often with an uncontrolled outcry at the onset.[13] The goals of epilepsy therapy can be considered at three levels: seizure control, overall epilepsy control, and ultimately the reversal of the process, seeking a cure for epilepsy.[14]

Frequently medications given in combination are used to treat a particular disease, such as quinidine and digoxin for atrial fibrillation or several AEDs to control seizures. Some drugs will induce a metabolic effect within hepatic mitochondria to lower the concentration of concurrent drug therapy. For example, levetiracetam

TABLE 14-2
Drug Trade and Generic Names for Anticonvulsants

Drug Generic Name	Trade Names
Phenytoin	Dilantin
Carbamazepine	Tegretol, Carbatrol, Atretol
Primidone	Mysoline
Valproic acid	Depakene, Depakote
Phenobarbital	Solfoton, Luminal

plasma concentrations tend to be lower than expected when given in conjunction with the medications phenytoin and phenobarbital, while valproic acid has no effect when given in combination.[15]

Case Scenario 14-3 Antiepileptic Medication Testing: Why Is She Still Having Seizures?

Follow-Up

The adult patient in the clinic is taking phenytoin and still suffers from occasional seizures. The physician considers prescribing a new antiepileptic drug, levetiracetam, along with phenytoin for seizure control. The current Dilantin level was within therapeutic range but not effectively controlling seizures, which most likely indicates that a change in drug dosage or schedule will be needed. Levetiracetam is a newer medication that can be used to control seizures, but it may be challenging to achieve therapeutic levels of both medications since phenytoin is likely to induce a faster metabolic rate of the newer medication. Thus additional TDM will be required until steady state is achieved, in order to achieve therapeutic levels of both drugs. ●

OTHER THERAPEUTIC DRUGS

Psychoactive Drugs

Psychoactive drugs, including lithium, have a long history of use in treating psychiatric disorders. Psychoactive drugs are those that affect the mind or behavior. It has been long recognized that some psychoactive drugs require frequent therapeutic monitoring. A classic therapeutic drug in this category is lithium, which has serious toxic side effects that begin when levels just exceed the upper limit of the therapeutic range. The traditional method of analysis for lithium, since it is a univalent metal, is by ion-selective electrode (ISE). Newer spectrophotometric methods provide a useful alternative to ISE and employ a more fully automated analyzer.[16]

Other common psychoactive drugs that require some therapeutic monitoring include tricyclic antidepressants, amitriptyline, desipramine, imipramine, and nortriptyline. Alternative psychoactive drugs are available on the market, but there is a lack of defined concentration-effect relationship for newer psychoactive drugs. Therefore, there is not much value in monitoring blood levels of these drugs.[17] For detailed information about these medications, please refer to the table in the appendix.

Antiasthmatic Drugs

Antiasthmatic drugs, such as theophylline and theobromine, are used for treatment of neonatal breathing disorders or of respiratory conditions that affect adults or children, such as asthma. Theophylline's action is in bronchodilation and smooth muscle relaxation. *Bronchodilation* is the term for respiratory airway opening. Antiasthmatic drugs are usually given intravenously for initial therapy, followed by a regimen of oral dosages. Toxicity causes nausea, vomiting, diarrhea, headache, cardiac rhythm problems, and seizures. Theophylline is commonly measured with immunoassay, while theobromine is generally measured by high-pressure liquid chromatography (HPLC).

Antineoplastic Drugs

Methotrexate is an antineoplastic agent that historically has been measured with TDM. It is a nonspecific cellular growth regulator that is useful in the treatment of various neoplasms as well as some severe chronic skin disorders. Methotrexate inhibits DNA synthesis in rapidly dividing tumor cells with some effect on certain healthy cells. Leucovorin is administered to counteract some of the side effects from methotrexate toxicity. This drug is generally given in a single high dose intravenously. Toxic effects include bone marrow suppression, GI inflammation, and hepatic cirrhosis. Methotrexate is commonly measured by immunoassay.

Immunosuppressive Drugs

Cyclosporin A is used for adult transplantation immunosuppression. It is usually monitored for optimized therapy in the first 2 to 4 hours postdose. In pediatric patients, blood levels of the drug may be monitored in the first 2 hours postdose.[18] Cyclosporin A and other immunosuppressant agents can be measured by immunoassay and chromatography. New immunosuppressant agents have low circulating concentrations and may need to be measured by more sensitive techniques such as HPLC–mass spectrometry.[19]

Toxicology

CASE SCENARIO 14-4

Acute Acetaminophen Overdose: A Child Gets Into the Medicine Cabinet

The emergency department laboratory receives a phone call looking for the STAT acetaminophen level on a 3-year-old patient named Susan Smith. A review of the computer log and received requisitions indicate that the specimen was collected by the attending nurse 15 minutes ago but not delivered yet. A short time later, the specimen is obtained and found to be properly labeled and in acceptable condition. It is placed on the instrument for STAT analysis. Acetaminophen is determined to be 175 μg/mL at the presumed time of exposure of 4 hours. The results were reported into the computerized hospital information system and phoned in to the attending physician.

ACETAMINOPHEN TOXICOLOGY

analgesics - medications that relieve pain

Most **analgesics**, such as salicylates, acetaminophen, and ibuprofen, do not require TDM because physicians and pharmacists are able to achieve and maintain therapeutic levels with standardized dosing intervals. There is generally a fairly wide therapeutic window for these over-the-counter analgesics. Patients are not prone to toxicity at typical doses. Because of the presumed safety of these medications, they are available without a prescription and sold as over-the-counter medications. However, if a patient exceeds the recommended dosage level as provided by the manufacturer, toxicity can occur.

Acetaminophen is a common over-the-counter analgesic. The elimination rate can vary such that the half-life of acetaminophen taken at toxic doses can be up to 15 hours. Toxicity generally occurs with plasma levels greater than 150 μg/mL within the first 8 hours after ingestion and results in metabolic acidosis and hepatotoxicity. Severe hepatic damage is the major concern in acetaminophen toxicity, particularly in that it can result in hepatic coma that occurs 72 hours after toxic ingestion. Plasma ammonia levels may be useful to monitor the degree of hepatic failure and likelihood of hepatic coma. Acetylcysteine treatment, such as Mucomyst, is effective in treatment when acetaminophen plasma levels exceed 150 μg/mL in the first 8 hours and may protect against hepatotoxicity.[3]

The Rumack-Matthew nomogram (Fig. 14–3), relates plasma acetaminophen levels in micrograms per milliliter to the likelihood of developing hepatotoxicity. It is useful only with blood levels starting at 4 hours after the acute dose and in single acute overdose rather than after multiple doses are taken.[20] This nomogram is a plot of time since single-dose exposure versus serum levels of acetaminophen in micrograms per milliliter. This nomogram is not useful if a reliable time of ingestion isn't available. However, several acetaminophen results from blood samples taken at 2- to 3-hour intervals have been used to estimate the $t\frac{1}{2}$ elimination rate of acetaminophen and relate it with patterns of toxicity.

Acetaminophen is typically analyzed using enzyme immunoassay, such as enzyme-mediated inhibition technique (EMIT), or fluorescent immunoassay, often by fluorescent polarization immunoassay (FPIA). One manufacturer of a dry-slide analysis system incorporates an enzyme-colorimetric method employing aryl acylamide amidohydrolase reagent. The reference method for acetaminophen is HPLC.

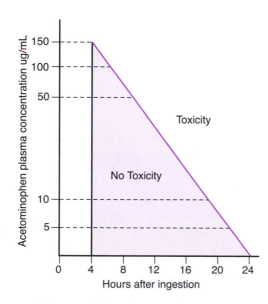

Figure 14–3. Rumack-Matthew curve.

TOXICITY OF OTHER ANALGESICS

antipyretics - medications that reduce fever

nonsteroidal anti-inflammatory drugs (NSAIDs) - drugs that reduce inflammation without the use of cortisone or other steroids

Salicylates are a group of organic acids used as painkillers (analgesics) and fever-reducing drugs **(antipyretics)** and to control inflammation and platelet function. They are called **nonsteroidal anti-inflammatory drugs (NSAIDs)**. An important example is acetylsalicylic acid (ASA). Also known as aspirin, ASA has a broad-range $t\frac{1}{2}$ of 2 to 20 hours depending on the amount taken. Small amounts of salicylate are excreted unchanged in urine while the majority is metabolized in the liver to organic acids before elimination. For treatment of severe inflammatory disease, the typical therapeutic level of salicylates is 150 to 300 μg/mL.

When analyzing serum or plasma salicylates, one must consider that overdose of salicylates usually occurs at levels greater than 300 μg/mL and toxicity results in acid-base disturbance. Respiratory alkalosis results from hyperventilation, the pharmacological action. Later, metabolic acidosis results from metabolic by-products, causing an increased anion gap. Children younger than 4 years of age tend to present with metabolic acidosis, while older children and adults tend to present with respiratory alkalosis or combined acid-base disturbances. Severe acid-base disturbance can result in coma and may be fatal. There is a nomogram, similar to the nomogram for acetaminophen toxicity, to relate degree of salicylate toxicity versus blood level and time since ingestion. This is helpful for clinicians in treating patients with overdoses. This nomogram is designed only for a single-dose toxic exposure and blood levels measured after at least 6 hours postdose. It is not useful if reliable time of ingestion isn't available.

Just as for therapeutic drugs, the most common methods for salicylate analysis use EMIT or FPIA. Both methods are easily automated and are competitive homogeneous systems. The classic method of salicylate analysis, and a method that continues to be fairly common in some analyzers, is spectrophotometric. It utilizes the principle reaction of salicylate with ferric nitrate, forming a purple chromogen that increases in spectrophotometric absorbance at 540 nm.

The reference method for salicylates is HPLC, which imparts a high level of specificity due to unique retention times in the column based on solubility in the mobile and stationary phases. High-pressure liquid chromatography can be moderate in cost, but more complex technology and training is required when compared to other automated systems. Turnaround time with HPLC can be longer than with other automated systems. Test Methodology 14–2 describes the analysis of salicylates with HPLC.

TEST METHODOLOGY 14-2.   HIGH-PERFORMANCE LIQUID CHROMATOGRAPHY FOR SALICYLATE ANALYSIS

The Reaction Principle

Serum plasma is first precipitated with acetonitrile, which contains *o*-methoxybenzoic acid as an internal standard. Salicylate, salicyluric acid, and gentisic acid are then separated with a octadecysilane reversed-phase chromatographic columns. Quantification is performed by calculating the ratio of peak height absorbance at 313 nm of the analyte versus that for the internal standard and then by comparing this ratio with appropriate calibrators.[21]

continued

TEST METHODOLOGY 14-2. HIGH-PERFORMANCE LIQUID CHROMATO-GRAPHY FOR SALICYLATE ANALYSIS *(continued)*

Equipment used includes a high-pressure liquid chromatograph with a 250 × 3.9-mm, 10-μm particle size, octadecylsilane-packed column, an ultraviolet detector, and a pump with a flow rate of 2.6 mL/min. Reagents include sodium azide stock solution, standard solutions of salicylic acid, salicyluric acid, and gentisic acid (2,4-dihydroxybenzoic acid), and an internal standard of *o*-methoxybenzoic acid dissolved in acetonitrile.

The Specimen

Heparinized plasma separated from cells promptly and stored at 4° to 6°C prior to analysis. Stability is enhanced for long-term storage at –20°C.

Therapeutic Range

150–300 μg/mL

Toxicity Cutoff

>300 μg/mL

Case Scenario 14-4 Acute Acetaminophen Overdose: A Child Gets Into the Medicine Cabinet

Follow-Up

The 3-year-old patient named Susan Smith has an acetaminophen of 175 μg/mL with a presumed time of exposure of 4 hours. The patient had accessed a medicine cabinet and ingested approximately 7 cherry-flavored children's cold tablets that contained 560 mg of acetaminophen, as well as antihistamine, cough suppressant, and nasal decongestant. Although there is concern for all medications, the hepatotoxicity resulting from acetaminophen is of most concern. The physicians used the Rumack-Matthew nomogram to compare the postingestion time frame of 4 hours with the blood level of 175 μg/mL, a value that indicated possible hepatic toxicity. If the level exceeds 200 μg/mL at 4 hours, it indicates probable hepatic toxicity. Either of these levels indicates the need to provide treatment to enhance hepatic clearance, monitor the acetaminophen level in 2-hour intervals to verify the elimination of acetaminophen, and possibly monitor liver function with plasma ammonia levels. ●

CASE SCENARIO 14-5

Medical and Legal Alcohol Testing: Was Alcohol Involved in the Accident?

There are two automobile accident victims in the ED. Mr. Brown is unconscious, suffering from multiple trauma wounds, and is in critical condition. A blood alcohol (ethanol) test is ordered for medical purposes prior to administration of certain medications and medical treatments. Due to the difficulty

continued

in obtaining venous samples because of the presence of multiple intravenous lines, the physician requests of the laboratory personnel that the alcohol level on Mr. Brown be determined from a previously collected specimen. The standard isopropanol wipes were used in collection of that specimen. Ethanol is currently being analyzed with a routine chemistry analyzer, but results are pending. The other patient, Mr. John Doe, was the driver in the automobile and had a breath alcohol test performed by police. Mr. Doe did not believe the breath test was accurate and exercised his legal rights to a more definitive alcohol test. He has now requested a legal blood alcohol test be obtained.

Here are some questions to consider in understanding the situation described with these two patients as we explore these concepts further:

1. How are samples collected and handled for these two methodologies?
2. What are the similarities and differences of these two methods of alcohol analysis?

ETHANOL AND ALCOHOL TESTING

Some key facts about ethanol and other toxic alcohols will be helpful to consider as you think about this case scenario. First, ethanol is the most common toxicological agent involved in medicolegal cases because it is legally obtained by adults and a common aspect of many social environments. It is a commonly measured analyte in the laboratory. Second, excessive exposure to ethanol can be lethal. It is often involved in automobile accidents and other legal situations, such as domestic violence.[22] Finally, ethanol, even in small amounts, can interfere or cause enhanced reactions with other medications such as hypnotics or analgesics, so that patients who are going to receive treatment such as surgery may need to have their alcohol level measured prior to administration of other medications.

Historical Aspects of Alcohol

Ethanol as a beverage, medicinal base, and intoxicating substance is not an invention of the 19th or 20th century. Records indicate that ethanol was obtained from fermented sugars in rice or wheat in ancient Egypt and China as far back as 1000 B.C. Ethyl alcohol is a legal drinking substance found in wine, beer, and spirits.

Physiological Effects of Alcohol Toxicity

Ethanol and other alcohols are small molecules that are soluble in water. Because they are easily distributed from the blood circulation to cerebrospinal fluid, disturbances to the CNS are common. Small amounts of alcohol depress the CNS and provide sensations of relaxation. Judgment, emotional release, reasoning, and recognition are all aspects controlled by cerebral functions, and these are affected by ethanol intake. Impaired cerebellar reflexes, including problems with balance and coordination as well as slower motor response times, occur when blood ethanol levels are 80 mg/dL or greater. The classic inability to walk in a straight line or balance on one foot has been used as a simple method to assess this type of impairment.

Laws and Limits

Alcohol is readily available from a variety of sources. A 12-ounce beer, a 5-ounce glass of wine, or a mixed drink containing one shot (1.5 oz.) of liquor all contain about 20 g of ethanol. Ethanol is regulated in terms of access for adults and minors, as defined by each state. In most states, the legal access to alcohol begins at 21 years of age and the limit to ingest is the amount that produces a blood level of 80 mg/dL (0.08 g/dL or 0.080 g%), particularly in regard to driving an automobile.

Toxicity of Ethanol

Toxicity and CNS disturbance increase proportionately with levels of alcohol. For example, blood ethanol concentrations of 10 to 100 mg/dL can cause diminished inhibitions, loss of self-control, and weakening of will power. Blood ethanol concentrations of 100 to 300 mg/dL are associated with problems walking, slurred speech, and dulled and distorted perceptions. Nausea and vomiting are usually triggered when alcohol toxicity begins. Severe CNS depression occurs with toxic levels of blood ethanol greater than or equal to 300 mg/dL.

Metabolism and Excretion of Ethanol

Small amounts of ethanol are metabolized in the gastric lining before absorption. Of the remaining ethanol, 90% is metabolized in the liver to acetaldehyde by hepatic alcohol dehydrogenase (ADH). The resulting acetaldehyde is converted to acetic acid by aldehyde dehydrogenase. In small or moderate amounts, the metabolites are nontoxic and readily excreted. Food contents in the stomach can slow absorption of alcohol, allow for more gastric metabolism of ethanol, and help to maintain lower blood alcohol concentrations. However, aspirin and gastric hyperacidity medication such as cimetidine can inhibit gastric ADH activity and thereby slow metabolism. ADH is not 100% specific for ethanol and can also metabolize other alcohols, including methyl alcohol.

Ten percent of the ethanol in circulation is not metabolized but is excreted unchanged in breath and urine. Thus ethanol can be tested in urine or in breath samples along with blood samples. Ethanol induces diuresis, helping in renal excretion of ethanol and its metabolites.

Specimen Handling for Forensic Blood Alcohol Testing

Test results that will be used as legal evidence must be collected following strict guidelines, including the transport, storage, and handling conditions and the personnel involved in each of these steps. Frequently the specimen is kept in a locked box until testing occurs. The specimen must have documentation called a **chain of custody**. This is additional documentation of the condition of a specimen, all procedures performed, and personnel who have encountered a test specimen. It is used to document the integrity of the legal evidence as obtained from the test result. This is also sometimes referred to as a chain of evidence. In addition, a **definitive test** method should be used rather than a **presumptive test** method of analysis. Presumptive tests are procedures with minimal complexity of instrumentation or personnel requirements so that the results can be quickly determined. Often presumptive tests have high sensitivity but lower specificity, and results must be veri-

CLINICAL CORRELATION
Medullary control of cardiac and respiratory function becomes depressed and death may result when blood alcohol levels are high. Blood alcohol concentrations that exceed 300 mg/dL are associated with apathy, cessation of autonomic nervous system function, stupor, coma, depression of respiration, subnormal temperature, and death.

CLINICAL CORRELATION
Metabolic acidosis can result from metabolic products of ethanol. Accumulation of acetic acid and depletion of bicarbonate contribute to the metabolic acidosis if excessive consumption of ethanol occurs. This can further complicate the toxicity.

chain of custody - additional documentation of the condition of a specimen, all procedures performed, and personnel who have encountered a test specimen

definitive test - highly sensitive and specific test in which results can be used as legal evidence

presumptive test - a procedure with minimal complexity, instrumentation, and personnel requirements so that the results can be quickly determined

fied by another methodology. A definitive test is a highly sensitive and specific test in which results can be used as legal evidence. Definitive test methodology is often the reference method, which requires more sophisticated instrumentation and personnel training.

For forensic blood alcohol testing in some states, a physician is required to draw a forensic specimen in the presence of the law enforcement officer, who will identify the patient and the specimen. In other situations, the officer of the law draws the specimen. The chain-of-custody documentation must be maintained. Prior to collection of the specimen for blood alcohol, cleaning of the skin puncture site should be performed with a nonalcoholic solution. The typical wipe contains isopropanol and should not be used. The sample must be collected in a closed system and may be arterial, venous, or capillary whole blood. The recommended sample tube is the 7-mL tube containing sodium fluoride and potassium oxalate as an anticoagulant. Some methods allow for use of serum. The container must be kept sealed until analysis. Lipemia, icterus, and hemolysis generally pose very little interference and are not considered problems in the collection phase. Some methods allow for use of freshly collected urine, maintained in a sealed container. As always, complete and accurate identification of the sample is important.

While enzymatic spectrophotometry is generally the method of analysis for medical testing of ethanol, a legal alcohol level is measured by gas-liquid chromatography (GLC), the reference method. Chromatography provides separation of ethanol from other alcohols within a low-temperature column using a carrier gas. Little or no sample preparation is required, and the sample includes the air above the meniscus of serum or plasma. This is referred to as headspace analysis. The resulting output is determined as a unique retention time when compared to standard alcohol solutions. This method is specific for all alcohols, including methanol.

Chromatography is a technique for separation and quantification of alcohol molecules in body fluids. Test Methodology 14–3 describes this method for ethanol testing. Chromatography involves the interaction of the sample mixture with a mobile phase, often a liquid or a gas, and a stationary phase, such as resin beads in a column. Detection of separated components can be achieved by using different solvents that selectively elute certain compounds, to be quantified spectrophotometrically or by flame ionization. Examples of other analytes that are separated and analyzed by chromatography include therapeutic drugs such as chloramphenicol and drugs of abuse.

✓ **Common Sense Check**

A medical alcohol test can be processed in a manner similar to other routine clinical chemistry tests, but a nonalcohol wipe prior to venipuncture is preferred.

✓ **Common Sense Check**

A specimen for a legal alcohol level must have a chain-of-custody document to accompany it at all times, and a more definitive test method is preferred to minimize analytical errors in a legal alcohol test.

⬡ **THE TEAM APPROACH**

Because a legal alcohol test needs to be collected, handled, and documented with special considerations, it is important that the test is ordered correctly. A legal alcohol test is generally analyzed by a reference method; a medical alcohol test is performed on routine clinical chemistry analyzers. Communication with the personnel placing the test order may be necessary prior to collection of samples.

TEST METHODOLOGY 14-3.   PRINCIPLE OF ALCOHOL TESTING BY GAS-LIQUID CHROMATOGRAPHY

The Reaction Principle

Patient and quality control samples are diluted with *n*-propanol, an internal standard. The solutions are placed in sealed vials for headspace analysis. Vials are capped, sealed, and swirled to ensure complete mixing. Vials of alcohol standard solutions are processed along with the patient and quality control vials. The sealed vials are heated at 40°C for 30 minutes. Using a tuberculin syringe, a portion of the headspace (air just above the liquid sample) is introduced into the gas chromatograph. The resolved components are

continued

TEST METHODOLOGY 14-3.   PRINCIPLE OF ALCOHOL TESTING BY GAS-LIQUID CHROMATOGRAPHY *(continued)*

detected using a flame ionization detector. Volatile alcohols elute from the column in the following order: 1) methanol at 0.94 minutes, 2) ethanol at 1.50 minutes, 3) isopropanol at 1.90 minutes, and 4) *n*-propanol at 3.90 minutes. Sources of error in gas chromatography include factors that can impede separation. For example, inadequate levels of carrier gas and incorrect column temperature can impede separation. Other sources of error include improperly identified or poorly preserved sample and improperly mixed or sealed test solution vials.[23]

The Specimen

Sodium fluoride and potassium oxalated whole blood or serum kept in a sealed container with minimal airspace. Prior to collection of the specimen for blood alcohol, cleaning of the skin puncture site should be performed with a nonalcoholic solution rather than the typical wipe, which contains isopropanol. The sample must be collected in a closed system and may be arterial, venous, or capillary whole blood.

Reference Range

0 mg/dL

A level of <80 mg/dL is considered legally acceptable for an adult; ≥80 mg/dL is intoxicated.

The more common method for measuring blood alcohol is a spectrophotometric method utilizing an enzyme that catalyzes the conversion of ethanol to measured product. This method is considered adequate for providing information for medical decisions, although it is not considered specific enough for forensic cases. In this commonly used method, as described in Test Methodology 14–4, alcohol dehydrogenase reagent reacts with ethanol to form a product measured spectrophotometrically.

TEST METHODOLOGY 14-4.   ENZYMATIC METHOD OF ETHANOL ANALYSIS

The Reaction

Ethanol + NAD—$\xrightarrow{(ADH)}$ acetaldehyde + NADH
NADH is measured at 340 nm as an increase in absorbance.

Alternative Second Reaction

NADH + fluorescent dye → NAD^+ + monotetrazolium dye (decrease in fluorescence)

This method is highly selective but not entirely specific for ethanol, with some interference (3% to 7%) from other alcohols, such as methanol, butanol, or *n*-propanol. It is also offered on routine chemistry analyzers that provide rapid turnaround time.[1] Therefore, it is acceptable for making decisions about medical condition but is not accurate for forensic, legal evidence.

continued

> **TEST METHODOLOGY 14-4. ENZYMATIC METHOD OF ETHANOL**
> **ANALYSIS** *(continued)*
>
> **The Specimen**
>
> Serum in a tightly capped container. Prior to collection of the specimen for blood alcohol, cleaning of the skin puncture site should be performed with a nonalcoholic solution. The typical wipe contains isopropanol and should not be used. The sample must be collected in a closed system and may be arterial, venous, or capillary whole blood.
>
> **Reference Range**
>
> A level >80 mg/dL (0.08 g/dL) is considered legally impaired in most states in the United States. A normal amount of ethanol is 0 mg/dL.

Case Scenario 14-5 Medical and Legal Alcohol Testing: Was Alcohol Involved in the Accident?

Follow-Up

The physician requested that the blood alcohol (ethanol) test for Mr. Brown be determined from a previously collected serum sample in which the standard isopropanol wipes were used. The ethanol method from a routine chemistry analyzer using alcohol dehydrogenase is highly selective but not entirely specific for ethanol. Since the sample had been exposed to isopropanol from the alcohol wipe, the physician needs to be informed of a possible 3% to 7% false elevation. This most likely would not deter making a correct medical decision, but the physician may decide to obtain a new blood specimen from an alternate site using a nonalcohol wipe to ensure better results. The other patient, Mr. James Doe, was the driver in the automobile and received a breath alcohol test, but now requested a legal blood alcohol test be obtained. Generally a law enforcement officer is expected to identify the patient for **forensic testing**. The blood sample may be obtained by the physician or laboratory personnel in the presence of the law officer. A chain of custody form must be used and the sample held in a secure place before and during testing. The definitive test for ethanol, particularly used for legal alcohol testing, is GLC. ●

forensic testing - testing in which results can be submitted to help answer a question of law or as evidence in a legal decision

OTHER ALCOHOLS

Toxicity also occurs from ingestion of other alcohols such as methanol, also known as wood alcohol. Methanol is a less common alcohol toxin. Sources of methanol include antifreeze and poorly distilled spirits (moonshine). Methanol is also used in some industrial circumstances.

Physiological effects of methanol toxicity are due to rapid absorption of the molecule and resulting nerve impairment. Effects are also due to the metabolic by-product, formic acid. Methanol toxicity results in severe metabolic acidosis, CNS disturbances, and blindness due to optic nerve damage. Treatment can help to prevent conversion of methanol to its toxic metabolites, and minimize the CNS and optical damage.

Analysis or detection of methanol by a screening method is through measuring osmolality by the freezing point depression (FDP) method and calculating the osmolal gap, or delta-osmolality. Increased osmolal gap is associated with potential presence of volatile organic substances, including alcohols such as ethanol and methanol, as well as other substances such as acetone, ethylene glycol, isopropanol, mannitol, and propylene glycol. Ethanol accounts for an increase of 21.7 mOsm/kg for each 100 mg/dL, and any remaining osmolal gap would be due to one of the other volatile substances mentioned.

The recommended formula for calculated osmolality when considering the effect of alcohol is

$$(1.86 \ Na^+ \ [mmol/L]) + (glucose \ [mg/dL]/18) + (urea \ N \ [mg/dL]/2.8) + 9$$

These numbers are used to convert milligrams per deciliter to molarity.

For example, let us calculate osmolality for a patient with serum levels of Na^+ = 135 mmol/L, glucose = 120 mg/dL, and urea N = 20 mg/dL. This would be calculated as

$$(1.86 \times 135) + (120/18) + (20/2.8) + 9$$
$$(251) + (6.7) + (7.2) + 9 = 273.9 \ or \ 274 \ mOsm/kg$$

The formula for osmolal gap is FDP osmolality – calculated osmolality. Normal osmolal gap is 0 ± 10 mOsmol/kg. An increase in osmolal gap could indicate the presence of a volatile substance such as methanol.

OSMOMETRY

Measuring the concentration of solute particles in solution is termed *osmometry*. The number of solute particles dissolved in the solution depends on ionization. For example, glucose or urea dissolves to form one osmotically active particle compared to sodium chloride, which dissociates to form two particles. Ethanol and methanol also form as one osmotically active particle. Osmometry is typically based on the changing colligative properties of a solution, depending on the total number of osmotically active particles. For example, osmotic pressure increases with increased concentration of solute particles, but vapor pressure is lowered when compared with a pure solution. Freezing point is also lowered when the solution has many solute particles compared to the pure solution. Due to the principle of analysis by vapor pressure osmometry, ethanol and other volatile substances are not effectively measured by this method. If volatile substances are suspected in the patient's sample, osmolality must be measured by the FDP method of osmometry.

Osmolality is the concentration in osmoles per kilogram of H_2O (osmol/kg H_2O), which is the more frequently used unit since temperature is negated in the mass of the solvent. The relationship of osmolality to concentration of the solution is such that the total number of particles multiplied by the concentration in moles per kilogram of H_2O and the osmotic coefficient for that solution equals the osmolality of the solution (in osmol/kg H_2O). Normally serum osmolality is around 290 mOsmol/kg H_2O. Osmolarity, while not used frequently with osmometry, is expressed in osmoles per liter of H_2O.

The reference method for methanol is GLC by headspace analysis, as described with ethanol. Gas chromatography for separation and quantification of formate metabolites can also be used with different column conditions. Due to the expertise and analytical time required, this method is generally only used in reference laboratories.

CLINICAL CORRELATION
In blood plasma or serum, the main substances that contribute most significantly to osmometry are sodium, glucose, and urea. Ethanol, when present, contributes significantly as well, but its detection is method dependent.

CASE SCENARIO 14-6

Volatile Organic Toxicity: Unexplained Intoxication

The laboratory technologist is asked to double-check the ethanol results from a patient in the emergency department with an ethanol level of 50 mg/dL and a preliminary diagnosis of intoxication. Quality control results and the sample integrity were acceptable. The physician requested that the laboratory personnel obtain a new sample to rerun ethanol along with additional laboratory tests.

Test	Patient	Reference Range
Lactic acid (mmol/L)	3.0	0.56–1.39
Osmolar gap (mOsm/kg)	40	<10
Osmolality (mOsm/kg)	340	275–290
Ethanol (mg/dL)	50	0 or below detection
Urine drugs of abuse	Negative	Negative

Volatile Organic Toxicity Screening

As noted with methanol testing, while waiting for gas chromatography to provide definitive results, presence of other alcohols such as methanol or ethylene glycol can be screened with osmolal gap. Ethanol can be included in the calculation by a correction factor to the calculated osmolality formula. This would help to eliminate an elevated osmolal gap due to ethanol.

Other volatiles such as isopropanol (rubbing alcohol) or ethylene glycol (antifreeze) can be measured by GLC if special sample treatment is applied. These alcohols can also be screened by osmolal gap as they will increase the measured osmolality by the FDP method. Clinical presentation and other diagnostic clues can also help the physician in arriving at a preliminary differential diagnosis and treatment plan while waiting for definitive results, such as chromatography.

Another screening method for ethylene glycol capitalizes on the interference with certain triglyceride methods that involve glycerol dehydrogenase as the indicator enzyme, due to the unusual presence of ethylene glycol. In this screening method, the sample can be pretreated with lipase to remove the native triglycerides. The sample is then analyzed by the lipase/glycerol dehydrogenase method. Ethylene glycol will be the measured product since triglycerides were removed in the pretreatment step.

Case Scenario 14-6 Volatile Organic Toxicity: Unexplained Intoxication

Follow-Up

Based on the earlier results of elevated osmolal gap but serum ethanol of 50 mg/dL, the physician ordered an alcohol screen for isopropanol, methanol, and ethylene glycol by chromatography. Results were pending while urinalysis and drug screen were being performed. The drug screen was found to be neg-

Case Scenario 14-6 Volatile Organic Toxicity: Unexplained Intoxication *(continued)*

ative for common drugs of abuse. When the urinalysis was completed, it was found that unusual microscopic results were reported, including 3 to 5 WBC/HPF (reference range, 0 to 2), 4 to 6 RBC/HPF (0 to 2), and 3 to 5 calcium oxalate crystals/LPF (0 to 2). Metabolites of ethylene glycol can enhance formation of calcium oxalate crystals in the urinary system. Appearance of calcium oxalate crystals may indicate ethylene glycol toxicity.

The patient also exhibited CNS disturbances with decreased responsiveness to pain and dilated pupils. Nystagmus or "lazy eye" and vision disturbances indicate toxicity of the optic nerve. These signs are characteristic of methanol and/or ethylene glycol toxicity.[13] Elevated lactic acid and calcium oxalate crystals also point toward ethylene glycol poisoning. Treatment was begun on the assumption of the presence of these toxins. The gas chromatography report later confirmed methanol and ethylene glycol poisoning. ●

CASE SCENARIO 14-7

Decision-Making: For Which Drugs of Abuse Should We Test?

At a rural hospital, the medical technologist has been asked to evaluate increasing the test menu to offer a screening method for drug-of-abuse testing. Currently all drug-of-abuse testing is sent to the reference laboratory, and quicker preliminary results are desired by the physicians. In consideration of drug testing methodology, the technologist needs to explore these four points:

1. Which drugs should be tested?
2. How sensitive and specific should the testing be?
3. Will specific information be available from the ordering physician?
4. What instrumentation should be used for drug testing?

DRUG-OF-ABUSE TESTING

Drug-of-abuse testing is ordered by physicians based on behaviors or signs exhibited by the patient. Since the patient may be uncooperative, a sample for drug testing should be relatively easy to obtain, such as urine or saliva, particularly if it is to be used for legal purposes. Blood or other body fluids may be analyzed also. Drugs of abuse are frequently involved in situations of trauma, including those involving legal situations. Motor-vehicular crimes are often associated with alcohol and drug-of-abuse intoxication.[22] Thus forensic testing for drugs of abuse is critical in providing legal evidence. Proper identification of the patient and sample, maintaining a chain of custody for the evidence, and following standardized procedures for maintaining the integrity of the sample during processing, testing, and reporting are critical in drug-of-abuse testing just as in legal alcohol testing.

There are thousands of potentially toxic drugs or toxins, and it is impossible to test for all of them. Consulting with the emergency department and the ordering physicians can determine what are the most important or likely drugs of abuse and toxins suspected for patients in the region. A negative result for a drug screen means that it is negative or below detectable levels only for the drugs that were tested. A good drug screen report should also list which drugs are tested for so that a negative result is not misleading.

Drugs of abuse are typically medications obtained without a prescription, or taken by a person other than the one for whom they were prescribed, or are illicit drugs. The most common drugs of abuse vary from region to region and change with current times. Currently throughout the country, marijuana and methamphetamine are common drugs of abuse, as are prescription drugs such as oxycodone (OxyContin) or diazepam (Valium).

Drugs of abuse are grouped by chemical similarity, methodology of analysis, and physiological effects. The following list groups common drugs of abuse within categories:

1. *CNS stimulants.* These drugs stimulate the CNS, raise heart and respiration rates, depress appetite, and give a feeling of euphoria. Drugs or drug classes commonly analyzed in this group include cocaine and its metabolite, benzoylecgonine, and amphetamines and methamphetamines. Methamphetamine use has been steadily rising and is common in rural and metropolitan areas. Drugs in this category taken in overdoses or over long periods of time cause serious nervous system and cardiac side effects.

2. *CNS depressants.* These drugs relax nerves, lower heart rate and respiratory rate, reduce pain, and give a feeling of euphoria. These include narcotics, hypnotics, sedatives, and tranquilizers. Drugs or drug classes in this group include barbiturates; methaqualone; benzodiazepines, including Valium; and oxycodone and other opiates, including morphine, heroin (which metabolizes to morphine), codeine (methylmorphine), and methadone. Drugs in this category taken in overdoses cause respiratory depression and acidosis.

3. *Hallucinogens or psychoactives.* Psychoactive drugs include cannabinoids and phencyclidine (PCP). Cannabinoids are drug forms derived from the cannabis plant such as marijuana and its active forms, Δ9-tetrahydrocannabinoid (THC) and 11-nor-Δ9-THC carboxylic acid. Long-term abuse of psychoactive drugs can cause memory loss.

4. *Antidepressants.* Antidepressants include lithium, tricyclic antidepressants, and others.

When considering how sensitive and specific drug testing should be, one needs to consider the intended use of the test results. Two main uses are for medical or for legal purposes. Often a quick and relatively simple method can be highly sensitive but less specific, with cross reaction with similar groups of drugs, but also have more analytical interferences. Drug-of-abuse screening tests require a high sensitivity, which often compromises analytical specificity, in order to provide quick turnaround time, low cost and low technological needs. Screening tests are considered presumptive and may be strictly qualitative (with positive or negative results). Confirmatory tests are needed for definitive results, especially for forensic or legal situations. Chain-of-custody considerations also must be made for results of legal concern.

The technologist needs to consider what instrumentation should be used for drug testing based on anticipated test volume, staffing, cost per test, and many other considerations. Some immunoassay methods have been incorporated into analyzers already in use. Other methods are simple spot tests that don't require sophisticated instruments but may require a confirmatory test before any results are reported. Thus all positive tests may need to be retested by an alternate method, which would slow down turnaround time and increase costs. The definitive or reference methods often utilize gas chromatography, which is time consuming and highly technical and is not likely to be a realistic consideration for many laboratories.

The standard for drug testing in clinical toxicology is an immunoassay screen conducted with a urine sample, followed by confirmation by gas chromatography with mass spectrometric detection. Qualitative results in the immunoassay method are determined based on federal guidelines for cutoff values. If a drug is present but determined to be below the recommended cutoff value based on a standard calibration curve, the positive result may be due to cross reactivity from similar drugs or chemicals. This would be considered a false positive for the drug and therefore not to be reported. Other screening tests for drugs of abuse include spot tests by ultraviolet (UV) spectrophotometry or enzyme-linked immunosorbent assay or by thin-layer chromatography (TLC). Drugs of abuse can also be presumptively quantified using immunoassays or HPLC or quantified by a definitive assay using gas chromatography. Column chromatography with mass spectrometry detection provides a high level of specificity and can be used for less common drugs that are not detected with routine immunoassays.[24]

Point-of-Care Drug Testing Devices

On-site urinalysis drug-testing devices have been used in emergency departments and clinics and for forensic purposes.[25] The false-negative rate for some of these point-of-care devices has been found to be less than 1% and the false-positive rate less than 1.75% for all drug classes, making them useful for impaired driving (DUI) investigations by law enforcement officers.[26] They tend to have a high cost per test but do not require purchase of new automated analyzers.

A commonly used point-of-care spot test is a competitive homogeneous immunoassay. In this method, the patient drug competes with a reagent drug complexed with colloidal gold for a limited amount of antibody. A second antibody, an anti-drug antibody, is bound to nylon membrane in a discrete zone and reacts with any residual drug–colloidal gold. Buffer is added, and a violet color indicates patient drug level that exceeded the threshold. Eight different drugs can be tested for in this system.[27] These methods do have some interference, with a likelihood of false positives due to cross reaction with similar chemicals. Spot tests use high-affinity monoclonal antibodies that are specific to drug classes, but cross reaction with related chemicals and over-the-counter medications are possible. For example, the spot test for pseudoephedrine may react positively with other amphetamines.

Automated Immunoassay Methods

Automated immunoassay techniques are often the method employed for drug screens, just as they are for therapeutic drugs. Considerable improvements in specificity and sensitivity have been made with newer generations of the immunoassays. The precision of several commercial immunoassay systems for drug-of-abuse screening is adequate to detect drugs below standardized lower limits of detection, but care should be used to interpret the results based on manufacturer's recommendations and federal guidelines for cutoff values. Knowledge of the positive predictive values of screening immunoassays at lower cutoff concentrations could enable efficient use of confirmatory testing resources and improved detection of illicit drug use.[27]

In a commonly employed enzyme immunoassay, enzyme-labeled drug competes with patient drug for a limited amount of specific antibody. Excess free enzyme-labeled drug reacts with substrate to form product. Color reaction is directly proportional to amount of patient drug. Thresholds are set so that qualitative results can be determined. Although monoclonal antibody is used with specificity to drug classes, cross reaction with similar drugs is possible. For example, in a test for an amphetamine, methamphetamine will enter into the reaction, as will other amphetamines, thus making this enzyme immunoassay a presumptive test.

Chromatography Methods

Thin-layer chromatography is also used as a presumptive screen for drugs of abuse. It can be used to screen for a variety of drugs in one process. In TLC, drugs migrate in a mobile phase on a silica gel support medium to a specific position depending on solubility in the two phases. Additional development of color or UV fluorescence provides further identification. Semiquantification of the drug may be achieved with densitometry. Although TLC separation is highly specific for drug classes, cross reaction with related chemicals is possible. For example, poppy seeds from food will often appear as a positive test for morphine. Therefore, TLC is a presumptive test that requires confirmation. It can often differentiate between types of amphetamine drugs and so may be used in conjunction with immunoassay methods to narrow the type of amphetamine drug class detected.

Results admissible for legal purposes must maintain scrupulous patient identification and follow specimen collection and handling protocols. Evidence chain of custody must be maintained. Definitive test methods, often the reference method, are required to assure the highest analytical specificity and sensitivity of results to be provided as legal evidence. Gas or liquid chromatography often is the definitive method for plasma ethanol and urinary drugs of abuse. Gas chromatography with mass spectrometry has even been adapted to detect and quantitate up to 18 common drugs of abuse or their metabolites in hair samples.[28,29]

Assessing patients with acute impairment often involves detecting large doses of drugs of abuse. However, sometimes the situation calls for monitoring of lingering doses or chronic use of drugs. In general, the detection time is longest in hair, followed by urine, sweat, oral fluid, and blood. In saliva, blood, or plasma, most drugs of abuse can be present for 1 or 2 days. In urine, the detection time of a single dose is 1.5 to 4 days.[30] In chronic users, most drugs of abuse can be detected in urine for approximately 1 week after last use, but up to 4 weeks for some drugs. Hair may be the sample of choice for monitoring chronic drug use since drugs can be detected over a longer time frame in hair samples.[28] Although the standard for drug testing in toxicology is conducted with urine samples, in recent years, more sensitive analytic techniques have enabled the analysis of drugs in saliva.[31,32] Saliva is becoming increasingly useful for the detection of drugs, since it is a noninvasive specimen to collect and, because collection is directly observed, it is difficult to adulterate. A point-of-collection oral fluid drug analysis kit has been developed for use in many drug-testing situations, including common drugs of abuse such as opiates, cannabinoids, and amphetamines.[33]

To determine the best specimen to collect and appropriateness of specific drug requests, specific information should be available from the ordering physician. For example, the time and date of suspected drug exposure help to determine the best specimen to collect. The suspected toxin or group of toxins for screening needs to be determined since drug-of-abuse panels are still limited to certain groups or categories. Sometimes other pertinent physical information is helpful as well.

Regardless of the type of testing employed by the laboratory for drug-of-abuse testing, a method validation and method comparison study must be completed prior to implementation. This should comply with guidelines established by the National Clinical Laboratory Standards Institute and meet Clinical Laboratory Improvement Amendments (CLIA) regulations. Refer to Chapter 2 (Quality Assessment), which addresses method validation.

In addition, a detailed operating procedure must be written and implemented along with training of personnel who will be involved in the specimen collection, transport, and preparation as well as analysis and reporting. This procedure should include maintenance and operation of equipment, when applicable, as well as quality control sample testing, documentation, and rules for corrective action, as well as other aspects of quality assessment.

Case Scenario 14-7 **Decision-Making: For Which Drugs of Abuse Should We Test?**

Follow-Up

To summarize the factors to consider in adding drug-of abuse testing in a rural site, we will consider four main points:

1. *Is it possible to measure the drugs requested by widely available methodologies?* Less frequently encountered drugs will need to be sent to reference laboratories that would have slower turnaround times and increased costs. Common drugs may be tested for with screening methods such as immunoassay found on common laboratory analyzers, particularly if forensic evidence won't be required.

2. *How sensitive and specific should the testing be?* Preliminary testing is often highly sensitive but lacks some specificity. This is useful for drug screening and for many medical considerations. These need confirmatory tests to enhance specificity. Confirmatory tests for medical purposes can be an alternate method such as HPLC or an alternative immunoassay procedure. The reference method with appropriate specimen chain-of-custody information should be used if forensic testing is required.

3. *What information will be needed?* Specific information that may be necessary to provide better drug testing results includes the time and date of suspected drug exposure and the suspected toxin or group of toxins to screen.

4. *What methods and instruments should be considered?* Different test methodologies and instrumentation needs to be considered including spot or point-of-care testing, routine analyzers, and reference methods such as chromatography. If preliminary testing is sufficient, screening methods can be utilized. Regardless of the type of testing employed by the laboratory for drug-of-abuse testing, a method validation and method comparison study must be completed prior to implementation. Refer to Chapter 2, which details the process of method validation. A summary of the advantages for three screening systems is as follows: Spot or point-of-care tests are the simplest techniques, with virtually no equipment costs involved but, depending on test volume, can be quite expensive based on

continued

Case Scenario 14-7 Decision-Making: For Which Drugs of Abuse Should We Test? *(continued)*

the test kits. Spot tests generally require less skilled training due to low technology involved and no need for instrumentation, but may require carefully timing and close supervision during the testing phase. Automated enzyme immunoassay has a higher initial cost for the automation if it isn't already present but, if test volume is higher, it may be the most cost effective. These assays are typically "walk away" systems in which the testing phase does not require close supervision. The amount of technologist time involved is especially noticed when multiple sample results can be obtained at once. Thin-layer chromatography can detect many more drugs than other screening method and is particularly good in situations in which it is difficult to determine to what the patient has been exposed. It requires only basic laboratory instrumentation but is moderately complex in skill required to perform and report the results. A considerable amount of technologist time is required throughout the testing phase. Cost is moderate, and only two samples can be analyzed at once. ●

HEAVY METAL TOXICITY

Heavy metal exposure, such as from mercury and lead, can be acute or chronic. Heavy metals can cause serious toxicological consequences that may be initially confused with drug-of-abuse or alcohol exposure due to behavioral and neurological manifestations. For example, high doses of lead can cause systolic hypertension and encephalopathy, while high or chronic exposure to mercury can cause psychotic behavior. *Encephalopathy* is a general term for disease of the brain, while *neuropathy* means disease of the nerves or neurons that may impair voluntary nerve function or functions of the brain. Psychosis, or confusion, complete disorientation, and loss of reasoning power, can be a result of heavy metal neurotoxicity. In addition, chronic low-dose exposure to heavy metals is a concern for proper neurological and other organ development in the young. Therefore, physical examination and history can be helpful in determining if heavy metal toxicity is suspected. Specific laboratory tests are required to confirm heavy metal toxicity. A detailed account of lead testing is found in Chapter 5 (Hemoglobin Production Disorders and Testing), since in typical doses lead exhibits hematologic changes. Table 14–3 lists common toxic metals, their clinical manifestations and a brief description of testing methods.

CASE SCENARIO 14-8

Mercury Poisoning: The Fish in the Sea

"Several environmental groups on Tuesday warned that fish caught by anglers, sold in local grocery stores, and served in restaurants could contain dangerously high levels of mercury. Fish caught along the beach tend to be safe, but the public is urged to use caution when eating large predator fish, in which mercury can accumulate. Coal-powered energy plants are the largest source of mercury in the area. Mercury is released into the air, is dropped to earth in rain, and works its way up the marine food chain." —*The Neighborhood News*

Case Scenario 14-8 **Mercury Poisoning: The Fish in the Sea** (*continued*)

This announcement in the local newspaper brought many concerned individuals to their physicians, who requested mercury screening on blood and urine specimens. One such patient, a fisherman, was anxious to know if he had come into contact with the contaminated fish. The laboratory technician instructed the patient on the proper collection of urine for mercury testing by stating, "A 24-hour collection must be placed into the metal-free container. Urine must not be allowed to come into contact with anything that may be contaminated in the environment." The technician had already drawn a blood sample into a metal-free, EDTA-containing tube for blood analysis for mercury.

TABLE 14-3

Toxic Heavy Metals

Metal	Pathology	Test Methodology
Aluminum	Pulmonary and nervous system impairment	Electrothermal atomic absorption spectroscopy (AAS)
Arsenic	Interferes with protein sulfhydryl group in protein coeznyemes, reduces oxidative phosphorylation and ATP production	AAS Qualitative tests: Gutzeit and Reinsch tests
Cadmium	Binds sulfhydryl groups to inhibit enzymes Pulmonary and nervous system impairment Affects kidney function, resulting in proteinuria	Electrothermal AAS
Lead	Binds sulfhydryl groups of proteins Symptom triad of colic, anemia, and encephalopathy	Anodic stripping voltammetry Electrothermal AAS Free erythrocyte protoporphyrin Erythrocyte zinc protoporphyrin Delta-aminolevulinic acid Delta-aminolevulinic acid synthetase Delta-aminolevulinic acid dehydratase
Mercury	Reacts with protein sulfhydryl groups Neurological, gastrointestinal, and renal impairment	AAS
Nickel	Pulmonary and nervous system impairment Dermatitis	Electrothermal AAS
Thallium	Has a great affinity for K and, thus, interrupts oxidative phosphorylation Binds sulfhydryl groups to inhibit enzymes	Electrothermal AAS
Iron	High doses of this mineral usually required to cause adverse effects Hemosiderosis and hepatic cirrhosis	Colorimetric, AAS

Mercury Exposure

Exposure to mercury can lead to neurological impairment, renal tubular acidosis, and gastrointestinal symptoms.[34] Mercury binds to structural and metabolic proteins to produce tissue impairment, such as renal tubular or myelin damage.[35] Clinically, patients present with symptoms of headache, tremor, abdominal cramps, diarrhea, neuropathy, proteinuria, and liver impairment.

Mercury may be found in the environment from mining and other industrial processes. The metal may also be found in seafood, thermometers, barometers, and dental amalgam. Mercury may be found in nonsymptomatic, healthy individuals as a result of diet and environmental exposure. Mercury exposure screening may not be appropriate for asymptomatic individuals or individuals without a history of recent exposure. Screening of individuals who have had occupational exposure may be appropriate.

Whole blood is the specimen of choice for recent exposure. A 12- or 24-hour timed urine collection in a mercury-free container is the specimen of choice for long-term exposure. The timed urine may be helpful in determining recent or long-term exposure and the need for therapy. Although there is no antidote to mercury, early chelation therapy may be used to lessen the effects of exposure. Dimercaprol has been used effectively as a chelator of inorganic and aryl organic mercury.

Laboratory analysis for mercury uses atomic absorption spectrophotometry (AAS) methodology. Tests for mercury are not generally available from the routine clinical laboratory. They are provided by reference laboratories. The toxic effects and laboratory testing methodologies for other potentially toxic heavy metals are listed in Table 14–3.[36]

Case Scenario 14-8 Mercury Poisoning: The Fish in the Sea

Follow-Up

An announcement in the local newspaper brought many concerned individuals, including one fisherman, to their physicians, who requested mercury screening on blood and urine specimens. The laboratory technician instructed the patient on the proper collection of urine for mercury testing. The technician had already drawn a blood sample in a metal-free, EDTA-containing tube for blood analysis for mercury.

The specimens were sent to a reference laboratory, where they were tested with AAS methodology, with the following results:

Test	Patient	Reference Range	Toxic Level
Blood mercury (μg/L)	4	<5	20–30
Urine mercury (μg/24 hours)	10	<20	>150
Organic mercury (μg/24 hours)	>200		
Inorganic mercury (μg/24 hours)	>150		

The results for this patient indicate exposure but not toxicity. The World Health Organization (WHO) suggests that mercury laboratory results should be interpreted on the basis of organic or inorganic exposure, exposure duration, and estimated time since exposure.[37] ●

SUMMARY

In this chapter, we explored some of the types of toxin and drug testing methods that are routinely employed in clinical laboratories. Working with toxicology and therapeutic drug monitoring testing in clinical laboratories involves many health-care personnel working together as a team, including physicians, pharmacists, nurses, blood collection staff, and other laboratory personnel. Drug testing can be requested for monitoring therapeutic drugs or for identifying and quantifying drugs of abuse. Likewise, serum or urinary heavy metal, ethanol, or other alcohol results may provide important information for the prognosis and treatment of patients. There are many similarities in the methodologies for these types of testing since immunoassay is commonly employed. Unique characteristics arise from specimen collection, timing, and handling. In addition, sophisticated instrumentation such as chromatography may provide definitive results of high specificity and sensitivity for drug of abuse or therapeutic drug monitoring. However, chromatography is often employed after simpler screening or presumptive tests have been utilized due to turnaround time and training issues. Newer test methods are continually being developed for improved specificity and sensitivity and for unusual samples such as saliva and hair.

EXERCISES

As you consider the scenarios presented in this chapter, answer the following questions:

1. What is a therapeutic range?

2. What is the specimen of choice for gentamicin TDM?

3. Describe the expected tobramycin trough level compared to the peak level obtained from an adult patient.

4. Describe the principle of EMIT enzyme immunoassay, including the role of the antibody, enzyme label, substrate, and source of antigen, in acetaminophen testing.

5. List the general drug source of Δ9-THC.

6. Describe the historical/classic spectrophotometric method for salicylate analysis.

7. Explain the likely toxic effects for acetaminophen overdose, using an appropriate nomogram.

8. List the legal ethanol threshold for intoxication in a 17-year-old male and a 37-year-old female in the state in which you reside.

9. Discuss two common heavy metal toxicities in terms of typical pathology and methods of analysis.

10. A patient has an elevated urine organic mercury level (125 μg/L). a. What is the typical reference range for urinary organic mercury in an adult? b. What are the proper collection criteria? c. What are some possible mechanisms by which this patient became exposed to mercury?

References

1. Hardman JG, et al (eds): *Goodman & Gilman's The Pharmacological Basis of Therapeutics*, ed 10. New York: McGraw-Hill, 2001.
2. Slaughter RL, Schneider PJ, Visconti JA: Appropriateness of the use of serum digoxin and digitoxin assays. *Am J Hosp Pharm.* 1978; 35:1376–1379.
3. McEvoy GK: *AHFS Drug Information 2003.* Bethesda, MD: American Society of Health-System Pharmacists, 2003.
4. Contopoulos-Ioannidis DG, et al: Extended-interval aminoglycoside administration for children: a meta-analysis. *Pediatrics* 2004; 114:e111–e118.
5. Quattrocchi F, et al: Effect of serum separator blood collection tubes on drug concentrations. *Ther Drug Monit* 1983; 5:359.
6. Smith TW: Digitalis toxicity: epidemiology and clinical use of serum concentration measurements. *Am J Med* 1975; 58:470–476..
7. Jolley ME, et al: Fluorescent polarization immunoassay: an automated system for therapeutic drug determination. *Clin Chem* 1981; 27:1575–1579.
8. Gupta A, et al: A case of nondigitalis cardiac glycoside toxicity. *Ther Drug Monit* 1997; 19:711–714.
9. Gowda RM, Cohen RA, Khan IA: Toad venom poisoning: resemblance to digoxin toxicity and therapeutic implications. *Heart* 2003; 89:e14.
10. Barrueto F Jr, et al: Cardioactive steroid poisoning from an herbal cleansing preparation. *Ann Emerg Med* 2003; 41:396–399.
11. Jaffe AM, Gephardt D, Courtemanche L: Poisoning due to ingestion of *Veratrum viride* (false hellebore). *J Emerg Med* 1990; 8:161–167.
12. Rich SA, Libera JM, Locke RJ: Treatment of foxglove extract poisoning with digoxin-specific Fab fragments. *Ann Emerg Med* 1993; 22:1904–1907.
13. Beers MH, Berkow RB: *The Merck Manual of Diagnosis and Therapy*, ed 17. Rahway, NJ: Merck & Co., 1999.
14. Steinhoff BJ, et al: The ideal characteristics of antiepileptic therapy: an overview of old and new AEDs. *Acta Neurol Scand* 2003; 107:87–95.
15. Contin M, et al: Levetiracetam therapeutic monitoring in patients with epilepsy: effect of concomitant antiepileptic drugs. *Ther Drug Monit* 2004; 26:375–379.
16. Lyon AW, Whitley C, Eintracht SL: Analytic evaluation and application of a novel spectrophotometric serum lithium method to a rapid response laboratory. *Ther Drug Monit* 2004; 26:98–101.
17. Bengtsson F: Therapeutic drug monitoring of psychotropic drugs: TDM "nouveau". *Ther Drug Monit* 2004; 26:145–151.
18. Members of the German Study Group on Pediatric Renal Transplantion: Cyclosporin A absorption profiles in pediatric renal transplant recipients predict the risk of acute rejection. *Ther Drug Monit* 2004; 26:415–424.
19. Taylor PJ: Therapeutic drug monitoring of immunosuppressant drugs by high-performance liquid chromatography-mass spectrometry. *Ther Drug Monit* 2004; 26:215–219.
20. Koda-Kimble MA, Young LY: *Applied Therapeutics: The Clinical Use of Drugs*, ed 7. Philadelphia: Lippincott, Williams & Wilkins, 2001.
21. Cham BE, et al: Simultaneous liquid-chromatographic quantitation of salicylic acid, salicyluric acid and gentisic acid in plasma. *Clin Chem* 1979; 25:1420–1425.
22. Orsay EM, et al: The impaired driver: hospital and police detection of alcohol and other drugs of abuse in motor vehicle crashes. *Ann Emerg Med* 1995; 25:430–431.
23. Sunshine I, Jatlow PI. *Methology for Analytical Toxicology*, vol 2. Boca Raton, FL: CRC Press, 1982.
24. Nordgren HK, Beck O: Multicomponent screening for drugs of abuse: direct analysis of urine by LC-MS-MS. *Ther Drug Monit* 2004; 26:90–97.
25. Phillips JE, et al: Signify ER Drug Screen Test evaluation: comparison to Triage Drug of Abuse Panel plus tricyclic antidepressants. *Clin Chim Acta* 2003; 328:31–38.
26. Crouch DJ, et al: A field evaluation of five on-site drug-testing devices. *J Anal Toxicol* 2002; 26:493–499.
27. Luzzi VI, et al: Analytic performance of immunoassays for drugs of abuse below established cutoff values. *Clin Chem* 2004; 50:717–722.

28. Paterson S, et al: Qualitative screening for drugs of abuse in hair using GC-MS. *J Anal Toxicol* 2001; 25:203–208.

29. Bourland JA, et al: Quantitation of cocaine, benzoylecgonine, cocaethylene, methylecgonine, and norcocaine in human hair by positive ion chemical ionization (PICI) gas chromatography-tandem mass spectrometry. *J Anal Toxicol* 2000; 24:489–495.

30. Verstraete AG: Detection times of drugs of abuse in blood, urine, and oral fluid. *Ther Drug Monit* 2004; 26:200–205.

31. Kintz P, Samyn N: Use of alternative specimens: drugs of abuse in saliva and doping agents in hair. *Ther Drug Monit* 2002; 24:239–246.

32. Kolbrich EA, et al: Cozart RapiScan Oral Fluid Drug Testing System: an evaluation of sensitivity, specificity, and efficiency for cocaine detection compared with ELISA and GC-MS following controlled cocaine administration. *J Anal Toxicol* 2003; 27:407–411.

33. Barrett C, Good C, Moore C: Comparison of point-of-collection screening of drugs of abuse in oral fluid with a laboratory-based urine screen. *Forensic Sci Int* 2001; 122:163–166.

34. Agency for Toxic Substance and Disease Registry: *Medical Management Guidelines for Mercury.* Atlanta: Division of Toxicology, Centers for Disease Control and Prevention, 2004.

35. Chunying C, et al: Increased oxidative DNA damage, as assessed by urinary 8-hydroxy-2'-deoxyguanosine concentrations, and serum redox status in persons exposed to mercury. *Clin Chem* 2005; 51:759–767.

36. Cannon DJ: Toxicology of heavy metals, parts 1 & 2. *TDM/Tox In-Service Training and Continuing Education* 13(2):7–11; 13(3):9–13, 1991.

37. Inter-Organization Programme for the Sound Management of Chemicals: *Elemental Mercury and Inorganic Mercury Compounds.* Geneva: World Health Organization. 2003.

Glossary

% v/v - number of milliliters per 100 mL

% w/v - number of grams per 100 mL

% w/w - number of grams per 100 g (mass/mass)

17-hydroxycorticosteroids (17-OHCS) - 21-carbon atoms with a hydroxyl group at the 17th carbon atom

A-a gradient - alveolar-to-arterial gradient, which assesses alveolar ventilation

absence seizures - mild, brief attacks with altered consciousness, eyelid fluttering, and abrupt stopping of activity with no memory of the attack

absorb - to take in or receive by chemical or molecular action

absorbance - the amount of light retained by a substance

absorptivity - the amount of absorbance specific for a certain substance

accreditation - the process by which an agency or an organization evaluates and recognizes a program of study or an institution as meeting certain predetermined qualifications or standards; applies only to institutions and programs

accuracy - how closely a measured value agrees with a true or expected value

acidosis - increase in the acidity of blood due to an accumulation of acids or an excessive loss of bicarbonate

acinar - granular tissue that makes up a gland such as the pancreas or prostate

acquired immunodeficiency syndrome (AIDS) - late stage of infection with the human immunodeficiency virus, which results in decreased immunity

activity - ability to produce motion or energy; for example, enzyme activity is the ability of the enzyme to influence the rate of a reaction

acute myocardial infarction (AMI) - sudden heart attack, resulting from dead heart muscle tissue unable to contract in rhythm

acyl - the radical derived from an organic acid when the hydroxyl group is removed

adenohypophysis - anterior lobe, or front portion, of the pituitary, sometimes called the master endocrine gland

adenoma - a benign tumor of glandular origin

adenomatous - referring to neoplasm of glandular cells

adrenergic - pertaining to the adrenal gland, especially the neuroendocrine tissues of the medulla

adsorb - attach to the surface of another material

alcohols - methanol (CH_3OH), isopropanol (($CH_3)_2CHOH$), and ethylene glycol (($CH_2OH)_2$), which are chemically similar to ethanol due to the –OH group

alkalosis - increase in blood alkalinity due to an accumulation of alkaline substances or reduction of acids

alpha-glucosidase inhibitor - blocks hydrolysis of an alpha glucoside for control of type 2 diabetes

alveolar PO_2 - PAO_2; the partial pressure of carbon dioxide gas in the alveolar sacs

alveolar ventilation - effective air exchange between alveoli and blood

alveoli - air sacs at the end of air ducts in the lungs and in contact with capillaries that allow gases to diffuse in or out (singular: alveolus)

Alzheimer's disease - progressive brain disorder with deterioration of mental capacity affecting memory and judgment

amniotic fluid - liquid that surrounds the fetus in the amniotic cavity

amperometry - measuring current in amperes, including coulometric methods

amyloidosis - metabolic disorder with starch accumulation in organs and tissues

anabolism - the constructive phase of metabolism

analgesics - medications that relieve pain

anaplasia - loss of cell differentiation and change in structure

anencephaly - a fatal congenital absence of or greatly reduced brain, particularly the cerebrum, resulting from failure of the neural tube to close during organ formation

angina - chest pain due to inadequate supply of oxygen to heart muscle

anion - an ion carrying a negative charge

anion gap - the unmeasured anions in plasma present with bicarbonate and chloride to balance sodium and potassium cations

anisocytosis - variation in sizes of red blood cells: smaller, larger, or both

anode - a positively charged electrode that attracts anions (negative ions)

anorexia - loss of appetite

antecubital fossa - area in the crook of the arm

anthropometric - literally means the "measure of man"; type of measurement also referred to as body composition analysis

antibody - an immunoglobulin produced by a B lymphocyte in response to a unique antigen

antibody titer - measure of the amount of antibody against a particular antigen present in the blood

antigen - a protein or oligosaccharide that elicits an antibody response

antipyretics - medications that reduce fever

antistreptolysin-O (ASO) titer - measurement of antibodies to a protein component of group A *Streptococcus* bacteria

apoferritin - the protein portion of ferritin, the storage form of iron

apoprotein - the protein portion of a lipoprotein

ARDS - respiratory distress syndrome of the adult; acquired respiratory failure

ascariasis - infection with the parasite *Ascaris lumbricoides*

ascites - accumulation of serous fluid in the abdomen

atelectasis - partial or complete lung collapse due to obstruction of the airway

atherosclerosis - fatty accumulation causing hardening and plugging in blood vessels

atrophy - decrease in size or function

automation - ability of an instrument to perform a laboratory test with minimal human involvement

azotemia - an elevated level of urea in the blood

basal metabolic rate - baseline rate of metabolism based on gender and weight (in kcal/24 hr)

base excess - concentration of titratable base in a solution with pH 7.40 and P_{CO_2} of 40 mm Hg

batch analysis - a group of samples are analyzed at the same time for the same test

Bence Jones protein - free light chains of the immunoglobulin molecule

benign - cell growth that doesn't spread and is cured with removal

benzoic acid analog - a compound that is structurally similar to $C_7H_6O_2$ and used for control of type 2 diabetes

beriberi - disease characterized by peripheral neurological, cerebral, and cardiovascular abnormalities; caused by deficiency of thiamine

biclonal - arising from two cell lines

biliary canaliculi - small ducts or tubes that carry bile out from the liver leading to the small intestine

biochemical marker - any biochemical compound, such as an antigen, antibody, abnormal enzyme, or hormone, that is sufficiently altered in a disease to serve as an aid in diagnosing or in predicting susceptibility to the disease

blastocyst - spherical shell enclosing fluid-filled cavity with the inner cell mass that will become the embryo at one pole and an outer layer of cells that will form the embryonic placenta

blood urea nitrogen (BUN) - urea concentration in the blood; historically, urea was measured as nitrogen remaining from a protein-free filtrate of the blood

blood-borne - carried or transmitted by blood

buffalo hump - fat accumulation on upper shoulders and collar bone causing the neck and head to jut forward

buffer - a mixture of chemicals that resist changes in pH by combining with free H^+ (proton acceptor) and OH^-, generally a strong salt and weak acid or base; human buffer systems include anionic proteins, deoxyhemoglobin, phosphate buffers, and bicarbonate/carbonic acid buffers

calculi - any abnormal concretion of precipitated inorganic materials, commonly called a stone, within the body (singular: calculus)

canalicular - within canals or small ducts

carbonic anhydrase inhibitors - compounds that reduce the secretion of H^+ ions through alkalinization of the urine; drugs that are commonly used to treat glaucoma

carboxypeptidase - a pancreatic enzyme that hydrolyzes peptides from the C-terminal end

cardiac catheterization - insertion of thin, flexible tube into the heart and coronary arteries for detecting blood pressure and flow and taking images

carryover - a sampling problem that occurs when remnants of a previous sample or test reaction product affect later samples

catabolism - the destructive phase of metabolism

catalyze - to accelerate the rate of a chemical reaction without being consumed

catecholamine metabolites - products of catecholamine metabolism (e.g., vanillylmandelic acid, homovanillic acid, metanephrine, normetanephrine)

catecholamines - biogenic amines that contain an aromatic catechol and an aliphatic amine (e.g., epinephrine, norepinephrine, dopamine)

cathode - a negatively charged electrode that attracts cations (positive ions)

cation - an ion carrying a positive charge

celiac sprue - malabsorption syndrome resulting from intolerance to dietary wheat proteins

centrifugal analysis - using centrifugal force to achieve chemical reaction and analysis

cerebrovascular accident - stroke or sudden loss of blood flow to the brain due to obstruction or clot in the blood vessels

certification - the process by which a nongovernmental agency or association grants recognition to an individual who has met certain predetermined qualifications specified by that agency or association

chain of custody - additional documentation of the condition of a specimen, all procedures performed, and personnel who have encountered a test specimen

chemiluminescence - light emitted by a chemical reaction

chief cells - secretory cells that line the gastric glands and secrete pepsin or its precursor, pepsinogen

cholecystokinin - hormone secreted by the upper small intestine that stimulates contraction of the gallbladder and pancreatic secretion

cholestasis - obstruction of the flow of bile; standing bile

choroid plexus - cavities in the cerebrum lined with thin membranes and blood vessels

chromatogram - record of molecular separation taking place in chromatography

chromatography - a technique for separating similar molecules based on differential absorption and elution

chromogen - colored product formed in a colorimetric reaction

chronic bronchitis - long-standing irritation and inflammation of the respiratory ducts

chylomicron - parcel of lipids and proteins made from dietary fats (especially triglycerides) during intestinal absorption

chymotrypsin - digestive enzyme produced by the pancreas that, with trypsin, hydrolyzes proteins to peptones or amino acids

clearance - the elimination of a substance, as related to its removal from the blood plasma by the kidneys

Clinical Laboratory Improvement Amendments of 1988 (CLIA) - quality standards for all clinical laboratories to ensure the accuracy, reliability, and timeliness of patient test results regardless of where the test was performed; the Centers for Medicare and Medicaid Services regulates all laboratory testing (except research) performed on humans in the United States

clones - genetically identical cells

closed reagent system - analytical system for which the reagents, in a unique container or format, are provided only by the manufacturer

cluster of differentiation (CD) - cell membrane molecules used to classify leukocyte subsets

colonoscopy - examination of the upper portion of the rectum with an instrument

colorimetric - determining analyte from visible light absorption of a colored product

competitive immunoassay - immunoassay in which patient antigen and labeled reagent antigen compete for the same binding site on the antibody

conductivity - the combined ability of ions to carry a charge

confirmatory test - using laboratory tests to verify that an initial test result is accurate; should be very specific

continuous flow analysis - each sample passes through the same stream and reactions as all other samples, with only a brief washout phase between samples

coproporphyrin - water-soluble tetrapyrrole precursor of heme found in urine and feces

cor pulmonale - right-sided heart failure

coronary arteries - three major blood vessels supplying blood and oxygen to the heart muscles

corpus luteum - yellow glandular mass that develops from an ovarian follicle following the release of a mature oocyte and secretes progesterone

coulometry - measuring aspects of current, including rate of electron flow; often used in titration of ions

coupled - chemical reactions that share a common intermediate

credentialing - the processes involved in identifying those institutions and individuals meeting acceptable standards in areas of accreditation, certification, or licensure

cretinism - growth deficiency and mental retardation

Crohn's disease - inflammatory disease of the gastrointestinal tract that can lead to intestinal obstruction

cryoglobulinemia - presence in the blood of an abnormal protein that forms gels at low temperatures

current - electrical charge (in coulombs/second); measured in units of amperes

cyanotic - characterized by bluish appearance due to lack of tissue oxygenation

cyclopentanoperhydrophenanthrene - an organic molecule with 17 carbon atoms composed of three six-sided rings (the phenanthrene portion) and one five-sided ring

deemed status - permission given to an external second party to act as the agent of the first party

definitive test - highly sensitive and specific test in which results can be used as legal evidence

dehydroepiandrosterone - 19-carbon molecule found in small amounts as a precursor to some estrogens in women and as a precursor to male sex steroids in men

delta check - comparison of concentration an analyte to values from previous specimens in the same patient; a form of quality assurance

densitometry - using colorimetry to determine the quantity of a dense region, such as in protein electrophoresis densitometry

dermatitis - an inflammatory rash

desensitization - lowering of responsiveness

detoxification - removal of waste or toxins from a fluid, rendering it harmless

dexamethasone - a synthetic glucocorticoid used to determine the cause of hypercortisolism

diabetes insipidus - lack of antidiuretic hormone output or response causing polyuria and potential dehydration

diabetic nephropathy - disease of the kidney, including inflammatory, degenerative, and sclerotic conditions, caused by diabetes

diagnostic sensitivity - the likelihood that, given the presence of disease, an abnormal test result predicts the disease

diagnostic specificity - the likelihood that, given the absence of disease, a normal test result excludes disease

diffuse - present over a large area

digital rectal examination - palpation of the prostate gland with a gloved finger inserted into the rectum

disaccharidases - enzymes that hydrolyze the glycolic bond of disaccharides

disaccharides - simple carbohydrates composed of two monosaccharides

discrete analysis - test reactions occur in separate compartments

diuretic - agent that promotes urine formation

diurnal variations - changes in chemical levels during the day, especially when comparing two different times

DNA - deoxyribonucleic acid; in the eukaryote and some prokaryotes, the chemical that transmits inherited characteristics of an organism to its progeny

downregulation - inhibition or suppression of the normal response of an organ or system

duodenum - the first part of the small intestine that is adjacent to the pyloric region of the stomach

eclampsia - coma and convulsive seizures of the mother between week 20 of pregnancy and the end of the first week after birth

ectoderm - the outermost of the three primary germ layers of an embryo forming neural tissue

ectopic - occurring outside the expected location

ectopic hormone secretion - production of hormones by nonendocrine cells

edematous - puffed up due to visible accumulation of fluids

Edwards' syndrome - congenital and fatal defect of the fetus (trisomy 18) causing severe multiorgan defects, including mental deficiency

ejaculation - ejection of sperm cells and seminal fluid at orgasm

elastase - an enzyme that dissolves elastin

electrocardiogram (ECG) - tracing of electrical activity of the heart

electrochemistry - measuring potential, current, or resistance to determine the activity of an analyte

electrode - a terminal that detects changes in current or voltage in response to changes in the environment

electrolytes - substances that ionize in solution and conduct electricity

electrophoresis - a separation technique of different charged molecules in solution in an electrical field of varying potential

electrostatic - producing electrical attractions within or between groups of molecules

eluate - the liquid obtained from a column during separation; derived from washing

elute - remove based on solubility

embryo - rapidly growing and developing human organism before the 10th week of gestation

emission - giving off or sending out

emphysema - chronic pulmonary disease marked by abnormal increase in the airspaces and destructive changes in their walls

encephalocele - congenital opening in the skull with protrusion of brain tissue

endogenous - originating inside the body

endometrium - lining of the uterus

endoplasmic reticulum - cell organelle that serves as a compartment for numerous chemical reactions

energy malnutrition - nutritional deficiency caused by inadequate intake of calories, protein, or both, seen in children under age 5 years or persons undergoing stress of major illness; also protein-calorie malnutrion

epilepsy - a recurrent disorder of cerebral function characterized by a variety of attacks caused by excessive discharge of cerebral neurons

epitopes - specific antibody binding sites found on an antigen

erythropoietic - pertaining to blood cell production

esophageal varices - tortuous dilatation of veins of the esophagus

essential nutrients - molecules that are required for metabolism but cannot be produced by the body; required in the diet

ester - compound formed by combination of an organic acid and an alcohol with elimination of water

estradiol - 18-carbon steroid molecule that is the main estrogen found in nonpregnant women

estriol - 18-carbon steroid molecule that is the main estrogen found in pregnant women

estrone - 18-carbon steroid molecule that is less active than other estrogens

ethanol - ethyl alcohol, CH_3CH_2OH

etiology - the cause of disease

euthyroid - showing normal clinical signs and normal thyroid function status despite the indications of dysfunction in some thyroid test results

ex vivo - outside of a living being

excretion - the elimination of waste products from the body

exocrine glands - glands that secrete externally through ducts

exogenous - originating outside an organ or part of the body

exophthalmos - protrusion of eyeballs due to accumulation of fluid and metabolic products

false negative - result below the decision limit in a patient who has the disease

false positive - result at or above the decision limit in a patient who does not have the disease

ferritin - the storage form of iron found in the liver, spleen, and bone marrow

fertilization - union of two gametes: male (sperm cell) and female (oocyte)

fetus - unborn but recognizable human organism between 10 weeks' and 40 weeks' gestation

filtration - the process of removing particles from a solution by passing the solution through a membrane or other barrier

FIO_2 - amount of oxygen available to breath

first-order (metabolic) kinetics - reaction in which velocity of metabolism by enzymes is proportional to the concentration of substrate (drug)

flatulence - excessive gas in the stomach and intestines

fluorescence - emission of low-energy light quickly after absorbing high-energy light; a type of luminescence

fluorometer - instrument that detects fluorescent emissions

focal - present in one small area

follicle - sac produced by the ovary containing an oocyte

follicular phase - first half of the female menstrual cycle leading up to maturity of one follicle and release of an oocyte

forensic testing - testing in which results can be submitted to help answer a question of law or as evidence in a legal decision

galactosemia - an inherited disorder marked by the inability to metabolize galactose due to a congenital absence of the enzyme galactose-1-phosphate uridyl transferase

gametocyte - sperm cell or oocyte

gammopathy - any disease in which serum immunoglobulins are increased

gastrectomy - surgical removal of part or all of the stomach

gastrinoma - gastrin-secreting tumor

gastritis - inflammation of the gastric mucosa

genome - the complete set of genetic information produced by the cell

glucocorticoids - adrenal cortical hormones primarily active in protecting against stress and affecting protein and carbohydrate metabolism

gluconeogenesis - formation of glucose from excess amino acids, fats, or other noncarbohydrate sources

glycemic - pertaining to control of blood glucose levels

glycogenesis - formation of glycogen

glycogenolysis - glycogen stored in the liver and muscles is converted to glucose 1-phosphate and then to glucose 6-phosphate

goiter - enlarged, usually hyperactive thyroid gland due to a variety of causes

gold standard method - test method that provides the best available approximation of a true value

gonads - reproductive organs: the testes in the male and ovaries in the female

gravimetric - measuring mass to relate to density or other concentration

half-life - one-half of the time between synthesis and degradation of a compound/time needed for the concentration of a drug to decrease by half

hapten - low molecular weight chemical coupled to a carrier protein to become a suitable immunogen

hematopoiesis - the production and development of blood cells

hemoconcentration - relative increase in the number of red blood cells resulting from a decrease in the volume of plasma

hemoglobinopathies - diseases that result in structural abnormalities of globin chains

hemolysis - rupture of erythrocyte cell membrane causing release of intracellular contents

hemosiderin - granular iron oxide found in the bone marrow or other cells

Henderson-Hasselbalch equation - equation that relates pH of blood plasma to equilibrium of salt (HCO_3^-) and weak acid (H_2CO_3)

hepatic - pertaining to the liver

hepatobiliary - relating to bile ducts and ducts within the liver

heterogeneous assay - immunoassay in which bound and free antibody must be separated before label is measured

homeostasis - the state of dynamic equilibrium of the internal environment of the body that is maintained by processes of feedback and regulation in response to external or internal changes

homogeneous assay - immunoassay in which bound and free antibody need not be separated before label is measured

human chorionic gonadotropin (hCG) - classic hormone marker of pregnancy produced by the placenta after the fertilized ooctye implants

human placental lactogen (hPL) - hormone produced by the placenta and involved in maternal glucose and fat metabolism and mammary gland function

hybridoma - a fused lymphocyte and myeloma cell used for making specific antibodies

hydrophobic - water insoluble

hydrops fetalis - stasis of fluids in tissue spaces, secondary to loss of albumin, leading to a condition in infants of hepatosplenomegaly and respiratory and circulatory distress

hyperkalemia - increased potassium in blood plasma

hypernatremia - increased sodium in blood plasma

hypernatriuric - exhibiting increased urinary sodium

hyperplasia - increase in cell mass, often with increased function

hypertension - in adults, blood pressure higher than 140 mm Hg systolic or 90 mm Hg diastolic on three separate readings recorded several weeks apart

hyperthermia - heat intolerance and higher than normal body temperature

hypertonicity - increased concentration of a body fluid due to increased solute compared to water in solution

hyperviscosity - gelatinous nature or excessive viscosity

hypochromic - having a large pale central area due to less hemoglobin (red blood cells)

hyponatremia - decreased sodium in blood plasma

hypo-osmolality - decreased concentration (tonicity) of a body fluid due to decreased solute compared to water in the solution

hypoperfusion - decreased passage of blood through vessels of an organ

hypophysectomy - resection or removal of the pituitary

hypophysis - pituitary or master endocrine gland

hypovolemia - decreased blood volume; may be caused by fluid losses or inadequate fluid intake

hypoxia - decreased oxygen supply to tissue despite adequate perfusion of the tissue

icterus - yellowish pigmentation in the blood due to increased bilirubin

idiopathic - without a recognizable cause

immunoassay - test tha measures the protein or protein-bound molecules concerned with the reaction of an antigen with its specific antibody

immunochemical - chemical that is able to enter into an antibody-antigen reaction

immunogen - high molecular weight molecule that stimulates antibody production; antigen

in utero - within the uterus

in vitro - pertaining to laboratory conditions, such as specimens in a test tube

inborn error of metabolism - an inherited metabolic disease that often causes deficiency of an enzyme

indices - plural of index; numbers used as indicators

inert - chemically nonreactive

infarction - dead muscle tissue often due to decreased blood flow from clogged coronary arteries

infiltration - deposition and accumulation of an external substance within a cell, tissue, or organ

insulin-like growth factor - peptide similar in chemical structure and activity to insulin

insulin-like growth factor binding protein - a soluble protein that binds insulin-like growth factors and affects them at the cellular level

intrinsic factor - glycoprotein that is secreted by the parietal cells of the gastric mucosa; necessary for the absorption of dietary vitamin B_{12} through the intestinal mucosa

ion-exchange chromatography - separating components of a mixture based on different solubility characteristics and attraction to an electrically charged solid substance

ionophore - substance that attracts charged molecules (ions)

ion-selective electrode (ISE) - electrode that measures the activity of one ion better than others

iontophoresis - introduction of a drug through intact skin by the application of a direct electric current

isoenzymes - forms of enzymes with different amino acid sequences giving unique properties but having the ability to catalyze similar chemical reactions

jaundice - bilirubin deposits in the skin, mucous membranes, and eyes giving tissues a yellow appearance

Joint Commission on Accreditation of Healthcare Organizations (JCAHO) - accreditation organization for health-care facilities in order to continuously improve safety and quality of health care

kernicterus - yellow staining of the lipid-rich meninges of the brain and spinal cord due to bilirubin infiltrates

ketoacidosis - the accumulation of keto acids in the blood causing metabolic acidosis

laser - light amplification by stimulated emission of radiation; device using a high-energy beam of electromagnetic radiation

law of mass action - the rate of any given chemical reaction is proportional to the product of the activities (or concentrations) of the reactants

lecithin:cholesterol acyltransferase - an enzyme that esterifies a fatty acid to cholesterol

Leydig cells - specialized interstitial cells of the testes surrounding the tubules that produce testosterone

libido - sexual desire

licensure - the process by which an agency of a state government grants permission to persons meeting predetermined qualifications to engage in a given occupation and/or to use a particular title; individuals who are not licensed cannot practice in that state

linearity - relation of independent and dependent data points that produces a straight line

lipemia - fatty accumulation in the blood giving cloudy appearance

lipogenesis - formation of fats

lipolysis - the catabolic degradation of triacylglycerol

lipoprotein - protein combined with lipid components

lipoprotein lipase - enzyme that catalyzes hydrolysis of triglycerides found on chylomicrons and VLDL

lobules - the microscopic functional units of the liver

lumen - space within a tube, such as a blood vessel or the esophagus

luminescence - production of light without the production of heat

luteal phase - second half of the female menstrual cycle following ovulation and the dominance of the corpus luteum

lytic - rupturing or breaking down cell membranes

M protein - paraprotein visible in protein electrophoresis causing a tall peak in the densitometry pattern, also called an M spike

macroglobulinemia - disease of plasma cells marked by excess production of immunoglobulin M (IgM)

macronutrient - a chemical element or substance, such as carbohydrates, proteins, and fats, required in relatively large quantities in the diet

macrosomia - increased size and weight of the fetus

malignant - characterized by completely unrestricted cell growth with a tendency to spread

malnutrition - disease-promoting condition resulting from either an inadequate or excessive exposure to nutrients

material safety data sheet - documents produced by the manufacturer of the chemical to provide safety information

median - the middle value of a population

medical decision level - concentration or limit at which test results are critically interpreted

medical decision limit - the value for a test result that is used in making the diagnosis

meningomyocele - congenital opening in the spinal cord membranes through which the cord protrudes; also called spina bifida

mesoderm - middle of the three primary germ layers of an embryo, the source especially of bone, muscle, connective tissue, and dermis

metabolic acidosis - acidosis resulting from increase in acids other than carbonic acid

metabolic alkalosis - alkalosis in which plasma bicarbonate is increased with a proportionate rise in the plasma concentration of carbon dioxide

metastasis - tumor appearance in a different body site than the primary tumor of the same cell line

metyrapone - metabolic hormone that inhibits biosynthesis of cortisol and corticosterone and is used to test for normal functioning of the pituitary gland; also known as metapyrone

micelle - ultramicroscopic particle

microalbuminuria - small amounts of albumin found in the urine, also called dipstick–negative increase in the excretion of albumin in urine

microcytic - of smaller than normal size (red blood cells)

micronutrient - organic compound, such as a vitamin, or chemical element essential in minute amounts in the diet

microvascular - pertaining to small blood vessels

Mie scatter - large particles scattering light predominently in the forward direction

mineralocorticoids - steroid molecules that influence blood electrolyte levels

minimum effective concentration - the lower limit of the therapeutic range

minimum toxic concentration - the lower limit of the toxicity range

miscarriage - sudden unplanned evacuation of the uterus, ending pregnancy

mixed venous oxygen saturation - capillary-to-venous exchange of gases

moiety - a portion of something that has been divided

monensin - sodium ionophore used for ISEs; made from *Streptomyces* species

monoclonal - arising from one cell line

monosaccharides - simple carbohydrates that cannot be broken down to further sugars by hydrolysis

morula - differentiated zygote that develops a cavity forming the blastocyst

motor nerves - nerves that control movement

mucin - a glycoprotein found in mucus, formed from mucigen and soluble in water

multichannel - able to perform a variety of tests at the same time with separate dedicated instrument components

multiple endocrine neoplasia - one of several inherited endocrine gland syndromes caused by a defect in tumor suppressor genes

multiple myeloma - a malignant disease characterized by the infiltration of bone and bone marrow by neoplastic plasma cells

multiple sclerosis - a progressive neurodegenerative disease affecting the axons of nerves in the area surrounding the ventricles of the brain but not the peripheral nerves

myelin - phospholipid protein sheath of nerve cells

myelodysplastic syndrome (MDS) - hematologic syndrome of inadequate bone marrow production of blood cells

myocardium - heart muscle

myxedema - puffiness in the face and surrounding the eyes

NAD - nicotinamide adenine dinucleotide

NADH - reduced nicotinamide adenine dinucleotide phosphate

NADP - nicotinamide adenine dinucleotide phosphate

NADPH - reduced nicotinamide adenine dinucleotide phosphate

necrosis - death of tissue

negative feedback - stabilizing a process by reducing its rate or output when its effects are too great

neoplasia - accelerated new cell growth, either benign or malignant

nephritis - inflammation of the kidney

nephrolithiasis - presence of calculi in the urinary tract; urate nephrolithiasis indicates the presence of uric acid in the stone

nephrotoxicity - damage to the kidneys

neurohypophysis - the posterior or back portion of the pituitary gland

nitrogen balance - difference between the amount of nitrogen ingested and that excreted

noncompetitive immunoassay - immunoassay that does not contain reagent antigen competing with patient antigen

nonprotein nitrogen - catabolites of protein and nucleic acid metabolism, including urea, ammonia, creatinine, creatine, and uric acid

nonsteroidal anti-inflammatory drugs (NSAIDs) - drugs that reduce inflammation without the use of cortisone or other steroids

nonwaived - complex tests that require skill to perform and interpret and are therefore regulated

nuclease - an enzyme that participates in the hydrolysis of nucleic acids

obesity - body mass index ≥ 30 kg/m^2

obstructive - causing blockage

oligoclonal - showing small discrete bands in cerebrospinal fluid electrophoresis indicating local production of immunoglobulin G (IgG)

oliguria - decreased urine output, < 400 mL of urine per day (a common sign of renal insufficiency)

oncologist - physician specializing in cancer detection and treatment

oocyte - female reproductive cell; ovum

open reagent system - analytical system that allows many sources for reagents

opsin - the protein portion of the rhodopsin molecule in the retina of the eye

osmometry - measurement of osmotic pressure from dissolved particles in a solution

osmotic pressure - pressure that develops when two solutions of different concentration are separated by a semipermeable membrane

osteoblasts - young active cells of the bone

osteoclasts - phagocytic cells in bone responsive to parathyroid hormone in bone breakdown

osteogenesis - production or formation of bone

osteomalacia - disease of bone in adults, characterized by soft or brittle bones; caused by vitamin D deficiency

osteopenia - decreased bone mass, or loss of bone density

ototoxicity - damage to the hearing of the patient

outcome - consequence, conclusion, or result

ovulation - cyclic release of an oocyte by the ovary

oxidation - combining with oxygen; increasing the positive valence of a molecule by loss of electrons/loss of electrons in a reaction; attraction of electrons produced in a reduction process at the anode

oxyhemoglobin (O_2Hb) - the combined form of hemoglobin with oxygen; a measure of the utilization of the potential oxygen transport capacity

p50 - the midway point of the hemoglobin-oxygen dissociation curve, representing the oxygen tension (in mm Hg) when the hemoglobin molecules are 50% saturated with oxygen

palpation - simple technique in which a physician presses lightly on the surface of the body to feel the organs or tissues underneath

pancreatitis - inflammation of the pancreas

paraprotein - an abnormal plasma protein, such as a macroglobulin, cryoglobulin, or immunoglobulin

parenchymal - part of the main structure of the organ

parenchymal cells - epithelial liver cells that make bile, bilirubin, and proteins and perform other duties; hepatocytes

parenteral - bypassing the gastrointestinal system to provide nutrients directly to the bloodstream

parietal cells - cells of the stomach that secrete hydrochloric acid and intrinsic factor

partial seizures - motor, sensory, or psychomotor phenomena without loss of consciousness

partial-complex seizures - brief loss of contact with surroundings; may accompany staring, automatic purposeless movements, and unintelligible sounds followed by motor activity and short-term confusion

pathogens - causative agents of disease

pCO_2 - partial pressure of dissolved carbon dioxide gas as related to carbonic acid (H_2CO_3); sometimes expressed as PCO_2

peak - the highest level of a particular drug found in the blood following administration of a dose

pectoris - chest

pellagra - deficiency of niacin characterized by cutaneous, gastrointestinal, mucosal, and neurological symptoms

perfusion - passage of blood through the vessels of a particular organ; designated as Q

peristalsis - wavelike movement that occurs involuntarily in hollow tubes of the body

pernicious anemia - autoimmune disease in which antibodies affect intrinsic factor and cause vitamin B_{12} deficiency

pharmacokinetics - the relationship of drug concentration to time

phlebotomy - opening of a vein to withdraw blood

phosphatidyl choline - phosholipid lung surfactant; also known as lecithin

phototherapy - exposure to sunlight or artificial ultraviolet light for therapeutic purposes, such as treating neonatal hyperbilirubinemia

pilocarpine - a muscarinic alkaloid drug that can induce sweating

plaque - accumulated deposits of fat and other substances in the blood vessels causing roughened and narrowed interior surface

pneumocytes - two types (I and II) of cells that form the alveoli of the lungs

poikilocytosis - unusual shape of red blood cells

point-of-care testing (POCT) - testing that does not require specimen preparation and provides rapid results at or near the patient's location

polarized light - light which vibrates in one plane

polarography - measurement of current flowing as electrons are formed in an oxidation-reduction system

polyclonal - arising from many cell lines

polydipsia - excessive thirst

polymerase - an enzyme that catalyzes the addition of nucleotides to the DNA chain

polyp - small tumor common to rectum or other vascular areas

polyphagia - excessive hunger

polysaccharides - complex carbohydrates composed of more than 20 monosaccharides

polyuric - exhibiting excessive urine output (>2.5 L/24 hr)

porcine - derived from swine (pigs)

porphyrinemia - condition in which the red blood cells contain excess protoporphyrin

porphyrinogen - tetrapyrrole that is a precursor of heme

porphyrins - cyclic compounds called tetrapyrroles that are formed by the linkage of four pyrrole rings

porphyrinuria - condition in which the urine contains excess coproporphyrin

positive feedback - enhancing the output when the effects are not at optimum

potential - force of electrical activity (in volts)

potentiometry - measuring electrical potential in voltage

precision - how closely measured results compare with each other

pre-eclampsia - a complication of pregnancy characterized by increasing hypertension, proteinuria, and edema

premature labor - labor that begins between 20 and 38 weeks' gestation

premature rupture of membranes - rupture of amniotic membrane prior to the time labor is expected

prepubescent - before sexual maturity

presumptive test - a procedure with minimal complexity, instrumentation, and personnel requirements so that the results can be quickly determined

primer - short piece of DNA that is a known sequence for DNA that is being replicated

proficiency testing - a method of monitoring accurate outcome in which test samples from an external source are analyzed and results compared to those of reference laboratories and scored for accuracy/a means of verifying the accuracy of tests; can include participation in an external assessment program, splitting samples with another laboratory, or blind testing of materials with known values

progesterone - steroid hormone produced by the corpus luteum and placenta that prepares the endometrium for blastocyst implantation and maintains pregnancy

prognosis - prediction of the course and end of a disease and estimate of chance for recovery

prostatism - the condition of partial or complete blockage of the urethra due to an enlarged prostate gland

protease inhibitor - a medication that inhibits the action of enzymes

proteome - the complete set of proteins produced by the cell

proteomics - analysis of the proteome

protocol - a formal plan or expectation concerning the actions of those involved in patient care

protomer - protein isomer in which the protein subunits have the same chemical formula but different spatial arrangements in the molecule

psychogenic - of mental origin, such as compulsive drinking of water in psychogenic water overload

punitive - relating to punishment

purity - number of parts per 100 parts

pyloric - pertaining to the distal portion of the stomach or to the opening between the stomach and duodenum

qualitative - giving either positive or negative test results (a binary response)

quality control sample - sample with a matrix similar to patient specimens with known concentration

quantitative - expressing test results by amount or concentration (a graded or proportional response)

Raleigh scatter - small particles scattering light in all directions with maximum scatter forward and backward

random access - test reactions can be programmed to occur in a variety of sequences

random error - error that occurs unpredictably due to poor precision

random (or casual) blood draw - blood collected at any time of day without regard to duration since last meal

Raynaud's syndrome - disease of small arteries and arterioles of unknown cause with exaggerated vasomotor response to cold or emotion

reabsorption - to absorb again, as related to the movement of particles through the nephron, the movement of particles from the renal filtrate back into blood

receiver operating characteristic (ROC) curve - a plot of the diagnostic specificity versus sensitivity of a test

reciprocal - opposite relationship

reduction - losing oxygen; increasing the negative valence of a molecule by gain of electrons/production of electrons and a positively charged ion; reaction at the cathode

reference method - a thoroughly investigated method with documented accuracy and precision

registration - the process by which qualified individuals are listed on an official roster maintained by a governmental or nongovernmental agency

regulatory - relating to rules or directives

remodeling - the overall effect of depositing and absorbing bone to remake new bone

renal failure - loss of renal function for control of water and electrolytes, decline in filtration and removal of wastes, and loss of nutrients

renal threshold - plasma level at which the kidneys no longer reabsorb a substance so that it is excreted into urine as waste

replication - duplication of DNA

resistance - opposing force to flow of electrons (in ohms)

resorption - to soak up or take in again

respiratory acidosis - acidosis caused by retention of carbon dioxide due to pulmonary insufficiency

respiratory alkalosis - alkalosis with an acute reduction of plasma bicarbonate and a proportionate reduction in plasma carbon dioxide

respiratory distress syndrome (RDS) - severe impairment of respiratory function in a preterm newborn due to immaturity of the enzymatic system essential for pulmonary surfactant production

rhodopsin - the glycoprotein opsin of the rods in the retina, which combines with retinal to form a functional photopigment responsive to light

rickets - disease of bone formation in children, most commonly caused by vitamin D deficiency

RNA - ribonucleic acid; serves as a messenger of inherited nucleic acid from the nucleus template and translates that message into protein; in some prokaryotes, it is the chemical that serves as the inherited message

rods - the slender sensory bodies in the retina of the eye, which respond to faint light

rouleaux - stickiness of erythrocytes causing a stacked coin appearance

sample - a portion of the specimen to be used in analysis

screening test - test to determine if patients have a disease before they present with symptoms; should be very sensitive

scurvy - disease of the skin and joints, caused by inadequate intake of ascorbic acid

secretin - hormone secreted by duodenal mucosa; stimulates sodium bicarbonate secretion by the pancreas and bile secretion by the liver

selective inactivation - process of rendering some chemicals nonfunctional while keeping the function of other similar chemicals

sensitivity - the ability to detect small concentrations of the measured analyte

sensitization - production of antibody as a response to antigen exposure

sensory nerves - nerves of the sensory organs

sequential analysis - performing a set of test reactions in a particular order on each sample in the order in which it is received

serological - studying serum components of the blood; making a serum titer for clinical laboratory testing, such as an antibody titer

Sertoli cells - specialized cells in the seminiferous tubules of the testis that produce inhibin and factors that help sperm maturation

shift - a sudden and sustained change in quality control results above the mean

shunt - passage between two natural channels, such as between blood vessels, that bypasses a particular organ

sideroblastic anemia - anemia characterized by ferritin-containing blast cells in bone marrow

sigmoidoscopy - examination of the lower portion of the colon (sigmoid portion) with an instrument

single-channel - able to perform only one test with a dedicated portion of the instrument

sinusoid - a large, permeable capillary

sinusoidal - forming a small channel for blood in the tissues of the liver or other organ

SO$_2$ - oxygen saturation; a measure of the utilization of the current oxygen transport capacity

solubility - the ability of a solute to dissolve in a solvent

solute - the substance that is dissolved in the solution

solution - a mixture of two or more substances

solvent - the substance that is used to dissolve the solute

spasms - twitching of muscles, which may accompany muscle ache

specificity - freedom from interference and cross reactivity, to determine solely the analyte purported to be measured

specimen - aliquot of body fluid or tissue from a patient

spectrophotometer - instrument that uses a photodetector to measure the amount of a specific wavelength of light transmitted through a test solution to determine concentration

sperm cell - male germinal cell

spider angioma - a form of tumor, usually benign, consisting of blood vessels or lymph vessels

STAT - immediately or at once

statin - medication used to control hypercholesterolemia by affecting metabolism of cholesterol

steady state - condition in which the average drug concentration remains in equilibrium after multiple intervals of drug dosage

steatorrhea - failure to digest or absorb fats in the gastrointestinal tract

steric - relating to the size of and distances between chemicals or side chains within the spatial arrangement of atoms in the chemical

steroids - high molecular weight compounds with carbon atoms in a four-ring structure similar to cholesterol

subarachnoid space - space between the membranes of the covering of the central nervous system that contains the cerebrospinal fluid

substrate - reactant in an enzyme-catalyzed reaction that is converted to product

sulfonylurea - one of a class of oral drugs used to control hyperglycemia in type 2 diabetes mellitus

surfactant - a substance that reduces the surface tension of the moist surfaces of solid tissue

sweat test - test for cystic fibrosis that involves measuring the subject's sweat for abnormally high sodium chloride content

systematic error - error that occurs predictably once a pattern of recognition is established; predictable errors of the same sign and magnitude

systemic lupus erythematosus - chronic autoimmune inflammatory disease involving multiple organ systems

tachometer - device that measures speed in revolutions per minute

tachycardia - racing heart rate

tagged - labeled with some component that allows detection or visualization

tared - adjusted a scale to zero, such as negating the mass of an empty vessel so that only the mass of an unknown is displayed

tertiary level - a third level in a hierarchy, such as the hypothalamus in the endocrine system

tetany - neuromotor irritability accompanied by muscular twitching and eventual convulsions

thalassemia - hereditary anemia caused by defective production of alpha or beta chain of hemoglobin/diseases resulting from decreased synthesis of globin chains

therapeutic drug monitoring - measuring serum levels of a drug to aid in adjusting drug dosage

therapeutic range - beneficial serum drug concentration levels, including a lower and an upper limit

thrombosis - formation or development of a blood clot (thrombus) in a blood vessel

thyrotoxicosis - acute illness due to hyperthyroidism

thyroxine (T_4) - main hormone synthesized in the thyroid gland, also known as 3,5,3'5'-tetraiodothyronine

tonic-clonic seizures - loss of consciousness and balance followed by contractions of the muscles of the extremities, trunk, and head, often with an uncontrolled outcry at the onset

tonometry - measurement of dissolved gases in a solution in order to standardize the partial pressure or tension of carbon dioxide and oxygen

total hemoglobin - a measure of potential oxygen transport capacity

tourniquet - band used on arm to cause the veins to distend

toxicity - poisoning due to exposure to a toxin, including drugs, gases, heavy metals, and alcohols

transcription - synthesis of RNA from a DNA template

transcutaneous - through the skin, not invading the body through a puncture; percutaneous

transferrin - a beta$_1$ globulin transport protein for carrying iron in blood plasma

translation - synthesis of protein

transmittance - the amount of light not retained but passed through a test solution

trend - a gradual but steady change in quality control results moving up or down away from the mean

triclonal - composed of three clones of plasma cell lines that each produce one type of identical antibody

triiodothyronine (T_3) - more potent thyroid hormone, also known as 3,5,3'-triiodothyronine

trisomy - three copies of a chromosome instead of the normal two

tropins - stimulating protein hormones

trough - the lowest level of a particular drug found in the blood following administration of a dose and just prior to the administration of the next dose, after a peak in drug level

true negative - result below the decision limit in a patient who does not have the disease

true positive - result at or above the decision limit in a patient who has the disease

truncal obesity - weight gain in the middle of the body rather than including the arms or legs

tubercular granuloma - a mass or nodule of chronically inflamed tissue with granulations that is usually associated with an infective process

tumor markers - surface molecules on tissue or proteins in serum that, in higher than normal quantities, are associated with the presence of malignancies

turbidity - cloudiness of solution due to presence of light-blocking particles or molecules such as fats

ultrafiltrate - filtrate formed under pressure, such as found in the choroid plexus

ultrasound - imaging technique that uses high frequency sound waves to create images of internal organs, tissue, and blood vessels

uremia - a toxic condition associated with renal insufficiency produced by the retention in the blood of nitrogenous substances normally excreted by the kidney

ureterosigmoidostomy - implantation of the ureter into the sigmoid colon to eliminate wastes when the urinary system is unable

uroporphyrin - highly water-soluble precursor of heme found in urine

uterus - hollow muscular organ located in the pelvic cavity of the woman in which the blastocyst implants and the fetus develops

ventilation - air exchange between lungs and gases inhaled and exhaled; designated as V

voltammetry - measuring the current at an electrode using a specific voltage generated at another electrode

waived - tests that are very simple or pose no reasonable risk of harm to the patient if the test is performed incorrectly

washout - water or wash solution flowing through a chamber after a sample has passed through in order to clean it out and prevent carryover

work of breathing - effort needed to inhale and exhale

xenobiotic - a biochemical that is not produced in the body

zero-order kinetics - catalyzed reaction with all active sites of the enzyme filled with substrate so reaction occurs at its fastest rate; also called saturation kinetics

zona fasciculata - middle of the three layers of the adrenal cortex that consists of radially arranged columnar epithelial cells

zona glomerulosa - outermost of the three layers of the adrenal cortex that consists of round masses of granular epithelial cells that stain deeply

zona reticularis - innermost of the three layers of the adrenal cortex that consists of irregularly arranged cylindrical masses of epithelial cells

zone electrophoresis - separating components of a mixture within a charged buffer solution by moving them through a porous filter based on electrical attractions

zygote - single cell formed from fertilization of the oocyte and sperm cell

Appendix

The Essential and Nonessential Amino Acids

Amino Acid	Essential/ Nonessential*	Diagnostic Use
Isoleucine	Essential	Maple syrup urine disease, in which a deficiency of the enzyme branched chain alpha–keto acid dehydrogenase complex results in accumulation of branch chain amino acids in body fluids Methylmalonic acidemia (see below)
Leucine	Essential	Maple syrup urine disease (see above)
Lysine	Essential	Cystinuria, in which a defect in renal tubular transport results in increased urinary excretion of cystine, lysine, arginine, and ornithine
Methionine	Essential	Methylmalonic acidemia, in which defect properties of the enzyme methylmalonyl coenzyme A mutase or defective binding of the enzyme to its cofactor cobalamin results in the inability to convert methylmalonyl coenzyme A to succinyl coenzyme A. Methylmalonyl coenzyme A is a product of the breakdown of some fatty acids and the amino acids isoleucine, valine, threonine, and methionine.
Phenylalanine	Essential	Phenylketonuria, in which a metabolic deficiency of the enzyme phenylalanine hydroxylase results in increased levels of reaction substrate phenylalanine
Threonine	Essential	Methylmalonic acidemia (see above)
Tryptophan	Essential	Hartnup disease, a defect of small intestine absorption of some amino acids, including trytophan. Deficiency of tryptophan leads to a deficiency of the vitamin niacin.
Valine	Essential	Maple syrup urine disease (see above) Methylmalonic acidemia (see above)
Alanine	Nonessential	
Arginine***	Nonessential	Cystinuria (see above)
Asparagine	Nonessential	
Aspartate	Nonessential	
Cysteine	Nonessential	
Glutamate	Nonessential	
Glutamine	Nonessential	
Glycine	Nonessential	
Histidine***	Nonessential	Histidinemia, in which a deficiency of the enzyme histidinase results in the accumulation of histidine and the absence of urocanate
Proline	Nonessential	
Serine	Nonessential	
Tyrosine	Nonessential	Tyrosinemia, in which a deficiency of one of the enzymes that metabolize tyrosine results in accumulation of tyrosine Alkaptonuria, in which a deficiency of the enzyme homogentistate oxidase, an enzyme of the catabolic pathway of tyrosine, results in the accumulation of homogentistate

*Essential: required in the diet; nonessential: not required in the diet, can be produced in the body.

**Diagnostic use: use for diagnosis or monitoring disease and health, or use for monitoring the efficacy of treatment.

*** Nonessential for adults; essential for infants.

TABLE A–2

Clinically Important Fatty Acids

Fatty Acid	Clinical Importance
Myristic acid	Associated with plasma membrane enzymes
Palmitic acid	First product of fatty acid synthesis
Palmitoleic acid	Component of glycerides of adipose tissue
Stearic acid	Component of phospholipids
Oleic acid	Component of phospholipids
Linoleic acid	Essential* fatty acid
	In deficiency, patients may exhibit growth failure, thrombocytopenia, and skin diseases
Linolenic acid	Essential* fatty acid
	In deficiency, patients may exhibit peripheral neuoropathy and vision problems
Arachidonic acid	Considered essential* in the diet; the body is able to make some arachidonic acid from linoleic acid
	A precursor in the biosynthesis of some prostaglandins

*Essential: required in the diet.

TABLE A–3

Common Carbohydrates

Saccharide	Structure	Clinical Importance
Glucose	Monosaccharide	Energy source
Fructose	Monosaccharide	Important energy source for sperm
Galactose	Monosaccharide	Used in the synthesis of lactose, glycolipids, some phospholipids, and glycoproteins
Lactose	Disaccharide	Composed of galactose and glucose
		Milk sugar
Maltose	Disaccharide	Composed of two glucose molecules
		Malt sugar
Sucrose	Disaccharide	Composed of glucose and fructose
		Cane or beet sugar
Starch	Polysaccharide	Glucose polymer
Cellulose	Polysaccharide	Glucose polymer
Glycogen	Polysaccharide	Glucose polymer

TABLE A–4

Additional Laboratory Tests Used in Carbohydrate Assessment

Name	Specimen	Testing Methodology	Clinical Use
Fructosamine	Whole Blood or serum	Affinity chromatography HPLC Photometric analysis	Measures glycosylated albumin, which has a half life of approximately 20 days Reflects glucose levels over a period of 2–3 wk
C-peptide	Serum or plasma	Chemiluminescence immunoassay	Inactive remnant of proinsulin Reflects the concentration of endogenous insulin
Islet cell antibody	Serum	Fluorescence immunoassay	Associated with autoimmune endocrine diseases and type 1 diabetes
Glutamic acid decarboxylase antibody	Serum	Immunoassay	Aids in the diagnosis and assessment of progression of type 1 diabetes

HPLC, high-pressure liquid chromatography.

TABLE A–5

Additional Enzymes of Clinical Significance

Enzyme	Abbreviation	Clinical Significance
Aldolase	ALD	Increased activity in skeletal muscle disease
Cholinesterase	CHE	Decreased activity in liver failure, following organophosphate poisoning and in some genetic variants
Creatinine kinsase isoenzymes	CK MM and CK MB	CK MM activity is elevated in skeletal muscular disorders such as muscular dystrophy; CK MB is elevated in myocardial infarction
Glucose-6-phosphate dehydrogenase	G6PD	Decreased red cell activity associated with oxidative stress–induced hemolytic anemia
Glutamate dehydrogenase	GLD	Increased activity of this hepatic mitochondrial enzyme correlates with severity of liver cell damage
5´-Nucleotidase	NTP	Increased activity of this hepatobiliary enzyme correlates with alkaline phosphatase
Pyruvate kinase	PK	Decreased red cell activity correlates with the most common cause of nonspherocytic hemolytic anemia
Trypsin-1	TRY-1	Decreased activity in children with cystic fibrosis; not diagnostic in neonates

TABLE A–6
Tumor Markers Summarized

Tumor Marker	Tissue Sources and Tumor Associations
ACTH	Cushing's syndrome and lung small cell
AFP	Liver, colon, stomach, and pancreas
BRCA1 gene mutation	Breast and ovary
BTA	Bladder
CA 15-3	Breast and ovary
CA 19-9	Liver and gastrointestinal tract
CA 125	Ovary and endometrium
Calcitonin	Thyroid (medullary carcinoma)
CEA	Colon, liver, stomach, and pancreas
c-erb B-2/Her-2	Breast and ovary
ER	Estrogen receptors in breast
hCG	Germinal tumors
HVA & VMA	Pheochromocytoma and neuroblastoma
MCA	Breast and ovary
M-spike/paraprotein	Myeloma
PSA	Prostate
Serotonin	Carcinoid enteroendocrine
tDT	Leukemia

TABLE A–7
Drugs of Abuse

Drug Name	Drug Class
Amphetamine/methamphetamine	Stimulant
Barbiturates	CNS sedative and hypnotic
Benzodiazepines (Valium)	CNS depressant and muscle relaxant
Cannabinoids	CNS depressant and relaxant
Cocaine	CNS stimulant
Gamma-hydroxybutyrate (GHB)	CNS depressant and relaxant, and used in drug-facilitated sexual assault
Ketamine	Anesthetic and sedative
Lysergic acid diethylamide (LSD)	Hallucinogen
Methylenedioxyamphetamine (MDA)	Designer amphetamines: stimulant
Methylenedioxymethamphetamine (MDMA)	Designer amphetamines: stimulant and hallucinogen
Opiates	Analgesic and CNS depressant
Phencyclidine (PCP)	Anesthetic and hallucinogen
Phenothiazines (Valium, etc.)	Neuroleptics; inhibit dopaminergic receptors

CNS, central nervous system.

TABLE A–8

Toxic Substances and Their Sources

Toxin	Sources
Aluminum	Bauxite or clay; some antacid medications
Arsenic	Inorganic forms in bedrock; pesticide
Carbon monoxide	Incomplete combustion of carbon
Cyanide	Urea foam insulation in buildings
Ethylene glycol	Antifreeze
Lead	Paint and varnish predating 1970; ceramics
Mercury	Industry; fungicide
Methanol	Solvent, antifreeze, and incomplete distillate of homemade alcohol
Nitrates/nitrites	Contaminated water, often from agriculture
Organophosphates	Insecticides (Malthion, Parathion, Diazinon)

TABLE A–9

Adult Therapeutic Drug Levels

Drug Level	Category	Therapeutic Range	Optimal Timing
Amikacin peak	Antimicrobial	20–35 µg/mL	1 hr after start of 30- to 60-min infusion
Amikacin trough	Antimicrobial	<5 µg/mL	Just prior to next dose
Carbamazepine trough	Anticonvulsant	4–12 µg/mL	Just prior to next dose
Cyclosporine trough	Immunosuppressant	50–300 ng/mL	Just prior to next dose
Digoxin	Cardioactive	0.8–2.2 ng/mL	Just prior to next dose
Ethosuximide trough	Anticonvulsant	40–100 µg/mL	Just prior to next dose
Gentamicin peak	Antimicrobial	5–10 µg/mL	1 hr after start of 30-to 60-min infusion
Gentamicin trough	Antimicrobial	<2 µg/mL	Just prior to next dose
Lidocaine	Cardioactive	1–5 µg/mL	4–8 hr after start of infusion
Lithium trough	Antimanic (bipolar disorder)	0.6–1.2 mEq/L	Just prior to first morning dose
NAPA	Cardioactive	10–30 µg/mL	Just prior to next procainamide dose
Phenobarbital trough	Anticonvulsant	15–40 µg/mL	Just prior to next dose
Phenytoin trough	Anticonvulsant	10–20 µg/mL	Just prior to next dose
Primidone trough	Anticonvulsant	5–12 µg/mL	Just prior to next dose
Procainamide	Cardioactive	4–8 µg/mL	Just prior to next dose
Quinidine	Cardioactive	1–4 µg/mL	Just prior to next dose
Theophylline	Antiasthmatic	5–15 µg/mL	8–12 hr after once-daily dose
Tobramycin peak	Antimicrobial	5–10 µg/mL	1 hr after start of 30-to 60-min infusion
Tobramycin trough	Antimicrobial	<2 µg/mL	Just prior to next dose
Valproic acid trough	Anticonvulsant	50–100 µg/mL	Just prior to next dose
Vancomycin trough	Antimicrobial	5–10 µg/mL	Just prior to next dose

NAPA, N-acetylprocainamide.

Index

Note: Page numbers followed by *f* indicate figures; page numbers followed by *t* indicate tables.